Operative Dictations in General and Vascular Surgery

Jamal J. Hoballah
Carol E.H. Scott-Conner
Editors

Operative Dictations in General and Vascular Surgery

Second edition

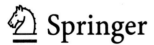
Springer

Editors
Jamal J. Hoballah, MD, MBA,
FACS
Professor and Chairman
Department of Surgery
American University of Beirut
Medical Center
Beirut, Lebanon

Professor of Surgery
Department of Surgery
Vascular Surgery Division
University of Iowa Carver
College of Medicine
Iowa City, IA, USA
jh34@aub.edu.lb

Carol E.H. Scott-Conner, MD, PhD,
MBA, FACS
Professor of Surgery
Department of Surgery
University of Iowa Carver College
of Medicine
Iowa City, IA, USA
carol-scott-conner@uiowa.edu

ISBN 978-1-4614-0450-7   e-ISBN 978-1-4614-0451-4
DOI 10.1007/978-1-4614-0451-4
Springer New York Dordrecht Heidelberg London

Library of Congress Control Number: 2011935376

Springer is part of Springer Science+Business Media (www.springer.com)

To Harry (CSC)
To Leila, Jawad, Nader and Wafa (JJH)

Preface

A SPECIAL WORD TO SURGICAL RESIDENTS AND FELLOWS

Surgeons love to operate, but nobody likes paperwork. The operative dictation, or "op note" as it is commonly called, is one of the most important pieces of paperwork that a surgeon creates. Accurately recording what happened in the operating room – what the indications were, what was found, what was done, who was there, what sutures and devices were used, what individual differences in anatomy were encountered – is a crucial skill that all surgeons must learn. Yet, surgical residents rarely receive detailed instruction in how to dictate concise, informative operative notes.

Quite simply, this is a book we wish we had had when we were residents. It is a book we want our residents to have and to use. Personalize your copy. Use the space labeled "notes" to take note of particular technical variations favored by the various attending surgeons with whom you scrub. Note their preferences in suture materials, patient positioning, and other small details. Make it your practice to review this material before scrubbing on a case. Surgery is made up of thousands of small details. Note what works well, and what is less useful. Sooner than you might believe, you will be facing your board exams and working independently. When you do, this book will help you recall everything you have learned, and help you to determine your own technical preferences.

We hope you will enjoy using this unique resource. We welcome your comments or suggestions.

Jamal J. Hoballah
Carol E.H. Scott-Conner

Introduction

The second edition of this book, once again, seeks to put a world of technical information in your pocket, or OR locker. A total of 60 new operations have been added, expanding the content by more than 35%. A large number of endovascular procedures have been added in the second edition, reflecting the changes in the management of vascular pathology.

The volume has two primary objectives. First, it is designed to serve as a source of model operative dictations that may be individualized and used as templates. Second, it is intended as an aide-memoir, giving the surgeon a short list of pertinent information about each procedure. Ample space is provided to allow each surgeon to add notes. By reviewing this introductory material before scrubbing on a procedure, the trainee surgeon will enter the operating room better prepared to participate actively and to learn as much as possible. At the end of training, this book, with the notes accumulated by the resident, will serve as an invaluable review resource analogous to the individualized notebooks many surgeons keep. The first edition was noted to be very valuable by graduating surgical trainees in preparation for the certifying exam of the American Board of Surgery.

This book is also intended for practicing surgeons, who may modify each template to reflect their own individual practice. It also serves as a concise reminder of essential steps in those operations that may be only rarely performed.

Here you will find concise summaries of 226 operations. This comprises the majority of procedures commonly performed by general and vascular surgeons. For each procedure, a list of common *indications* is given. This list is by no means exhaustive, but is intended to cover 95% of the situations in which a particular procedure will be used.

A list of *essential steps* follows. These can be used to mentally rehearse the procedure before it is performed. The next heading, *Note these technical variations*, introduces a list that is intended to prompt the surgeon for particular things to note and dictate within the template. These particular things must be individualized – they range from fundamental variations such as a stapled vs. sutured anastomosis, through such details as type of suture or whether an autotransfusion device was used. A list of *possible complications* that are typically associated with that particular surgical procedure follows. Complications (such as myocardial infarction, bleeding, infection) which can follow any operative intervention are not listed unless they are characteristically more common after that operation.

Finally, a *template operative dictation* is provided. We believe that paper is cheap and time is precious, and have assumed that the reader of this part of the chapter wants completeness and convenience. We have minimized the need to refer to other chapters by including all the parts of the operative note regardless of duplication across chapters. To this end, we have included common opening and terminating sequences (for example, how to enter and close the abdomen) in all laparotomy dictations. (Although fundamental to any operative notes, comments regarding blood loss, fluid replacement, and instrument counts were not included in these templates to avoid redundancy.) More complicated procedures are more prone to variation, and we have tried to strike a balance between conciseness and completeness. Thus, under operative findings, we have enumerated those most pertinent to the procedure in question and prompted for additional findings.

These surgery operative dictations are intended to be used in conjunction with the following texts by the editors:

Scott-Conner CEH (ed). Chassin's Operative Strategy in General Surgery, 3rd edition, Springer-Verlag, New York, 2001. This detailed review of strategy in general surgery includes almost all of these procedures. The sections of the present book correspond directly to the sections of this text.

Scott-Conner CEH (ed). Chassin's Operative Strategy in Colon and Rectal Surgery. Springer-Verlag, New York, 2006. This provides additional information on laparoscopic colorectal procedures.

Scott-Conner CEH (ed). The SAGES Manual: Fundamentals of Laparoscopy and GI Endoscopy. Springer-Verlag, New York, 2nd edition, 2006. Endoscopic and laparoscopic procedures are discussed in detail.

Scott-Conner CEH, Cuschieri A, Carter AF. Minimal Access Surgical Anatomy. Lippincott Williams & Wilkins, Philadelphia, 2000. This text covers the anatomy of laparoscopic surgery in color plates and line drawings.

Scott-Conner CEH, Dawson DL. Operative Anatomy, 3rd edition. Lippincott Williams & Wilkins, Philadelphia, 2009. The anatomy and technique of common procedures, including thoracic, vascular, and transplant, is covered.

Lumley JSP, Hoballah JJ. Vascular Surgery. Springer Surgery Atlas Series. Springer, Heidelberg (forthcoming 2010).

Hoballah, JJ. Vascular Reconstructions: Anatomy, Exposures, and Techniques. Springer-Verlag, New York, 2000. Step-by-step review of all common vascular reconstructions, along with basics of exposure and access, and technical tips.

The vast majority of these chapters were written by surgical residents at the University of Iowa College of Medicine or the American University of Beirut. These residents are introduced to you on the pages which follow. The virtues of this book must accrue to them; any faults rest squarely with the section editor. The hard work and assistance of Ms. Katherine Carolan, the encouragement of Laura Gillan who saw the first edition to fruition, and Richard Hruska and Elizabeth Orthmann who shepherded this second edition along, and the input of residents and colleagues is gratefully acknowledged.

Contents

Section IV   Large Intestine

Section XVI Aortoiliac Occlusive Disease

Section XVII Infrainguinal Occlusive Disease

Section XX   Venous Disorders

Contributors

Maher A. Abbas, MD Regional Colon and Rectal Surgery, SCPMG Director, Permanente National Center of Excellence Chair, Center for Minimally Invasive Surgery, Los Angeles, CA, USA

Ahmed M. Abou-Zamzam, MD Department of Cardio Vascular and Thoracic Surgery, Loma Linda University Medical Center, Loma Linda, CA, USA

Maen S. Aboul Hosn, MD Department of Surgery, American University of Beirut Medical Center, Beirut, Lebanon

Mark Adelman, MD Department of Surgery, NYU Langone Medical Center, New York, NY, USA

Abdi Ahari, MD General Surgery, Mason City Clinic, Mason City, IA, USA

Houssein Haidar Ahmad, MD Department of Surgery, American University of Beirut Medical Center, Beirut, Lebanon

Mohamad H. Alaeddine, MD Department of Surgery/Division of General Surgery, American University of Beirut Medical Center, Beirut, Lebanon

Parth B. Amin, MD Department of Vascular Surgery, University of Iowa Hospitals and Clinics, Iowa City, IA, USA

Evgeny V. Arshava, MD Department of Surgery, University of Iowa, Iowa City, IA, USA

Jeffrey L. Ballard, MD Division of Vascular Surgery, Loma Linda University Medical Center, Loma Linda, CA, USA

Hisham Bassiouny, MD Department of Surgery, University of Chicago, Chicago, IL, USA

Ross Bengtson, MD Department of General Surgery, St. Joseph's Medical Center, Brainerd, MN, USA

Christian Bianchi, MD Division of Vascular Surgery, Loma Linda University Medical Center, Loma Linda, CA, USA

Kelly S.A. Blair, MD Department of Surgery, Section of Vascular Surgery, University of Chicago, Chicago, IL, USA

Michael Bonebrake, MD Department of Surgery, University of Iowa Hospitals and Clinic, Iowa City, IA, USA

Kevin A. Bridge, MD, MSPH Department of General Surgery, University of Iowa Hospitals and Clinics, Iowa City, IA, USA

Christopher Bunch, MD Department of Vascular Surgery, Essentia Health System/Duluth Clinic, Duluth, MN, USA

John C. Byrn, MD Department of Surgery, University of Iowa Hospital and Clinics, Iowa City, IA, USA

Keith D. Calligaro, MD Department of Surgery, Division of Vascular Surgery, University of Pennsylvania Hospital, Philadelphia, PA, USA

Daniel Calva-Cerqueira, MD Department of Surgery, University of Iowa Hospitals & Clinics, Iowa City, IA, USA

Gregory A. Carlson, MD Memorial Health System, Colorado Springs, CO, USA

Cassius Iyad Ochoa Chaar, MD, MS Department of Vascular Surgery, University of Pittsburgh Medical Center, Pittsburgh, PA, USA

Roderick T.A. Chalmers, MD Vascular Surgical Service, Royal Infirmary of Edinburgh, Edinburgh, UK

Edward Y. Chan, MD Department of Surgery, Mount Sinai Hospital, New York, NY, USA

Edward H. Chin, MD Department of Surgery, Mount Sinai School of Medicine, New York, NY, USA

Jason Chiriano, DO Department of Surgery, Loma Linda University Medical Center, Loma Linda, CA, USA

Sung Woon Chung, MD Department of Thoracic and Cardiovascular Surgery, Pusan National University Hospital, Busan, Korea

Brian A. Coakley, MD Department of Surgery, The Mount Sinai Medical Center, New York, NY, USA

Thomas E. Collins, MD Department of Surgery, University of Iowa Hospitals and Clinics, Iowa City, IA, USA

Michael S. Connors III, MD Division of Vascular Surgery, Department of Surgery, Ochsner Clinic, New Orleans, LA, USA

David C. Corry, MD Department of Vascular/Endovascular Surgery, Memorial Health System, Colorado Springs, CO, USA

John W. Cromwell, MD Department of Surgery, University of Iowa Carver College of Medicine, Iowa City, IA, USA

Roy R. Danks, DO School of Medicine, St. Lukes Health System, Cushing Memorial Hospital, Leavenworth, KS, USA

R. Clement Darling III, MD Department of Vascular Surgery, Division of Vascular Surgery, Albany Medical Center Hospital, Albany, NY, USA

Celia M. Divino, MD Department of Surgery, The Mount Sinai Medical Center, New York, NY, USA

Matthew J. Dougherty, MD Department of Surgery, Division of Vascular Surgery, University of Pennsylvania Hospital, Philadelphia, PA, USA

Laura Doyon, MD Department of Surgery, The Mount Sinai Hospital, New York, NY, USA

Walid Faraj, MD, FRCS Department of Surgery, American University of Beirut-Medical Center, Beirut, Lebanon

Michael C. Fraterelli, MD Department of Surgery, Medical Center of Aurora, Aurora, CO, USA

Julie Freischlag, MD Department of Surgery, Johns Hopkins University School of Medicine, Baltimore, MD, USA

Joshua R. French, MD Department of Surgery, University of Iowa Hospitals and Clinics, Iowa City, IA, USA

Peter C. Fretz, MD Department of Urology, Elkhart General Hospital, Elkhart, IN, USA

Nabil Fuleihan, MD Department of Otolaryngology-Head and Neck Surgery, American University of Beirut, Beirut, Lebanon

Julie Guidroz, MD Department of Surgery, University of Iowa Hospitals and Clinics, Iowa City, IA, USA

Fady F. Haddad, MD Department of Surgery,
American University of Beirut Medical Center, Beirut, Lebanon

Susan Skaff Hagen, MD, MSPH Department of Surgery,
University of Iowa Hospital and Clinics, Iowa City, IA, USA

Mazen M. Hashisho, MD Department of Surgery,
Stony Brook University Hospital, Northport VA Medical Center,
Northport, NY, USA

Jamal J. Hoballah, MD, MBA Department of Surgery,
American University of Beirut Medical Center, Beirut, Lebanon;
Department of Surgery, Vascular Surgery Division,
University of Iowa Carver College of Medicine, Iowa city, IA, USA

Mohammad A. Hojeij, MD Department of Surgery/Division
of General Surgery, American University of Beirut Medical Center,
Beirut, Lebanon

Hisakazu Hoshi, MD Department of Surgery,
Division of Endocrine and Surgical Oncology, University of Iowa
Hospitals and Clinics, Iowa City, IA, USA

Rabih Houbballah, MD Department of Vascular
and Endovascular Surgery, Henri Mondor Hospital, Creteil, France

James Howe, MD Department of Surgery, University of Iowa
Hospitals and Clinics, Iowa City, IA, USA

Jennifer E. Hrabe, MD Department of Surgery,
University of Iowa, Iowa City, IA, USA

Mohammad K. Jamal, MD Department of Surgery,
University of Iowa Hospitals and Clinics, Iowa City, IA, USA

Faek R. Jamali, MD Department of Surgery,
American University of Beirut Medical Center, Beirut, Lebanon

Bellal A. Joseph, MD Department of Surgery Section of Trauma,
Critical Care, and Emergency Surgery, University of Arizona,
Tucson, AZ, USA

Sergy Khaitov, MD Division of Colon and Rectal Surgery,
Department of Surgery, The Mount Sinai Hospital,
New York, NY, USA

Ismail Mohamad Khalil, MD Department of Surgery,
American University of Beirut Medical Center, Beirut, Lebanon

Mohammad Khreiss, MD Department of Surgery, University of Arizona, Tucson, AZ, USA

Prashant Khullar, MD Department of Surgery, University of Iowa Hospitals and Clinics, Iowa city, IA, USA prashant-khullar@uiowa.edu

John Lane, MD Department of Surgery, University of California, Irvine, Orange, CA, USA

Chad Laurich, MD Department of Surgery, University of Iowa Hospital and Clinics, Iowa City, IA, USA

Yi-Horng Lee, MD Department of Surgery, University of Iowa Hospitals and Clinics, Iowa City, IA, USA

Timothy D. Light, MD Department of Surgery, University of Iowa Hospitals and Clinics, Iowa City, IA, USA

Danny Liu, MD Department of Surgery, University of Iowa Hospitals and Clinics, Iowa City, IA, USA

Shauna Lorenzo-Rivero, MD Department of Surgery, University of Tennessee School of Medicine, Chattanooga, TN, USA

Catherine Madorin, MD Department of Surgery, The Mount Sinai Hospital, New York, NY, USA

Dale Maharaj, MBBS Caribbean Vascular and Vein Clinic, St. Clair Medical Center, St. Clair, Trinidad

Michel S. Makaroun, MD Department of Vascular Surgery, University of Pittsburgh Medical Center, Pittsburgh, PA, USA

Samy Maklad, MD Department of General Surgery, University of Iowa Hospitals and Clinics, Iowa City, IA, USA

Elizabeth A. Marshall, MD University of Iowa Hospital and Clinics, Iowa City, IA, USA

Mario Martinasevic, MD Department of Surgery, University of Iowa Hospital and Clinics, Iowa City, IA, USA

Manish Mehta, MD, MPH The Institute for Vascular Heath and Disease, Albany Medical Center Hospital, Albany, NY, USA

Samuel R. Money, MD Department of Surgery, Division of Vascular Surgery, Ochsner Clinic, New Orleans, LA, USA

Charles H. Mosher, MD University Medical Center, University of Arizona, Tuscon, AZ, USA

Munier M.S. Nazzal, MD Department of Surgery, University of Toledo Medical Center, Toledo, OH, USA

Scott Q. Nguyen, MD Department of Surgery, Mount Sinai School of Medicine, New York, NY, USA

Kathleen J. Ozsvath, MD Department of Vascular Surgery, Albany Medical Center Hospital, Albany, NY, USA

F. Ezequiel Parodi, MD Department of Vascular Surgery, University of South Florida, Tampa, FL, USA

Graeme Pitcher, MBBCh University of Iowa Hospital and Clinics, Iowa City, IA, USA

Simon Roh, MD Department of Surgery, University of Iowa Hospital and Clinics, Iowa City, IA, USA

Bassem Y. Safadi, MD Department of Surgery/Division of General Surgery, American University of Beirut Medical Center, Beirut, Lebanon

Jean Salem, MD Department of Surgery, American University of Beirut Medical Center, Beirut, Lebanon

Carol E.H. Scott-Conner, MD
Department of Surgery, University of Iowa Carver College of Medicine, Iowa City, IA, USA

Pierre Sfeir, MD Department of Surgery, American University of Beirut Medical Center, Beirut, Lebanon

Murray L. Shames, MD Division of Vascular and Endovascular Surgery, University of South Florida, Tampa, FL, USA

Mark Shapiro, MD Department of Cardiothoracic Surgery, The Mount Medical Center, New York, NY, USA

Mel J. Sharafuddin, MD Department of Surgery and Radiology, University of Iowa Hospitals and Clinics, Iowa City, IA, USA

William J. Sharp, MD Department of Surgery, University of Iowa Hospitals and Clinics, Iowa City, IA, USA

Rajesh Shetty, MD Organ Transplant Centre, University of Iowa Hospitals and Clinics, Iowa City, IA, USA

Joel Shilyansky, MD Division of Pediatric Surgery, Department of Surgery, University of Iowa Children's Hospital, Iowa City, IA, USA

Kristen C. Sihler, MD, MS Departments of General Surgery, Trauma, and Critical Care, Maine Medical Center, Portland, ME, USA

Jessica K. Smith, MD Department of Surgery, University of Iowa Hospitals and Clinics, Iowa City, IA, USA

Lori K. Soni, MD Department of Surgery, University of Iowa Hospitals and Clinics, Iowa City, IA, USA

Philip M. Spanheimer, MD Department of Surgery, University of Iowa Hospitals and Clinics, Iowa City, IA, USA

Amy Bobis Stanfill, MD Department of Pediatric Surgery, Children's Hospital of Illinois, University of Illinois College of Medicine, Peoria, IL, USA

Emily Steinhagen, MD Department of Surgery, The Mount Sinai Medical Center, New York, NY, USA

Sujata Subramanian, MD Department of Surgery, Division of Vascular Surgery, University of Pennsylvania Hospital, Philadelphia, PA USA

Raphael C. Sun, MD Department of Surgery, University of Iowa Hospital and Clinics, Iowa City, IA, USA

Gary William Swain, Jr., MD Department of Surgery, Mount Sinai Hospital, New York, NY, USA

Theodore H. Teruya, MD Department of Vascular Surgery, Loma Linda University Medical Center, Loma Linda, CA, USA

Vassiliki Liana Tsikitis, MD Department of Surgery, University of Arizona, Tucson, AZ, USA

Georgios Tsoulfas, MD Department of Surgery, Aristoteleion University of Thessaloniki, Thessaloniki, Greece

Kaare Weber, MD Department of Surgery, The Mount Sinai Hospital, New York, NY, USA

Jessemae L. Welsh, MD Department of Surgery, University of Iowa Hospitals and Clinics, Iowa City, IA, USA

Eanas S. Yassa, MD Department of Surgery, University of Iowa Hospitals and Clinics, Iowa City, IA, USA

John W. York, MD Division of Vascular Surgery, Department of Surgery, Ochsner Clinic, New Orleans, LA, USA

Ahmad Zaghal, MD Department of Surgery, American University of Beirut-Medical Center, Beirut, Lebanon

Linda P. Zhang, MD Department of General Surgery, Mount Sinai School of Medicine, New York, NY, USA

Section I
Esophagus

Chapter 1

Esophagectomy: Right Thoracotomy and Laparotomy with Thoracic Anastomosis

Carol E.H. Scott-Conner, M.D.

INDICATIONS

- *Carcinoma/high-grade dysplasia* of the *lower third of the esophagus/gastric cardia.*
- Rarely: benign stricture, severe neuromuscular dysfunction, or perforation.

ESSENTIAL STEPS

1. Single lung ventilation via double-lumen endotracheal tube. Collapse right lung.
2. Right posterolateral thoracotomy through the fifth or sixth intercostal space.
3. Divide the azygous vein (if needed).
4. Incise the pleura and mobilize the esophagus.
5. Take care to avoid injury to the recurrent laryngeal nerves.
6. Divide the esophagus.
7. Upper midline abdominal incision.
8. Divide the gastrocolic ligament, preserve the right gastroepiploic artery, and ligate the left gastroepiploic artery and short gastric arteries.
9. Dissect the lesser curvature via the lesser sac; preserve the right gastric and aberrant left hepatic artery if present.
10. Ligate the left gastric vessels.
11. Circumferentially free the esophagus at hiatus.
12. Perform a generous Kocher maneuver.

2

J.J. Hoballah and C.E.H. Scott-Conner (eds.), *Operative Dictations in General and Vascular Surgery*, DOI 10.1007/978-1-4614-0451-4_1,
© Springer Science+Business Media, LLC 2012

13. Gastric drainage procedure (pyloromyotomy or pyloroplasty) to prevent delayed emptying.
14. Withdraw the distal esophagus into the abdomen.
15. Divide the stomach.
16. Advance the distal stomach into the chest.
17. Stapled/sutured anastomosis.
18. Wrap the proximal stomach around anastomosis and tack to the apex of pleura.
19. Close hiatus around the distal stomach.
20. *Feeding jejunostomy.*
21. Close the chest with thoracostomy tube drainage.
22. Close the abdomen.

NOTE THESE VARIATIONS

- Stapled vs. sutured anastomosis (size of stapler and type of suture).
- Pyloromyotomy vs. pyloroplasty.

COMPLICATIONS

- Injury to the tracheobronchial tree.
- Recurrent laryngeal nerve injury.
- Splenic injury.
- Gastric necrosis.
- Pneumothorax.
- Chylothorax.
- Anastomotic leak.
- Empyema/mediastinitis.
- Delayed gastric emptying.
- Dumping syndrome.
- Herniation of the abdominal viscera through the diaphragmatic hiatus.
- Anastomotic stricture.
- Reflux esophagitis.

TEMPLATE OPERATIVE DICTATION

Preoperative diagnosis: *Carcinoma/high-grade dysplasia* of the *lower third of the esophagus/gastric cardia/other.*

Procedure: Esophagectomy via right thoracotomy and laparotomy with thoracic anastomosis.

Postoperative diagnosis: Same.

Indications: This ___-year-old *male/female* had developed dysphagia and on workup was found to have *dysplasia/carcinoma of the esophagus* *extending from ___ to ___ cm/other. (If carcinoma, detail preoperative staging and any neoadjuvant chemotherapy and radiation therapy given.)* Esophagectomy was indicated.

Description of procedure: Following smooth induction of general anesthesia, the patient was intubated with a double-lumen endotracheal tube, placed in a modified left decubitus position, and padded appropriately. The right chest and abdomen were prepped and draped in the usual sterile fashion. A time-out was completed verifying correct patient, procedure, site, positioning, and implant(s) and/or special equipment prior to beginning this procedure.

A standard right posterolateral thoracotomy was performed through the fifth intercostal space. Single lung ventilation was established, allowing for anterior retraction of the lung and exposure of the mediastinum. The chest was explored, confirming no evidence of metastatic disease. The azygous vein was identified, dissected, ligated, and divided. The pleura was then incised along the azygous vein and inferior pulmonary ligament divided, allowing the esophagus to be circumferentially mobilized from the level of the hiatus to the thoracic inlet. Esophageal artery branches were identified and ligated with vascular clips. Lymphatic tissues were mobilized en bloc with the esophagus. The vagus nerves were identified proximally, clipped, and divided to minimize risk of recurrent laryngeal nerve injury. Any in-dwelling esophageal tubes were withdrawn. Two traction sutures were placed and the esophagus was divided at its proximal margin *with a linear cutting stapler/with electrocautery.* Moist laparotomy pads were placed on the thoracic field *and the Finochetto retractor released.*

The operating table was then tilted with the left side up. The abdomen was opened via a midline incision extending from the xiphoid to umbilicus. Abdominal exploration yielded no evidence of metastatic spread to the liver or other organs. The greater curvature of the stomach was identified with a palpable gastroepiploic vessel. The gastrocolic ligament was then divided by ligating and dividing the left gastroepiploic and short gastric vessels. The right gastroepiploic pedicle was carefully preserved. Attention was then turned to the lesser curvature via the lesser sac by gentle cephalad traction of the stomach. The right gastric artery was preserved; the left gastric artery was similarly identified. No anomalous left hepatic artery was identifiable; therefore, the left gastric artery was ligated and divided. Next, having dissected the lesser curvature to the pylorus, the duodenum was mobilized with a Kocher maneuver. A *pyloromyotomy/pyloroplasty* was performed to avoid postoperative outlet obstruction.

Attention was then turned to the hiatus. The phrenic vein was doubly ligated and the esophagus mobilized circumferentially. A silk suture was placed in the proximal specimen and the entire esophagus was advanced into the abdomen. A linear cutting stapler was used to divide the stomach below the gastroesophageal junction, establishing a distal margin 8 cm distal to the tumor.

The stomach was then advanced atraumatically into the chest, taking care to avoid torsion. It reached easily to the site of the proposed anastomosis without tension and appeared viable.

[Choose one:]

If stapled with linear stapler: The esophagus and gastric conduit were then aligned and a gastrotomy performed. Two sutures of 3-0 silk were placed to maintain alignment. A limb of a linear cutting stapler was placed down both the cervical esophagus and gastric fundus. The stapler was fired, creating a side-to-side functionally end anastomosis. A nasogastric tube was advanced through the anastomosis with the end resting distal to the pylorus. The remaining enterotomy was closed with a linear stapler/in two layers with running 3-0 Vicryl and interrupted 3-0 silk.

If stapled with circular stapler: Sizers were used to establish that a ___-mm circular stapler could be accommodated within the esophagus. A purse-string suture of 3-0 prolene was placed through all layers of the esophagus and the anvil inserted. The purse-string suture was tied. A gastrostomy was then made and the circular stapler inserted into the stomach. It was advanced through the anterior wall in a region that reached easily to the esophagus. The stapler was closed and fired. It was withdrawn and two complete donuts were noted. The nasogastric tube was advanced through the anastomosis and down through the pylorus. The gastrotomy was closed with a linear stapler/in two layers with running 3-0 Vicryl and interrupted 3-0 silk.

If sutured: A two-layer anastomosis was constructed between the distal esophagus and the stomach using an inner layer of running 3-0 Vicryl and an outer layer of 3-0 silk. The nasogastric tube was advanced through the anastomosis and down through the pylorus.

The anastomosis was checked and found to be patent and intact. The stomach was wrapped around the anastomosis and tacked to the apex of the pleura with interrupted sutures of 3-0 silk.

The pyloromyotomy site was reinforced with omentum in a patch fashion. The hiatus was closed around the stomach with interrupted sutures of 2-0 silk. *A feeding jejunostomy was created approximately 20 cm from the ligament of Treitz in the usual fashion, utilizing a Witzel tunnel and multiple abdominal wall tacking sutures.*

The abdomen was then irrigated and hemostasis checked. (*Optional: Multiple interrupted through-and-through retention sutures of* ____ *were placed.*) The fascia was closed with *a running suture of* ____/*a Smead-Jones closure of interrupted* ____. The skin was closed with *skin staples/subcuticular sutures of* ___/*other.*

The chest was irrigated, hemostasis checked, and closed in layers with sutures. Two ___ French thoracostomy tubes were placed.

The patient tolerated the procedure well and was taken to the postanesthesia care unit in stable condition.

ACKNOWLEDGMENT

This chapter was contributed by Benjamin E. Schneider, MD in the first edition.

NOTES

Chapter 2

Esophagectomy: Right Thoracotomy and Laparotomy with Cervical Anastomosis

Carol E.H. Scott-Conner, M.D.

INDICATIONS

- *Carcinoma/high-grade dysplasia* of the *middle/lower third of the esophagus/gastric cardia.*
- Rarely: benign stricture, severe neuromuscular dysfunction, or perforation.

ESSENTIAL STEPS

Thoracic Dissection

1. Single lung ventilation via double-lumen endotracheal tube. Collapse right lung.
2. Right posterolateral thoracotomy through the fifth or sixth intercostal space.
3. Divide the azygous vein (if needed).
4. Incise the pleura and mobilize the esophagus.
5. Take care to avoid injury to the recurrent laryngeal nerves.
6. Close the chest with thoracostomy tube drainage.

Abdominal Dissection

1. Upper midline abdominal incision.
2. Divide the gastrocolic ligament, preserve the right gastroepiploic artery, and ligate the left gastroepiploic artery and short gastric arteries.
3. Dissect the lesser curvature via the lesser sac; preserve the right gastric and aberrant left hepatic artery if present.

J.J. Hoballah and C.E.H. Scott-Conner (eds.), *Operative Dictations in General and Vascular Surgery*, DOI 10.1007/978-1-4614-0451-4_2,
© Springer Science+Business Media, LLC 2012

4. Ligate the left gastric vessels.
5. Circumferentially free the esophagus at hiatus.
6. Perform a generous Kocher maneuver.
7. Gastric drainage procedure (pyloromyotomy or pyloroplasty) to prevent delayed emptying.
8. Feeding jejunostomy, if desired.
9. Close hiatus.

Cervical Dissection
1. Incision through the platysma.
2. Dissect anterior to the sternocleidomastoid.
3. Mobilize the esophagus.
4. Avoid traction injury or cautery injury to the recurrent laryngeal nerve.
5. Cervical anastomosis *stapled/sutured*.
6. Close wound with drainage.

NOTE THESE VARIATIONS
- *Stapled/sutured* anastomosis.
- *Pyloromyotomy/pyloroplasty.*
- *Feeding jejunostomy.*

COMPLICATIONS
- Injury to the tracheobronchial tree.
- Recurrent laryngeal nerve injury.
- Splenic injury.
- Gastric necrosis.
- Pneumothorax.
- Chylothorax.
- Anastomotic leak.
- Empyema/mediastinitis.
- Delayed gastric emptying.
- Dumping syndrome.
- Herniation of the abdominal viscera through the diaphragmatic hiatus.
- Anastomotic stricture.
- Reflux esophagitis.

TEMPLATE OPERATIVE DICTATION
Preoperative diagnosis: *Carcinoma/high-grade dysplasia* of the *lower/middle third of the esophagus/gastric cardia/other.*
Procedure: Esophagectomy via right thoracotomy and laparotomy with cervical anastomosis.

Postoperative diagnosis: Same.

Indications: This ___-year-old *male/female* had developed dysphagia and on workup was found to have *dysplasia/carcinoma of the esophagus extending from ___ to ___ cm/other. (If carcinoma, detail preoperative staging and any neoadjuvant chemotherapy and radiation therapy given.)* Esophagectomy was indicated.

Description of procedure: Following smooth induction of general anesthesia, the patient was intubated with a double-lumen endotracheal tube, placed in a modified left decubitus position, and padded appropriately. The right chest was prepped and draped in the usual sterile fashion.

A time-out was completed verifying correct patient, procedure, site, positioning, and implant(s) and/or special equipment prior to beginning this procedure.

A standard right posterolateral thoracotomy was performed through the fifth intercostal space. Single lung ventilation was established, allowing for anterior retraction of the lung and exposure of the mediastinum. The chest was explored, confirming no evidence of metastatic disease. The azygous vein was identified, dissected, ligated, and divided. The pleura was then incised along the azygous vein and inferior pulmonary ligament divided, allowing the esophagus to be circumferentially mobilized from the level of the hiatus to the thoracic inlet. Esophageal artery branches were identified and ligated with vascular clips. Lymphatic tissues were mobilized en bloc with the esophagus. The vagus nerves were identified proximally, clipped, and divided to minimize risk of recurrent laryngeal nerve injury. The chest was then irrigated, hemostasis confirmed, and two thoracostomy tubes placed in the usual fashion. The chest was closed in layers and the skin approximated with surgical staples. Sterile dressings were applied and the patient turned to a supine position for the abdominal and cervical portions of the procedure.

Again, the patient was padded appropriately and positioned such that the left neck and abdomen could be accessed. The abdomen and left neck were prepped and draped in the usual sterile fashion. The abdomen was opened via a midline incision extending from the xiphoid to umbilicus. Abdominal exploration yielded no evidence of metastatic spread to the liver or other organs. The greater curvature of the stomach was identified with a palpable gastroepiploic vessel. The gastrocolic ligament was then divided by ligating and dividing the left gastroepiploic and short gastric vessels. The right gastroepiploic pedicle was carefully preserved. Attention was then turned to the lesser curvature via the lesser sac by gentle cephalad traction of the stomach. The right gastric artery was preserved; the left gastric artery was similarly identified. No anomalous left hepatic artery was identifiable; therefore, the left gastric artery was ligated and divided. Next, having dissected the lesser curvature to the pylorus, the duodenum was mobilized with a Kocher maneuver. A *pyloromyotomy/pyloroplasty* was performed.

Attention was then turned to the hiatus. The phrenic vein was doubly ligated and the esophagus mobilized circumferentially. Moist laparotomy pads were placed on the abdominal incision and the retractors withdrawn.

The skin was incised obliquely along the medial border of the left sternocleidomastoid muscle extending from the level of the thyroid cartilage to the sternal notch. Dissection was then carried out dividing the platysma and omohyoid and ligating the middle thyroid vein. Blunt dissection was extended to the prevertebral fascia and tracheoesophageal groove. The sternocleidomastoid muscle and carotid artery were gently retracted laterally; care was taken to avoid medial retraction to the recurrent laryngeal nerve. The cervical esophagus was then bluntly freed with care taken to avoid injury to the trachea. All in-dwelling esophageal tubes were withdrawn.

With the esophagus now free of its distal attachments, a linear cutting stapler was fired, creating the distal margin. The abdominal field was again entered. A silk suture was placed in the proximal specimen and the entire esophagus was advanced into the abdomen. A linear cutting stapler was used to divide the stomach below the gastroesophageal junction, establishing a distal margin 8 cm distal to the tumor. The previously placed silk was tied to the inflation port of a 30-cc Foley catheter, allowing the catheter to be placed with the balloon end within the abdomen and the port end exiting the cervical incision. The balloon was then placed within an arthroscopy bag and affixed with a tie. Placing the stomach within the bag-vacuum device, a Yankauer suction catheter was applied to the Foley end. The entire apparatus was advanced, bringing the gastric fundus out through the cervical incision with care taken to avoid torsion of the stomach.

[Choose one:]

If stapled with linear stapler: The esophagus and gastric conduit were then aligned and a gastrotomy performed. Two sutures of 3-0 silk were placed to maintain alignment. A limb of a linear cutting stapler was placed down both the cervical esophagus and gastric fundus. The stapler was fired, creating a side-to-side functionally end anastomosis. A nasogastric tube was advanced through the anastomosis with the end resting distal to the pylorus. The remaining enterotomy was closed with a linear stapler/in two layers with running 3-0 Vicryl and interrupted 3-0 silk.

If *sutured*: *A two-layer anastomosis was constructed between the distal esophagus and the stomach using an inner layer of running 3-0 Vicryl and an outer layer of 3-0 silk. The nasogastric tube was advanced through the anastomosis and down through the pylorus.*

The anastomosis was checked and found to be patent and intact. The stomach was tacked to the soft tissues in such a way as to avoid tension on the anastomosis. The cervical incision was irrigated, hemostasis was checked, and a *closed suction/small Penrose* drain was placed near the anastomosis. The incision was closed in layers with interrupted 3-0 Vicryl. The skin was closed with *skin staples/a subcuticular suture of running 4-0 monocryl.*

The pyloromyotomy site was reinforced with omentum in a patch fashion. The hiatus was closed around the stomach with interrupted sutures of 2-0 silk. *A feeding jejunostomy was created approximately 20 cm from the ligament of Treitz in the usual fashion utilizing a Witzel tunnel and multiple abdominal wall tacking sutures.*

The abdomen was then irrigated and hemostasis checked. (*Optional: Multiple interrupted through-and-through retention sutures of ____ were placed*). The fascia was closed with *a running suture of ____/a Smead-Jones closure of interrupted ____*. The skin was closed with *skin staples/subcuticular sutures of ___/other.*

The patient tolerated the procedure well and was taken to the postanesthesia care unit in stable condition.

ACKNOWLEDGMENT

This chapter was contributed by Benjamin E. Schneider, MD in the first edition.

NOTES

Chapter 3
Esophagogastrectomy

Elizabeth A. Marshall, M.D.

INDICATIONS
- *Carcinoma/high-grade dysplasia* of the *distal esophagus/ gastric cardia.*
- Rarely: benign stricture.

ESSENTIAL STEPS
1. Single lung ventilation via double-lumen endotracheal tube. Collapse L lung.
2. Left thoracoabdominal incision through the sixth intercostal space.
3. Ligate and divide the internal mammary artery.
4. Extend the incision onto the abdomen *obliquely/obliquely to midline and then down.*
5. Incise the diaphragm, avoiding the phrenic nerve.
6. Explore the abdomen and chest for metastases.
7. Incise the pleura and mobilize the esophagus with wide lymph node dissection. Divide vagal trunks.
8. Divide the esophagus.
9. Incise the phrenoesophageal ligament.
10. Progress down the greater curvature, taking greater omentum with the specimen.
11. Divide greater omentum; preserve the right gastroepiploic artery and ligate the left gastroepiploic artery and short gastric vessels.
12. Enter the lesser sac, lift stomach and divide the L gastric vessels.

J.J. Hoballah and C.E.H. Scott-Conner (eds.), *Operative Dictations in General and Vascular Surgery*, DOI 10.1007/978-1-4614-0451-4_3,
© Springer Science+Business Media, LLC 2012

13. Divide the stomach with cutting linear stapler and remove the specimen.
14. Perform a generous Kocher maneuver.
15. Gastric drainage procedure (pyloromyotomy or pyloroplasty) to prevent delayed emptying.
16. Advance the distal stomach into the chest.
17. *Stapled/sutured* anastomosis – two layer.
18. Close the hiatus around the distal stomach.
19. *Feeding jejunostomy.*
20. Close the chest with thoracostomy tube drainage.
21. Close the diaphragm and abdomen.

NOTE THESE VARIATIONS

- Two separate incisions (laparotomy and left thoracotomy) rather than thoracoabdominal incision.
- *Stapled* vs. *sutured* anastomosis (size of stapler and type of suture).
- *Pyloromyotomy/pyloroplasty.*

COMPLICATIONS

- Inadequate proximal resection margin.
- Injury to the tracheobronchial tree.
- Recurrent laryngeal nerve injury.
- Splenic injury.
- Injury to the tail of the pancreas.
- Gastric necrosis.
- Chylothorax.
- Anastomotic leak.
- Empyema/mediastinitis.
- Delayed gastric emptying.
- Dumping syndrome.
- Diaphragmatic hernia.
- Anastomotic stricture.
- Reflux esophagitis.

TEMPLATE OPERATIVE DICTATION

Preoperative diagnosis: *Carcinoma/high-grade dysplasia* of the *distal esophagus/gastric cardia/other.*
Procedure: Esophagogastrectomy.
Postoperative diagnosis: Same.
Indications: This ___-year-old *male/female* with *dysplasia/carcinoma limited to the distal esophagus/proximal stomach/other* on work up for _____. *(If carcinoma, detail preoperative staging*

and any neoadjuvant chemotherapy and radiation therapy given.) Esophagogastrectomy was indicated.

Description of procedure: Following induction of general anesthesia, the patient was intubated with a double-lumen endotracheal tube, placed in a modified right decubitus position, and padded appropriately. The left chest and abdomen were prepped and draped in the usual sterile fashion. A time-out was completed verifying correct patient, procedure, site, positioning, and implant(s) and/or special equipment prior to beginning this procedure. Preoperative antibiotics were given as indicated.

A posterolateral thoracotomy incision was made through the sixth intercostal space and extended medially through the costal margin *in an oblique direction/obliquely to the midline and then down the midline* as a thoracoabdominal incision. The internal mammary vessels were doubly ligated and divided. A circumlinear incision was made in the diaphragm, taking care to spare the phrenic nerve. The chest and abdomen were thoroughly explored and *no evidence of metastatic disease/(other: detail findings)* was found.

Single lung ventilation was established, allowing for anterior retraction of the lung and exposure of the mediastinum. The tumor was palpated *(detail location, findings)*. The pleura was incised and the inferior pulmonary ligament divided, exposing the distal esophagus. The esophagus was circumferentially mobilized en bloc with overlying pleura and periesophageal areolar and lymphatic tissues. Esophageal artery branches were identified and ligated with vascular clips. The vagus nerves were identified proximally, clipped, and divided. Two traction sutures were placed and the esophagus was divided at its proximal margin *with a linear cutting stapler/with electrocautery* at a distance of ___ cm above any obvious tumor. The phrenoesophageal membrane was incised.

Dissection then progressed along the greater curvature of the stomach. Greater omentum was dissected from the splenic flexure and removed with the specimen. A point of division was selected on the greater curvature. Omentum was serially divided with clamps and ligated, including a branch of the gastroepiploic arcade. Dissection progressed similarly along the lesser curvature, including nodal tissue along the lesser curvature and celiac axis. The right gastric and right gastroepiploic arteries were preserved.

The stomach was divided with a linear cutting stapler ___ cm beyond any obvious tumor and the specimen removed. Margins were checked by pathology *and determined to be clear/additional tissue was resected at the proximal/distal margin to obtain a free margin.*

The duodenum was mobilized with a Kocher maneuver. A *pyloromyotomy/pyloroplasty* was performed. The stomach was then advanced into the chest, taking care to avoid torsion. It reached easily to the site of the proposed anastomosis without tension and appeared viable.

If stapled with linear stapler: *The esophagus and gastric conduit were then aligned and a gastrotomy performed. Two sutures of 3-0 silk were placed to maintain alignment. A limb of a linear cutting stapler was placed down both the cervical esophagus and gastric fundus. The stapler was fired, creating a side-to-side functionally end anastomosis. A nasogastric tube was advanced through the anastomosis with the end resting distal to the pylorus. The remaining enterotomy was closed with a linear stapler/in two layers with running 3-0 Vicryl and interrupted 3-0 silk.*

If stapled with circular stapler: *Sizers were used to establish that a ___-mm circular stapler could be accommodated within the esophagus. A purse-string suture of 3-0 prolene was placed through all layers of the esophagus and the anvil inserted. The purse-string suture was tied. A gastrostomy was then made and the circular stapler inserted into the stomach. It was advanced through the anterior wall in a region that reached easily to the esophagus. The stapler was closed and fired. It was withdrawn and two complete donuts were noted. The nasogastric tube was advanced through the anastomosis and down through the pylorus. The gastrotomy was closed with a linear stapler/in two layers with running 3-0 Vicryl and interrupted 3-0 silk.*

If sutured: *A two-layer anastomosis was constructed between the distal esophagus and stomach using an inner layer of running 3-0 Vicryl and an outer layer of 3-0 silk. The nasogastric tube was advanced through the anastomosis and down through the pylorus.*

The anastomosis was checked and found to be patent and intact and hemostatic.

The pyloromyotomy site was reinforced with omentum in a patch fashion. The hiatus was closed around the stomach with interrupted sutures of 2-0 silk. *A feeding jejunostomy was created approximately 20 cm from the ligament of Treitz in the usual fashion utilizing a Witzel tunnel and abdominal wall tacking sutures.* Operative field was irrigated and examined for hemostasis.

The thoracoabdominal incision was then closed in stages: The diaphragm was closed with interrupted figure of eight sutures of ____. The thoracic portion was closed in layers in the usual fashion. Two thoracostomy tubes were placed in proximity to the anastomosis. The diaphragm was closed with interrupted figure-of-eight sutures of ___. The fascia was closed with *a running interrupted suture of* _____. The skin was closed with *skin staples/ subcuticular sutures of* ___.

The patient tolerated the procedure well and was taken to the postanesthesia care unit in stable condition.

ACKNOWLEDGMENT
This chapter was contributed by Natisha Busick, MD in the first edition.

NOTES

Chapter 4
Transhiatal Esophagectomy

Carol E.H. Scott-Conner, M.D.

INDICATIONS

- *Carcinoma/high-grade dysplasia* of the *lower third of the esophagus/gastric cardia.*
- Rarely: benign stricture, severe neuromuscular dysfunction, or perforation.

ESSENTIAL STEPS

1. Midline abdominal incision.
2. Divide the gastrocolic ligament.
3. Preserve the right gastroepiploic artery, ligate the left gastroepiploic artery, and ligate the short gastric arteries.
4. Dissect the lesser curvature.
5. Preserve the right gastric and *aberrant left hepatic artery if present*.
6. Ligate the left gastric vessels.
7. Dissect the hiatus, mobilizing the esophagus from below.
8. Kocher maneuver.
9. *Gastric drainage procedure to prevent delayed emptying.*
10. Oblique neck incision.
11. Dissect anterior to the sternocleidomastoid.
12. Avoid traction injury or cautery injury to the recurrent laryngeal nerve.
13. Mobilize the cervical esophagus.
14. Divide the esophagus in the neck and stomach in the abdomen.

J.J. Hoballah and C.E.H. Scott-Conner (eds.), *Operative Dictations in General and Vascular Surgery*, DOI 10.1007/978-1-4614-0451-4_4,

15. Pull the specimen down through the abdomen and remove.
16. Pull the stomach up into cervical incision.
17. Cervical anastomosis: *sutured/stapled.*
18. Place closed suction drain adjacent to the anastomosis in the neck.
19. Close the hiatus around the stomach.
20. Check hemostasis and close wounds.

COMPLICATIONS

- Major hemorrhage.
- Injury to the tracheobronchial tree.
- Recurrent laryngeal nerve injury.
- Splenic injury.
- Gastric necrosis.
- Pneumothorax.
- Chylothorax.
- Anastomotic leak.
- Empyema/mediastinitis.

TEMPLATE OPERATIVE DICTATION

Preoperative diagnosis: *Carcinoma/high-grade dysplasia* of the *lower third of the esophagus/gastric cardia/other.*
Procedure: Transhiatal esophagectomy.
Postoperative diagnosis: Same.
Indications: This ___-year-old *male/female* had developed dysphagia and on workup was found to have *dysplasia/carcinoma of the esophagus extending from ___ to ___ cm/other. (If carcinoma, detail preoperative staging and any neoadjuvant chemotherapy and radiation therapy given.)* Esophagectomy was indicated.
Description of procedure: The patient was taken to the operating room and general anesthesia was induced. The abdomen and left neck were prepped and draped in the usual sterile fashion. A time-out was completed verifying correct patient, procedure, site, positioning, and implant(s) and/or special equipment prior to beginning this procedure. An upper midline incision was made and the abdomen explored. *No evidence of metastatic disease was found/other.*

Attention was then turned to the greater curvature of the stomach, where a palpable gastroepiploic vessel was identified. The left gastroepiploic and short vessels were ligated with 2-0 silk and divided. The right gastroepiploic pedicle was carefully preserved.

When the greater curvature was fully mobilized, attention was turned to the lesser curvature. Gentle cephalad traction was placed on the stomach and the lesser sac was entered. The right gastric artery was preserved and the left gastric artery was similarly identified. No anomalous left hepatic artery was identifiable; therefore, the left gastric artery was ligated and divided. The dissection of the lesser curvature was continued to the pylorus. An extensive Kocher maneuver was performed.

Attention was then turned to dissection of the hiatus. The phrenic vein was doubly ligated and divided; the phrenoesophageal ligament was divided using sharp and blunt dissection. The mediastinum was entered anterior to the esophagus. The left triangular ligament was divided and the esophagus mobilized circumferentially. *A pyloromyotomy/pyloroplasty was performed to avoid postoperative outlet obstruction.*

The skin was incised obliquely along the medial border of the left sternocleidomastoid muscle extending from the level of the thyroid cartilage to the sternal notch. Dissection was then carried out dividing the platysma and omohyoid and ligating the middle thyroid vein. Blunt dissection was extended to the prevertebral fascia and tracheoesophageal groove. The sternocleidomastoid muscle and carotid artery were gently retracted laterally; care was taken to avoid medial retraction to the recurrent laryngeal nerve. The cervical esophagus was then bluntly mobilized, taking care to avoid injury to the trachea. With the esophagus now free of its distal attachments, a linear cutting stapler was fired, creating the distal margin. A silk suture was placed in the proximal specimen and the entire esophagus was advanced into the abdomen. A linear cutting stapler was used to divide the stomach below the gastroesophageal junction, establishing a distal margin 8 cm distal to the tumor. The previously placed silk was tied to the inflation port of a 30-cc Foley catheter, allowing the catheter to be placed with the balloon end within the abdomen and the port end exiting the cervical incision. The balloon was then placed within an arthroscopy bag and affixed with a tie. Placing the stomach within the bag-vacuum device, a Yankauer suction catheter was applied to the Foley end. The entire apparatus was advanced, bringing the gastric fundus out through the cervical incision with care taken to avoid torsion of the stomach.

[Choose one:]

If stapled anastomosis: The esophagus and gastric conduit were then aligned and a gastrotomy performed. A limb of a linear cutting stapler was placed down both the cervical esophagus and gastric fundus.

The stapler was fired, creating a side-to-side functionally end anastomosis. A nasogastric tube was advanced through the anastomosis with the end resting distal to the pylorus. The remaining enterotomy was closed with a linear stapler/in two layers with running 3-0 Vicryl and interrupted 3-0 silk.

If sutured: *A two-layer anastomosis was constructed between the distal esophagus and stomach using an inner layer of running 3-0 Vicryl and an outer layer of 3-0 silk. The nasogastric tube was advanced through the anastomosis and down through the pylorus.*

A closed suction drain was placed in the cervical bed and the incision irrigated and closed in the usual fashion. *The pyloromyotomy/pyloroplasty site was reinforced with omentum in a patch fashion.* The hiatus was reapproximated around the stomach and secured with interrupted 2-0 silk suture. *A feeding jejunostomy was created approximately 20 cm from the ligament of Treitz in the usual fashion utilizing a Witzel tunnel and multiple abdominal wall tacking sutures.*

(*Optional: Multiple interrupted through-and-through retention sutures of* ____ *were placed*). The fascia was closed with *a running suture of* ____/*a Smead-Jones closure of interrupted* ____. The skin was closed with *skin staples/subcuticular sutures of* ___/*other.* The cervical incision was irrigated, hemostasis was checked, and the incision was closed in two layers with interrupted 3-0 Vicryl. The skin was closed with *skin staples/subcuticular sutures of* ___/*other.* The drain was secured.

The patient tolerated the procedure well and was taken to the postanesthesia care unit in stable condition.

ACKNOWLEDGMENT

This chapter was contributed by Benjamin E. Schneider, MD in the previous edition.

NOTES

Chapter 5
Thoracoscopic Esophagectomy

Edward Y. Chan, M.D. and Edward H. Chin, M.D.

INDICATIONS
- Surgically resectable esophageal cancer.
- High-grade dysplasia of the esophagus.
- Massive esophageal dilatation due to benign disease (end-stage achalasia, Chagas' disease).

ESSENTIAL STEPS
1. Esophagogastroduodenoscopy *and bronchoscopy.*
2. Double-lumen endotracheal tube.
3. Left lateral decubitus position with right arm secured above head.
4. Deflate right lung.
5. Insert thoracoscopic ports in right chest.
6. Thoracoscopic exploration of the chest *and send biopsies for frozen section.*
7. Place suture in central tendon of right diaphragm.
8. Divide inferior pulmonary ligament.
9. Dissect around esophagus, pass penrose drain around esophagus for retraction.
10. Divide the azygos vein.
11. Dissect the esophagus cephalad toward the thoracic inlet, including all lymph nodes en-bloc, and caudad to the crus of the diaphragm.
12. Free the esophagus from the thoracic duct and aorta, dividing branches as needed.

J.J. Hoballah and C.E.H. Scott-Conner (eds.), *Operative Dictations in General and Vascular Surgery*, DOI 10.1007/978-1-4614-0451-4_5,
© Springer Science+Business Media, LLC 2012

13. Place penrose in thoracic inlet for later retrieval during cervical dissection.
14. Inject local anesthetic into intercostal spaces, place chest tube for drainage.
15. Close thoracoscopic port sites.
16. Position patient supine and reprep the abdomen for laparoscopy.
17. Exchange double-lumen endotracheal tube for single lumen tube.
18. Insert laparoscopic ports.
19. Insert self-retaining liver retractor to retract left lobe of liver.
20. Divide the hepatogastric ligament exposing the right crus and dissect to the left crus.
21. Continue dissection in retroesophageal window cephalad, taking care not to enter the thoracic cavity.
22. Divide the phrenogastric attachments.
23. Divide the short gastric vessels along the greater curvature.
24. Divide the hepatoduodenal ligaments.
25. Perform Kocher maneuver to fully mobilize pylorus.
26. Divide retrogastric attachments.
27. Identify and mobilize lymph nodes and fatty tissue of the celiac axis.
28. Divide left gastric vessels with endovascular stapler or LigaSure vessel sealing device.
29. Place additional 11-mm port in right lower quadrant to facilitate the retraction of stomach during creation of gastric tube.
30. Create gastric tube by stapling parallel to greater curvature while gently retracting the stomach cephalad and caudad.
31. Perform a pyloroplasty or pyloromyotomy by dividing the pylorus along the anterior wall, suction the gastric tube, then close the incision transversely.
32. Create jejunostomy tube by needle catheter technique or using 14 French catheter.
33. Suture the tip of the gastric tube to the lesser curvature of the specimen.
34. Make a low cervical incision with dissection down through the platysma to the deep prevertebral fascia.
35. Dissect the cervical esophagus laterally and retrieve the penrose drain.

36. While insufflating the abdomen to maintain direct visualization, pull the gastric tube through the hiatus into the neck using the penrose drain, maintaining appropriate orientation.
37. Perform esophageal anastomosis using an EEA stapler or hand-sewn technique.
38. Insert nasogastric tube across the anastomosis with end in the gastric tube.
39. Resect the distal end of the gastric tube with a linear stapler.
40. Retract the distal end of the gastric tube to align the conduit while observing the neck anastomosis.
41. Affix gastric tube to diaphragmatic hiatus.
42. Close laparoscopic port sites and neck incision.
43. *Toilet bronchoscopy.*

NOTE THESE VARIATIONS

- Type of suture, use of pledgets.
- Type and size of stapling device.
- Laparoscopic or thoracoscopic staging prior to operation.
- Confirmation of jejunostomy tube placement with contrast X-ray.
- If the hiatal opening appears narrowed, incisions may be made in the crura to relieve tension on the gastric tube.
- Esophageal anastomosis with alternative technique: hand-sewn or side-to-side stapled.
- Bronchoscopy before and after the operation.
- Decision to start with laparoscopic portion prior to thoracoscopic.
- Decision to create a narrow gastric tube vs. leave stomach intact.
- Pyloroplasty vs. pyloromyotomy as gastric drainage procedure.

COMPLICATIONS

- Injury to the lungs, esophagus, aorta, spleen, transverse colon, trachea, bronchi, vagus, and recurrent laryngeal nerves.
- Chylothorax from thoracic duct injury.
- Damage to, twisting of, or devascularization of the gastric tube.
- Anastomotic leak either in the neck or in the thoracic cavity.

TEMPLATE OPERATIVE DICTATION

Preoperative diagnosis: Esophageal cancer *or end-stage achalasia, Chagas' disease.*

Postoperative diagnosis: Same.

Procedure: Thoracoscopic and laparoscopic esophagectomy.

Indications: This ___-year-old *male/female* presented with _____ and was subsequently diagnosed with esophageal cancer/*end-stage achalasia*. A staging workup was undertaken with *CT scan/PET scan/endoscopic ultrasound/needle biopsy* that demonstrated surgically resectable disease. After a discussion of the risks, benefits, and alternatives to surgery, the patient elected to undergo thoracoscopic esophagectomy.

Description of procedure: *A thoracic epidural catheter was placed by anesthesia for postoperative pain control.* A time-out was completed verifying correct patient, procedure, site, positioning, and implant(s) and/or special equipment prior to beginning this procedure. Esophagogastroduodenoscopy was performed to assess the extent of the tumor. *Given the mid-thoracic location of the tumor, bronchoscopy was also performed.* Following induction of general anesthesia, the patient was intubated with a double-lumen endotracheal tube and placed in the left lateral decubitus position with the right arm raised and padded appropriately. The right chest was prepped and draped in the usual sterile fashion.

A 10-mm camera port was inserted in the *eighth/ninth* intercostal space anterior to the midaxillary line. Another 10-mm port was placed at the *eighth/ninth* intercostal space in the posterior axillary line. Two 5-mm ports were placed inferior to the tip of the scapula and anterosuperiorly in the fifth intercostal space. Single lung ventilation was established, allowing for anterior retraction of the lung and exposure of the mediastinum. The chest was explored and no abnormalities found *(detail abnormalities* and *biopsies taken)*. A suture was placed in the costophrenic recess anteriorly to provide traction on the diaphragm and provide exposure of the distal thoracic esophagus. The inferior pulmonary ligament was divided and the lung retracted cephalad.

The mediastinal pleura overlying the esophagus was incised to the level of the azygos vein. The esophagus was then encircled with a Penrose drain to assist with retraction. The azygos vein was divided using a vascular load stapler. The mediastinal pleura superior to the azygos was preserved to aid in sealing the mediastinum around the gastric tube. The esophagus was gently mobilized from the diaphragm to above the carina with care taken to include surrounding lymph nodes and fat en bloc.

The recurrent laryngeal nerves were identified superiorly and protected. The thoracic duct was identified and lymphatic attachments to the esophagus were clipped and divided. Branches between the aorta and esophagus were also clipped and divided *(or coagulated with a harmonic scalpel)*. The remainder of the thoracic esophagus was mobilized circumferentially from the thoracic inlet to the level of the diaphragm. No bleeding, air leaks, or chyle leaks were visualized. The Penrose drain was placed in the thoracic inlet for later retrieval. One to two mL of bupivicaine was injected into the intercostal space, and a 28 French thoracostomy tube placed. The right lung was reinflated and the airway and lung were examined for air leaks. The thoracic ports were closed.

The patient was turned to the supine position. The double-lumen endotracheal tube was exchanged for a single-lumen endotracheal tube. The abdomen was reprepped and draped in the standard surgical manner. An 11-mm port was placed in the right epigastrium. Two 5-mm ports were placed along the right costal margin for liver retraction, one 5-mm port in the left costal margin, and one 5-mm port in the left epigastrium opposite the 11-mm port. The left lobe of the liver was retracted using a self-retaining system.

The hepatogastric ligament was divided toward the right crus of the diaphragm, with the dissection of the right and left crura. Dissection of the esophageal hiatus was continued to the top of the left crus and the phrenogastric attachments were divided in this area. Care was taken not to enter the thoracic cavity and to maintain the phrenoesophageal attachments to preserve abdominal pneumoperitoneum.

The stomach was mobilized by division of the short gastric vessels along the greater curve and the gastrocolic omentum. Care was taken to avoid the gastroepiploic vessels and arcade, and attention was paid to avoid injury to the transverse colon. The hepatoduodenal attachments were divided along the lateral duodenum and the stomach was mobilized superiorly. Care was taken not to handle the stomach directly to avoid damaging the vascular supply. The lymph nodes and fat around the celiac axis were dissected and mobilized. The left gastric artery was divided with a vascular stapler *(or Ligasure vessel sealing system)*.

Another 11-mm port was inserted in the right lower quadrant and an atraumatic grasper was used to retract the pylorus inferiorly. An endoscopic stapler was placed above the right gastric artery and fired perpendicular to the lesser curve with attention paid to preserving the first arterial arcades. __ staple loads were used to create the gastric tube as the stapling progressed cephalad parallel to the greater curve. Throughout the stapling, cephalad and caudad traction was maintained to limit inadvertant twisting or shortening of the gastric tube.

After creation of the gastric tube, a pyloroplasty *(or pyloromyotomy)* was performed. Stay sutures were first placed above and below the anterior aspect of the muscle. The muscle was opened from the duodenal side along the length of the pyloric channel using harmonic scalpel. The gastric tube was suctioned clean through the pyloroplasty, and the incision was then closed using intracorporeal suturing, in two layers.

A feeding jejunostomy was placed using a needle catheter system (or 14 French catheter). A loop of jejunum was identified approximately 30 cm distal to the ligament of Treitz. The jejunum was tacked to the abdominal wall in the left *mid/lower* quadrant using intracorporeal suturing *(or automated suturing device)*. The needle and guidewire were inserted through the abdominal wall into the jejunum, with insufflation of 10 mL of air confirming proper placement of the catheter. The loop of jejunum was tacked to the abdominal wall circumferentially covering the entry site. An additional stitch was placed several centimeters away to secure the bowel loop and avoid torsion.

The phrenoesophageal membrane was circumferentially mobilized at the hiatus and the end of the gastric tube was sutured to the lower edge of the specimen. The abdomen was deflated and the laparoscopic equipment was withdrawn.

A cervical collar incision was made at this point and taken down through the platysma to the prevertebral fascia. The penrose drain that had previously been left in the thoracic inlet was retrieved and the cervical esophagus was dissected free. The recurrent laryngeal nerves were again visualized and care was taken not to damage them.

The laparoscope was reinserted and the abdomen was reinsufflated. The esophageal specimen was withdrawn through the neck, while the gastric tube was pulled into the hiatus under direct laparoscopic vision. The appropriate alignment of gastric tube was confirmed with the gastroepiploic arcade toward the left crus. *Incisions were made in the left and right crura to relieve tension on the gastric tube through the hiatal opening.*

The esophageal anastomosis was performed in the neck by dividing the cervical esophagus 2 cm below the cricopharyngeus using an automatic purse-string device. An end-to-side anastomosis was performed with a 25-mm EEA stapler between the cervical esophageal stump and the fundic tip of the gastric tube *(anastomotic techniques may vary)*. The EEA rings were inspected and found to be intact. A nasogastric tube was inserted and passed across the anastomosis with its tip in the gastric tube. The distal tip of the gastric tube was resected with a linear stapler.

The laparoscope was reinserted and the gastric tube was gently retracted to ensure that there was no redundancy of the conduit. The anastomosis was carefully observed through the cervical incision as the tube was retracted and no tension or dehiscence of the anastomosis was noted. The gastric tube was sutured to the hiatus laparoscopically to prevent later development of a hiatal hernia and to maintain orientation. The greater curve of the stomach was secured to the left crus, the anterior aspect of the tube was secured to the anterior crus, and the lesser curve of the tube was secured to the right crus.

The liver retractor was withdrawn and the 11-mm port defects were closed under direct vision. The abdomen was deflated and the skin was closed with a *subcuticular suture of* ___. The skin of the cervical incision was reapproximated without closure of the platysma. *Bronchoscopy was performed prior to extubation.* The patient tolerated the procedure well and was taken to the postanesthesia care unit in satisfactory condition.

NOTES

Chapter 6

Transabdominal Nissen Fundoplication

Linda P. Zhang, M.D. and Scott Q. Nguyen, M.D.

INDICATIONS

- Chronic GERD unresponsive to medical treatment.
- Chronic GERD in patients desiring discontinuation of medical therapy.
- Aspiration.
- Complications of GERD not responding to medical therapy.
  - Barrett's esophagus.
  - Esophagitis.
  - Stricture.
- Paraesophageal hernia with GERD.
- Children with severe esophagitis, pulmonary compromise, or failure to thrive.

ESSENTIAL STEPS

1. Decompress the stomach with an orogastric tube.
2. Upper midline incision.
3. Explore the abdomen and confirm pathology.
4. Incise the phrenoesophageal membrane.
5. Dissect both crura, encircling the esophagus.
6. Identify and preserve both vagus nerves.
7. *Close the hiatus if enlarged.*
8. Divide the short gastric vessels to mobilize the fundus.
9. Calibrate the wrap with esophageal bougie.
10. Create the loose floppy wrap involving the anterior and posterior aspects of the fundus.

J.J. Hoballah and C.E.H. Scott-Conner (eds.), *Operative Dictations in General and Vascular Surgery*, DOI 10.1007/978-1-4614-0451-4_6,
© Springer Science+Business Media, LLC 2012

11. Suture to the esophagus to prevent the wrap from sliding.
12. Check hemostasis.
13. Close the abdomen.

NOTE THESE VARIATIONS

- Hiatal closure.
- Vagus nerves encircled in wrap/excluded from wrap.
- Use of bougie.
- Use of pledgets during wrap.

COMPLICATIONS

- Esophageal perforation.
- Gastric perforation.
- Dysphagia.
- Wrap too loose.
- Wrap too tight or too long.
- Hiatal closure too tight, causing esophageal obstruction.
- Hiatal closure too loose, permitting paraesophageal herniation and dysphagia.
- Injury to the vagus nerve.
- Slipped wrap.

TEMPLATE OPERATIVE DICTATION

Preoperative diagnosis: *Reflux esophagitis/barrett's esophagus/ aspiration due to reflux/other.*

Procedure: Transabdominal Nissen fundoplication.

Postoperative diagnosis: Same.

Indications: This is a ____old *male/female* with *reflux/biopsy-proven reflux esophagitis/other. This had been treated medically with* _____ *in the past with improvement. The patient wished to minimize the need for long-term medication in the future.*

Description of procedure: After the patient was placed in a supine position, general endotracheal anesthesia was induced. A time-out was completed verifying correct patient, procedure, site, positioning, and implant(s) and/or special equipment prior to beginning this procedure. Lower extremity sequential compression devices were applied. *A Foley catheter was inserted under sterile conditions.* An orogastric tube was also placed. A midline vertical incision was made from the umbilicus up past the left edge of the xiphoid. The subcutaneous tissue and fascia was divided using electrocautery. The abdomen was entered with care under direct vision. *Any adhesions were carefully dissected off of the abdominal wall.*

The abdomen was explored. The hiatus of the abdominal esophagus, as well as the bilateral crura, were visualized. The hiatus appeared *enlarged/normal*. For adequate visualization, fixed retractors were used to retract the liver and abdominal wall. The gastrohepatic ligament was incised over the caudate lobe of the liver. *Care was taken to identify and preserve an aberrant left hepatic artery*. The phrenoesophageal membrane was carefully opened over the left crus and dissected off of the esophagus circumferentially. Care was taken to avoid injuring the anterior and posterior vagus nerves. A Penrose drain was then used to encircle the esophagus at the hiatus.

At the greater curve of the stomach, the short gastric vessels were identified and divided between 2-0 silk ties. These short gastric vessels were divided to the level of the angle of *His*, completely mobilizing the gastric fundus. Care was taken not to avulse the vessels from their attachments to the spleen. The crural opening was then closed with interrupted 2-0 silk sutures, approximately 1 cm apart. At the end of this reapproximation, the crus was snug around the esophagus.

The orogastric tube and all esophageal monitors/probes were removed. A 56 French bougie was passed through the esophagogastric junction under direct vision and palpation. The fundoplication was subsequently constructed over this bougie.

To create the 360° wrap around the esophagus, the fundus was brought around the posterior aspect of the esophagus, to form the medial aspect of the wrap. A position on the greater curve of the stomach was chosen to make the lateral portion of the wrap. The wrap was able to rest behind the esophagus without slipping back to its original position even when not held by instruments. 2-0 silk sutures were used to approximate the margins of the wrap, also taking a muscular bite of the esophagus anteriorly. A total of three sutures were used spaced 1 cm apart so that the length of the wrap was approximately 2–3 cm. These sutures were placed carefully to avoid injuring the vagus nerves or penetrating the esophageal and stomach lumen. The bougie was then removed, and the tightness of the wrap was checked using a finger inserted between the wrap and esophagus. The area was irrigated, and hemostasis was checked.

The fascia was closed using _____ *sutures in a running/interrupted fashion*. After the subcutaneous tissue was irrigated, skin was closed using *staples/subcuticular sutures of* ____. The patient tolerated the procedure well and *was extubated. S/he* was brought to the recovery room in stable condition.

ACKNOWLEDGMENT

This chapter was contributed by Kevin F. Satisky, MD in the first edition.

NOTES

Chapter 7

Laparoscopic Nissen Fundoplication

Jessica K. Smith, M.D.

INDICATIONS

- Reflux esophagitis unresponsive to maximal medical treatment and confirmed with 24-h pH probe.
- History of aspiration and/or recurrent pneumonias.
- Complications of longstanding reflux: erosive esophagitis, vocal cord changes, esophageal stricture, Barrett's esophagus.
- Unwillingness or inability to remain on lifelong acid suppression therapy.
- Symptomatic paraesophageal hernia with reflux.
- Children with severe esophagitis, recurrent pneumonia, or failure to thrive.

ESSENTIAL STEPS

1. Supine or modified lithotomy with a steep reverse Trendelenburg position.
2. Foley catheter and nasogastric or orogastric tube.
3. Induce pneumoperitoneum.
4. Mark xiphoid and bilateral costal margins.
5. Place the first 12-mm trocar just to the left of midline 12–15 cm below the xiphoid depending on the height of the patient.
6. Inspect the abdomen with a 30°, 10-mm laparoscope.
7. Place four additional trocars:
   - Operating ports: Two 12-mm trocars are placed in the bilateral subcostal margins in the midclavicular line.

J.J. Hoballah and C.E.H. Scott-Conner (eds.), *Operative Dictations in General and Vascular Surgery*, DOI 10.1007/978-1-4614-0451-4_7,
© Springer Science+Business Media, LLC 2012

- Assistant port: One 12-mm trocar is placed in the left anterior axillary line at the same level as the camera port.
- Liver retractor: Depending on the retractor to be used, one 5- or 10-mm trocar is placed in the right midaxillary line at the same level as the camera port. (Note: If a Nathanson retractor is used, a 5 mm incision is made just below the xiphoid to accommodate the instrument).

8. Elevate the left lobe of the liver to expose the hiatus.
9. Downward traction on the stomach to reduce hernia if present, held in place by the assistant.
10. Open the gastrohepatic ligament at the pars flaccida to expose the caudate lobe and right crus.
11. Develop the medial plane between the right crus and the esophagus.
12. Continue peritoneal incision over the hiatus.
13. Expose the left crus and decussation.
14. Complete atraumatic circumferential dissection of the esophagus.
15. Create a large enough retroesophageal window such that there is excellent visualization of the left upper quadrant looking from the right side.
16. Identify and preserve both vagus nerves.
17. Encircle esophagus including vagus nerves with 1/4″ wide 6″ long penrose drain or other retracting device.
18. Close the crura.
19. Divide the short gastric vessels to mobilize the fundus.
20. Pass an esophageal bougie under direct visualization with the laparoscope. Use 56 Fr for men, 52 Fr for women, adjust to the size of the patient.
21. Create a loose floppy wrap by passing the fundus behind the esophagus and performing the "shoeshine" maneuver.
22. Suture the fundus to itself with the first stitch to size the wrap.
23. Withdraw the bougie under direct visualization with the laparoscope.
24. Place two additional sutures in the fundoplication which include the anterior esophageal wall and create a wrap length of 2 cm.
25. Perform the following gastropexy stitches: A stitch at the 3 o'clock position of the wrap which includes the wrap, esophagus, and left crus. A posterior stitch which includes the wrap and the crural repair. A third stitch at

the 9 o'clock position which includes the wrap, esophagus, and the right crus.

26. Ensure hemostasis.
27. Remove the liver retractor under direct visualization and inspect for bleeding.
28. Remove ports under direct visualization, closing any dilated fascial defects.
29. Release pneumoperitoneum.
30. Proceed with skin closure.

VARIATIONS
- Position of the patient.
- Size of the esophageal bougie.
- Type of liver retractor.
- Type of suture.
- Suturing device, intra- or extracorporeal knot tying.
- Gastropexy sutures.
- 30 or 45° laparoscope.

COMPLICATIONS
- Trocar injuries to the vessels or viscera.
- Injury to the esophagus.
- Injury to the spleen or stomach.
- Wrap too loose or too tight causing recurrent reflux or dysphagia.
- Hiatal closure too tight, causing esophageal obstruction.
- Hiatal closure too loose, permitting paraesophageal herniation or wrap slippage.
- Injury to the vagus nerves.
- Pneumothorax or tension pneumothorax.

TEMPLATE OPERATIVE DICTATION

Preoperative diagnosis: *Reflux esophagitis/Barrett's esophagus/ aspiration due to reflux/other.*

Procedure: Laparoscopic Nissen fundoplication.

Postoperative diagnosis: Same.

Indications: This ___-year-old *male/female* had *biopsy-proven reflux esophagitis/Barrett's esophagus/aspiration due to reflux/other. This had been refractory to medical management/the patient did not want to remain on lifelong acid suppression therapy/other.* The decision was made to proceed with laparoscopic Nissen fundoplication.

Description of procedure: The patient was placed on the operating table on a secured vacuum beanbag in the supine position. General anesthesia was induced. A time-out was completed verifying correct patient, procedure, site, positioning, and implant(s) and/or special equipment prior to beginning this procedure. *A Foley catheter and nasogastric/orogastric tubes were placed. The legs were placed in stirrups with appropriate padding.* The right arm was tucked to accommodate the liver retractor. *The beanbag was placed to suction to secure the patient.* The abdomen was prepped and draped in the usual sterile fashion. The xiphoid and costal margins were marked with a marking pen. A point 12 cm from the xiphoid just to the left of midline was chosen for the camera port. A transverse incision was made to accommodate a 12-mm trocar.

[Choose one:]

    For Veress needle: The fascia was elevated and the Veress needle inserted. Proper position was confirmed by aspiration and saline meniscus test. A 11/12-mm trocar was then inserted.

    For Hassan cannula: The fascia was elevated and incised. Entry into the peritoneum was confirmed visually and no bowel was noted in the vicinity of the incision. Two figure-of-eight sutures of 2-0 Vicryl were placed and the Hassan cannula inserted under direct vision. The sutures were anchored around the cannula.

The abdomen was insufflated with carbon dioxide to a pressure of 15 mmHg. The patient tolerated the pneumoperitoneum well. The 30°, 10-mm laparoscope was inserted and the abdomen inspected. No injuries from Veress needle or initial trocar placement were noted. Additional trocars were then inserted under direct vision in the following locations: Two 12-mm trocars were placed in the bilateral subcostal margins in the midclavicular line. An assistant port using a 12-mm trocar was placed in the left anterior axillary line at the same level as the camera port. The final fifth 12-mm trocar was placed in the right midaxillary line at the same level as the camera port for the liver retractor. No injuries were noted during port placement.

The patient was placed in reverse Trendelenburg position. A liver retractor was introduced in the right subcostal port to elevate the left lobe of the liver and expose the hiatus. A 10-mm endoscopic Babcock clamp was introduced through the left assistant port and used to grasp the stomach and gently pull it toward the left lower quadrant.

The gastrohepatic ligament was opened with the *ultrasonic shears/electrocautery* beginning at the pars flaccida. The peritoneum was incised anteriorly over the hiatus to the left crus. The right crus was identified and cleared of investing tissue and the medial plane between the right crus and esophagus was developed and the crural decussation visualized. The dissection was then carried over the arch of the crura. The left crus was similarly dissected and the phrenoesophageal ligament divided. The vagus nerves were identified and protected. The esophagus was gently elevated with a closed grasper and dissection progressed underneath the esophagus until the esophagus was fully mobilized and a large retroesophageal window had been created.

An *esophageal retractor/penrose drain* was then passed under the esophagus. The esophagus was encircled to include the vagus nerves and the penrose secured with large endoscopic ligaclips. The assistant then released the stomach and grasped the penrose to maneuver the esophagus.

Attention was then directed to the hiatus. *Two/three* simple interrupted sutures of *0 dacron* were placed to approximate the hiatus behind the esophagus, leaving an approximately 1 cm space posteriorly and allowing the esophagus to rest in its normal position. At least 2 cm of intra-abdominal esophagus was observed.

The short gastric vessels were divided with ultrasonic shears and the fundus of the stomach was completely mobilized. The nasogastric/orogastric tube was removed. With the esophagus and stomach in a neutral position, a 56 Fr bougie was slowly passed under direct visualization with the laparoscope.

With the esophagus gently retracted anteriorly, a grasper was passed behind the esophagus and the fundus grasped and pulled over to the right side behind the esophagus. It passed easily and the proper orientation was ensured by performing the "shoeshine" maneuver. The wrap was approximated to itself without tension using a 2-0 silk suture, creating a 360° floppy wrap around the distal esophagus. The esophageal bogie was then removed. Two additional sutures were placed in the wrap which included a partial-thickness bite of esophagus to anchor the wrap. A wrap length of 2 cm was formed.

Three additional gastropexy sutures were placed using 2-0 silk suture. The first stitch was placed at the 3 o'clock position of the wrap which included the wrap, esophagus, and left crus. A posterior stitch which included the wrap and the crural repair was placed. A third stitch was placed at the 9 o'clock position which included the wrap, esophagus, and the right crus.

Hemostasis was achieved. The liver retractor was removed under direct visualization and the liver inspected for any bleeding. The trocars were removed one at a time and the fascial openings carefully inspected. Any dilated defects were reapproximated with a transfascial suture. Pneumoperitoneum was released, the laparoscope was withdrawn and the umbilical trocar removed. The skin was closed with subcuticular sutures of ___ and steristrips/skin adhesive. The patient tolerated the procedure well and was taken to the postanesthesia care unit in satisfactory condition.

ACKNOWLEDGMENT

This chapter was contributed by Kevin F. Satisky, MD in the first edition.

NOTES

Chapter 8

Transthoracic Collis Gastroplasty and Nissen Fundoplication

Mark Shapiro, M.D. and Edward H. Chin, M.D.

INDICATION

- Gastroesophageal reflux disease with inadequate intra-abdominal esophagus for fundoplication.

ESSENTIAL STEPS

1. Intubation with double-lumen endotracheal tube, and deflate the left lung.
2. Place the patient in the right lateral decubitus position.
3. Perform a left posterolateral thoracotomy in the sixth intercostal space.
4. Incise the mediastinal pleura overlying the esophagus.
5. Divide the inferior pulmonary ligament for additional exposure.
6. Mobilize the esophagus from the level of the carina to the diaphragm, dividing aortic branches as necessary.
7. Identify and preserve the vagus nerves.
8. Place a Penrose drain around the esophagus for traction.
9. Dissect the hernia sac from the right and left crura.
10. Divide the phrenoesophageal membrane and enlarge the hiatus bluntly.
11. Incise the gastrohepatic ligament in an avascular plane.
12. Divide the short gastric vessels *using harmonic scalpel/ with 2-0 silk ties*.
13. Reapproximate the right and left crura posteriorly with *two to four* permanent sutures; leave untied until gastroplasty

J.J. Hoballah and C.E.H. Scott-Conner (eds.), *Operative Dictations in General and Vascular Surgery*, DOI 10.1007/978-1-4614-0451-4_8,
© Springer Science+Business Media, LLC 2012

and fundoplication completed. Pledget reinforcement of the sutures can be used as well.

14. Retract the fundus of the stomach into the chest.
15. Pass 56 French esophageal bougie into the stomach along the lesser curvature.
16. Divide the fundus with a gastrointestinal anastomosis (GIA) stapler parallel to the lesser curvature.
17. Oversew gastric staple lines with running 2-0 silk suture.
18. Create 360° floppy Nissen fundoplication around the neoesophagus.
19. Secure the wrap with *two/three* interrupted sutures of 2-0 silk, with each suture incorporating a partial thickness bite of anterior esophagus, or neoesophagus.
20. Remove bougie.
21. Gently reduce the wrap into the abdomen.
22. Tie previously placed crural sutures.
23. Confirm that the index finger passes through the hiatus next to the esophagus.
24. *If hiatal hernia defect was very large, consider Surgisis reinforcement in onlay manner.*
25. Place 28 French thoracostomy tube.
26. Close thoracotomy incision.

NOTE THESE VARIATIONS

- Surgisis™ reinforcement of hiatal closure.
- Division of short gastric vessels with harmonic scalpel ™ or silk ties.
- Number of sutures used to close hiatus, and to create gastric wrap. Use of pledget reinforcement of the sutures used to close hiatus.

COMPLICATIONS

- Leakage from gastric staple lines.
- Ischemic necrosis of gastroplasty tube.
- Injury to esophagus, vagus nerves, stomach, and spleen.
- Dysphagia due to excessively tight wrap, or hiatal closure.
- Recurrent hiatal hernia, reflux.

TEMPLATE OPERATIVE DICTATION

Preoperative diagnosis: Gastroesophageal reflux disease with short esophagus.
Postoperative diagnosis: Same.

Procedure: Transthoracic Collis gastroplasty with Nissen fundoplication.

Indications: The patient is a ___-year-old *male/female* with long-standing gastroesophageal reflux refractory to medical management, who has elected for surgical management. *Her/his* preoperative endoscopy and UGI series demonstrated a short esophagus. Collis gastroplasty with Nissen fundoplication was planned.

Description of procedure: *A thoracic epidural catheter was placed by anesthesia for perioperative pain control.* After general anesthesia was induced, the patient was intubated with a double-lumen endotracheal tube, placed in the right lateral decubitus position, and padded appropriately. A time-out was completed verifying correct patient, procedure, site, positioning, and implant(s) and/or special equipment prior to beginning this procedure. The operating table was flexed to distract the ribs. The left chest was prepped and draped in the standard sterile fashion.

After single lung ventilation was established, a standard left posterolateral thoracotomy was performed through the sixth intercostal space. The latissimus dorsi was divided. The chest cavity was then entered. The inferior pulmonary ligament was divided with electrocautery to the level of the inferior pulmonary vein to assist with exposure.

The mediastinal pleura overlying the esophagus was longitudinally incised, and the distal esophagus circumferentially dissected, dividing aortic branches as necessary. The esophagus was encircled with a Penrose drain for gentle retraction. The right and left vagus nerves were identified and carefully preserved. Dissection was continued inferiorly to expose the right and left crura.

The esophagus was retracted anteriorly to expose the phrenoesophageal membrane, which was divided with blunt and sharp dissection. The left crus was then retracted laterally and the hiatus was spread to better visualize the stomach. The cardia of the stomach was freed circumferentially from the hiatus. The gastrohepatic ligament was identified and divided in an avascular plane. The short gastric vessels were coagulated using the harmonic scalpel, taking care to avoid excessive traction on the spleen. *Alternatively, these vessels can be ligated with 2-0 silk sutures.*

The crura were approximated posterior to the esophagus with *two to four* interrupted sutures of 0-Ethibond and left untied Pledget reinforcement of the sutures can be used as well. The length of the esophagus was confirmed be too short for proper fundoplication, and Collis gastroplasty necessary. The fundus of the stomach was delivered into the chest using a Babcock clamp.

A 56 French bougie was placed to size the neoesophagus diameter. The bougie tip was advanced to the distal stomach and placed along the lesser curvature. The fundus was then divided parallel to the lesser curvature with a 60-mm gastrointestinal anastomosis (GIA) stapler loaded with 3.5-mm staples, resulting in an approximately 4–5 cm neoesophagus. Both staple lines were oversewn with running 2-0 silk suture in a seromuscular fashion.

Then, a 360° floppy Nissen fundoplication was constructed using *two/three interrupted 2-0 silk sutures*. Each suture incorporated the left and right side of fundus, and an anterior bite of the esophagus or neoesophagus. Care was taken to avoid the anterior vagus nerve.

The bougie was then removed, and the stomach returned to the abdomen. The crural sutures were tied down, ensuring that a finger could still be passed behind the esophagus. The chest was irrigated and appropriate hemostasis obtained. The divided mediastinal pleura was reapproximated with a running 3-0 Vicryl suture. A 28 French thoracostomy tube was placed and the thoracotomy incision was closed with several layers of Vicryl suture. The skin was closed with *staples/a running subcuticular suture of* ___. The procedure was well-tolerated, and the patient was extubated and then taken to the postanesthesia care unit in stable condition.

ACKNOWLEDGMENT

This chapter was contributed by Natisha Busick, MD, in the first edition.

NOTES

Chapter 9
Laparoscopic Collis Gastroplasty and Nissen Fundoplication

Mohamad H. Alaeddine, M.D. and Bassem Y. Safadi, M.D.

INDICATIONS
- Gastroesophageal (GE) reflux disease with short esophagus.
- Paraesophageal hiatal hernia with short esophagus.

ESSENTIAL STEPS
1. Position the patient in modified lithotomy with reverse Trendelenburg for better exposure of the GE junction.
2. Place five ports in the upper abdomen: The first (camera) port should be high around 12–15 cm below the Xiphoid process.
3. Place the two working ports a "hands-breadth" away from the camera port in the upper abdomen on each side of the midline.
4. Place a 5-mm port on the left side in the anterior axillary line.
5. Retract the liver.
6. Open the pars flaccida and divide all peritoneal covers over the crura and esophagus.
7. Identify the posterior vagus nerve and develop a retrogastric window.
8. Divide the short gastric vessels and mobilize the fundus.
9. Release all mediastinal attachments of the distal esophagus.
10. If after all the mobilization the GE junction does not rest at least 2 cm below the crura, a Collis gastroplasty is warranted.

J.J. Hoballah and C.E.H. Scott-Conner (eds.), *Operative Dictations in General and Vascular Surgery*, DOI 10.1007/978-1-4614-0451-4_9,
© Springer Science+Business Media, LLC 2012

11. Perform intraoperative endoscopy to accurately identify the GE junction and mark the exact location on the serosal side with the aid of the endoscope.
12. Place a 48-Fr bougie transorally into the stomach.
13. Exchange the left-sided 5-mm port for a 12-mm port.
14. Introduce an angulated laparoscopic stapler via the left-sided port and staple transversely across the fundus to reach the bougie around 3 cm below the GE junction (more than one fire may be needed).
15. Fire another staple line vertically snugly along the bougie to the angle of His (thus excising a wedge of the fundus and creating a 3-cm extension of the GE junction).
16. Complete the procedure as a standard fundoplication: closure of the crura and the creation of a 360° wrap around the neo-esophagus.
17. Take care to place the fundic flaps at and above the level of the GE junction.
18. Remove the Bougie and check the integrity of the staple line with endoscopy or Methylene Blue.

NOTE THESE VARIATIONS

■ A combined laparoscopic/thoracoscopic approach can be done with the endoscopic stapler placed from the chest oriented alongside the esophagus to lengthen it. Both right- and left-sided thoracoscopic approaches have been described.
■ Another approach is to use a circular stapler similar to the vertical banded gastroplasty approach. The circular stapler is fired 3–4 cm below the GE junction creating window that allows the firing of the vertical stapler.

COMPLICATIONS

■ Bleeding.
■ Dysphagia.
■ Staple line leak.
■ Pulmonary embolism.

TEMPLATE OPERATIVE DICTATION

Preoperative diagnosis: Gastroesophageal reflux disease.
Procedure: Laparoscopic Collis gastroplasty with fundoplication.
Postoperative diagnosis: Same, with short esophagus.
Indications: Gastroesophageal reflux disease refractory to medical therapy with short esophagus.

Description of procedure: The patient was placed in the modified lithotomy position and general endotracheal anesthesia was induced. Preoperative antibiotics were given. The abdomen was prepped and draped in the usual sterile fashion. A time-out was completed verifying correct patient, procedure, site, positioning, and implant(s) and/or special equipment prior to beginning this procedure.

A 10 mm incision was made 12 cm below the Xiphoid process to the left of midline. Then under direct vision, a 10-mm trocar was inserted and the abdomen was inflated with CO_2 till 14 mmHg. Then under direct laparoscopic vision, a 10-mm trocar was inserted into the left subcostal area in the epigastric region to be used as the right hand working port, and another 10-mm trocar was inserted into the right subcostal area for the left hand. Another 5-mm trocar was inserted into the left anterior axillary line at the umbilical level for the assistant.

The operating table was placed in reverse Trendelenburg position and the left lobe of the liver was retracted laterally to expose the esophageal hiatus using a Nathanson fixed liver retractor through a 5 mm subxiphoid incision.

Then using the Ligasure® or Ultracision® the gastrohepatic ligament (pars flaccida) was then divided. The right diaphragmatic crus was identified and the peritoneum at its border was incised all the way to reach the phreno-esophageal membrane anteriorly. That was divided from the right to the left to reach the left crus of the diaphragm. Then with blunt dissection along an avascular plane the stomach was separated from the crura posteriorly to create a retrogastric tunnel allowing us to place a Penrose around the proximal stomach just below the GE junction. The short gastric vessels were then sealed and divided and the fundus was well mobilized. With gentle traction on the esophagus all mediastinal attachments and small vessels were divided allowing adequate mobilization of the distal esophagus. Despite that we felt that the GE junction remained *at/above* the level of the crura.

To confirm our suspicion intraoperative flexible endoscopy confirmed the location of the GE junction. With transillumination the squamo-columnar junction was identified and a point 3 cm distal to that on the cardia was marked with a suture.

At this stage, we decided to proceed with a lengthening gastroplasty. The most lateral 5-mm port on the left was exchanged with a 12-mm port. Then we introduced the 12-mm roticulating Endoscopic stapler 45 mm with 3.8 mm cartridge and with downward traction on the fundus a transverse application of the stapler was fired aiming to the marking suture placed 3 cm below the GE junction. We placed a 48-Fr OG bougie transorally and into the stomach. Another transverse application of the EndoGIA 45-mm stapler was done to reach the bougie level. The stapler was then applied parallel to the bougie and snug to it aiming to the GE junction until a wedge of the fundus was excised and a "wedge lengthening Collis gastroplasty" was done. There was no significant bleeding from the staple line. The bougie was pulled back into the esophagus and with gentle traction on the esophagus the crura of the diaphragm were outlined. There was a 3-cm posterior defect that was approximated with three interrupted 0-Ethibond sutures with pledgets. We then passed the fundus in the retrogastric tunnel from left to right under minimal tension. The bougie was re-introduced and the two flaps of fundus were sutured together anteriorly with 2-0 m\nonabsorbable suture. Using that suture for traction the fundoplication was pushed up above the GE junction and two more sutures incorporated the anterior wall of the esophagus. The fundus was secured posteriorly to the crural pillars of the diaphragm using a nonabsorbable suture. The bougie was removed and an orogastric tube was placed. Methylene blue filling of the tube showed no leak.

Hemostasis was secured. The trocars were removed under vision. The abdomen was deflated. The fascia defects at the 10- and 12-mm trocar sites were closed with absorbable sutures. The wounds were closed with 4-0 monocryl continuous subcuticular sutures.

The patient tolerated the procedure well and left the operating room in good condition.

NOTES

Chapter 10

Cricopharyngeal Myotomy and Operation for Pharyngoesophageal (Zenker's) Diverticulum

Nabil Fuleihan, M.D.

INDICATION

- Symptomatic Zenker's diverticulum: dysphagia, aspiration, regurgitation, halitosis, malnutrition, and dehydration due to fear of inability to eat or drink.

ESSENTIAL STEPS

1. Endotracheal intubation, tube shifted to left side.
2. Perform esophagoscopy and identify the diverticulum.
3. Pack the diverticulum with gauze to help identify it during transcervical surgical exposure.
4. Insert an esophageal dilator into the esophagus under direct vision to assist in cricopharyngeal myotomy and to minimize the risk of esophageal stenosis.
5. Insert NG to be used after surgery for feeding.
6. Create a transverse incision along a skin crease between the hyoid and clavicle 4 cm above the edge of the clavicle.
7. Elevate subplatysmal flaps.
8. Retract sternocleidomastoid muscle laterally.
9. Divide fascial attachments along the anterior border.
10. Retract the strap muscles anteromedially.
11. Divide the anterior belly of the omohyoid muscle inferiorly (specially in large diverticulae).
12. Identify the recurrent laryngeal nerve as blunt dissection is carried out to expose the posterior aspect of the pharynx, larynx, and esophagus, and protect it before

J.J. Hoballah and C.E.H. Scott-Conner (eds.), *Operative Dictations in General and Vascular Surgery*, DOI 10.1007/978-1-4614-0451-4_10,
© Springer Science+Business Media, LLC 2012

ligation of the thyroid vessels if needed, depending on mobility on the thyroid lobe.

13. Retract the trachea, strap muscles, and thyroid gland medially. Take a stay suture at the neck of the diverticulum for retraction.
14. Identify the diverticulum and free it from the surrounding tissues down to its base attachment to the esophagus.
15. Perform a long cricopharyngeal myotomy.
16. Excise the pouch or invert it, or suspended by a suturing or stapling technique.
17. Check hemostasis.
18. Close the wound.

NOTE THESE VARIATIONS

- Sutured or stapled resection of diverticulum.
- Diverticulopexy technique. After a cricopharyngeal myotomy and freeing of the diverticulum, the sac is tacked with 2-0 silk sutures superiorly to the prevertebral fascia.

COMPLICATIONS

- Fistula.
- Wound infection.
- Bleeding.
- Recurrence.
- Recurrent laryngeal nerve palsy.
- Pneumomediastinum.
- Mediastinitis.

TEMPLATE OPERATIVE DICTATION

Preoperative diagnosis: Symptomatic Zenker's diverticulum.
Procedure: Transcervical diverticulectomy.
Postoperative diagnosis: Same.
Indications: This____-year-old *male/female* with large symptomatic Zenker diverticulum requiring diverticulectomy for management.
Description of procedure: The patient was placed in the supine position and general endotracheal anesthesia was induced. Preoperative antibiotics were given. A time-out was completed verifying correct patient, procedure, site, positioning, and implant(s) and/or special equipment prior to beginning this procedure.

Esophagoscopy was performed and the diverticulum was identified and packed with gauze to assist during surgical exposure. Then an esophageal dilator and a nasogastric feeding tube were inserted under direct vision. The neck was prepped and draped in the usual sterile fashion. A transverse incision was done along a skin crease between the hyoid and clavicle. It was deepened through the subcutaneous tissues and hemostasis was achieved with electrocautery. Then subplatysmal flaps were elevated and the sternocleidomastoid muscle retracted laterally for better exposure. The fascial attachments along the anterior border were divided and the strap muscles retracted anteromedially. The anterior belly of the omohyoid muscle was divided inferiorly. The attention was turned to identify the recurrent laryngeal nerve. It was successfully identified to avoid injuring it as blunt dissection was carried out to expose the posterior aspect of the pharynx, larynx, and esophagus, and to protect it before the thyroid vessels were ligated. Then the trachea and thyroid gland were retracted medially. The diverticulum was then identified and freed it from the surrounding tissues down to its base attachment to the esophagus. A long cricopharyngeal myotomy was performed and the pouch was then *excised with a linear stapler/excised and closed in layers with sutures/inverted and tacked to the precervical fascia so that the mouth of the diverticulum was dependent*.

Hemostasis was achieved and the fascia was closed with ____. The skin was closed with *skin staples/subcuticular sutures of* ____.

The patient tolerated the procedure well and was taken to the postanesthesia care unit in stable condition.

ACKNOWLEDGMENT

This chapter was contributed by Benjamin E. Schneider, MD, in the first edition.

NOTES

Chapter 11

Transoral Surgery for Zenker's Diverticulum

Nabil Fuleihan, M.D.

INDICATION

- Symptomatic Zenker's diverticulum: dysphagia, aspiration, malnutrition, and dehydration due to the fear of inability to eat or drink.

ESSENTIAL STEPS

1. Place a dental guard to protect the maxillary teeth.
2. Insert a bivalved laryngoscope or a diverticuloscope into the oral cavity to expose the common wall between the esophagus and the diverticulum (with the endotracheal tube anterior to the anterior flange of the scope).
3. Advance the lower flange of the diverticuloscope until it inserts in the diverticulum and the upper flange in the esophagus.
4. Remove food debris in the diverticulum if present.
5. Use a rigid 0 or 30° telescope connected to a video camera to magnify the view.
6. Examine the diverticular pouch carefully for any lesions.
7. Biopsy any suspicious lesions.
8. Abort the procedure in case of malignancy.
9. Expose the diverticular common wall with the flanges of the scope.
10. Divide the diverticular common wall with a disposable ENDO GIA stapler by placing the blade containing the cartridge into the esophageal lumen, and the opposite blade into the diverticulum.

J.J. Hoballah and C.E.H. Scott-Conner (eds.), *Operative Dictations in General and Vascular Surgery*, DOI 10.1007/978-1-4614-0451-4_11,

11. Approximate the blades around the common wall, and confirm their position using the scope.
12. Activate the stapler (repeated firing may be needed).
13. Use the scope again to examine the diverticulum, esophagus, and the incision for any perforation or foreign bodies.
14. Remove the diverticuloscope under vision.

NOTE THESE VARIATION

- CO_2, KTP laser, or cautery can be used instead of the stapler for the cricopharyngeal myotomy.

COMPLICATIONS

- Esophageal perforation.
- Bleeding.
- Foreign body sensation.
- Odynophagia.
- Recurrence.
- Mediastinitis.

TEMPLATE OPERATIVE DICTATION

Preoperative diagnosis: Symptomatic Zenker's diverticulum.
Procedure: Transoral operation for Zenker's diverticulectomy.
Postoperative diagnosis: Same.
Indications: This ___-year-old *male/female* with a symptomatic Zenker diverticulum requiring diverticulectomy for management.
Description of procedure: The patient was placed in the supine position and general endotracheal anesthesia was induced. Preoperative antibiotics were given. The neck was hyperextended. A time-out was completed verifying correct patient, procedure, site, positioning, and implant(s) and/or special equipment prior to beginning this procedure.

A dental guard was placed to protect the maxillary teeth. A diverticuloscope was inserted to identify the diverticulum and the common wall between the esophagus and the diverticulum. The diverticuloscope was inserted until its lower flange rested in the diverticulum and its upper one in the esophagus. Food debris was suctioned. Using a rigid 0/30° scope connected to a video camera, the diverticular pouch was carefully examined and was found to be free of any lesions. Using an ENDO GIA, the diverticular common wall was divided by placing the stapler blade containing the stapler cartridge into the esophageal lumen, and the opposite blade into the diverticulum. The position of the blades was confirmed using the scope. The stapler was fired ___times to ensure complete cricopharyngeal myotomy. The scope was used again to examine the esophagus, diverticulum, and incised common wall for any perforation foreign bodies or bleeding. The diverticuloscope was removed under vision.

The patient tolerated the procedure well and was taken to the postanesthesia care unit in stable condition.

NOTES

Chapter 12

Esophagomyotomy for Achalasia and Diffuse Esophageal Spasm

Carol E.H. Scott-Conner, M.D.

INDICATIONS

- Achalasia.
- Diffuse esophageal spasm.

ESSENTIAL STEPS

1. Left posterolateral thoracotomy through the sixth or seventh interspace.
2. Incise the inferior pulmonary ligament and retract the lung cephalad.
3. Incise the pleura overlying the esophagus.
4. Mobilize the esophagus.
5. Longitudinal incision through muscular layers to expose the submucosa.
6. Extend the myotomy for the entire length of hypertrophied segment proximally and onto the stomach distally.
7. Check hemostasis and integrity of the mucosa.
8. Close the pleura over the esophagus.
9. Close the chest with thoracostomy tube drainage.

NOTE THESE VARIATION

- Length of myotomy, both proximally and distally.

J.J. Hoballah and C.E.H. Scott-Conner (eds.), *Operative Dictations in General and Vascular Surgery*, DOI 10.1007/978-1-4614-0451-4_12,
© Springer Science+Business Media, LLC 2012

COMPLICATIONS
- Inadequate myotomy.
- Esophageal or gastric perforation.
- Gastroesophageal reflux.

TEMPLATE OPERATIVE DICTATION
Preoperative diagnosis: *Achalasia/diffuse esophageal spasm*.
Procedure: Esophagomyotomy via left thoracotomy.
Postoperative diagnosis: Same.
Indications: This ___-year-old *male/female* had developed dysphagia and on workup was found to have *achalasia/diffuse esophageal spasm*. The decision was made for esophagomyotomy.
Description of procedure: Following smooth induction of general anesthesia, the patient was intubated with a double-lumen endotracheal tube, placed in a right lateral decubitus position, and padded appropriately. A time-out was completed verifying correct patient, procedure, site, positioning, and implant(s) and/or special equipment prior to beginning this procedure. The left chest was prepped and draped in the usual sterile fashion.

A standard left posterolateral thoracotomy was performed through the seventh intercostal space. Single-lung ventilation was established, allowing for anterior retraction of the lung and exposure of the mediastinum. No abnormalities were noted. The inferior pulmonary ligament was incised to allow the lung to be retracted cephalad, exposing the mediastinal pleura overlying the esophagus.

A longitudinal incision was made in the mediastinal pleura and the esophagus was exposed and gently mobilized. It was encircled with a Penrose drain and elevated, delivering the hypertrophied distal segment and several centimeters of proximal stomach into the operative field.

A longitudinal incision was made from just above the hypertrophied segment extending down onto the stomach. This was deepened through the hypertrophied circular muscle layer until submucosa was encountered. All hypertrophied circular muscle fibers were carefully divided. Proximally the myotomy extended beyond the hypertrophied segment and distally onto the stomach for approximately *1 cm/other*. The myotomy measured___ cm in length. The submucosa pouted out adequately. Hemostasis was achieved by cautious use of *electrocautery/fine sutures* of 4-0 silk. Mucosal integrity was demonstrated by instillation of air into the nasogastric tube; *no bubbles were observed in a saline-filled field/ bubbles were observed to come from the (specify location)*.

If inadvertent mucosal injury: The injury was repaired with interrupted sutures of 4-0 Vicryl to the mucosa and the muscular layers closed with interrupted 3-0 silk. The esophagus was rotated and a myotomy made in a fresh location on the opposite side in a similar manner.

The Penrose drain was removed and the esophagus allowed to return to its normal location. The mediastinal pleura was closed with a running suture of 3-0 Vicryl, leaving a small gap at the inferior aspect.

The chest was irrigated, hemostasis checked, and closed in layers with ___ sutures. Two ___ French thoracostomy tubes were placed.

The patient tolerated the procedure well and was taken to the postanesthesia care unit in stable condition.

NOTES

Chapter 13
Laparoscopic Esophagomyotomy with Partial Fundoplication

Carol E.H. Scott-Conner, M.D.

INDICATION
- Achalasia.

ESSENTIAL STEPS
1. Induce the pneumoperitoneum and place ports.
2. Place a liver retractor.
3. Incise the phrenoesophageal ligament; avoid injury to the anterior vagus.
4. Mobilize the anterior mediastinal attachments of the esophagus.
5. Perform a myotomy.
6. Check the distal esophagus for integrity and lack of spasm.
7. Perform a partial fundoplication.

NOTE THESE VARIATION
- Toupet (posterior) or Dor (anterior) partial fundoplication.

COMPLICATIONS
- Esophageal perforation/leak.
- Pneumothorax.
- Gastroesophageal reflux.
- Inadequate myotomy.
- Injury to vagus nerves.

J.J. Hoballah and C.E.H. Scott-Conner (eds.), *Operative Dictations in General and Vascular Surgery*, DOI 10.1007/978-1-4614-0451-4_13,
© Springer Science+Business Media, LLC 2012

TEMPLATE OPERATIVE DICTATION

Preoperative diagnosis: Achalasia.

Procedure: Laparoscopic myotomy with *anterior/posterior* partial fundoplication.

Postoperative diagnosis: Same.

Indications: This ___-year-old *male/female* developed progressive dysphagia and on workup was found to have achalasia. Laparoscopic myotomy with *anterior/*posterior partial fundoplication was chosen for management.

Description of procedure: The patient was brought to the operating room and general anesthesia was induced. The patient was then placed in the lithotomy position. A Foley catheter was placed. Endoscopy was performed to clear the esophagus of secretions and identify the gastroesophageal junction. The abdomen was then prepped and draped in the usual sterile fashion. A time-out was completed verifying correct patient, procedure, site, positioning, and implant(s) and/or special equipment prior to beginning this procedure.

An incision was made in a natural skin line *above/below* the umbilicus. The fascia was elevated and the Veress needle inserted. Proper position was confirmed by aspiration and a saline meniscus test. The abdomen was insufflated with carbon dioxide to a pressure of 15 mm. A trocar was then inserted superior to and 3 cm to the left of the umbilicus. A 10-mm left subcostal port was placed under direct vision. A right subcostal (5-mm) port was placed for the introduction of the liver retractor. Two additional epigastric ports were placed.

The liver was retracted cephalad and laterally. The gastric fundus was grasped and gently retracted caudally. The hepatogastric ligament was left intact; *an anomalous hepatic artery was identified and protected*. The phrenoesophageal fat pad was dissected and removed using *ultrasonic shears/electrocautery*. Dissection of the phrenoesophageal ligament was limited to the space anterior to the esophagus. The mediastinum was entered bluntly by gentle medial traction upon the lateral aspects of the hiatus anterior to the esophagus. The anterior vagus nerve was identified, freed from the surface of the esophagus, and thus mobilized out of harm's way. Approximately 7 cm of esophagus was easily visualized.

The anterior fibers of the esophagus were then scored in a longitudinal fashion with hook cautery and the myotomy performed, exposing intact submucosa. Dissection was carried out approximately 1 cm distal to the squamocolumnar junction.

The abdomen was irrigated with saline and no leak was noted upon endoscopic insufflation. The lower esophageal sphincter opened easily upon gentle insufflation, confirming an adequate myotomy. The endoscope was withdrawn.

[Choose one:]

If Dor fundoplication: A mobile region of the fundus was then grasped and rolled up over the myotomy and tacked in place with several interrupted sutures of ___.

If Toupet fundoplication: The mobile fundus was then pulled behind the esophagus and tacked to the edges of the myotomy on both sides with interrupted ___ sutures.

Hemostasis was checked. Secondary trocars were removed under direct vision. *No bleeding was noted/trocar site bleeding was controlled by electrocautery/suture placement.* The laparoscope was withdrawn and the umbilical trocar removed. The abdomen was allowed to collapse. All trocar sites greater than 5 mm were closed with ___. The skin was closed with subcuticular sutures of ___ and steristrips.

The patient tolerated the procedure well and was taken to the postanesthesia care unit in satisfactory condition.

ACKNOWLEDGMENT

This chapter was contributed by Benjamin E. Schneider, MD in the first edition.

NOTES

Section II

Stomach and Duodenum

Chapter 14
Gastrojejunostomy

Lori K. Soni, M.D.

INDICATIONS
- Gastric outlet obstruction from unresectable cancer of the pancreas or duodenum or periampullary origin.
- Peptic ulcer disease.

ESSENTIAL STEPS
1. Upper midline incision.
2. Explore the abdomen and confirm pathology.
3. Identify the mobile portion of the greater curvature of stomach and loop of proximal jejunum.
4. *If antecolic:*
   - *Measure jejunum 30 cm from the ligament of Treitz and bring antecolic (pull omentum to right and pass jejunum to left of bulk of omentum).*
5. *If retrocolic:*
   - *Create a window in the transverse mesocolon to the left of the middle colic vessels.*
   - *Measure jejunum 30 cm from the ligament of Treitz and bring the loop retrocolic.*
6. *If stapled:*
   - *Align the loop and chosen region of greater curvature with two stay sutures of 3-0 silk.*
   - *Create gastrostomy and jejunostomy, use suction/sponge forceps to remove any leftover particles of food and fiber from the stomach.*
   - *Insert linear cutting stapler and fire.*

J.J. Hoballah and C.E.H. Scott-Conner (eds.), *Operative Dictations in General and Vascular Surgery*, DOI 10.1007/978-1-4614-0451-4_14,
© Springer Science+Business Media, LLC 2012

- *Check staple line for hemostasis.*
- *Close enterotomies with linear stapler/two-layered sutured closure.*

7. *If sutured:*
   - *Align the loop and chosen region of greater curvature of stomach.*
   - *Place back wall of interrupted 3-0 silk Lembert sutures.*
   - *Open the stomach and jejunum use suction/sponge forceps to remove any leftover particles of food and fiber from the stomach; achieve hemostasis.*
   - *Place an inner layer of continuous 3-0 Vicryl to posterior and anterior walls.*
   - *Place an outer layer of 3-0 silk Lembert sutures.*

8. Check the anastomosis for integrity and patency of both limbs (afferent and efferent).
9. Place omentum over the gastrojejunostomy.
10. *Suture the stomach to the transverse mesocolon (if retrocolic).*
11. Check hemostasis.
12. Close the abdomen in the usual fashion.

NOTE THESE VARIATIONS
- Biopsy tumor if no tissue diagnosis previously obtained.
- Antecolic vs. retrocolic.
- Stapled vs. sutured.
- Jejunojejunostomy may be added to avoid bile reflux.

COMPLICATIONS
- Failure to empty.
- Stricture.
- Anastomotic leak.

TEMPLATE OPERATIVE DICTATION
Preoperative diagnosis: Gastric outlet obstruction due to *unresectable carcinoma of pancreas/duodenum/ampulla/peptic ulcer disease/other*.
Procedure: Gastrojejunostomy.
Postoperative diagnosis: Same.
Indications: This ___-year-old *male/female* developed gastric outlet obstruction due to *unresectable carcinoma of pancreas/duodenum/ampulla/peptic ulcer disease/other*. Gastrojejunostomy was indicated to bypass the obstruction.

Description of procedure: *An epidural catheter was placed by anesthesia prior to the start of the operation.* The patient was placed in the supine position and general endotracheal anesthesia was induced. Preoperative antibiotics were given. A Foley catheter and nasogastric tube were placed. The abdomen was prepped and draped in the usual sterile fashion. A time-out was completed verifying correct patient, procedure, site, positioning, and implant(s) and/or special equipment prior to beginning this procedure.

A vertical midline incision was made from xiphoid to just below the umbilicus. This was deepened through the subcutaneous tissues and hemostasis was achieved with electrocautery. The linea alba was identified, grasped and elevated, incised and the peritoneal cavity entered. Care was taken not to injure the abdominal contents below. The abdomen was explored. *Adhesions were lysed sharply under direct vision with Metzenbaum scissors. Tumor was identified in the following locations (detail). Biopsy of ___ was performed and submitted for pathology.*

[Choose one:]

If antecolic: A mobile loop of jejunum 30 cm distal to the ligament of Treitz was identified and passed to the left of the omentum and brought to lie comfortably adjacent to the greater curvature of the stomach.

If retrocolic: An opening was created in the transverse mesocolon. The transverse colon was retracted upward and the ligament of Treitz was identified. The transverse mesocolon was carefully incised to the left of the middle colic vessels and near the ligament of Treitz and care was taken to avoid the large vessels of the arcade. A mobile loop of jejunum 30 cm distal to the ligament of Treitz was identified and passed through the window in the transverse mesocolon. It was brought to lie comfortably adjacent to the greater curvature of the stomach.

If stapled: The jejunum and gastric wall were approximated with two stay sutures of 3-0 silk. A gastrotomy and jejunostomy were made and the linear cutting stapler inserted, closed, and fired. The staple line was inspected for hemostasis. The stomach had retained particles of food and/or fiber. These were removed with suction irrigation and/or a sponge forceps. The enterotomy was closed with a linear stapler/a two-layer sutured closure of 3-0 Vicryl and 3-0 silk.

If sutured: A two-layered sutured anastomosis was then constructed using interrupted 3-0 silk Lembert sutures for the outer layer and running 3-0 Vicryl for the inner layer.

The anastomosis was tested for integrity and patency of both the afferent and efferent limbs. The nasogastric tube was confirmed to be in a good position.

If retrocolic: The mesocolon was sutured to the gastric wall with interrupted sutures of 3-0 silk to prevent herniation.

Omentum was placed over the gastrojejunostomy. Hemostasis was checked. *(Optional: Multiple interrupted through-and-through retention sutures of ____ were placed.)* The fascia was closed with *a running suture of ____/a Smead-Jones closure of interrupted ____.* The skin was closed with *skin staples/subcuticular sutures of ___/ other.*

The patient tolerated the procedure well and was taken to the postanesthesia care unit in stable condition.

ACKNOWLEDGMENT

This chapter was contributed by Natisha Busick, MD in the first edition.

NOTES

Chapter 15
Proximal Gastric Vagotomy

Carol E.H. Scott-Conner, M.D.

INDICATIONS

- Peptic ulcer disease refractory to medical management.
- Noncompliance with medical management.
- Adjunct to plication of perforated peptic ulcer in noncompliant patient.

ESSENTIAL STEPS

1. Upper midline incision.
2. Abdominal exploration for unexpected findings.
3. Place the table in reverse Trendelenburg position.
4. Retract the left lobe of the liver upward (divide triangular ligament and reflect left lobe to right if necessary).
5. Place fixed retractors.
6. Gently retract the stomach toward left lower quadrant.
7. Divide the peritoneum overlying the abdominal esophagus.
8. Extend the peritoneal incision to expose crura.
9. Gently encircle the esophagus with an index finger.
10. Separate each vagal trunk gently from the esophageal wall, pulling the vagal trunk toward the right and esophagus to the left.
11. Encircle each vagal trunk with a silastic loop.
12. Bring silastic loops out to the right of the esophagus.
13. Pass the left index and middle fingers through an avascular area of the gastrohepatic omentum and enter the lesser sac.

J.J. Hoballah and C.E.H. Scott-Conner (eds.), *Operative Dictations in General and Vascular Surgery*, DOI 10.1007/978-1-4614-0451-4_15,
© Springer Science+Business Media, LLC 2012

14. Identify crow's foot (terminal branches of the nerve of Latarjet).
15. Working from below upward, sequentially doubly clamp, divide, and ligate neurovascular bundles in the anterior leaflet of the gastrohepatic omentum, staying close to the gastric wall.
16. Continue dissection until the anterior vagus is reached.
17. Preserve this trunk (and its hepatic branches) by retracting it toward the patient's right with a silastic loop.
18. Begin a second pass through middle and posterior leaflets of the gastrohepatic ligament; start below, at the crow's foot, and work cephalad.
19. *A third pass may be needed if lesser omentum is very thick.*
20. Dissect the posterior aspect of the esophagus from the posterior vagus nerve to 7 cm above the esophagogastric junction.
21. Divide any tiny fibers resembling nerve tissue throughout the circumference of lower 7 cm of the esophagus.
22. Imbricate the lesser curvature with interrupted 4-0 silk Lembert sutures.
23. Check hemostasis.
24. Close the abdomen.

NOTE THESE VARIATION

- None of significance.

COMPLICATIONS

- Incomplete vagotomy.
- Injury to the vagal trunks.
- Injury to the spleen.
- Necrosis of the lesser curvature of the stomach.

TEMPLATE OPERATIVE DICTATION

Preoperative diagnosis: Peptic ulcer disease refractory to medical management.
Procedure: Proximal gastric vagotomy.
Postoperative diagnosis: Same.
Indications: This ___-year-old *male/female* with peptic ulcer disease *refractory to/noncompliant with* medical therapy required proximal gastric vagotomy for management.
Description of procedure: *An epidural catheter was placed by anesthesia prior to the start of the operation.* The patient was placed

in the supine position and general endotracheal anesthesia was induced. A time-out was completed verifying correct patient, procedure, site, positioning, and implant(s) and/or special equipment prior to beginning this procedure. Preoperative antibiotics were given. A Foley catheter and nasogastric tube were placed. The abdomen was prepped and draped in the usual sterile fashion. A vertical midline incision was made from xiphoid to just below the umbilicus. This was deepened through the subcutaneous tissues and hemostasis was achieved with electrocautery. The linea alba was identified and incised and the peritoneal cavity entered. The abdomen was explored. *Adhesions were lysed sharply under direct vision with Metzenbaum scissors.*

The operating table was placed in reverse Trendelenburg position and *the left lobe of the liver was retracted cephalad/the triangular ligament divided with electrocautery and the left lobe of the liver retracted to the right.* Fixed retractors were placed to expose the esophageal hiatus. The peritoneum overlying the esophagus was incised to expose the esophagus and left and right crura. The esophagus was gently encircled by blunt dissection and a Penrose drain passed behind it. Both vagal trunks were identified, gently dissected free of the esophagus, and retracted to the patient's right with silastic loops. The esophagus was retracted to the left by the Penrose drain.

An avascular portion of the lesser omentum was entered. The crow's foot termination of the anterior nerve of Latarjet was identified and the terminal branches preserved. Beginning just above these terminal branches, the anterior leaflet of the lesser omentum was sequentially divided between clamps and the neurovascular branches to the lesser curvature were secured with ties of 3-0 silk. Care was taken to avoid damage to the nerves of Latarjet or the lesser curvature of the stomach. This dissection progressed cephalad until the anterior vagus was encountered. The anterior vagus and its hepatic branches were preserved. The remaining lesser omentum, including the posterior leaflet, was sequentially divided in a similar fashion. At the conclusion of this dissection, the main vagal trunks were intact and separated from the distal 7 cm of esophagus, the distal esophagus was circumferentially cleaned of any apparent nerve fibers, and the lesser curvature was noted to be intact.

The lesser curvature of the stomach was imbricated with interrupted 3-0 silk Lembert sutures. The nasogastric tube was positioned. Hemostasis was checked.

(Optional: Multiple interrupted through-and-through retention sutures of ____ were placed). The fascia was closed with *a running*

suture of ____/a Smead-Jones closure of interrupted ____. The skin was closed with *skin staples/subcuticular sutures of ___/other.*

The patient tolerated the procedure well and was taken to the postanesthesia care unit in stable condition.

NOTES

Chapter 16
Truncal Vagotomy and Pyloroplasty

Carol E.H. Scott-Conner, M.D.

INDICATIONS
- Refractory peptic ulcer disease.
- As adjunct to oversewing of bleeding duodenal ulcer.

ESSENTIAL STEPS
1. Upper midline incision.
2. Abdominal exploration for unexpected findings.
3. *If bleeding: Place two 2-0 silk stay sutures on the pylorus.*
4. *Longitudinal incision across the pylorus.*
5. *Identify the bleeding vessel in the ulcer crater.*
6. *Suture ligate three points (superior, inferior, and medial).*
7. *Confirm hemostasis.*
8. *Pack pyloroplasty and change gloves.*
9. Place the table in reverse Trendelenburg position.
10. Retract the left lobe of the liver upward (divide triangular ligament and reflect the left lobe to right if necessary).
11. Place fixed retractors.
12. Gently retract the stomach toward the left lower quadrant.
13. Divide the peritoneum overlying the abdominal esophagus.
14. Extend this peritoneal incision to expose the crura.
15. Gently encircle the esophagus with the right index finger.
16. Pass a Penrose drain around the esophagus and apply downward traction.

J.J. Hoballah and C.E.H. Scott-Conner (eds.), *Operative Dictations in General and Vascular Surgery*, DOI 10.1007/978-1-4614-0451-4_16,
© Springer Science+Business Media, LLC 2012

17. Identify the two main vagal trunks by inspection and palpation.
18. Pass a right-angle clamp behind the anterior vagal trunk and gently dissect from the esophagus for a distance of 1–1.5 cm.
19. Elevate the anterior vagal trunk; clip proximal and distal with hemostatic clips and excise the segment.
20. Send the excised segment for frozen section confirmation.
21. Roll the esophagus to expose the posterior vagal trunk.
22. Similarly, excise the posterior vagal trunk and submit separately for frozen section.
23. Carefully inspect and palpate the esophagus and paraesophageal tissues; excise and submit any possible nerve tissue.
24. Place packs in region of the hiatus.
25. *If elective: Place two 2-0 silk stay sutures on the pylorus.*
26. *Longitudinal incision through the pylorus.*
27. *If for bleeding: Remove pack from the duodenum and verify hemostasis.*
28. Close pyloroplasty transversely in a single layer with interrupted 2-0 silk.
29. Place omentum over the pyloroplasty.
30. Remove packs from the hiatus and check hemostasis.
31. Close the abdomen in the usual fashion.

NOTE THESE VARIATIONS

- In a situation of active bleeding, first open the pyloroplasty and control the bleeding. Then perform vagotomy. Pyloroplasty incision is closed last to allow confirmation of hemostasis.
- In an elective situation, vagotomy is done first (because it is the clean part of the operation), then pyloroplasty.

COMPLICATIONS

- Injury to the esophagus.
- Injury to the spleen.
- Incomplete vagotomy.
- Delayed gastric emptying.
- Gastroesophageal reflux due to disruption of the hiatus.
- Recurrent bleeding if inadequate suture ligature of the gastroduodenal artery.

TEMPLATE OPERATIVE DICTATION

Preoperative diagnosis: *Refractory/bleeding* duodenal ulcer.

Procedure: Vagotomy and pyloroplasty *with suture ligation of bleeding ulcer.*

Postoperative diagnosis: Same.

Indications: This ___-year-old *male/female* with *refractory ulcer disease/bleeding duodenal ulcer* required vagotomy and pyloroplasty *with suture ligation of bleeding ulcer as an emergency procedure.*

Description of procedure: *An epidural catheter was placed by anesthesia prior to the start of the operation.* The patient was placed in the supine position and general endotracheal anesthesia was induced. A time-out was completed verifying correct patient, procedure, site, positioning, and implant(s) and/or special equipment prior to beginning this procedure. Preoperative antibiotics were given. A Foley catheter and nasogastric tube were placed. The abdomen was prepped and draped in the usual sterile fashion. A vertical midline incision was made from xiphoid to just below the umbilicus. This was deepened through the subcutaneous tissues, and hemostasis was achieved with electrocautery. The linea alba was identified and incised and the peritoneal cavity entered. The abdomen was explored. *Adhesions were lysed sharply under direct vision with Metzenbaum scissors.*

[Choose one:]

If bleeding duodenal ulcer: Two stay sutures of 2-0 silk were placed at the pylorus. A longitudinal incision was made across the pylorus and the duodenal bulb inspected. A posterior duodenal ulcer with active arterial bleeding was identified. Hemostasis was achieved with three sutures of 2-0 silk placed to control the gastroduodenal artery superiorly, inferiorly, and medially. All clot was suctioned and the duodenum packed lightly proximally and distally. Gloves were changed and attention was directed to the hiatus.

The table was placed in reverse Trendelenburg position. *The left triangular ligament of the liver was incised and the left liver lobe retracted toward the right/the left lobe of the liver was retracted upward.* Fixed retractors were placed to expose the hiatus. The stomach was gently retracted and the peritoneum overlying the abdominal esophagus was incised. The esophagus was gently mobilized and encircled with a Penrose drain. The anterior and posterior vagus were identified, dissected free from the esophagus, doubly clipped, and a segment excised and submitted for frozen section confirmation. Frozen section returned peripheral nerve. *Additional nerve fibers were identified and submitted separately.* At the conclusion of this dissection, all neural tissue had been divided and the esophagus was intact. A pack was placed in the region of the hiatus.

Attention was then turned to the region of the pylorus.

If bleeding: *The duodenal ulcer crater was again inspected and hemostasis noted to be secure.*

If elective: *Two stay sutures of 2-0 silk were placed at the pylorus. A longitudinal incision was made across the pylorus and the duodenal bulb inspected.* The pyloroplasty incision was closed in a transverse fashion with a single layer of interrupted 2-0 silk sutures. The closure was noted to be intact, with a patent lumen, at the conclusion of this. The nasogastric tube was positioned. Omentum was placed in the vicinity of the pyloroplasty. The pack was removed from the region of the hiatus and hemostasis confirmed.

(Optional: Multiple interrupted through-and-through retention sutures of ____ were placed.) The fascia was closed with *a running suture of ____/a Smead-Jones closure of interrupted ____.* The skin was closed with *skin staples/subcuticular sutures of ___/other.*

The patient tolerated the procedure well and was taken to the postanesthesia care unit in stable condition.

NOTES

Chapter 17

Partial Gastrectomy with Billroth I Reconstruction

Roy R. Danks, D.O.

INDICATIONS
- Gastric ulcer.
- Prepyloric ulcer.
- Recurrent ulcer of stomach and duodenum (after vagotomy).
- Early gastric or antral carcinoma or other gastric malignancy (see Chap. 23).

ESSENTIAL STEPS
1. Upper midline incision.
2. Confirm pathology.
3. Identify probable points of division of the stomach on the greater and lesser curvature.
4. Create an opening in the gastrocolic omentum close to the gastric wall near the point of division.
5. Create a similar window in lesser omentum.
6. Serially clamp, divide, and ligate branches of the gastroepiploic vessels with 2-0 silk, progressing toward the duodenum.
7. Similarly divide lesser omentum, taking care to identify and protect the common bile duct.
8. Perform a Kocher maneuver.
9. Circumferentially dissect the duodenum, taking care to protect the common bile duct, gastroduodenal artery, and pancreas.
10. Place bowel clamps across the duodenum and divide it.

J.J. Hoballah and C.E.H. Scott-Conner (eds.), *Operative Dictations in General and Vascular Surgery*, DOI 10.1007/978-1-4614-0451-4_17,
© Springer Science+Business Media, LLC 2012

11. Divide the stomach with 90-mm linear stapler and remove the specimen.
12. Amputate the greater curvature tip of the gastric remnant.
13. Approximate the duodenum to gastric remnant.
14. Construct a two-layer anastomosis.
15. Check hemostasis.
16. Close the abdomen.

NOTE THESE VARIATIONS
- Stapled anastomosis is also possible.
- Early division of the stomach facilitates difficult duodenal dissection.
- Biopsy gastric ulcer (if not previously done) to exclude malignancy.

COMPLICATIONS
- Anastomotic leak.
- Recurrent ulcer.
- Injury to the common bile duct or pancreas.

TEMPLATE OPERATIVE DICTATIONS
Preoperative diagnosis: Gastric ulcer.
Procedure: Partial gastrectomy with Billroth I reconstruction.
Postoperative diagnosis: Same.
Indications: This ___-year-old *male/female* had a nonhealing gastric ulcer despite ___ weeks of maximal medical therapy. Partial gastrectomy was indicated.
Description of procedure: *An epidural catheter was placed by anesthesia prior to the start of the operation.* The patient was placed in the supine position and general endotracheal anesthesia was induced. Preoperative antibiotics were given. A Foley catheter and nasogastric tube were placed. The abdomen was prepped and draped in the usual sterile fashion. A time-out was completed verifying correct patient, procedure, site, positioning, and implant(s) and/or special equipment prior to beginning this procedure. A vertical midline incision was made from xiphoid to just below the umbilicus. This was deepened through the subcutaneous tissues and hemostasis was achieved with electrocautery. The linea alba was identified and incised and the peritoneal cavity entered. The abdomen was explored. *Adhesions were lysed sharply under direct vision with Metzenbaum scissors.*

A self-retaining retractor was then placed and the abdominal wall was retracted laterally, inferiorly, and superiorly. The small bowel and colon were then packed inferiorly with wet laparotomy pads and held in place with retractors. This afforded adequate exposure of the stomach and duodenum. The pancreas was then gently examined by palpation and determined to be *normal/abnormal (detail)*. The gallbladder was palpated and found to *be normal/contain gallstones*.

The gastrocolic ligament was incised at the midpoint of the greater curvature of the stomach. This allowed good exposure of the omental bursa. Next, an opening was made in the lesser omentum and a Penrose drain was placed around the stomach for retraction. The dissection was continued along the greater curvature toward the duodenum. Gastroepiploic vessels were clamped, sharply divided, and ligated with 2-0 silk ties. Once the duodenum was reached, a Kocher maneuver was undertaken by sweeping the second limb of the duodenum from medial to lateral, sharply dividing the duplicated peritoneal reflection. Blunt and sharp dissection was used to free the duodenum until it was adequately mobilized.

The stomach was then retracted in a left cephalad direction to facilitate circumferential duodenal mobilization. This was accomplished by proceeding from the left, medial duodenal wall, posteriorly to the back wall, and laterally to the hepatoduodenal ligament. The gastroduodenal artery was identified and kept out of harm's way.

The dissection was continued along the lesser curvature of the stomach to the level of the third vein. Vessels were clamped, transected, and tied with 2-0 silk sutures. Guy sutures were placed on the lateral aspects of the duodenum. Bowel clamps were then applied across the duodenum and it was sharply transected. The stomach was transected by placing a TA90 stapling device across the proximal resection margin at a 45° angle to the lesser curvature and firing the stapler. The specimen was passed off the operative field.

A gastrotomy was then created by placing a clamp across the lower corner of the gastric remnant, at a width adequate to receive the duodenum, and removing the corner. A posterior row of interrupted 3-0 silk Lembert sutures was placed, followed by an inner layer of running 4-0 Vicryl and an anterior row of interrupted 3-0 silk Lembert sutures. The stoma was palpably patent and intact at the conclusion of the procedure.

The vascular pedicles of the stomach were then secured to the ligated gastric pedicles of the duodenum with 4-0 silk sutures. Hemostasis was checked. The gastric tube was seen to lie in a comfortable position. It was covered with omentum.

(Optional: Multiple interrupted through-and-through retention sutures of ____ were placed.) The fascia was closed with *a running suture of ____/a Smead-Jones closure of interrupted ____*. The skin was closed with *skin staples/subcuticular sutures of ___/other*.

The patient tolerated the procedure well and was taken to the postanesthesia care unit in stable condition.

NOTES

Chapter 18

Partial Gastrectomy with Billroth II Reconstruction

Roy R. Danks, D.O.

INDICATIONS
- Duodenal ulcer disease.
- Gastric ulcer.
- Failed Billroth I operation.

ESSENTIAL STEPS
1. Upper midline incision.
2. Confirm pathology.
3. Identify probable points of division of the stomach on the greater and lesser curvature.
4. Create an opening in the gastrocolic omentum close to the gastric wall near the point of division.
5. Create a similar window in lesser omentum.
6. Serially clamp, divide, and ligate branches of the gastroepiploic vessels with 2-0 silk, progressing toward the duodenum. Vessels may also be divided with harmonic shears or Ligasure device.
7. Similarly divide lesser omentum, taking care to identify and protect the common bile duct.
8. Perform a Kocher maneuver.
9. Circumferentially dissect the duodenum, taking care to protect the common bile duct, gastroduodenal artery, and pancreas.
10. Pull the nasogastric tube back into the distal esophagus.

J.J. Hoballah and C.E.H. Scott-Conner (eds.), *Operative Dictations in General and Vascular Surgery*, DOI 10.1007/978-1-4614-0451-4_18,
© Springer Science+Business Media, LLC 2012

11. *Place bowel clamps across the duodenum/staple the duodenum with linear stapler* and divide it.
12. *If sutured duodenal stump closure:*
    - *Close the duodenal stump with an inner layer of 3-0 Vicryl placed as a running Connell suture, followed with an outer layer of interrupted 3-0 silk.*
13. *If sutured gastrojejunostomy:*
    - *Divide the stomach with bowel clamps across the greater curvature.*
    - *Divide the lesser curvature to within 3–4 cm of the esophagus with a linear stapler.*
14. *If stapled gastrojejunostomy:*
    - *Divide the stomach with a linear stapler from the chosen point on the greater curvature to within 3–4 cm of the esophagus on the lesser curvature.* Trace jejunum to the ligament of Treitz; identify mobile loop of jejunum close to the ligament of Treitz.
    - Pass jejunum antecolic/through window in transverse mesocolon and place adjacent to the gastric remnant.
15. *If sutured:*
    - *Create two-layered gastrojejunostomy, with the inner layer running 3-0 Vicryl and the outer layer interrupted 3-0 silk Lembert sutures.*
    - *Three-corner stitch at the angle of sorrows.*
16. *If stapled:*
    - *Approximate posterior wall of the stomach and jejunum with two 3-0 silk sutures.*
    - *Create gastrotomy and jejunotomy and insert a linear cutting stapler.*
    - *Fire the stapler.*
    - *Check the staple line for hemostasis.*
    - *Close enterotomies with a linear stapler/in two layers with running 3-0 Vicryl and interrupted 3-0 silk.*
17. Check anastomosis for integrity and patency of both afferent and efferent limbs.
18. *If retrocolic:*
    - *Close the transverse mesocolon by suturing to the gastric remnant with interrupted 3-0 silk sutures.*
19. Position the nasogastric tube.
20. Bring omentum up to lie over the duodenal stump and gastrojejunostomy.
21. Check hemostasis.
22. Close abdomen.

NOTE THESE VARIATIONS

- Divide the stomach early if duodenal dissection is difficult.
- Extent of resection dictated by pathology.
- Stapled vs. sutured closure of the duodenal stump.
- Stapled vs. sutured gastrojejunostomy.
- Antecolic vs. retrocolic.

COMPLICATIONS

- Anastomotic leak.
- Injury to the common bile duct, pancreas, or spleen.
- Recurrent ulcer.
- Bile reflux gastritis.
- Afferent limb syndrome.
- Herniation through transverse mesocolon defect (retrocolic).

TEMPLATE OPERATIVE DICTATION

Preoperative diagnosis: *Gastric/duodenal* ulcer refractory to medical therapy.

Procedure: Subtotal gastrectomy with Billroth II reconstruction.

Postoperative diagnosis: Same.

Indications: This ___-year-old *male/female* had a nonhealing gastric ulcer despite ___ weeks of maximal medical therapy. Partial gastrectomy was indicated.

Description of procedure: *An epidural catheter was placed by anesthesia prior to the start of the operation.* The patient was placed in the supine position and general endotracheal anesthesia was induced. Preoperative antibiotics were given. A Foley catheter and nasogastric tube were placed. The abdomen was prepped and draped in the usual sterile fashion. A time-out was completed verifying correct patient, procedure, site, positioning, and implant(s) and/or special equipment prior to beginning this procedure. A vertical midline incision was made from xiphoid to just below the umbilicus. This was deepened through the subcutaneous tissues and hemostasis was achieved with electrocautery. The linea alba was identified and incised and the peritoneal cavity entered. The abdomen was explored. *Adhesions were lysed sharply under direct vision with Metzenbaum scissors. Adhesions not involved with viscera were divided with electrocautery/Ligasure/harmonic shears.*

A self-retaining retractor was then placed and the abdominal wall was retracted laterally, inferiorly, and superiorly. The small bowel and colon were then packed inferiorly with moist laparotomy pads and held in place with retractors. This afforded adequate exposure of the stomach and duodenum. The pancreas was then gently examined by palpation and determined to be *normal/abnormal (detail)*. The gallbladder was palpated and found to *be normal/contain gallstones*.

The gastrocolic ligament was incised at the midpoint of the greater curvature of the stomach. This allowed good exposure of the omental bursa. Next, an opening was made in the lesser omentum and a Penrose drain was placed around the stomach for retraction. The dissection was continued along the greater curvature toward the duodenum. Gastroepiploic vessels were clamped, sharply divided, and ligated with 2-0 silk ties/divided with harmonic shears/Ligasure device. Once the duodenum was reached a Kocher maneuver was undertaken by sweeping the second limb of the duodenum from medial to lateral, sharply dividing the duplicated peritoneal reflection. Blunt and sharp dissection was used to free the duodenum until it was adequately mobilized.

The stomach was then retracted in a left cephalad direction to facilitate circumferential duodenal mobilization. This was accomplished by proceeding from the left, medial duodenal wall, posteriorly to the back wall, and laterally to the hepatoduodenal ligament. The gastroduodenal artery was identified and kept out of harm's way.

The dissection was continued along the lesser curvature of the stomach to within 3–4 cm of the esophagus. Vessels were clamped, transected, and tied with 2-0 silk sutures/divided with harmonic shears/Ligasure device.

[Choose one:]

If stapled duodenal stump closure: A linear stapler was then used to divide the duodenum just beyond the pylorus.

If sutured duodenal stump closure: The duodenum was divided just beyond the pylorus with bowel clamps. The duodenal stump was closed in two layers: an inner running layer of 3-0 Vicryl placed as a Connell suture and an outer layer of interrupted 3-0 silk Lembert sutures.

The duodenal stump closure was inspected and found to be satisfactory.

If sutured gastrojejunostomy: The stomach was then divided by placing bowel clamps at right angles across the greater curvature for a length of 4–5 cm and sharply transecting it. A linear stapler was fired along the lesser curvature to complete the resection to within 3–4 cm of the esophagus.

If stapled gastrojejunostomy: The stomach was divided with a linear stapler placed across it from the chosen point of division on the greater curvature to a point within 3–4 cm of the esophagus on the lesser curvature.

The specimen was removed. The ligament of Treitz was palpated and a mobile loop of jejunum as close as possible to the ligament of Treitz was identified. It was passed in an *antecolic fashion/ through a window in the transverse mesocolon* and brought to lie comfortably adjacent to the gastric remnant.

If sutured gastrojejunostomy: *A two-layered sutured gastrojejunostomy was then constructed with an inner layer of running 3-0 Vicryl and an outer layer of interrupted 3-0 silk Lembert sutures. A three-point suture was placed at the angle of sorrows.*

If stapled gastrojejunostomy: *The jejunum was approximated to the posterior wall of the stomach with two sutures of 3-0 silk. A gastrotomy and a jejunotomy were then made and the linear cutting stapler inserted and fired. The staple line was inspected for hemostasis. The enterotomies were closed with a linear stapler/in two layers using 3-0 Vicryl and 3-0 silk.*

The anastomosis was checked for integrity and patency of both the afferent and efferent limbs. It was noted to lie comfortably without tension or torsion in the left upper quadrant. *The transverse mesocolon was approximated to the gastric remnant with interrupted 3-0 silk sutures to prevent herniation.*

Hemostasis was checked. The nasogastric tube was positioned. Omentum was brought up and made to lie over the duodenal stump and gastrojejunostomy site.

(Optional: The abdominal cavity was lavaged with ___ liters of sterile saline solution. As much of the irrigant as possible was removed with suction. Laparotomy pad and instrument counts were completed and reported as correct).

(Optional: Multiple interrupted through-and-through retention sutures of ___ were placed.) The fascia was closed *with a running suture of ___/a Smead-Jones closure of interrupted ___.*

The skin was closed with *skin staples/subcuticular sutures of ___/other.*

The patient tolerated the procedure well and was taken to the postanesthesia care unit in stable condition.

NOTES

Chapter 19

Plication of Perforated Peptic Ulcer

Georgios Tsoulfas, M.D.

INDICATION
- Perforated duodenal ulcer.

ESSENTIAL STEPS
1. Upper midline incision.
2. Culture and aspirate any peritoneal fluid.
3. Explore the abdomen with special attention to the stomach and duodenum and identify perforation.
4. Place interrupted sutures across margins of perforation.
5. Bring healthy omentum over the defect and secure in place by tying previously placed sutures.
6. Lavage the peritoneal cavity with large volumes of normal saline.
7. Check position of the nasogastric tube.
8. Check hemostasis.
9. Close the abdomen.

NOTE THESE VARIATIONS
- Decision to plicate rather than resect or excise and close as pyloroplasty is based on size and location of perforation, patient's risk and hemodynamic status, and surrounding tissue condition.
- Pack skin open if significant contamination.

J.J. Hoballah and C.E.H. Scott-Conner (eds.), *Operative Dictations in General and Vascular Surgery*, DOI 10.1007/978-1-4614-0451-4_19,
© Springer Science+Business Media, LLC 2012

COMPLICATIONS

- Subphrenic abscess.
- Gastrointestinal bleeding.
- Recurrence of ulcer.

TEMPLATE OPERATIVE DICTATION

Preoperative diagnosis: Acute abdomen and perforated viscus.
Procedure: Plication of perforated duodenal ulcer.
Postoperative diagnosis: Perforated duodenal ulcer.
Indications: ____-year-old *male/female* developed *acute abdomen/ epigastric pain/leukocytosis* with free air on *upright chest X-ray/ lateral decubitus abdominal film/computed tomography scan of abdomen.*
Description of procedure: *An epidural catheter was placed by anesthesia prior to the start of the operation.* The patient was placed in the supine position and general endotracheal anesthesia was induced. A time-out was completed verifying correct patient, procedure, site, positioning, and implant(s) and/or special equipment prior to beginning this procedure. Preoperative antibiotics were given. A Foley catheter and a nasogastric tube were placed. The abdomen was prepped and draped in the usual sterile fashion. A vertical midline incision was made from xiphoid to just below the umbilicus. This was deepened through the subcutaneous tissues and hemostasis was achieved with electrocautery. The linea alba was identified and incised and the peritoneal cavity entered. The abdomen was explored. *Adhesions were lysed sharply under direct vision with Metzenbaum scissors.* A large quantity of *bilious/ turbid* fluid was suctioned from the peritoneal cavity and cultured. The stomach and duodenum were inspected and palpated and a small anterior perforation of a duodenal ulcer was found just distal to the pylorus. Because of the patient's *age/condition/absence of previous ulcer history*, the decision was made to proceed with plication rather than resection.

Three interrupted sutures of 2-0 silk were placed through healthy duodenal tissue in such a fashion as to span the perforation. These were left untied for now. A mobile portion of viable omentum was brought up, placed over the perforation, and secured in place by tying the previously placed sutures over it in such a manner as to completely close the hole in the duodenum. Care was taken to avoid excess tension.

Hemostasis was checked. The position of the nasogastric tube was verified. The abdomen was copiously lavaged with warm saline. *(Optional: Multiple interrupted through-and-through retention sutures of* ____*were placed.)* The fascia was closed with *a running suture of* ____*/a Smead-Jones closure of interrupted* ____. The skin was *packed open/closed with skin staples/subcuticular sutures of* ____*/other.*

The patient tolerated the procedure well and was taken to the postanesthesia care unit in stable condition.

NOTES

Chapter 20
Laparoscopic Plication of Perforated Ulcer

Roy R. Danks, D.O.

INDICATIONS

- Perforated ulcer with adequate laparoscopic access.
- Patient able to tolerate laparoscopic procedure with above findings.

ESSENTIAL STEPS

1. Monitors at the head.
2. Nasogastric tube and Foley to decompress the stomach and bladder.
3. Induce the pneumoperitoneum.
4. Insert the first trocar below the umbilicus.
5. Inspect the abdomen.
6. Second and third trocars (5 mm) form an isosceles triangle with laparoscope.
7. Aspirate and culture fluid.
8. Identify the perforation.
9. Place three interrupted sutures across the perforation and leave untied.
10. Bring omentum up and tie sutures over the perforation.
11. Test with air under saline.
12. Irrigate the abdomen.
13. Close 10/11-mm trocar site.

J.J. Hoballah and C.E.H. Scott-Conner (eds.), *Operative Dictations in General and Vascular Surgery*, DOI 10.1007/978-1-4614-0451-4_20,
© Springer Science+Business Media, LLC 2012

NOTE THESE VARIATIONS

- Open vs. closed entry with Veress needle.
- 30° laparoscope will, in general, give the best visualization. The decision to plicate rather than resect or excise and close as pyloroplasty is based on size and location of perforation, patient's risk and hemodynamic status, and surrounding tissue condition.
- Exclude malignancy if gastric ulcer.
- Closed suction drain in subhepatic space.

COMPLICATIONS

- Leakage from plication site.
- Subphrenic abscess.
- Gastrointestinal bleeding.
- Duodenal stenosis.

TEMPLATE OPERATIVE DICTATION

Preoperative diagnosis: Pneumoperitoneum due to perforated ulcer.

Procedure: Laparoscopic plication of perforated ulcer.

Postoperative diagnosis: Same, perforated *gastric/duodenal* ulcer.

Indications: _____-year-old *male/female* developed *acute abdomen/ epigastric pain/leukocytosis* with free air on *upright chest X-ray/ lateral decubitus abdominal film/computed tomography scan of abdomen.*

Description of procedure: The patient was placed on the operating table in the supine position. General anesthesia was induced. A Foley catheter and a nasogastric tube were placed. The abdomen was prepped with (Chloraprep/Betadine/etc.) and draped in the usual sterile fashion. A time-out was completed verifying correct patient, procedure, site, positioning, and implant(s) and/or special equipment prior to beginning this procedure.

Local anesthetic was infiltrated in the skin and subcutaneous tissues. An incision was made in a natural skin line below/above the umbilicus.

[Choose one:]

For Veress needle: The umbilical raphe grasped with a Kocher and elevated and the Veress needle inserted. Proper position was confirmed by aspiration and saline meniscus test. Opening intra-abdominal pressure was ____ mmHg. Pneumoperitoneum was created with sterile CO_2. A 10/11-mm trocar was they inserted [alternatively: 5 *(or 10) mm 0° (or 30°) laparoscopic through viewing trocar was advanced into the peritoneum under video-visualization].*

For Hassan cannula: *The fascia was elevated and incised. Entry into the peritoneum was confirmed visually and no bowel was noted in the vicinity of the incision. Two figure-of-eight sutures of 2-0 Vicryl were placed and the Hassan cannula inserted under direct vision. The sutures were anchored around the cannula.* The abdomen was insufflated with carbon dioxide to a pressure of 12–15 mmHg. The patient tolerated insufflation well.

The laparoscope was inserted and the abdomen inspected. No injuries from initial trocar placement were noted. Two additional 5-mm trocars were then inserted in the following locations: subxiphoid to the right of the midline and right subcostal. The trocars were placed under video visualization, after instillation of local anesthetic.

Next, the laparoscope was switched to a 30° laparoscope and an intra-abdominal survey was completed. No other pathology was appreciated. A moderate amount of bilious fluid was suctioned and cultured. *A fourth trocar was placed under video visualization, in the right subcostal region at the anterior axillary line and a liver retractor inserted.* The liver was gently elevated and the site of perforation identified on the *anterior wall of the first portion of the duodenum/anterior gastric wall.*

The table was placed in a head-up, left-rotated position. The ulcer was clearly identified and the perforation delineated by removing fibropurulent material with the suction irrigator. The perforation measured approximately _____ mm in maximum diameter.

The nasogastric tube was pulled back. Three interrupted sutures of were then placed across the perforation *but not tied/the perforation was closed with interrupted sutures of _____.*

Omentum was brought up and laid over the perforation. The previously placed sutures were tied in such a fashion as to pull the omentum snugly over the perforation. The closure was tested with air insufflation under saline and found to be intact. All four quadrants of the peritoneum were then irrigated with warm sterile saline until clear. The saline was aspirated. Hemostasis was checked. *A closed suction drain was placed in the subhepatic space.*

Secondary trocars were removed under direct vision. *No bleeding was noted/trocar site bleeding was controlled by electrocautery/suture placement.* The laparoscope was withdrawn and the umbilical trocar removed. All instruments were removed and pneumoperitoneum was allowed to egress. All trocar sites greater than

5 mm were closed at the fascial layer with _____. (Alternatively: Laparoscopic fascial closure device and transfascial suture passer were utilized to place _____ sutures of _____ in the fasical of the 10/11 port sites.) The skin incisions were lavaged with sterile saline and *packed open with small wicks/closed with subcuticular sutures of* _____ *and steristrips. Sterile dressings were applied.*

The patient tolerated the procedure well and was taken to the postanesthesia care unit in satisfactory condition.

NOTES

Chapter 21
Gastrostomy

Philip M. Spanheimer, M.D.

INDICATIONS

- Need for prolonged enteral support when percutaneous endoscopic gastrostomy or feeding tube not feasible.
- Need for prolonged enteral decompression.
- Adjunct to complex abdominal procedures.

ESSENTIAL STEPS

1. Short upper midline incision.
2. Identify the stomach.
3. Pass a tube through the abdominal wall at desired site.
4. Purse-string suture on the anterior surface of the stomach.
5. Insert tube into stomach.
6. Tie purse-string suture, inkwelling the stomach around the catheter.
7. Place and tie a second outer purse-string suture.
8. Tack the stomach to the abdominal wall at catheter entrance site.
9. Check for torsion, tension.
10. Close the abdomen.
11. Secure the catheter.

NOTE THESE VARIATION

- Type and size of catheter.

J.J. Hoballah and C.E.H. Scott-Conner (eds.), *Operative Dictations in General and Vascular Surgery*, DOI 10.1007/978-1-4614-0451-4_21,

COMPLICATIONS
- Insertion into the colon.
- Distal migration of the catheter causing pyloric obstruction.
- Leakage around catheter.
- Tube dislodgement.

TEMPLATE OPERATIVE DICTATION

Preoperative diagnosis: *Head and neck malignancy/other* with need for prolonged enteral *nutrition/decompression/other*.

Procedure: Stamm gastrostomy.

Postoperative diagnosis: Same.

Indications: This ___-year-old *male/female* required prolonged enteral *nutrition/decompression* because of *head and neck malignancy/other* and was unable to tolerate other routes of access due to ___. Stamm gastrostomy was chosen as the route of *nutritional support/decompression*.

Description of procedure: The patient was placed in the supine position and general endotracheal anesthesia was induced. A time-out was completed verifying correct patient, procedure, site, positioning, and implant(s) and/or special equipment prior to beginning this procedure. Preoperative antibiotics were given. The abdomen was prepped and draped in the usual sterile fashion. A short upper midline incision was made and deepened through the subcutaneous tissues with electrocautery. Hemostasis was assured. The linea alba was incised and the peritoneal cavity entered. The abdomen was explored. *Adhesions were lysed sharply under direct vision with Metzenbaum scissors.*

The stomach was identified and a location on the anterior wall near the greater curvature was selected. That site was approximated to the chosen exit site and found to reach without tension. A small incision was made and the ___ *-French mushroom catheter/ Malecot tube/Foley catheter/other* was passed through the anterior abdominal wall and into the field.

A purse-string suture of ___-0 *silk/proline* was placed on the anterior surface of the stomach and an enterotomy was made with electrocautery in the center of the suture. The catheter was inserted into the lumen of the stomach. The purse-string suture was secured in place in such a manner as to inkwell the stomach around the catheter. A second, outer concentric pursestring was placed in a similar manner and tied to further inkwell the stomach.

The stomach was then tacked to the anterior abdominal wall at the catheter entrance site with several ___-0 *silk/proline* sutures in such a manner as to prevent leakage or torsion. The catheter was secured to the skin with a 3-0 nylon suture.

Hemostasis was checked and omentum was brought adjacent to the surgical field. The fascia was closed with *a running suture of ___/a Smead-Jones closure of interrupted ___*. The skin was closed with *skin staples/subcuticular sutures of ___/other*.

The patient tolerated the procedure well and was taken to the postanesthesia care unit in stable condition.

NOTES

Chapter 22
Percutaneous Endoscopic Gastrostomy

Carol E.H. Scott-Conner, M.D.

INDICATION
- Need for prolonged enteral nutrition.

ESSENTIAL STEPS
1. Sedation and topical analgesia of the oropharynx.
2. Pass endoscope into the stomach and insufflate with air.
3. Identify light reflex on skin of the anterior abdominal wall and indent skin with a finger to confirm position of fundus of the stomach.
4. Local anesthesia at chosen site.
5. Make small incision.
6. Pass snare down biopsy channel of endoscope and position.
7. Pass introducer needle into the stomach and through loop of snare, under direct endoscopic visual control.
8. Pass guide wire into the stomach.
9. Tighten snare around guide wire and withdraw endoscope, snare, and guide wire.
10. Attach gastrostomy tube.
11. Pull retrograde into the stomach and out through the abdominal wall.
12. Reinsert gastroscope and inspect site; confirm position of bumper of gastrostomy.
13. Secure tube to skin.

J.J. Hoballah and C.E.H. Scott-Conner (eds.), *Operative Dictations in General and Vascular Surgery*, DOI 10.1007/978-1-4614-0451-4_22,
© Springer Science+Business Media, LLC 2012

NOTE THESE VARIATIONS

- On occasion done as Seldinger technique with introducer and placement of Foley catheter ("push technique").
- Variations exist that allow gastroscope to be replaced over guide wire.
- PEG-PEJ tube allows tube to be passed through pylorus.
- T-bars may be placed to secure stomach to anterior abdominal wall.

COMPLICATIONS

- Premature tube dislodgement, resulting in peritonitis.
- Leakage around tube.
- Necrosis of gastric wall.
- Perforation of the intervening transverse colon.

TEMPLATE OPERATIVE DICTATION

Preoperative diagnosis: *Head and neck malignancy/other* with need for prolonged enteral nutrition.

Procedure: Percutaneous endoscopic gastrostomy.

Postoperative diagnosis: Same.

Indications: This ___-year-old *male/female* required prolonged enteral nutrition because of *stroke/neuromuscular disorder/head and neck malignancy/other*. Percutaneous endoscopic gastrostomy was chosen as the route of nutritional support.

Description of procedure: The patient was taken to the *procedure suite/operating room*. Topical analgesia of the oropharynx was induced using ___. *He/she* was sedated with ___.

A time-out was completed verifying correct patient, procedure, site, positioning, and implant(s) and/or special equipment prior to beginning this procedure.

After adequate sedation, a mouthpiece was placed in the patient's mouth and the endoscope was passed down into the stomach. No abnormalities were noted. The stomach was insufflated with air and the endoscope positioned in the midportion and directed toward the anterior abdominal wall. With the room darkened and intensity turned up on the endoscope, a good light reflex was noted on the skin of the abdominal wall in the left upper quadrant. Finger pressure was applied at the light reflex with adequate indentation on the stomach wall on endoscopy. A polypectomy snare was passed into the stomach, opened fully, and positioned so that the loop encircled the point of demonstrated finger indentation.

The overlying skin was anesthetized with lidocaine and a 1.0-cm incision was made at the chosen site. The introducer needle with overlying catheter was passed through this incision and into the stomach under visualization with the gastroscope. The needle and catheter were gently captured by the endoscopic snare. The guide wire was passed and snared. The endoscope, snare, and guide wire were then withdrawn and pulled back out of the mouth. The gastrostomy tube was attached to the loop of the guide wire and the whole thing pulled back into the stomach until the ___-cm mark of the gastrostomy tube was noted at skin level.

The gastroscope was reintroduced and adequate placement of the gastrostomy tube was identified and a picture was taken. The gastrostomy tube end was cut to length and the clamping appendage was placed. A collecting bag was applied.

The patient tolerated the procedure well and was taken to the postanesthesia care unit in good condition.

ACKNOWLEDGMENT

This chapter was contributed by Mazen M. Hashisho, MD in the first edition.

NOTES

Chapter 23
Distal Gastrectomy with D2 Nodal Dissection, Roux-en-Y Reconstruction for Cancer

Hisakazu Hoshi, M.D.

INDICATION
■ Carcinoma of the distal stomach.

ESSENTIAL STEPS
1. Upper midline incision.
2. Explore the abdomen and confirm pathology and stage.
3. Separate the greater omentum from the transverse colon.
4. Subpyloric nodal dissection and ligation of the right gastroepiploic vessels.
5. Suprapyloric nodal dissection and ligation of the right gastric vessels.
6. Divide the duodenum.
7. *If stapled duodenal closure:*
   • *Fire linear stapler across the duodenum.*
8. *If sutured duodenal stump closure:*
   • *Divide the duodenum between intestinal clamps.*
   • *Close the duodenal stump in two layers with an inner row of running 3-0 Vicryl and an outer row of interrupted 3-0 silk Lembert sutures.*
9. Dissect nodes along the common hepatic artery.
10. Dissect nodes around the celiac axis and the proximal splenic artery.
11. Ligate the left gastric artery at the celiac axis.
12. Dissect nodes along the lesser curvature toward GE junction.

J.J. Hoballah and C.E.H. Scott-Conner (eds.), *Operative Dictations in General and Vascular Surgery*, DOI 10.1007/978-1-4614-0451-4_23,
© Springer Science+Business Media, LLC 2012

13. Ligate the left gastroepiploic vessels.
14. Dissect nodes along the greater curvature.
15. Pull the nasogastric tube back into the distal esophagus.
16. Divide stomach at least 3 cm for differentiated and 5 cm for poorly differentiated carcinoma from the tumor.
17. *If sutured gastrojejunostomy:*
    - *Divide the stomach with bowel clamps across the greater curvature.*
    - *Divide the lesser curvature to within 3–4 cm of the esophagus with a linear stapler.*
18. *If stapled gastrojejunostomy:*
    - *Divide the stomach with a linear stapler from the chosen point on the greater curvature to within 3–4 cm of the esophagus on the lesser curvature.*
19. Trace jejunum to the ligament of Treitz; identify mobile loop of the jejunum close to the ligament of Treitz.
20. Divide loop of the jejunum with a linear stapler.
21. Pass the distal jejunum antecolic/retrocolic for Roux-en-Y reconstruction and place adjacent to the gastric remnant.
22. *If sutured:*
    - *Create one-layer gastrojejunostomy: interrupted Gambee sutures.*
23. *If stapled:*
    - *Approximate the posterior wall of the stomach and the jejunum with two 3-0 silk sutures.*
    - *Create gastrotomy and jejunotomy and insert a linear cutting stapler.*
    - *Fire stapler.*
    - *Check the staple line for hemostasis.*
    - *Close the enterotomies with a linear stapler/in two layers with running 3-0 Vicryl and interrupted 3-0 silk.*
24. Check the anastomosis for integrity and patency.
25. Create a stapled jejunojejunostomy.
26. Check hemostasis.
27. Position nasogastric tube.
28. Close the abdomen without drainage.

NOTE THESE VARIATIONS

- Stapled or sutured duodenal stump closure.
- Stapled or sutured gastrojejunostomy.
- Billroth I or Billroth II reconstruction.
- En bloc resection of contiguous structures.

COMPLICATIONS
- Recurrence.
- Anastomotic leak.
- Injury to the common bile duct, pancreas, or spleen.
- Bile reflux gastritis (rare in Rou-en-Y reconstruction).
- Afferent limb syndrome.
- Herniation through transverse mesocolon defect (retrocolic).

TEMPLATE OPERATIVE DICTATION
Preoperative diagnosis: Adenocarcinoma of the stomach (T_, N_, M_ stage __).
Procedure: Distal gastrectomy with D2 nodal dissection, Roux-en-Y reconstruction.
Postoperative diagnosis: Same.
Indications: This ___-year-old *male/female* developed symptoms of *early satiety/gastrointestinal bleeding/epigastric pain* and on evaluation was found to have adenocarcinoma of the distal stomach. Distal gastrectomy with D2 nodal dissection was indicated for *treatment*.
Description of procedure: An epidural catheter was placed by anesthesia prior to the start of the operation. A time-out was completed verifying correct patient, procedure, site, positioning, and implant(s) and/or special equipment prior to beginning this procedure. The patient was placed in the supine position and general endotracheal anesthesia was induced. Preoperative antibiotics were given. A Foley catheter and a nasogastric tube were placed. The abdomen was prepped and draped in the usual sterile fashion.

A vertical midline incision was made from the xiphoid to just below the umbilicus. This was deepened through the subcutaneous tissues and hemostasis was achieved with electrocautery. The linea alba was identified and incised and the peritoneal cavity entered. The abdomen was explored. *Adhesions were lysed sharply under direct vision with Metzenbaum scissors.* No liver metastasis and peritoneal involvement was seen. Wash cytology was obtained in the upper abdomen. Tumor was *limited to the stomach/found in (detail locations)*. The stomach was mobile and the decision was made to proceed with distal gastrectomy.

The spleen was gently elevated from the diaphragm with abdominal laparotomy pads behind it. The dissecting the greater omentum from the transverse colon was performed first, by starting dissection at the avascular plain near the splenic flexure. Dissection was advanced toward the hepatic flexure and then advanced along the anterior leaf of the transverse mesocolon into the lesser sac. The anterior leaf of the transverse mesocolon was dissected toward the head of the pancreas until identification of the accessory right colic vein at its insertion point into the right gastroepiploic vein. The right gastroepiploic vein was ligated just proximal to the insertion of the accessory right colic vein with silk ligatures. The right gastroepiploic artery was also identified, ligated with silk ligatures, and reinforced with a silk stick tie. All lymphatic tissue at subpyloric area was separated from the duodenal wall toward the pylorus.

In the left side of the hepatoduodenal ligament peritoneum was incised and the origin of the right gastric artery was exposed. The artery was ligated with 2-0 silk ties and divided. All the node baring tissue in the suprapyloric area was separated from the duodenum. The pylorus was identified. The duodenum was then transected with a GIA stapler utilizing a blue load 1 cm distal to the pylorus. We then over-sewed the staple line with 3-0 silk Lembert stitches. This allowed the stomach to be reflected in a cephalad manner. This exposed the head of the pancreas, the common hepatic artery, and the origin of the celiac axis. The nodal tissue adjacent to the head of the pancreas along the common hepatic artery was dissected by sharp and blunt fashion. The lesser omentum was then divided toward the GE junction with electrocautery just inferior to its attachment with the inferior border of the liver. Then the retroperitoneal dissection advanced up to the right crus of the diaphragm. The left gastric vein and the left gastric artery were identified. The left gastric vein was ligated with silk ties. The left gastric artery was then ligated with silk sutures and further reinforced with a silk stick tie. The plane was developed in between the left gastric artery and the aorta. Proximal splenic nodes were dissected toward the specimen. Soft tissue in between diaphragmatic crura in front of the aorta was dissected toward specimen.

Starting at the GE junction, soft tissue around the left gastric artery located along the lesser curvature of stomach was then dissected off the adjacent wall of the stomach with a combination of blunt dissection, silk ligature, and Harmonic scalpel. Dissection was advanced in this manner toward the pylorus until our planned level of transection on the stomach. This allowed dissection of paracardial and lesser curvature nodes.

Attention was next turned to the greater curvature of the stomach. The origin of the left gastroepiploic artery was identified in the gastrosplenic ligament, from its takeoff of the splenic artery. The gastroepiploic artery was further isolated, ligated with silk suture, and reinforced with a silk stick tie. The short gastric arteries were preserved. Dissection was advanced along the greater curvature close to the wall of the stomach with a combination of blunt dissection, silk ligatures, and Harmonic scalpel to dissect the nodes along the gastroepiploic artery and the greater omentum. This was continued toward the pylorus until our planned line of transection. The lesion within the stomach was palpated in the antrum. A 5 cm margin was measured from the proximal extent of the lesion for a line of transection.

If sutured gastrojejunostomy: With a Kocher clamp on the specimen side and a gastric clamp on the remnant side, the stomach was half way divided from the greater curvature side and the lesser curvature side was divided with a TA stapler slightly cut back toward the GE junction. This was oversewn with 3-0 silk Lembert stitches.

If stapled gastrojejunostomy: The stomach was divided with a linear stapler placed across it from the chosen point of division on the greater curvature to a point within 3–4 cm of the esophagus on the lesser curvature.

The stomach, the greater omentum, and nodal stations as described above were then passed off the table to Pathology. The stomach was everted on the back table to identify the tumor and to ensure adequate margins of resection.

If Roux-en-Y reconstruction: A segment of jejunum approximately 20 cm downstream from the ligament of Treitz was selected. A window in the mesentery was created, the bowel loop was divided with a linear stapler. The distal part of the intestine was then brought up in front of/through the mesenteric defect behind the transverse colon to the gastric remnant. A gastrojejunostomy was created with 3-0 absorbable Gambee stitches for a single-layer anastomosis. The anastomosis was then checked for patency. It appeared to be patent and without any areas of apparent concern for leakage.

If two layered sutured gastrojejunostomy: A two-layered sutured gastrojejunostomy was then constructed with an inner layer of running 3-0 absorbable suture and an outer layer of interrupted 3-0 silk Lembert sutures. A three-point suture was placed at the angle of sorrows.

If stapled gastrojejunostomy: The jejunum was approximated to the posterior wall of the stomach with two sutures of 3-0 silk. A gastrotomy and a jejunotomy were then made and the linear cutting stapler inserted and fired. The staple line was inspected for hemostasis. The enterotomies were closed with a linear stapler/in two layers using 3-0 absorbable suture and 3-0 silk.

Then anastomosis was created between the pancreatobiliary end of the jejunum and approximately 45 cm down from the gastrojejunostomy to perform a Roux-en-Y jejunojejunostomy anastomosis. This was done in a side-to-side fashion, tacking stitches of 3-0 silk were placed. Enterotomy was then placed in both bowels and the two limbs of a GIA stapler were then introduced into both these enterotomy sites. The GIA stapler was fired. No bleeding was seen from staple line. The enterotomies were then closed with a TA stapler and oversewn with 3-0 silk Lembert stitches.

After ensuring adequate hemostasis, the fascia was closed with *a running suture of* ____. The skin was closed with *skin staples/ subcuticular sutures of* ____*/other*.

The patient tolerated the procedure well and was taken to the postanesthesia care unit in stable condition.

ACKNOWLEDGMENT

This chapter was contributed by Mazen M. Hashisho, MD, Roy R. Danks, DO, and Mario Martinasevic, MD in the first edition.

NOTES

Chapter 24

Total Gastrectomy with D2 Nodal Dissection, Roux-en-Y Reconstruction, Feeding Tube Jejunostomy

Hisakazu Hoshi, M.D.

INDICATION

- Gastric cancer.

ESSENTIAL STEPS

1. Upper midline incision.
2. Explore the abdomen and confirm pathology and stage.
3. Separate greater omentum from the transverse colon.
4. Dissect subpyloric nodes and ligate right gastroepiploic vessels.
5. Dissect suprapyloric nodes and ligate right gastric vessels.
6. Divide the duodenum.
7. *If stapled duodenal closure: Fire linear stapler across the duodenum.*
8. *If sutured duodenal stump closure:*
   - *Divide the duodenum between intestinal clamps.*
   - *Close the duodenal stump in two layers with an inner row of running 3-0 absorbable suture and an outer row of interrupted 3-0 silk Lembert sutures.*
9. Dissect nodes along the common hepatic artery.
10. Dissect nodes around the celiac axis and the proximal splenic artery.
11. Ligate left gastric artery at the celiac axis.

J.J. Hoballah and C.E.H. Scott-Conner (eds.), *Operative Dictations in General and Vascular Surgery*, DOI 10.1007/978-1-4614-0451-4_24,
© Springer Science+Business Media, LLC 2012

12. Ligate of short gastric vessels and divide gastrosplenic ligament.
13. Dissect around the abdominal part of esophagus.
14. Transect esophagus and remove specimen.
15. Identify the ligament of Treitz and identify a loop of upper jejunum.
16. *If retrocolic:*
    • *Create a window in the transverse mesocolon adjacent to the ligament of Treitz.*
17. Create Roux-en-Y limb.
18. Pass jejunum *anterior to colon/through window in the transverse mesocolon and bring adjacent to the esophagus.*
19. *Stapled/sutured* esophagojejunal anastomosis.
20. Roux-en-Y jejunojejunostomy.
21. *Feeding jejunostomy.*
22. *Closed suction drains in vicinity of the hiatus.*
23. Position the nasogastric tube.
24. Check hemostasis.
25. Close the abdomen.

NOTE THESE VARIATIONS
- Stapled or sutured duodenal stump closure.
- Antecolic vs. retrocolic passage of jejunal limb.
- *Creation of jejunal pouch optional.*
- *Feeding tube jejunostomy.*

COMPLICATIONS
- Injury to the left replaced hepatic.
- Anastomotic leak.
- Injury to the esophagus.
- Duodenal stump leak.
- *Small bowel obstruction caused by feeding jejunostomy.*

TEMPLATE OPERATIVE DICTATION
Preoperative diagnosis: Adenocarcinoma of the stomach (T_, N_, M_ stage __).
Procedure: Total gastrectomy with D2 nodal dissection, Roux-en-Y reconstruction, *feeding tube jejunostomy.*
Postoperative diagnosis: Same.
Indications: This ___-year-old *male/female* developed symptoms of *early satiety/gastrointestinal bleeding/epigastric pain* and on evaluation was found to have gastric adenocarcinoma. A total gastrectomy was indicated for *treatment.*

Description of procedure: An epidural catheter was placed by anesthesia prior to the start of the operation. The patient was placed in the supine position and general endotracheal anesthesia was induced. A time-out was completed verifying correct patient, procedure, site, positioning, and implant(s) and/or special equipment prior to beginning this procedure. Preoperative antibiotics were given. A Foley catheter and a nasogastric tube were placed. The abdomen was prepped and draped in the usual sterile fashion.

A vertical midline incision was made from the xiphoid to just below the umbilicus. This was deepened through the subcutaneous tissues and hemostasis was achieved with electrocautery. The linea alba was identified and incised and the peritoneal cavity entered. The abdomen was explored. *Adhesions were lysed sharply under direct vision with Metzenbaum scissors.* Tumor was *limited to the stomach/found in (detail locations).* No liver metastasis and peritoneal involvement was seen. Wash cytology was obtained in the upper abdomen. The stomach was mobile and the decision was made to proceed with total gastrectomy.

The spleen was gently elevated from the diaphragm with abdominal laparotomy pads behind it. The dissecting the greater omentum from the transverse colon was performed first, by starting dissection at the avascular plain near the splenic flexure. Dissection was advanced toward the hepatic flexure and then advanced along the anterior leaf of the transverse mesocolon into the lesser sac. The anterior leaf of the transverse mesocolon was dissected toward the head of the pancreas until identification of the accessory right colic vein at its insertion point into the right gastroepiploic vein. The right gastroepiploic vein was ligated just proximal to the insertion of the accessory right colic vein with silk ligatures. The right gastroepiploic artery was also identified, ligated with silk ligatures, and reinforced with a silk stick tie. All the lymphatic tissue at subpyloric area was separated from duodenal wall toward pylorus.

In the left side of the hepatoduodenal ligament peritoneum was incised and origin of the right gastric artery was exposed. The artery was ligated with 2-0 silk ties and divided. All the node-baring tissue in the suprapyloric area was separated from the duodenum. The pylorus was identified. The duodenum was then transected with a GIA stapler utilizing a blue load 1 cm distal to the pylorus. We then over-sewed the staple line with 3-0 silk Lembert stitches. This allowed the stomach to be reflected in a cephalad manner. This exposed the head of the pancreas, the common hepatic artery, and the origin of the celiac axis. The nodal tissue adjacent to the head of the pancreas along the common hepatic artery was dissected by sharp and blunt fashion. The lesser omentum was then divided toward GE junction with electrocautery just inferior to its attachment with the inferior border of the liver. Then the retroperitoneal dissection advanced up to the right crus of the diaphragm. The left gastric vein and the left gastric artery was identified. The left gastric vein was ligated with silk ties and divided. The left gastric artery was then ligated with silk sutures, further reinforced with a silk stick tie and divided. The plane was developed in between left gastric artery and aorta. The proximal splenic artery nodes were dissected toward the specimen. Soft tissue in between the diaphragmatic crura in front of the aorta was dissected toward the specimen.

Attention was next turned to the greater curvature of the stomach. The origin of the left gastroepiploic artery was identified in the gastrosplenic ligament, from its takeoff of the splenic artery. The gastroepiploic artery was further isolated, ligated with silk suture, and reinforced with a silk stick tie. The short gastric arteries were serially ligated at the hilum of the spleen. Nodal tissue around the distal splenic artery was dissected. *Posterior gastric artery was identified, dissected, ligated, and divided.* Entire fundus was mobilized from retroperitoneum toward esophagus.

Retractors were placed and attention was directed to the region of the hiatus. An incision was made in the peritoneum overlying the abdominal esophagus. The esophagus was gently mobilized by sharp and blunt dissection and encircled by a Penrose drain. The anterior and posterior vagus nerve was identified, ligated, and divided. A purse string clamp was applied just oral to the GE junction and a purse string suture was placed. The anterior wall of the esophagus was opened and __ mm circular stapler anvil was placed within the esophagus. The purse string suture was tied around the esophagus and the posterior wall of the esophagus was divided. The stomach and nodal tissue were removed en bloc.

The ligament of Treitz was identified and the small bowel was transected approximately 20 cm distal to it with the linear cutting stapler. *An arcade in the small bowel mesentery was ligated and transected to allow for further mobilization of the small bowel.* The distal limb of this jejunum was brought up to the esophagus *in an antecolic/through a window in the transverse mesocolon in a retrocolic* fashion and brought to lie comfortably without tension or torsion adjacent to the esophagus.

The circular stapler was then introduced into the open end of the jejunum and the spike driven out through the antemesenteric border approximately ___ cm from the end. The stapler was assembled and fired. Intact donuts were retrieved. The open end of jejunum was then closed with a linear stapler.

If sutured: Single layer esophagojejunostomy was created with interrupted 3-0 absorbable sutures.

The anastomosis was inspected and found to be intact. NG tube was guided through the anastomosis and placed distally.

The Roux-en-Y jejunojejunostomy was then constructed 45 cm distal to the esophagojejunostomy.

If stapled: The two limbs of jejunum were approximated with 3-0 silk sutures. Enterotomies were then made and the stapler was introduced and fired. The staple line was checked for hemostasis and the enterotomy closed with a linear stapler/two layers of sutures.

If sutured: A hand-sewn two-layer anastomosis was then made between the end of one limb of jejunum and the side of the jejunum using running 3-0 Vicryl and 3-0 silk. The anastomosis was checked for integrity and was noted to be widely patent in all three directions.

A feeding jejunostomy was then made a comfortable distance distal to the Roux-en-Y anastomosis. A pursestring suture was then placed within the jejunum 20 cm distal to the jejunal anastomosis. An enterotomy was made at the center of the purse string. A ___ French red Robinson catheter was placed within the lumen of the jejunum and the pursestring suture was tightened. 3-0 silk Lembert sutures were then placed to create a Witzel tunnel and bury the jejunostomy tube without compromising the lumen. A subsequent stab incision was made to the left of the midline incision and a hemostat was placed through the rectus fascia and the red rubber catheter was grasped and brought out through the stab incision. The jejunum was sutured to the anterior abdominal wall with four-quadrant sutures through the anterior abdominal wall and seromuscular bites on the jejunum. These were securely tied, affixing the jejunum and jejunostomy tube up to the anterior abdominal wall. The exit site of the tube was sutured with 3-0 nylon sutures and the jejunostomy feeding tube was secured in place.

Hemostasis was checked. *One closed suction drain was placed in the vicinity of the hiatus and brought out through separate stab wounds.*

The fascia was closed with *a running suture of ___*. The skin was closed with *skin staples/subcuticular sutures of ___/other.*

The patient tolerated the procedure well and was taken to the postanesthesia care unit in stable condition.

ACKNOWLEDGMENT

This chapter was contributed by Mario Martinasevic, MD in the first edition.

NOTES

Chapter 25
Vertical Banded Gastroplasty

Carol E.H. Scott-Conner, M.D.

INDICATION
- Morbid obesity.

ESSENTIAL STEPS
1. General anesthesia: Avoid postoperative epidural analgesia to avoid masking clinical assessment of possible gastric leak.
2. Upper midline incision.
3. Reverse Trendelenburg position.
4. Note the location of the pylorus (prepyloric veins of Mayo).
5. Identify and divide the falciform ligament.
6. Identify the gastrohepatic ligament (be aware that the right hepatic artery sometimes arises from the superior mesenteric artery).
7. Anesthesia passes 32 French Ewald tube down into the stomach.
8. Incise the peritoneum over the esophagus and mobilize it.
9. Encircle the esophagus with a Penrose drain.
10. Enter the lesser sac approximately 6 cm inferior to the gastroesophageal junction and over the pancreas lateral to the lesser curvature vessels.
11. Mark a point 3 cm from the lesser curve and 6 cm from the angle of His, where a circular stapled defect will be created.

J.J. Hoballah and C.E.H. Scott-Conner (eds.), *Operative Dictations in General and Vascular Surgery*, DOI 10.1007/978-1-4614-0451-4_25,
© Springer Science+Business Media, LLC 2012

12. Create a circular defect with a circular stapling device, centered at the mark point.
13. Place a Penrose drain through the circular defect and around the lesser curvature.
14. Pass a red rubber catheter through the circular defect and bring it out over the angle of His to guide a stapler.
15. Connect the circular stapling defect with the left side of gastroesophageal junction with a TA 90-D stapler (Autosuture Corp.); do not divide the stomach.
16. Cover Marlex mesh with an omentum.
17. A 32 French Ewald tube is removed.
18. Pouch volume is measured to be <20 mL at 60-cm water pressure.
19. TA 90-D stapler is now fired.
20. A 7 × 1.5-cm piece of Marlex mesh is placed around the pouch outlet and sutured in place with three serially placed 3-0 prolene sutures to approximate the overlapped ends.
21. Check hemostasis.
22. Close the abdomen.

COMPLICATIONS
- Staple line leak.
- Injury to the vagus nerves.
- Injury to the right hepatic artery.
- Injury to the esophagus.

TEMPLATE OPERATIVE DICTATION
Preoperative diagnosis: Morbid obesity.
Procedure: Vertical banded gastroplasty.
Postoperative diagnosis: Same.
Indications: This ___-year-old *male/female* underwent thorough evaluation for morbid obesity (BMI ___) and had failed medical management.
Description of procedure: The patient was placed in the supine position and general endotracheal anesthesia was induced. Preoperative antibiotics were given. A Foley catheter and nasogastric tube were placed. The abdomen was prepped and draped in the usual sterile fashion. A time-out was completed verifying correct patient, procedure, site, positioning, and implant(s) and/or special equipment prior to beginning this procedure.

A vertical midline incision was made from xiphoid to the umbilicus. This was deepened through the subcutaneous tissues and hemostasis was achieved with electrocautery. The linea alba was identified and incised. Preperitoneal fat was dissected from the peritoneum and subsequent access was gained into the peritoneal cavity. A wound protector was inserted and wound retractors were applied using an Omni. The abdomen was explored. *Adhesions were lysed sharply under direct vision with Metzenbaum scissors.* The falciform ligament was divided and ligated with 2-0 silk.

Attention was turned to the stomach and the gastrohepatic ligament was divided, gaining access to the lesser sac. The anterior plane between the esophagus and the crus of the diaphragm was opened by gently inserting two fingers superiorly to disrupt the phrenoesophageal ligament. The lower end of the esophagus, including the posterior vagus nerve, was encircled with a finger, and a Penrose drain was passed around it.

The nasogastric tube was removed and a 32 French Ewald tube was passed from the mouth by the anesthesiologist and placed in the stomach. The lesser omentum was opened adjacent to the stomach at a point approximately 6 cm inferior to the gastroesophageal junction. A Penrose drain was passed through this opening. Three centimeters from the lesser curve and 6 cm from the angle of His, a point was marked on the anterior wall of the stomach. A 5-mm trocar was passed through the anterior and posterior walls of the stomach at this point. A grasper was passed through this and used to position the anvil of a 28-mm EEA stapler within this region of the stomach.

The Ewald tube was mobilized so it would lie along the lesser curvature of the stomach and the EEA stapling device was used to create a circular stapled defect at the site. Two intact donuts were obtained. The second Penrose drain was then passed through this defect. By blunt finger dissection, a canal was then created behind the stomach connecting the lesser sac to the gastroesophageal junction on the left side. A red rubber catheter was passed from the left gastroesophageal junction along the posterior aspect of the stomach and through the circular stapled defect. A TA 90-D stapler was inserted into the flanged end of the red rubber catheter and passed superiorly using this catheter as a lead. The stapler was closed and the two Penrose drains were tightened to occlude the inlet and outlet and allow measurement of the gastric pouch. Saline was instilled by anesthesia into the Ewald tube to confirm that the pouch measured <20 mL at 60-cm water pressure. The Ewald tube was pulled back in esophagus and the TA stapler was then fired, connecting the circular stapling defect to the left side of the gastroesophageal junction without dividing the stomach.

A 7×1.5-cm piece of Marlex mesh was placed around the pouch outlet and sutured in place with three serially placed 3-0 prolene sutures to approximate the overlapped ends.

The omentum was brought up and made to lie comfortably over the mesh. It was affixed in place with interrupted sutures of 3-0 silk. All Penrose drains were removed and the upper abdomen was filled with normal saline. Air was instilled into the Ewald tube by anesthesiology. No leaks were identified. The saline was aspirated from the abdomen. Hemostasis was achieved.

The abdominal wall and fascia were reapproximated using a running suture of #1 looped PDS. The skin was closed with *skin staples/subcuticular sutures* of ___.

The patient tolerated the procedure well and was transferred to the postanesthesia care unit in satisfactory condition.

ACKNOWLEDGMENT

This chapter was contributed by Mario Martinasevic, MD in the first edition.

NOTES

Chapter 26

Laparoscopic Adjustable Gastric Banding for Obesity

Mohammad A. Hojeij, M.D. and Bassem Y. Safadi, M.D.

INDICATIONS

■ Morbid obesity with body mass index (BMI) greater or equal to 40 kg/m².
■ Morbid obesity with BMI greater than 35 kg/m² with serious co-morbidities.
■ The patient should have tried but failed supervised medical weight loss program, and should have had a multidisciplinary assessment in a bariatric surgical program preoperatively.

ESSENTIAL STEPS

1. The procedure is done via four or five laparoscopic ports placed in the upper abdomen.
2. We prefer to use an optical trocar to facilitate initial port placement in these patients.
3. Place the first port, which will be used for the laparoscope, high – around 15 cm below the xiphoid process to ensure.
4. Pass the band through a retrogastric tunnel that is created by blunt dissection connecting these two points:
   • The Angle of His on the left.
   • A window created through the Pars Flaccida just anterior to the right crus of the diaphragm at the inferior edge of the lesser omentum.

J.J. Hoballah and C.E.H. Scott-Conner (eds.), *Operative Dictations in General and Vascular Surgery*, DOI 10.1007/978-1-4614-0451-4_26,
© Springer Science+Business Media, LLC 2012

5. Wrap the gastric band around the upper part of the stomach in such a manner as to lie below the esophago-gastric (EG) junction and partition the stomach into a small 15 cc. proximal gastric pouch separate from the rest of the stomach.
6. Calibrate the pouch using a balloon-tipped oro-gastric tube that is placed in the stomach and pulled back toward the EG junction. With experience this step becomes unnecessary.
7. Lock the band into position.
8. Secure the band posteriorly by intact retroperitoneal gastroesophageal attachments and anteriorly by plicating the fundus around the band to the upper gastric pouch.
9. Tunnel the tubing to exit through the abdominal wall at an oblique angle and then to the subcutaneous pocket that will house the band reservoir.
10. Test the band for leakage with Methylene Blue.

NOTE THESE VARIATIONS

- Hiatal hernias if detected should be repaired by approximating the crura prior to band passage.
- The technique of band placement has transitioned from a peri-gastric to a "Pars Flaccida" approach because of less risk of slippage and erosion.

COMPLICATIONS

- Bleeding.
- Esophageal perforation.
- Gastric perforation.
- Band slippage.
- Pulmonary embolus.

OPERATIVE DICTATION

Preoperative diagnosis: Morbid obesity.
Procedure: Laparoscopic adjustable gastric band placement.
Postoperative diagnosis: Same.
Indications: *BMI above 40 kg/m²/BMI above 35 kg/m² with serious co-morbidities.*
Description of procedure: The patient was placed in the supine position with the legs in stirrups. General endotracheal anesthesia was induced. The patient received *Heparin 5,000 units subcutaneous/other* and *1 g Cefazolin/other* prior to induction. The abdomen was prepped and draped in the usual sterile fashion.

A time-out was completed verifying correct patient, procedure, site, positioning, and implant(s) and/or special equipment prior to beginning this procedure.

A 10 mm incision was made 15 cm below the Xyphoid process to the left of midline. A 10 mm _____ optical port was placed under direct vision without complications. The peritoneal cavity was insufflated to a pressure of 14 mmHg. The patient was placed in the reverse Trendelenburg position. The liver was noted to have fatty infiltration and the left lateral segment of the liver was large. A 5-mm port was inserted via a subxiphoid incision and a grasper was used to effectively retract the liver and expose the esophagogastric junction. Three additional ports were placed under direct vision, one 5 mm in the right upper quadrant, a 15-mm port left subcostal at the midclavicular line and a 5-mm port at the anterior axillary line in left upper quadrant.

The peritoneum at the level of angle of His was incised and the plane between the stomach and the diaphragm was bluntly dissected to expose the left crus of the diaphragm. Then the pars flaccida was opened. The right crus of the diaphragm was identified, and the peritoneum overlying the right crus was opened at the inferior edge of the lesser omentum. With blunt dissection, a forceps was passed behind the stomach toward the angle of His without any resistance. Then the band with tubing attached was introduced through the 15-mm port. The tubing was grasped with the forceps and passed around the stomach. The tubing was gently pulled to allow the band to pass circumferentially around the stomach leaving a proximal gastric pouch with an estimated volume of 15 ml. The tubing was then passed through the band buckle and the band was locked in place. An anterior fundoplication was done bringing the fundus to the upper pouch of the stomach with two interrupted Prolene sutures. Once this part was done the tubing was exteriorized from the subxyphoid incision. The 15-mm port was removed and the tubing was passed through a subcutaneous tunnel to the 15-mm port incision. A subcutaneous pocket for the reservoir was created by blunt dissection of the fat above the fascia. The band reservoir was then connected to the tubing and fixed to the fascia with nonabsorbable sutures. Laparoscopic re-exploration was done to make sure the tubing was not kinked. We injected the band reservoir with saline and Methylene blue to make sure there was no leakage in the band system. Once that was done the remaining ports were removed. The skin was closed with absorbable sutures. The patient tolerated the procedure well and was extubated and transferred to the recovery room in stable condition. The instrument and sponge counts were reported to be correct.

NOTES

Chapter 27
Roux-en-Y Gastric Bypass for Obesity

Yi-Horng Lee, M.D.

INDICATION

- Severe obesity (body mass index of 40 kg/m² or above without co-morbidities or body mass index of ³35 kg/m² for those with co-morbid conditions) refractory to dietary changes and medical treatment.

ESSENTIAL STEPS

1. Sequential compression stocking and administer subcutaneous fractionated low-molecular weight heparin.
2. General anesthesia.
3. Administer antibiotic prophylaxis.
4. Upper midline incision.
5. Reverse Trendelenburg position.
6. Explore the abdomen.
7. Assess the gallbladder.
8. Mobilize the distal esophagus and gastroesophageal junction.
9. Create a proximal gastric pouch of 15–30 mL.
10. Divide jejunum 50 cm distal to the ligament of Treitz.
11. Create a window in the transverse mesocolon anterolateral to the ligament of Treitz that is large enough to enable the retrocolic passage of distal jejunum (Roux limb) to lie adjacent to the gastric pouch.
12. Create a stapled jejunojejunostomy 45 cm along the Roux limb.

137

J.J. Hoballah and C.E.H. Scott-Conner (eds.), *Operative Dictations in General and Vascular Surgery*, DOI 10.1007/978-1-4614-0451-4_27,
© Springer Science+Business Media, LLC 2012

13. Create 1-cm side-to-side sutured anastomosis between the proximal gastric pouch and the Roux limb.
14. Test for leaks.
15. Manually guide the nasogastric tube through the gastrojejunostomy.
16. Close all mesenteric defects with running 3-0 Vicryl.
17. Close the transverse mesocolon to Roux limb.
18. *If the gallbladder is abnormal and the procedure has gone well, perform cholecystectomy.*
19. Check hemostasis.
20. Close fascia with running #1 looped PDS.
21. Close skin.

NOTE THESE VARIATIONS

- Cholecystectomy is performed after bypass if gallbladder is abnormal.
- Jejunojejunostomy may be made 150 cm (rather than 45 cm) distal to the gastrojejunostomy in patients whose BMI is $^{3}50$ kg/m^2.

COMPLICATIONS

- Anastomotic leak.
- Injury to the vagus nerves, esophagus, or spleen.

TEMPLATE OPERATIVE DICTATION

Preoperative diagnosis: Severe obesity.
Procedure: Roux-en-Y gastric bypass.
Postoperative diagnosis: Same.
Indications: This ___-year-old *male/female* has severe obesity with BMI of ___ kg/m^2 that is refractory to dietary changes and medical management.
Description of procedure: The patient was placed in the supine position and general endotracheal anesthesia was induced. Preoperative antibiotics were given. A Foley catheter and nasogastric tube were placed. The abdomen was prepped and draped in the usual sterile fashion. A time-out was completed verifying correct patient, procedure, site, positioning, and implant(s) and/or special equipment prior to beginning this procedure.

A vertical midline incision was made from xiphoid to the umbilicus. This was deepened through the subcutaneous tissues and hemostasis was achieved with electrocautery. The linea alba was identified and incised. Preperitoneal fat was dissected from the peritoneum and subsequent access was gained into the peritoneal cavity.

A wound protector was inserted and wound retractors were applied using an Omni. The abdomen was explored. *Adhesions were lysed sharply under direct vision with Metzenbaum scissors.* The gallbladder was *normal/abnormal (list any additional abnormalities noted).* The falciform ligament was divided and ligated with 2-0 silk.

The liver was first reflected superiorly to expose the lesser omentum. The lesser sac was entered by bluntly dissecting the lesser omentum overlying the caudate lobe of the liver. Care was taken to avoid the left hepatic artery. The incision was extended over the gastroesophageal junction and the distal esophagus was gently mobilized. It was then encircled with a Penrose drain. With downward traction on the Penrose drain, phrenoesophageal ligament was taken down and the distal esophagus fully mobilized. Care was taken not to injure the short gastric vessels in this process.

After the gastroesophageal junction was clearly defined, the Penrose drain was lifted anteriorly and a finger was passed through the lesser sac onto the posterior aspect of the stomach. An opening was created bluntly in the mesentery adjacent to the lesser curvature of the stomach between the first and second branches of the left gastric artery. A right-angle clamp was passed from the angle of His to this mesenteric opening and a 28 French red rubber catheter pulled through. The open end of the red rubber catheter was attached to the tip of a TA stapler. Traction on the red rubber catheter was then employed to position the TA stapler in such a manner as to create a proximal gastric pouch that measured ___ mL. The nasogastric tube was removed and the stapler was fired and removed.

The ligament of Treitz was then identified and jejunum was transected 45–50 cm distal to the ligament of Treitz using a linear cutting stapler. A window was made in the transverse mesocolon just anterolateral to the ligament of Treitz. The mesentery was divided sufficiently so that the distal jejunal loop could pass retrocolic through this window and reach the proximal gastric pouch without tension.

The proximal jejunal stump was then brought down distally to approximately *45 cm/150 cm (if superobese)* along the Roux limb, and a side-to-side stapled jejunojejunostomy was created in the usual fashion.

A 1-cm side-to-side anastomosis was then created between the proximal gastric pouch and the Roux limb with an outer layer of interrupted 3-0 silk and an inner layer of continuous 3-0 PDS sutures. The anastomoses were all checked and found to be patent and not to leak air when tested under saline.

The nasogastric tube was then replaced and the tip was manually guided through the gastrojejunostomy just beyond the suture line. All mesenteric defects were then closed with continuous 3-0 Vicryl sutures and the Roux limb of jejunum was sutured to the transverse mesocolon to prevent a Petersen hernia.

If cholecystectomy performed: *Attention was then turned to the gallbladder, which had been found to be abnormal/to contain stones during initial exploration. It was removed in the usual fashion, taking care not to injure the common duct or other adjacent structures. The cystic duct and cystic artery were ligated with ____. The region was checked for hemostasis.*

Hemostasis was checked. The abdomen was closed using running #1 looped PDS sutures and skin edges were approximated with *staples/a running subcuticular suture of ___.*

The patient tolerated the procedure well and was taken to the postanesthesia care unit in stable condition.

NOTES

Chapter 28

Laparoscopic Antecolic Roux-en-Y Gastric Bypass for Obesity

Mohammad K. Jamal, M.D.

INDICATIONS

- Morbid obesity refractory to dietary changes and medical treatment.
- Current NIH guidelines suggest these qualifications for surgical weight loss procedures:
  - BMI ^{3} 35 kg/m^2 with obesity-related co-morbidities, or
  - BMI ^{3} 40 kg/m^2 without any medical conditions.

ESSENTIAL STEPS

1. Supine position, with appropriate tubes (Foley catheter and OG tube) placed and prophylactic antibiotics and subcutaneous heparin given preoperatively.
2. Carefully pad all pressure points and place a padded foot board on the operating table.
3. Create a 15 mmHg pneumoperitoneum using Veress needle (upper abdominal quadrant insertion preferred).
4. Place trocars in the following locations: 12 mm port in left paraumbilical location for the 10 mm laparoscope, 12 mm port in the right midclavicular line, a 5 mm port in the lateral subcostal location, and two 5 mm ports in the left midclavicular and left subcostal position. The ports should resemble a "smiley face configuration."
5. Perform a diagnostic laparoscopy to verify that no iatrogenic injury has occurred during Veress or port entry.
6. Retract greater omentum and transverse colon superiorly to expose the ligament of Treitz.

J.J. Hoballah and C.E.H. Scott-Conner (eds.), *Operative Dictations in General and Vascular Surgery*, DOI 10.1007/978-1-4614-0451-4_28,

7. Divide the jejunum with a linear cutting endoscopic stapler (2.5 mm, 60 mm) approximately 30 cm from the ligament of Treitz.

8. Divide the jejunal mesentery with two applications of a linear cutting endoscopic stapler (2.0 mm/45 mm) loaded with staple line re-inforcement.

9. Mark the distal cut end of small bowel with a silk stitch.

10. Measure the Roux limb 75 cm distally and align the two limbs in a side-to-side fashion.

11. Make enterotomies in both limbs with the ultrasonic shears.

12. Insert the linear cutting endoscopic stapler (2.5/45 mm), approximate, and fire it to create the entero-enterostomy.

13. Check hemostasis at the staple line.

14. Align and staple the common enterotomy site closed with another firing of the linear cutting stapler (2.5/60 mm).

15. Close the jejunal mesenteric defect with a running nonabsorbable stitch.

16. Divide the omentum underneath the falciform ligament to allow the antecolic Roux limb to reach the supracolic compartment.

17. Suture the proximal end of the Roux limb to the greater curvature of the stomach.

18. Place the patient in steep reverse Trendelenburg position and ask the Anesthesiologist to remove all tubes from the esophagus and stomach.

19. Elevate the left lateral segment of the liver with a 5-mm Nathanson liver retractor placed in the subxiphoid location to expose the hiatus.

20. Retract the stomach and omentum inferiorly.

21. Excise the gastroesophageal fat pad with ultrasonic shears and define the angle of His.

22. Create a window into the lesser sac at a point adjacent to the gastric wall high on the lesser curvature of the stomach.

23. Insert an endoscopic linear stapler (2.5/60 mm) to divide the lesser curvature vessels below the left gastric artery.

24. Apply and fire the stapler three to four times to staple and create the gastric pouch using linear cutting stapler (3.5/60 mm).

25. Align the Roux limb and the gastric pouch side by side.

26. Suture the back wall of the anastomosis with a running nonabsorbable suture from an appropriately marked site on the staple line to the lesser curvature in a tension-free fashion.

27. Make enterotomies in the proximal gastric pouch and the Roux limb with the ultrasonic shears.
28. Use the endoscopic cutting linear stapler (3.5/45 mm) to make a measured 2.5-cm anastomosis.
29. Check hemostasis.
30. Pass an Ewald tube orally into the gastric pouch under direct visualization.
31. Close the common enterotomy in two layers.
32. Clamp the distal Roux limb with a bowel clamp.
33. With the Ewald tube in the gastric pouch, test the anastomosis with air insufflation under saline.
34. Remove the Ewald tube.
35. Place a closed suction drain just posterior to the gastrojejunostomy anastomosis.
36. Desufflate the abdomen.
37. Close all large port sites and skin.

NOTE THIS VARIATION
- Size and exact locations of trocars varies with size of instruments used and individual patient physique.

COMPLICATIONS
- Anastomotic leak.
- Injury to the esophagus or spleen.
- Torsion of the Roux limb.
- Pulmonary embolism.

TEMPLATE OPERATIVE DICTATION
Preoperative diagnosis: Morbid obesity with co-morbidities.
Operation performed: Laparoscopic Roux-en-Y gastric bypass, antecolic, 75 cm roux loop, 30 cm bilio-pancreatic limb.
Postoperative diagnosis: Same.
Indications: This patient was diagnosed with morbid obesity with a BMI of ___ and significant co-morbidities including ___. The patient was counseled extensively in the Bariatric Outpatient Clinic and after a thorough explanation of the risks and benefits of surgery (including death from complications, bowel leak, infection such as peritonitis and/or sepsis, internal hernia, bleeding, need for blood transfusion, bowel obstruction, organ failure, pulmonary embolus, deep venous thrombosis, wound infection, incisional hernia, skin breakdown, marginal ulceration, stomal stenosis, and others entailed on the consent form) and after a

compliant diet and exercise program, the patient was scheduled for an elective laparoscopic Roux-en-Y gastric bypass.

Description of operation: Following informed consent, the patient was taken to the operating room and placed on the operating table in the supine position. The patient had previously received prophylactic antibiotics and subcutaneous heparin for DVT prophylaxis in the pre-op holding area. After induction of general endotracheal anesthesia by the anesthesiologist, the patient underwent placement of sequential compression devices, Foley catheter and orogastric tube. The patient was adequately padded at all pressure points and placed on a footboard to prevent slippage from the OR table during extremes of position during surgery. The left arm was extended on an armboard and the right arm was tucked in. The surgical field was prepped and draped in the usual sterile fashion. A time-out was completed verifying correct patient, procedure, site, positioning, and implant(s) and/or special equipment prior to beginning this procedure.

Using a Veress needle in the left upper quadrant, a carbon dioxide pneumoperitoneum up to a pressure of 15 mmHg was obtained after retracting the anterior abdominal wall upwards. A 12 mm laparoscopic port was placed in the right upper quadrant and then using a 45°, 10-mm scope, other ports were placed under direct visualization as follows – two 5 mm left upper quadrant, a 5 mm right upper quadrant, and another 12 mm umbilical port for the surgeon and assistant.

The organs were inspected for injury during entry and none was seen. The transverse colon and greater omentum were reflected toward the supracolic compartment and the ligament of Treitz was identified. The jejunum was measured 30 cm from the ligament of Treitz and transected at this point using a linear cutting stapler (2.5/45 mm) whereas the small bowel mesentery was divided to the root using two firings of the linear cutting stapler (2.5/45 mm) loaded with staple line re-inforcement. The distal cut end of the bowel was identified with a suture. From this point, 75 cm of small bowel were measured and the proximal cut end of jejunum was anastomozed at the 75 cm site using a side-to-side stapled anastomosis using a linear cutting stapler (2.5/45 mm) and the common enterotomy was closed with another firing of the linear cutting stapler (2.5/60 mm). An anti-obstruction Brolins silk stitch was applied and the mesenteric defect was closed with a continuous running nonabsorbable suture. A crotch silk stitch was also applied to stabilize the anastomosis. Hemostasis was found to be satisfactory and there was no evidence of leakage at the completed jejunojejunostomy site. The Roux limb was then placed underneath the transverse mesocolon for identification and later anastomosis to the gastric pouch.

The greater omentum was then divided into two halves along the midline starting at the antimesenteric border of the transverse colon and extending up to the free edge of the greater curvature of the stomach. Between the two halves of the greater omentum, the distal cut end of jejunum was brought up in an antecolic fashion into the supracolic compartment and temporarily sutured to the greater curvature of the stomach to prevent slippage into the pelvis. Care was taken to prevent twisting of the mesentery while bringing the Roux limb toward the supracolic compartment.

Attention was then turned to the gastric portion of the operation. The patient was placed into steep reverse Trendelenburg position and the anesthesiologist was asked to empty the stomach and then remove ALL tubes (including the orogastric tube and the esophageal temperature probe) from the patient's GI tract. A liver retractor was applied to retract the left lobe of the liver anteriorly and expose the Angle of His. The lesser omentum was transected near the lesser curve using a linear cutting stapler (2.5/60 mm) loaded with staple line re-inforcement and then the stomach was transected using several firings of the linear cutting stapler (3.5/60 mm) to create a small proximal gastric pouch.

Hemostasis was found to be excellent and then a side-to-side gastrojejunostomy was performed in four layers using the posterior wall of the stomach. The first layer was a continuous hand sewn layer using nonabsorbable suture, the next two layers were a stapled gastrojejunostomy using a linear cutting stapler (3.5/45 mm), and the gastrotomy and enterotomy were closed with a hand sewn continuous suture, and the final fourth layer was the anterior hand sewn continuous suture, both using nonabsorbable suture. The anastomosis was checked for leaks under water after turning the patient back into the supine position, clamping the distal jejunum with a bowel clamp and insufflating air through an Ewald tube that was placed into the Roux limb via the gastric pouch through the transesophageal route. No leaks were identified at the gastrojejunostomy anastomosis. The Ewald tube and the bowel clamp were removed and a 10 mm closed suction drain was placed posterior to the gastrojejunostomy and brought out through the right lateral-most port site and anchored onto the skin using a 3-0 Nylon suture. All ports were removed under direct visualization ensuring hemostasis.

The 12 mm ports, one on either side of the midline, did not require closure, as only blunt ports were used throughout the procedure. The skin was approximated using 4-0 absorbable subcuticular sutures followed by application of Steri-strips. *This was followed by injection of a total of 50 cc of local anesthetic (including 25 cc of 1% Lidocaine containing 1:100,000 epinephrine mixed with 25 cc of 0.25% Marcaine containing 1:100,000 epinephrine) at the port sites.*

The patient was then extubated and transferred to the recovery room in a stable condition. The sponge and instrument counts were correct at the end of the operation.

ACKNOWLEDGMENT

This chapter was contributed by Yi-Horng Lee, MD in the first edition.

NOTES

Chapter 29
Laparoscopic Sleeve Gastrectomy

Mohamad H. Alaeddine, M.D. and Bassem Y. Safadi, M.D.

INDICATIONS

- Morbid Obesity with body mass index greater than 40 kg/m^2.
- Morbid obesity with BMI greater than 35 kg/m^2 with serious co-morbidities.
- Super obesity (BMI > 50 kg/m^2) as a first stage of the duodenal switch.
- Patients should have been evaluated in a multidisciplinary bariatric surgical program and deemed appropriate for such surgical intervention.

ESSENTIAL STEPS

1. Place the patient in the supine position; split leg position is optional.
2. Reverse Trendelenburg positioning helps expose the esophago-gastric (EG) junction.
3. Initial port placement in obese patients is facilitated by the use of an optical port. Place this first port high, about 18 cm below the Xiphoid process for adequate visualization.
4. Place four to six ports in the upper abdomen.
5. Retract the left lateral segment of the liver.
6. Identify the pylorus.
7. Identify the anterior vagal branches along the lesser curvature and Crow's feet.
8. Start sealing and dividing all the vessels along the greater curvature of the stomach from a point around 6 cm proximal to the Pylorus and all the way to the angle of His.

J.J. Hoballah and C.E.H. Scott-Conner (eds.), *Operative Dictations in General and Vascular Surgery*, DOI 10.1007/978-1-4614-0451-4_29,
© Springer Science+Business Media, LLC 2012

9. Lift the stomach and divide all posterior attachments to the pancreas.
10. Expose the EG junction well to ensure there are no missed hiatal hernias. Excising the EG junction fat pad aids in the exposure.
11. Ask the anesthesiologist to place an orogastric tube or bougie (34–42 Fr) into the esophagus and lying along the lesser curve to the antrum.
12. Alongside the tube, staple and divide the stomach in a vertical fashion aiming to the Angle of His. Approximately 60–120 ml of gastric volume should remain.
13. Align these staple lines parallel. Avoid crossed staple lines.
14. Extract the stomach in a bag.
15. Test the "sleeved" stomach by filling it with Methylene blue or by intraoperative endoscopy.
16. Close the fascia at the gastric extraction with nonabsorbable sutures.

NOTE THESE VARIATIONS

- Hiatal hernias can be repaired simultaneous with the sleeve gastrectomy.
- An alternate approach is to perform the stapling and division of the stomach first followed by gastric resection.

COMPLICATIONS

- Bleeding.
- Staple line leak with resultant abscess or fistula.
- Pulmonary embolism.
- Gastroesophageal reflux.

OPERATIVE DICTATION

Preoperative diagnosis: Morbid obesity.
Procedure: Laparoscopic sleeve gastrectomy.
Postoperative diagnosis: Same.
Indications: This _____ -year-old *female/male* had morbid obesity with *BMI above 40 kg/m²/BMI above 35 kg/m² with significant co-morbidities* and failure of medical weight loss.
Description of procedure: The patient was placed in the supine position and general endotracheal anesthesia was induced. Preoperative antibiotics were given. The patient received 5,000 units of Heparin subcutaneously prior to induction. The abdomen was prepped and draped in the usual sterile fashion. A time-out

was completed verifying correct patient, procedure, site, positioning, and implant(s) and/or special equipment prior to beginning this procedure. A 12 mm incision was made 18 cm below the Xyphoid process and a 12-mm "optical" port was placed under direct vision without any complication. Then under direct vision two 12-mm trocar were inserted in the left upper quadrant along the midclavicular and anterior axillary lines. A 15-mm port was placed in the right upper quadrant at the midclavicular line just above the umbilical level.

The operating table was placed in reverse Trendelenburg position and the left lobe of the liver was retracted cephalad using a fixed retractor "Nathanson" through a 5 mm subxiphoid incision to expose the esophageal hiatus.

Using an energy device (Ligasure®, Harmonic scalpel®, or Ultrasonic Shears®) the lipoma of the gastroesophageal junction was excised and the peritoneum overlying the cardia was incised and the plane between the cardia and left crus of the diaphragm was bluntly opened to expose the left diaphragmatic crus. Then the pylorus was identified and a point 6 cm proximal to the pylorus along the greater curvature of the stomach was marked with cautery. This corresponded to the Incisura Angularis just proximal to Crow's foot of Latarjet's nerve. Then all the vessels along the greater curvature and all the short gastric vessels were sealed and divided completely freeing up the greater curvature and the fundus of the stomach. The stomach was lifted up and all posterior attachments to the pancreas were divided sharply. Then a 36-Fr. Orogastric tube was placed by the anesthesiologist and oriented toward the antrum snug along the lesser curvature. Alongside the tube the stomach was stapled and divided sequentially in a vertical fashion heading toward the Angle of His. We used a total of six cartridges 60 mm in length with 4.8 mm staple height with staple line re-enforcement. There was no bleeding from the staple line. Intraoperative endoscopy revealed no areas of stenosis and no leak along the staple line. The stomach was placed in a plastic bag and was extracted from the left upper quadrant port which was widened a bit. The port site was closed with three interrupted sutures that were passed through the abdominal wall using the suture passer. Then the other ports and liver retractor were removed under vision. The abdomen was deflated. The wounds were closed with 4-0 monocryl continuous subcuticular sutures. Patient tolerated the procedure well and left the operating room in good condition.

NOTES

Chapter 30
Simple Excision of Duodenal Diverticulum

Roy R. Danks, D.O.

INDICATION

■ Complications of the duodenal diverticulum, which is not in close proximity to the head of the pancreas or ampulla of Vater, including bleeding, obstruction of the common bile duct, perforation, and diverticulitis.

ESSENTIAL STEPS

1. Upper midline incision.
2. Wide Kocher maneuver.
3. Confirm that the diverticulum is distant from the ampulla of Vater and pancreas.
4. Place a *bowel clamp/linear stapler* across base.
5. Reconfirm that the ampulla of Vater is not in the vicinity.
6. *Fire the stapler and* remove the diverticulum.
7. *If sutured: Close the duodenum in two layers.*
8. *Perform any needed biliary tract surgery.*
9. Check hemostasis.
10. Place omentum over the staple line.
11. Close the abdomen.

NOTE THESE VARIATIONS

■ Convert to transduodenal excision if the diverticulum is in proximity to the ampulla of Vater, embedded in the pancreas, or if anatomy is in doubt.

J.J. Hoballah and C.E.H. Scott-Conner (eds.), *Operative Dictations in General and Vascular Surgery*, DOI 10.1007/978-1-4614-0451-4_30,
© Springer Science+Business Media, LLC 2012

- *Stapled/sutured* closure.
- Gallstones and/or common duct stones may coexist, requiring cholecystectomy and/or common bile duct exploration.

COMPLICATIONS

- Injury to the common duct, pancreas, or ampulla of Vater.
- Pancreatitis.
- Leak from duodenal staple line.

TEMPLATE OPERATIVE DICTATION

Preoperative diagnosis: Duodenal diverticulum with *bleeding/ obstruction/perforation/inflammation.*

Procedure: Simple excision of the duodenal diverticulum *(list any additional biliary tract procedures).*

Postoperative diagnosis: Same.

Indications: This ____-year-old *male/female* developed *gastrointestinal bleeding/obstruction/perforation/inflammation* and on workup was found to have a duodenal diverticulum. Excision was required for management.

Description of procedure: An epidural catheter was placed by anesthesia prior to the start of the operation. The patient was placed in the supine position and general endotracheal anesthesia was induced. Preoperative antibiotics were given. A Foley catheter and nasogastric tube were placed. The abdomen was prepped and draped in the usual sterile fashion. A time-out was completed verifying correct patient, procedure, site, positioning, and implant(s) and/or special equipment prior to beginning this procedure. A vertical midline incision was made from xiphoid to just below the umbilicus. This was deepened through the subcutaneous tissues and hemostasis was achieved with electrocautery. The linea alba was identified and incised and the peritoneal cavity entered. The abdomen was explored. *Adhesions were lysed sharply under direct vision with Metzenbaum scissors/divided with harmonic shears/divided with Ligasure device.*

A self-retaining retractor was then placed and the abdominal wall was retracted laterally, inferiorly, and superiorly. The small bowel and colon were then packed inferiorly with wet laparotomy pads and held in place with retractors. This afforded adequate exposure of the stomach and duodenum. The pancreas was then gently examined by palpation. The gallbladder was palpated and *gallstones/no gallstones* were noted. A duodenal diverticulum located approximately ____ cm from the palpated ampulla of Vater was noted. *There was no pancreatic involvement, nor there were signs of perforation/there was surrounding inflammation.*

A wide Kocher maneuver was undertaken by sweeping the second limb of the duodenum from medial to lateral, sharply dividing the peritoneal reflection. Blunt and sharp dissection was used to free the duodenum until it was fully mobilized.

The diverticulum was identified and completely isolated. Small branches of the pancreaticoduodenal artery were clamped, cut, and ligated with 4-0 silk ties/divided with harmonic shears/divided with Ligasure device to allow complete exposure of the diverticulum. The diverticulum was completely isolated. A *small bowel clamp/linear stapler* was applied across the base of the diverticulum. The position of the *clamp/stapler* relative to the ampulla was confirmed by palpation before the *diverticulum was sharply removed/stapler was fired and the diverticulum removed* and passed off the operative field.

If sutured: *The resulting defect was then closed in two layers – an inner layer of running 3-0 Vicryl placed as a Connell suture and an outer layer of interrupted 3-0 silk Lembert sutures.* At the conclusion, the duodenum was intact with a patent lumen and the common bile duct, ampulla, and pancreas appeared normal to inspection and palpation.

Detail any additional biliary tract surgery performed.

The abdomen was thoroughly irrigated with warm, sterile saline solution, suctioned until clear, and the self-retaining retractor and all sponges removed. Hemostasis was checked and omentum was brought up and made to lie over the operative field.

(Optional: Multiple interrupted through-and-through retention sutures of ____ *were placed.)* The fascia was closed with *a running suture of* ____/*a Smead-Jones closure of interrupted* ____.

Subcutaneous tissues were lavaged with ____ *ml of sterile saline solution.*

The skin was closed with *skin staples/subcuticular sutures of* ____/*other.*

The patient tolerated the procedure well and was taken to the postanesthesia care unit in stable condition.

NOTES

Chapter 31
Transduodenal Excision of Duodenal Diverticulum

Roy R. Danks, D.O.

INDICATION

- Complications of the duodenal diverticula in close proximity to the ampulla or embedded in the head of the pancreas, including the following: bleeding, obstruction of the common bile duct or duodenum, perforation, and diverticulitis.

ESSENTIAL STEPS

1. Upper midline incision.
2. Extensive Kocher maneuver.
3. Longitudinal duodenotomy opposite the site of the diverticulum.
4. Identify and protect the ampulla of Vater.
5. *Cannulate the ampulla and perform a cholangiogram if necessary.*
6. Evaginate the diverticulum.
7. Place a clamp across the base and excise.
8. Close mucosa with a full-thickness running suture of 3-0 Vicryl.
9. Reassess the ampulla of Vater.
10. Close the duodenotomy transversely (if possible) in two layers.
11. *Perform any needed biliary tract surgery.*
12. Check hemostasis.
13. Place omentum over the duodenotomy and into the operative field.
14. Close the abdomen.

J.J. Hoballah and C.E.H. Scott-Conner (eds.), *Operative Dictations in General and Vascular Surgery*, DOI 10.1007/978-1-4614-0451-4_31,
© Springer Science+Business Media, LLC 2012

NOTE THESE VARIATIONS

- Cannulation of the ampulla and cholangiography may be needed in difficult cases.
- Gallstones and/or common bile duct stones may coexist, requiring cholecystectomy and/or common bile duct exploration.

COMPLICATIONS

- Injury to the common bile duct, pancreas, or ampulla of Vater.
- Pancreatitis.
- Leak from the duodenal suture line.

TEMPLATE OPERATIVE DICTATION

Preoperative diagnosis: Duodenal diverticulum with *bleeding/ obstruction/perforation/inflammation.*

Procedure: Transduodenal excision of the duodenal diverticulum *with operative cholangiogram (list any additional biliary tract procedures).*

Postoperative diagnosis: Same.

Indications: This ____-year-old *male/female* developed *gastrointestinal bleeding/obstruction/perforation/inflammation* and on workup was found to have a duodenal diverticulum. Excision was required for management.

Description of procedure: An epidural catheter was placed by anesthesia prior to the start of the operation. The patient was placed in the supine position and general endotracheal anesthesia was induced. Preoperative antibiotics were given. A Foley catheter and nasogastric tube were placed. The abdomen was prepped and draped in the usual sterile fashion. A time-out was completed verifying correct patient, procedure, site, positioning, and implant(s) and/or special equipment prior to beginning this procedure. A vertical midline incision was made from xiphoid to just below the umbilicus. This was deepened through the subcutaneous tissues and hemostasis was achieved with electrocautery. The linea alba was identified and incised and the peritoneal cavity entered. The abdomen was explored. *Adhesions were lysed sharply under direct vision with Metzenbaum scissors/with harmonic shears/with Ligasure device.*

A self-retaining retractor was then placed and die abdominal wall was retracted laterally, inferiorly, and superiorly. The small bowel and colon were then packed inferiorly with wet laparotomy pads and held in place with retractors. This afforded adequate exposure of the stomach and duodenum. The pancreas was then gently examined by palpation. The gallbladder was palpated and *gallstones/no gallstones* were noted. A periampullary diverticulum was identified. *There was no pancreatic involvement, nor there were signs of perforation/there was surrounding inflammation.*

A wide Kocher maneuver was undertaken by sweeping the second limb of the duodenum from medial to lateral, sharply dividing the peritoneal reflection. Blunt and sharp dissection was used to free the duodenum until it was fully mobilized.

The diverticulum was identified and completely isolated. It lay in close relation to the head of the pancreas, *but did not directly involve the pancreas/and appeared embedded in the pancreas.* A longitudinal anterior duodenotomy was created with electrocautery at a point opposite the diverticulum. The orifice of the diverticulum was identified. A curved hemostat was placed into the diverticulum and the sac grasped and invaginated into the duodenum. The ampulla of Vater was identified and *was distant from/in close proximity to* the invaginated specimen.

If cannulation of ampulla and/or cholangiogram: *Because of the intimate involvement of the ampulla and diverticulum, the orifice of the ampulla was identified and gently cannulated with a ____ tube. Cholangiograms were obtained/a stent was left in the ampulla to protect it during the subsequent dissection.*

A small bowel clamp was then applied across the base of the diverticulum and the diverticulum was cut away sharply with a #15 scalpel blade. The specimen was removed from the operative field. The mucosa was then reapproximated with a running full-thickness suture of 3-0 Vicryl. At the conclusion of this portion of the procedure, the *ampulla was again visually inspected/cholangiogram was repeated* and the common bile duct noted to be intact.

The duodenotomy was then closed *transversely/longitudinally* with an inner running layer of 3-0 Vicryl placed as a Connell suture. This was followed by an outer seromuscular layer of interrupted 3-0 silk Lembert sutures. At the conclusion of the procedure the duodenum was noted to be intact, with a widely patent lumen. The ampulla, common bile duct, and pancreas appeared uninjured.

Detail any additional biliary tract surgery performed.

The abdomen was thoroughly irrigated with warm, sterile saline solution, suctioned until clear, and the self-retaining retractor and all sponges removed. Hemostasis was checked.

(Optional: Multiple interrupted through-and-through retention sutures of ____ were placed.) The fascia was closed with *a running suture of ____/a Smead-Jones closure of interrupted ____.*

The subcutaneous layer was lavaged with ____ ml of warm, sterile saline solution.

The skin was closed with *skin staples/subcuticular sutures of ____/other.*

The patient tolerated the procedure well and was taken to the postanesthesia care unit in stable condition.

NOTES

Section III

Small Intestine and Appendix

Chapter 32

Small Bowel Resection

Ross Bengtson, M.D.

INDICATIONS

- Ischemia.
- Tumor.
- Trauma.
- Stricture.
- Obstruction.

ESSENTIAL STEPS

1. Perform Timeout.
2. Midline incision.
3. Explore the abdomen.
4. Mobilize the bowel to be resected (lyse adhesions if necessary).
5. Create a window in the mesentery at the resection edges in the avascular area.
6. Divide the mesentery.
7. Clamp/staple and divide the bowel.
8. Remove the specimen *(mark proximal/distal ends)*.
9. *Stapled anastomosis:*
   - *Create enterotomy at stapled ends for anastomosis.*
   - *Approximate enterotomies.*
   - *Fire linear cutting stapler.*
   - *Inspect lumen for bleeding.*
   - *Close enterotomies (staple/suture).*
   - *(Or sutured anastomosis.)*

J.J. Hoballah and C.E.H. Scott-Conner (eds.), *Operative Dictations in General and Vascular Surgery*, DOI 10.1007/978-1-4614-0451-4_32,
© Springer Science+Business Media, LLC 2012

10. Check the anastomosis for patency and integrity.
11. Close the mesenteric defect.
12. Check hemostasis.
13. Make sure sponge needle and instrument count is correct.
14. Close the abdomen.

NOTE THESE VARIATIONS
- Extent of resection, length of the remaining bowel (if extensive).
- Stapled vs. sutured anastomosis.

COMPLICATIONS
- Anastomotic leak.
- Intra-abdominal abscess.
- Enterocutaneous fistula.
- Obstruction.
- Malabsorption/short gut syndrome.
- Hernia.

TEMPLATE OPERATIVE DICTATION
Preoperative diagnosis: *Intestinal ischemia/tumor/trauma/other.*
Procedure: Exploratory laparotomy with small bowel resection.
Postoperative diagnosis: Same.
Indications: The patient is a ____-year-old *man/woman* with signs and symptoms of *(list)* and a preoperative diagnosis of *(detail)*. Small bowel resection indicated for management of *ischemia/tumor/trauma/other.*
Description of procedure: *An epidural catheter was placed by anesthesia prior to the start of the operation.* The patient was placed in the supine position and general endotracheal anesthesia was induced. A timeout was completed verifying correct patient, procedure, site, positioning, and implant(s) and/or special equipment prior to beginning this procedure. Preoperative antibiotics were given. A Foley catheter and nasogastric tube were placed. The abdomen was prepped and draped in the usual sterile fashion. After a timeout was performed, a vertical midline incision was made from xiphoid to just below the umbilicus. This was deepened through the subcutaneous tissues and hemostasis was achieved with electrocautery. The linea alba was identified and incised and the peritoneal cavity entered. The abdomen was explored *(list any abnormal findings). Adhesions were lysed sharply under direct vision with Metzenbaum scissors.*

[Choose one:]

If ischemia: The segment of nonviable small bowel was ____ cm long and *began ____ cm from the ligament of Treitz/ended ____ cm from the ileocecal valve.* The margins were determined to be viable by arterial Doppler.

If tumor or trauma: The *region of the tumor/perforation or stricture* was identified and the extent of resection determined so as to *achieve an adequate margin and allow resection of a fan-shaped portion of mesentery with accompanying lymph nodes/allow anastomosis to be performed in a region of normal bowel.*

A window was created by using a curved hemostat to separate the mesentery from the bowel at each resection margin. The mesentery was scored and serially divided with hemostats, and the vessels were then ligated with 3-0 silk ties.

If stapled anastomosis: The bowel was divided with a cutting linear stapler at each resection margin and passed off the table as a specimen *(label proximal and distal margins for ischemia or tumor).* The antimesenteric angles of the proximal and distal segments were then approximated with two sutures of 3-0 silk placed approximately 5 cm apart. Enterotomies were made at the antimesenteric borders and the cutting linear stapler inserted and fired. The lumen was inspected for hemostasis. The enterotomies were closed with *a single firing of a linear stapler/in two layers with 3-0 Vicryl and 3-0 silk.*

If sutured anastomosis: A pair of noncrushing bowel clamps were placed on the bowel at each resection margin. The small bowel was then transected between clamps with a #10 scalpel and passed off the table as a specimen *(label proximal and distal ends for tumor or ischemia).* The small bowel was then brought together approximating the ends. A two-layer anastomosis was created with an inner layer of running 3-0 Vicryl and an outer layer of interrupted 3-0 silk Lembert sutures completely imbricating the inner layer.

The anastomosis was then inspected for patency and integrity. The mesenteric defect was closed with a running 3-0 Vicryl suture. The abdomen was irrigated with 2 L of saline. *The remaining small bowel appeared viable.* The resection site was ____ cm from the *ileocecal valve/ligament of Treitz,* and the patient had ____ cm of small bowel remaining.

After the sponge needle and instrument count was correct, (optional: *multiple interrupted through-and-through retention sutures of* ____ *were placed.)* The fascia was closed with *a running suture of* ____/*a Smead-Jones closure of interrupted* ____. The skin was closed with *skin staples/subcuticular sutures of* ____/*other.*

The patient tolerated the procedure well and was taken to the postanesthesia care unit in stable condition.

NOTES

Chapter 33
Laparoscopic Small Bowel Resection

Walid Faraj, M.D., F.R.C.S. and Ahmad Zaghal, M.D.

INDICATIONS

- Small intestinal neoplasm.
- Resection of nonviable bowel in the context of intestinal obstruction.
- Ischemic small bowel.
- Stricture.

ESSENTIAL STEPS

1. Foley catheter, nasogastric tube insertion.
2. Induce pneumoperitoneum (Veress needle or Hassan cannula).
3. Place trocars – supraumbilical 10 mm for laparoscope; then one in each midclavicular line, left and right, approximately 6–7 cm from umbilicus (also 10 mm), taking due consideration of location of old scars to avoid adhesions.
4. Explore the abdomen.
5. Lyse any adhesions.
6. Identify segment to resect.
7. Create a window in the mesentery at the resection margins.
8. Divide the mesentery.
9. Deliver the resected segment.
10. Restore bowel continuity.
11. Close the mesenteric defect.
12. Check hemostasis.
13. Close wounds.

J.J. Hoballah and C.E.H. Scott-Conner (eds.), *Operative Dictations in General and Vascular Surgery*, DOI 10.1007/978-1-4614-0451-4_33,
© Springer Science+Business Media, LLC 2012

NOTE THESE VARIATIONS

- Extent of resection.
- Stapled or sutured anastomosis.
- Placement of incision to deliver bowel.
- Use of second-look operation for intestinal ischemia.
  - Anastomosis may be delayed until second operation in this case.
- Length of the remaining bowel.

COMPLICATIONS

- Anastomotic leak.
- Intra-abdominal abscess.
- Wound infection.
- Enterocutaneous fistula.
- Intestinal obstruction.
- Short bowel syndrome.
- Bleeding.
- Internal hernia.
- Incisional hernia at trocar site.

TEMPLATE OPERATIVE DICTATION

Preoperative diagnosis: *Intestinal tumor/ischemia/other.*

Procedure: Exploratory laparoscopy, with *lysis of adhesions and* laparoscopic small bowel resection.

Postoperative diagnosis: Same.

Indications: This ___-year-old *male/female* presented with signs and symptoms of ___, work up confirmed the diagnosis of___, and the decision was to proceed with laparoscopic segmental small bowel resection.

Description of procedure: The patient was placed supine on the operating table, anesthesia placed appropriate lines and induced and intubated the patient without complications, preoperative antibiotics were given. Foley catheter and nasogastric tube were inserted and the patient's anterior abdomen was prepped and draped in the usual sterile fashion. A timeout was completed verifying correct patient, procedure, site, positioning, and implant(s) and/or special equipment prior to beginning this procedure.

A *supraumbilical 10 mm trocar was inserted under direct vision, using Hasson technique/a Veress needle was used to insufflate the abdomen and a 10 mm trocar was placed in the supraumbilical location.* Abdominal exploration revealed *no incidental findings/ the following incidental findings (detail).* This was followed by insertion of two trocars, one on the left and the other on the right side; at the midclavicular line 6–7 cm from the umbilicus, 10 mm each, respectively.

Adhesions were lysed sharply under direct vision.

[Choose one:]

If ischemia: the segment of nonviable small bowel was ___ cm long, ___ from the ligament of Treitz. An arterial Doppler probe was used to determine arterial mesenteric pulsation to aid the laparoscopic inspection.

The bowel was found to be gangrenous, and the decision was to proceed with laparoscopic small bowel resection with anastomosis/second-look operation with delayed reconstruction, after extensive normal saline irrigation of the abdomen.

If tumor/stricture: the region of the tumor/stricture was identified, and the resection planned to get enough surgical margins, and include the nodal basin via a wide resection margin in the mesentery.

A window was created at the junction points between the mesentery and the borders of bowel resection, a V-shaped portion of the mesentery suspending the bowel segment was scored using electrocautery, then ligaSure was used to divide the mesentery, then the resection borders of the selected bowel segment were cut using a cutting linear stapler.

A separate incision was made in the left lower quadrant and the specimen was placed in a laparoscopic specimen bag and delivered through this incision.

Then attention was drawn toward restoring the continuity of the bowel.

The antimesenteric angles of the proximal and distal margins were then approximated using stay silk sutures, enterotomies were made using electrocautery at the antimesenteric borders and the cutting linear endo-GIA inserted and fired. Lumen was then inspected for bleeding points.

The enterotomies were then closed with *endo-GIA/using two layers of 3-0 Vicryl or PDS sutures.*

The mesenteric defect was then closed using running suture of 3-0 PDS.

Abdomen was irrigated extensively with normal saline.

The remaining of the bowel looked viable.

Hemostasis secured.

Trocar sites were then closed in layers, with O/PDS for the fascia, and 4/0 monocryl continuous subcuticular sutures for the skin.

The left lower abdominal incision was also closed in layers, 0/PDS interrupted sutures for the fascia, and 3-0 nylon interrupted sutures for the skin.

The patient tolerated the procedure well and was transferred to the postanesthesia care unit in stable condition.

NOTES

Chapter 34
Enterolysis for Intestinal Obstruction

Carol E.H. Scott-Conner, M.D.

INDICATIONS
- Small bowel obstruction.
- Adjunct to other surgical procedures (previously operated abdomen).

ESSENTIAL STEPS
1. Midline incision.
2. Enter the abdomen above or below the old scar if possible.
3. Apply traction to adherent loops and divide the adhesions sharply under direct vision.
4. Identify point(s) of obstruction.
5. Ascertain viability of the bowel.
6. Run the small bowel.
7. Confirm absence of additional areas of obstruction, injuries, or compromised bowel.
8. Repair deserosalized areas or inadvertent enterotomies.
9. Check hemostasis.
10. Close the abdomen.

NOTE THIS VARIATION
- Repair of enterotomies.

J.J. Hoballah and C.E.H. Scott-Conner (eds.), *Operative Dictations in General and Vascular Surgery*, DOI 10.1007/978-1-4614-0451-4_34,
© Springer Science+Business Media, LLC 2012

COMPLICATIONS

- Recurrent obstruction.
- Enterocutaneous fistula.

TEMPLATE OPERATIVE DICTATION

Preoperative diagnosis: Small bowel obstruction.
Procedure: Exploratory laparotomy and enterolysis.
Postoperative diagnosis: Same.
Indications: The patient is a _____-year-old *male/female* with his-tory of *appendectomy/hysterectomy/other abdominal procedure,* who presented _____ *days ago with picture consistent with partial small bowel obstruction that progressed to complete bowel obstruction unresponsive to conservative measures/complete bowel obstruction/ bowel obstruction with tenderness and clinical deterioration/other.*
Description of procedure: *An epidural catheter was placed by anesthesia prior to the start of the operation.* The patient was placed in the supine position and general endotracheal anesthesia was induced. Preoperative antibiotics were given. The abdomen was prepped and draped in the usual sterile fashion. A timeout was completed verifying correct patient, procedure, site, position-ing, and implant(s) and/or special equipment prior to beginning this procedure.

A vertical midline incision was made from *above the previous laparotomy incision down to its most inferior extent/xiphoid to just below the umbilicus/other.* This was deepened through the subcu-taneous tissues and hemostasis was achieved with electrocautery. The linea alba was identified and incised *in a region above the old incision/in the upper abdomen/other* and the peritoneal cavity entered with care.

Upon entering the abdominal cavity, there are extensive adhe-sions of omentum and bowel *to the underside of the old incision/ more prominent in (specify location).* Omentum and loops of bowel were carefully dissected from the underside of the abdominal wall using sharp dissection with Metzenbaum scissors. Careful explora-tion of the abdomen was then performed *(detail findings).*

The small bowel was run from the ligament of Treitz to the ileocecal valve. The bowel was noted to be dilated proximally and collapsed distally with a zone of transition *(describe location). An adhesive band was noted/multiple adhesions were noted* to be obstructing the distal small bowel. All adhesions were divided sharply and all small bowel loops carefully separated. The entire small bowel was then inspected for viability and the absence of any additional obstructing bands. *A small patch/patches of deserosalized bowel was imbricated with 3-0 silk Lembert sutures. An inadvertent enterotomy was repaired/enterotomies were repaired in two layers with 3-0 Vicryl and 3-0 silk.* Small bowel content was milked proximally to be aspirated by the nasogastric tube and distally into the colon, again confirming patency and integrity throughout its entire length. The abdominal cavity was copiously washed with saline and hemostasis was obtained.

(Optional: Multiple interrupted through-and-through retention sutures of ____*were placed.)* The fascia was closed with *a running suture of* ____*/a Smead-Jones closure of interrupted* ____. The skin was closed with *skin staples/subcuticular sutures of* ____*/other.*

The patient tolerated the procedure well and was taken to the postanesthesia care unit in stable condition.

ACKNOWLEDGMENT

This chapter was contributed by Mazen M. Hashisho, MD, in the first edition.

NOTES

Chapter 35

Laparoscopic Enterolysis for Small Bowel Obstruction

Mohamad H. Alaeddine, M.D. and Bassem Y. Safadi, M.D.

INDICATIONS

- Acute small bowel obstruction with moderate bowel dilation and expectation of limited adhesions based on previous surgical history (example appendectomy, tubal ligation, C-section, etc.).
- Subacute or recurrent intestinal obstruction with a well-defined transition zone on preoperative imaging.
- Suspicion of internal hernia after laparoscopic bariatric surgery (particularly laparoscopic Roux-y-gastric bypass).

ESSENTIAL STEPS

1. Position the patient supine with both arms to the side.
2. Enter the abdomen away from the previous incisions using open Hasson technique.
3. Insert all trocars under direct laparoscopic vision away from location of suspected pathology.
4. Manipulate the table position (e.g., Trendelenburg position) to serve exposure.
5. Lyse adhesions to the anterior abdominal with sharp dissection. Minimize use of energy sources.
6. Retract the omentum cephalad along with the transverse colon and mesocolon.
7. Handle the bowel gently, and use intestinal graspers.
8. Run the small intestine from the ligament of treitz or the ileocecal area. If the bowels are edematous and dilated, it is safer to start distally.

J.J. Hoballah and C.E.H. Scott-Conner (eds.), *Operative Dictations in General and Vascular Surgery*, DOI 10.1007/978-1-4614-0451-4_35,
© Springer Science+Business Media, LLC 2012

9. Dissect all adhesions sharply.
10. After laparoscopic ante-colic gastric bypass procedures, inspect two potential defects for internal hernias; that is Petersen's defect and the mesenteric defect at the jejuno-jejunostomy.
11. After laparoscopic retro-colic gastric bypass the, inspect the mesocolic window as well.

NOTE THESE VARIATIONS
- Dense diffuse adhesions with massive bowel distention should prompt the surgeon to convert to open early on avoid intestinal injury.
- Small intestinal obstruction in the setting of large incisional hernias are best approached open since the defects need to be repaired as well.

COMPLICATIONS
- Bleeding.
- Intestinal injury.
- Recurrent bowel obstruction.

OPERATIVE DICTATION
Preoperative diagnosis: Small bowel obstruction.
Procedure: Laparoscopic adhesiolysis and release of small bowel obstruction.
Postoperative diagnosis: Same.
Indications: A ___ -year-old *male/female* patient with a remote history *open appendectomy/C-section/hysterectomy/other* has clinical and radiographic features of partial small bowel obstruction. *He/she* failed to improve with naso-gastric decompression. A clear transition point at the level of distal small bowel was seen on CT imaging in *the right iliac fossa/pelvis/other location*.
Description of procedure: The patient was placed in the supine position and general endotracheal anesthesia was induced. Preoperative antibiotics were given. The abdomen was prepped and draped in the usual sterile fashion. A urinary catheter was placed in the urinary bladder using sterile technique. A timeout was completed verifying correct patient, procedure, site, positioning, and implant(s) and/or special equipment prior to beginning this procedure.

A 10-mm trocar was inserted under direct vision using open Hasson technique and the abdomen was inflated with CO_2 till 14 mmHg. Then under direct laparoscopic vision, two 5-mm trocars were inserted in the left upper and left lower quadrants. Immediately upon exploration we noted loops of bowel that were dilated and others that were decompressed. There were *adhesions between omentum/loops of small intestines adherent to the anterior abdominal wall at the previous appendectomy site in the right lower quadrant/other.* The adhesions to abdominal wall were sharply incised carefully releasing the omentum and intestines from the abdominal wall. There was no evidence of any incisional hernia. Once the adhesions to the abdominal wall were released it became clear that the transition point was at the level of distal ileum and was due to a fibrous adhesive band. There was no ischemia or necrosis of the bowel. The adhesive band was sharply incised totally releasing the obstruction. Other than that there were no significant adhesions.

The small bowel was then examined from the ileocecal valve to the Ligament of Treitz. We added a 5-mm port in the right upper quadrant to help retract the transverse colon cephalad to aid in the exposure.

At this stage, we were satisfied that the obstruction was resolved. The trocars were removed under vision. The abdomen was deflated. The fascia defect at the 10-mm trocar was closed with an absorbable suture. The incisions were closed with 4-0 monocryl subcuticular sutures. The patient tolerated the procedure well and left the operating room in good condition.

NOTES

Chapter 36
Feeding Jejunostomy

Carol E.H. Scott-Conner, M.D.

INDICATIONS
- Need for prolonged enteral support when gastrostomy or feeding tube not feasible.
- Frequently done as adjunct to complex upper-abdominal procedures.

ESSENTIAL STEPS
1. Short midline incision.
2. Identify the ligament of Treitz.
3. Trace distally to the mobile loop of the proximal jejunum.
4. Pass a tube through the abdominal wall at the desired site.
5. Pursestring suture on the antimesenteric border of the jejunum.
6. Insert a tube and manually pass it distally as far as possible.
7. Tie a pursestring suture.
8. Create a Witzel tunnel with interrupted 3-0 silk Lembert sutures.
9. Tack the jejunum to the abdominal wall at the catheter entrance site.
10. Check for torsion and tension.
11. Close the abdomen.
12. Secure the catheter to the abdominal wall.

J.J. Hoballah and C.E.H. Scott-Conner (eds.), *Operative Dictations in General and Vascular Surgery*, DOI 10.1007/978-1-4614-0451-4_36,
© Springer Science+Business Media, LLC 2012

NOTE THIS VARIATION

- Needle-catheter jejunostomy sometimes used when need is temporary.

COMPLICATIONS

- Insertion into the ileum rather than jejunum.
- Obstruction of the lumen by Witzel tunnel and catheter.
- Torsion of the bowel.
- Leakage of succus into the abdomen.
- Tube dislodgement.

TEMPLATE OPERATIVE DICTATION

Preoperative diagnosis: *Head and neck malignancy/other* with need for prolonged enteral nutrition.

Procedure: Feeding jejunostomy.

Postoperative diagnosis: Same.

Indications: This ____-year-old *male/female* required prolonged enteral nutrition because of *head and neck malignancy/other* and was unable to tolerate other routes of access due to ____. Feeding jejunostomy was chosen as the route of nutritional support.

Description of procedure: The patient was placed in the supine position and general endotracheal anesthesia was induced. Preoperative antibiotics were given. The abdomen was prepped and draped in the usual sterile fashion. A timeout was completed verifying correct patient, procedure, site, positioning, and implant(s) and/or special equipment prior to beginning this procedure.

A short midline incision was made and deepened through the subcutaneous tissues. Hemostasis was achieved with electrocautery. The linea alba was identified and incised and the peritoneal cavity entered. The abdomen was explored. *Adhesions were lysed sharply under direct vision with Metzenbaum scissors.*

The ligament of Treitz was identified. A loop of proximal jejunum was delivered into the wound. It was confirmed to be sufficiently mobile to reach the chosen site without tension.

A pursestring suture of 3-0 silk was placed on the antimesenteric border of the bowel at 20 cm from the ligament of Treitz, and an incision was made with electrocautery in the intestinal wall in the center of the pursestring suture. A *14-French feeding tube/other* was passed through the anterior abdominal wall and inserted into the lumen of the jejunum and advanced distally. The pursestring suture was secured in place. A Witzel tunnel was then constructed with 3-0 silk Lembert sutures in such a manner as to completely cover the entry site into the jejunum and to extend proximally, completely covering the catheter, for approximately 5 cm. The jejunum was noted to have a patent lumen at the conclusion of this procedure.

The jejunum was then tacked to the anterior abdominal wall at the catheter entrance site with several 3-0 silk sutures in such a manner as to prevent torsion. The catheter was secured to the skin with a 3-0 nylon suture.

Hemostasis was checked and omentum was brought adjacent to the surgical field. The fascia was closed with *a running suture of* ____*/a Smead-Jones closure of interrupted* ____. The skin was closed with *skin staples/subcuticular sutures of* ____*/other.*

The patient tolerated the procedure well and was taken to the postanesthesia care unit in stable condition.

ACKNOWLEDGMENT

This chapter was contributed by Mazen M. Hashisho, MD, in the first edition.

NOTES

Chapter 37

Appendectomy

Lori K. Soni, M.D.

INDICATIONS

- Acute appendicitis.
- Interval appendectomy.
- Benign tumor of the appendix.

ESSENTIAL STEPS

1. Right lower quadrant incision over McBurney's point or the point of maximum tenderness that was marked prior to induction of anesthesia *(rarely, the incision is made in the lower midline or right paramedian).*
2. Divide each muscular and aponeurotic layer parallel to fibers to achieve a muscle splitting incision.
3. Enter the peritoneum, note any discoloration or malodor of the peritoneal fluid. Send the peritoneal fluid for gram stain and culture.
4. Expose the cecum, pulling it into the wound and elevating it with a moist pad.
5. *Divide the lateral peritoneal attachments of the cecum (may be required for better exposure).*
6. Protect the wound with moist pads.
7. Deliver the appendix into the wound.
8. If the appendix appears normal, check the terminal ileum and pelvis. Check for any fluid in the right paracolic gutter which may arise from another pathology such as perforated peptic ulcer *(convert to laparotomy if necessary).*

J.J. Hoballah and C.E.H. Scott-Conner (eds.), *Operative Dictations in General and Vascular Surgery*, DOI 10.1007/978-1-4614-0451-4_37,
© Springer Science+Business Media, LLC 2012

9. Divide and carefully ligate the appendiceal mesentery to the base of the appendix.
10. Crush the stump of the appendix with a clamp; then, move the clamp 1 cm toward the tip of the appendix.
11. Ligate the proximal edge of the crushed appendix.
12. Take a *pursestring suture/z-stitch* in the wall of the cecum at the base of the appendix.
13. Transect the appendix above the ligature and remove it.
14. Invaginate the stump and tie the *pursestring suture/z-stitch.*
15. Place omentum over the site.
16. Aspirate any purulent material, cautiously irrigate and gently suction to minimize bleeding.
17. *Drain if a well-formed abscess cavity is encountered.* Remove all fibrinous material lining the abscess cavity and send for culture.
18. Check hemostasis.
19. Close the incision in three layers: transversalis fascia and peritoneum, internal then external oblique.
20. *Close the subcutaneous tissue and skin/pack the wound open.*

NOTE THESE VARIATIONS
- Choice of incision.
- Incision of the peritoneum to mobilize the cecum.
- Location of the appendix.
- Method of stump inversion.
- Degree of purulence, whether drain used.

COMPLICATIONS
- Pelvic abscess.
- Stump leak.
- Missed other pathology (e.g., perforated ulcer).
- Small bowel obstruction.

TEMPLATE OPERATIVE DICTATION
Preoperative diagnosis: Acute appendicitis.
Procedure: Appendectomy.
Postoperative diagnosis: *Same/mesenteric adenitis/Crohn's disease/pelvic inflammatory disease/other.*
Indications: Choose one: *If acute appendicitis:* This ____-year-old *male/female* presented with right lower quadrant pain of ____ duration, fever, elevated WBC count. *Computed tomography scan/ultrasound/physical examination* was consistent with acute

appendicitis. *If interval appendectomy:* This ____-year-old *male/ female* had appendiceal abscess treated by percutaneous drainage and antibiotics ____ weeks earlier and now presents for interval appendectomy.

Description of procedure: The patient was placed in the supine position and general endotracheal anesthesia was induced. The abdomen was prepped and draped in the usual sterile fashion. A timeout was completed verifying correct patient, procedure, site, positioning, and implant(s) and/or special equipment prior to beginning this procedure.

A skin incision was made in a natural skin line centered *over McBurney's point/over the palpable mass in the right lower quadrant/over the point of maximum tenderness.* Subcutaneous tissues were divided until the aponeurosis of the external oblique was encountered. This was opened in a direction parallel to its fibers, extended medially toward the rectus sheath, and extended laterally to the iliac crest, and the underlying internal oblique aponeurosis exposed. The transversus abdominus was then encountered and similarly split. The transversalis fascia is entered, the peritoneum lifted with forceps and entered, and care taken not to injure the bowel below. *Turbid fluid was encountered and cultured.* Moist pads were placed to protect the edges of the wound. The cecum was identified and pulled into the wound and held in place using a moist pad. *The appendix came into view/it was necessary to incise the lateral peritoneal attachment of the cecum to mobilize the cecum and display the appendix.* The appendix was noted to be *free/retrocecal and inflamed/gangrenous/perforated/normal. [If normal: The terminal ileum was then run for ____ ft and found to be normal/ inflamed. Pelvic viscera were inspected and found to be ____. A presumptive diagnosis of Crohn's disease/mesenteric adenitis/inflamed Meckel's diverticulum/pelvic inflammatory disease was made. The decision was made to proceed with appendectomy (detail other procedures performed).]*

The mesentery of the appendix was divided between clamps and ligated with 3-0 silk. The base of the appendix was crushed in a clamp and the clamp was then advanced 1 cm toward the tip of the appendix. The appendix was then ligated at the proximal edge of the crushed portion with a 0 chromic ligature. A *pursestring suture/z-stitch* was taken in the wall of the cecum. The appendix was held upward, cut distal to the ligature, and removed. The stump was *(cauterized and)* then invaginated into the cecum using forceps and the *pursestring suture/z-stitch* was tied in such a manner as to completely invert and cover the stump. Hemostasis was checked. Omentum was placed on the site of the operation.

All purulent material was aspirated and the field gently irrigated with normal saline. *An abscess was/was not encountered and a swab was sent for gram stain and culture. The abscess was well formed, its entire lining of fibrinous material was removed and sent to the lab for culture. A closed suction drain was placed in the abscess cavity.* The incision was closed in layers in the following fashion: Peritoneum and transversalis fascia were closed with a running suture of ____. The opening in the rectus sheath and the internal oblique was then closed with a *running/interrupted* suture of ____. The external oblique was closed with interrupted ____. *Subcutaneous tissues and skin were closed with ____/the wound was packed open with fine mesh gauze.*

The patient tolerated the procedure well and was taken to the postanesthesia care unit in satisfactory condition.

ACKNOWLEDGMENT

This chapter was contributed by Mohamad Allam, MD, in the first edition.

NOTES

Chapter 38

Laparoscopic Appendectomy

Georgios Tsoulfas, M.D.

INDICATIONS

- Acute appendicitis or right lower quadrant pain, especially if: atypical presentation, obesity, female of child-bearing age, need for rapid return to activities.
- Interval appendectomy after the treatment of appendiceal abscess.

ESSENTIAL STEPS

1. Tuck the left arm.
2. Monitors at the foot.
3. Nasogastric tube and Foley catheter to decompress the stomach and bladder.
4. Induce the pneumoperitoneum.
5. Insert the first trocar above the umbilicus.
6. Inspect the abdomen.
7. Second 11/12-mm cannula above the symphysis pubis below the hairline or in the left lower quadrant lateral to the rectus muscle.
8. Third 5-mm cannula in the right upper quadrant between the umbilicus and right costal margin.
9. Trendelenburg position with table rotated right side up.
10. Grasp the cecum with Babcock forceps and pull toward the left upper quadrant.
11. Dissect away omentum if necessary.
12. Atraumatic grasper in right upper quadrant port to identify and elevate the appendix.

J.J. Hoballah and C.E.H. Scott-Conner (eds.), *Operative Dictations in General and Vascular Surgery*, DOI 10.1007/978-1-4614-0451-4_38,
© Springer Science+Business Media, LLC 2012

13. Develop a window at the base of the mesoappendix next to the cecum.
14. *If stapled:*
    - *Endoscopic linear cutting stapler across base of the appendix.*
    - *Endoscopic linear cutting stapler with vascular cartridge across the mesoappendix.*
15. *If pretied ligature:*
    - *Serially divide the mesentery with clips/cautery/ultrasonic shears.*
    - *Doubly ligate the base of the appendix with pretied ligature.*
    - *Transect with endoscopic shears.*
16. Remove the appendix through trocar or place into an endoscopic retrieval pouch.
17. Short bursts of electrocautery to the base as needed.
18. Irrigate and assure hemostasis.
19. *Closed suction drain if well-formed abscess cavity encountered.*
20. Close.

NOTE THESE VARIATIONS

- Veress needle or Hassan cannula.
- Stapler or pretied ligature.
- Location of the appendix (retrocecal) and pathology.
- If retrocecal, mobilize the cecum.
- Drain if well-formed abscess encountered.

COMPLICATIONS

- Stump leak.
- Dropped/lost fecalith or appendix.
- Bowel, bladder, or vascular trocar injury.

TEMPLATE OPERATIVE DICTATION

Preoperative diagnosis: Acute appendicitis.
Procedure: Laparoscopic appendectomy.
Postoperative diagnosis: *Same/mesenteric adenitis/Crohn's disease/pelvic inflammatory disease/other.*
Indications: *Acute appendicitis:* This ___-year-old *male/female* presented with right lower quadrant pain of ___ duration, fever, elevated WBC. Computed tomography *scan/ultrasound/physical examination* was consistent with acute appendicitis. *Interval appendectomy:* This ___-year-old *male/female* had appendiceal

abscess treated by percutaneous drainage and antibiotics ___ weeks earlier and now presents for interval appendectomy. The decision was made to proceed with a laparoscopic, possibly open, appendectomy.

Description of procedure: The patient was placed on the operating table in the supine position. General anesthesia was induced. A time-out was completed verifying correct patient, procedure, site, positioning, and implant(s) and/or special equipment prior to beginning this procedure. *A Foley catheter and nasogastric/orogastric tubes were placed.* The abdomen was prepped and draped in the usual sterile fashion.

An incision was made in a natural skin line above the umbilicus.

[Choose one:]

If **Veress needle:** *The fascia was elevated and the Veress needle inserted. Proper position was confirmed by aspiration and saline meniscus test. A 10/11-mm trocar was then inserted.*

If **Hassan cannula:** *The fascia was elevated and incised. Entry into the peritoneum was confirmed visually and no bowel was noted in the vicinity of the incision. Two figure-of-eight sutures of 2-0 Vicryl were placed and the Hassan cannula inserted under direct vision. The sutures were anchored around the cannula.*

The abdomen was insufflated with carbon dioxide to a pressure of 12–15 mmHg. The patient tolerated insufflation well.

The laparoscope was inserted and the abdomen inspected. No injuries from initial trocar placement were noted. *Turbid fluid was noted in the right lower quadrant/other.* Under direct visualization, an *11/12-mm trocar (if stapled)/5-mm trocar (if ligated)* was inserted *above the symphysis pubis and below the hairline/in the left lower quadrant lateral to the rectus muscle.* Care was taken to avoid injury to the bladder or inferior epigastric vessels. A 5-mm port was then placed in the right upper quadrant, between the umbilicus and the right costal margin. The table was placed in the Trendelenburg position with the right side elevated.

The cecum was gently grasped with an endoscopic Babcock forceps and pulled toward (the left upper quadrant). An atraumatic grasper was then passed through the right upper quadrant port and omentum was dissected away until the appendix was identified. The appendix was then grasped and elevated. It was noted to be *normal/inflamed/gangrenous/perforated.*

If **retrocecal:** *The appendix was not seen. The lateral peritoneal attachment was incised and the cecum mobilized until a retrocecal appendix was visualized.* A window was developed in the mesoappendix at a point between the base of the appendix and the cecum.

If stapled: An endoscopic linear cutting stapler was then used to divide and staple the base of the appendix. It was reloaded with a vascular cartridge and the mesoappendix similarly divided.

If ligated: The mesentery was serially divided with clips/cautery/ ultrasonic shears. A pretied endoscopic ligature was then passed over the appendix and snugged tight at the base. A second ligature was similarly placed and the appendix divided.

The appendix was *withdrawn into the 11/12-mm trocar/placed in an endoscopic retrieval bag* and removed.

The appendiceal stump was then irrigated and hemostasis was assured. Fluid was suctioned and no other pathology was identified. *A closed suction drain was placed in the abscess cavity and withdrawn through the ___ trocar site.*

Secondary trocars were removed under direct vision. *No bleeding was noted/trocar site bleeding was controlled by electrocautery/ suture placement.* The laparoscope was withdrawn and the umbilical trocar removed. The abdomen was allowed to collapse. All trocar sites greater than 5 mm were closed with ___. The skin was closed with subcuticular sutures ___ of and steristrips.

The patient tolerated the procedure well and was taken to the postanesthesia care unit in satisfactory condition.

ACKNOWLEDGMENT

Natisha Busick, MD coauthored this chapter with Dr. Tsoulfas in the first edition.

NOTES

Chapter 39
Resection of Meckel's Diverticulum

Ross Bengtson, M.D.

INDICATIONS
- Bleeding.
- Inflammation.
- Volvulus.
- Littre's hernia.
- Intussusception.
- Incidental finding during laparotomy.

ESSENTIAL STEPS
1. Perform time-out.
2. Lower midline incision.
3. Mobilize Meckel's and adjacent ileum.
4. *Lyse adhesions if necessary.*
5. Clamp, transect, and ligate the mesentery of the diverticulum near the ileal mesentery.
6. *Clamp Meckel's with two noncrushing bowel clamps transversely near its takeoff from the ileum/apply cutting linear stapler to base.*
7. *Transect Meckel's between the two clamps and* pass off as specimen.
8. *(If sutured: Close enterotomy transversely in two layers with running 3-0 Vicryl and interrupted 3-0 silk Lembert sutures.)*
9. Check *suture line/staple line* for integrity and the terminal ileum for adequate lumen.

J.J. Hoballah and C.E.H. Scott-Conner (eds.), *Operative Dictations in General and Vascular Surgery*, DOI 10.1007/978-1-4614-0451-4_39,
© Springer Science+Business Media, LLC 2012

10. Check hemostasis.
11. Irrigate the abdomen.
12. Perform sponge, needle, and instrument count.
13. Close in the usual fashion.

NOTE THESE VARIATIONS
- Simple diverticulectomy as described here vs. small bowel resection (see Chap. 27).
- Stapled vs. sutured closure.

COMPLICATIONS
- Anastomotic leak.
- Enterocutaneous fistula.
- Abscess.
- Small bowel obstruction.

TEMPLATE OPERATIVE DICTATION
Preoperative diagnosis: *Bleeding/peritonitis/small bowel obstruction/ other.*
Procedure: Resection of Meckel's diverticulum.
Postoperative diagnosis: *Same, due to Meckel's diverticulum/ incidental Meckel's diverticulum/other.*
Indication: The patient is a ___-year-old *male/female* with *bleeding/peritonitis/other. He/she* was brought to the operating room for exploration to alleviate this condition.
Description of procedure: An epidural catheter was placed by anesthesia prior to the start of the operation. The patient was placed in the supine position and general endotracheal anesthesia was induced. A time-out was completed verifying correct patient, procedure, site, positioning, and implant(s) and/or special equipment prior to beginning this procedure. Preoperative antibiotics were given. A Foley catheter and nasogastric tube were placed. The abdomen was prepped and draped in the usual sterile fashion. A time-out was performed, then a vertical midline incision was made from xiphoid to just below the umbilicus. This was deepened through the subcutaneous tissues and hemostasis was achieved with electrocautery. The linea alba was identified and incised and the peritoneal cavity entered. The abdomen was explored. *Adhesions were lysed sharply under direct vision with Metzenbaum scissors.*

A survey of the abdomen revealed *(detail findings)* including a Meckel's diverticulum approximately ___ cm from the ileocecal valve. *If incidental Meckel's diverticulectomy, dictate primary procedure here.*

The Meckel's diverticulum was mobilized with lysis of surrounding adhesions. The mesodiverticulum was gently dissected at its takeoff from the ileal mesentery in an avascular plane with a curved hemostat and then clamped, transected, and ligated with 3-0 silk. *A linear cutting stapler was placed across the base of the diverticulum in such a manner as to preserve the lumen of the ileum and then fired/two noncrushing bowel clamps were placed transversely across the junction of the diverticulum and small bowel. The diverticulum was transected with a scalpel and passed off the table as a specimen. The enterotomy was then closed in two layers: an inner layer of running 3-0 Vicryl and an outer layer of interrupted 3-0 silk Lembert sutures. The remaining bowel clamp was removed.* The integrity of the *staple line/suture line* and adequate patency of the terminal ileum were confirmed.

Hemostasis was checked and the abdomen was irrigated with normal saline. The omentum was placed over the operative site and under the incision. The sponge, needle, and instrument count were correct. *(Optional: Multiple interrupted through-and-through retention sutures of were placed.)* The fascia was closed with *a running suture of ___/a Smead-Jones closure of interrupted ___.* The skin was closed with *skin staples/subcuticular sutures of ___/other.*

The patient tolerated the procedure well and was taken to the postanesthesia care unit in stable condition.

NOTES

Section IV
Large Intestine

Chapter 40
Right Hemicolectomy

Simon Roh, M.D. and John C. Byrn, M.D.

INDICATIONS
- Cancer.
- Ischemia.
- Right-sided diverticular disease.
- Bleeding from the right colon.
- Cecal volvulus/bascule.

ESSENTIAL STEPS
1. Long midline incision.
2. *Explore the abdomen for metastatic disease (liver and peritoneum and ovaries in female).*
3. Incise the line of Toldt and mobilize the colon toward midline.
4. Identify and protect both ureters and the duodenum.
5. Divide the colon proximally and distally.
6. Ligate the mesenteric vessels.
7. Remove the specimen (tag proximal and distal ends).
8. Anastomose the colon.
9. Check the anastomosis for patency and integrity.
10. Close the abdomen.

NOTE THESE VARIATIONS
- Stapled or sutured anastomosis.
- Size/type of stapler and type of sutures.

J.J. Hoballah and C.E.H. Scott-Conner (eds.), *Operative Dictations in General and Vascular Surgery*, DOI 10.1007/978-1-4614-0451-4_40,
© Springer Science+Business Media, LLC 2012

- Ligation of the main trunk vs. right branch of the middle colic artery.
- Presence/extent of metastatic disease.

COMPLICATIONS
- Injury to the ureter.
- Injury to the duodenum.
- Anastomotic leak.

TEMPLATE OPERATIVE DICTATION

Preoperative diagnosis: *Carcinoma of ascending colon/ischemia/diverticular disease/bleeding.*

Procedure: Right hemicolectomy with primary anastomosis.

Postoperative diagnosis: Same *(enumerate any metastatic disease found).*

Indications: This ____-year-old *male/female* with *abdominal pain/bleeding/obstructive symptoms/recurrent bouts of diverticulitis* was found to have *carcinoma/ischemia/diverticular disease/bleeding* involving the ascending colon. *Elective/emergency* resection was indicated.

Description of procedure: *An epidural catheter was placed by anesthesia prior to the start of the operation.* The patient was placed in the supine position and general endotracheal anesthesia was induced. Sequential pneumatic compression devices were placed on lower extremities. Preoperative antibiotics were given. A Foley catheter and nasogastric tube were placed. The abdomen was prepped and draped in the usual sterile fashion. A time-out was completed verifying correct patient, procedure, site, positioning, and implant(s) and/or special equipment prior to beginning this procedure.

A vertical midline incision was made from xiphoid to just above the pubis. This was deepened through the subcutaneous tissues and hemostasis was achieved with electrocautery. The linea alba was identified and incised and the peritoneal cavity entered.

The abdomen was explored. *Adhesions were lysed sharply under direct vision with Metzenbaum scissors. A mass was palpated in the ascending colon. The liver, omentum, peritoneum, and ovaries (if present) were inspected for the evidence of metastatic disease. Metastatic disease was noted ____/no metastatic disease was noted.*

The small bowel was inspected and retracted to the left using a moist gauze and self-retaining retractor. Using electrocautery, the colon was freed from its peritoneal attachments along the avascular line of Toldt from the cecum to the hepatic flexure. Additional lateral peritoneal coverings were incised to further mobilize the colon. The dissection was extended across the ileocolic junction and terminal ileum was mobilized. Both ureters were identified and protected, as were the duodenum, right kidney, and gonadal vessels. The hepatic flexure was carefully mobilized by dividing the peritoneum in the hepatorenal fossa.

Points of transection were selected proximally and distally *(specify locations)*. The bowel was divided with the linear cutting stapler. The peritoneum overlying the mesentery was then scored with electrocautery and the ileocolic artery was identified, double ligated with 2-0 silk sutures, and transected. The *right branch/main trunk* of the middle colic and right colic arteries were similarly identified and ligated. Remaining mesentery and all associated nodal tissue was divided and swept down with the specimen. The specimen was removed, proximal and distal ends tagged, and sent to pathology. Hemostasis was checked in the operative field. The two ends of bowel were checked and found to be viable, with excellent blood supply.

If stapled anastomosis: *The proximal and distal segments were brought into apposition and found to lie comfortably next to each other. Two stay sutures of 3-0 silk were placed to approximate the antimesenteric borders of the bowel segments. Enterotomies were made on the antimesenteric corner of the staple line on the ileum and transverse colon and the linear cutting stapler inserted and fired. Hemostasis was checked on the staple line. The enterotomies were then closed with a linear stapler/a two-layer sutured closure of running 3-0 Vicryl and interrupted 3-0 silk Lembert sutures.*

If sutured: *The fat was gently cleared from the terminal 2–3 mm of the bowel ends. The ileum and transverse colon ends of bowel were brought into apposition and found to lie comfortably without excessive tension. A Cheatle slit was made in the antimesenteric border of the ileum to equalize the caliber of the two pieces of bowel. A two-layer hand-sewn end-to-end anastomosis was then constructed using an outer layer of interrupted 3-0 silk Lembert sutures and an inner running layer of 3-0 Vicryl.*

The anastomosis was checked and found to be intact and widely patent. Mesenteric defect was closed with interrupted 3-0 Vicryl. The abdominal cavity was then copiously irrigated and hemostasis was checked.

(Optional: Multiple interrupted through-and-through retention sutures of ____were placed.) The fascia was closed with *a running suture of ____/a Smead-Jones closure of interrupted ____.* The skin was closed with *skin staples/subcuticular sutures of____/other.*

The patient tolerated the procedure well and was taken to the postanesthesia care unit in stable condition.

NOTES

Chapter 41
Laparoscopic Right Hemicolectomy

Faek R. Jamali, M.D.

INDICATIONS

- Right-sided colonic dysplastic polyps or malignancy.
- Appendiceal neoplasms (carcinoids >2 cm or with positive nodes; mucinous neoplasm).
- Resection of specific benign conditions of the ascending and transverse colon (arteriovenous malformations, diverticular disease, and ischemic strictures).
- Cecal volvulus.
- Severe appendicitis with involvement of the cecum in the inflammatory process.
- Right colon involvement in inflammatory bowel disease (primarily Crohn's disease).

ESSENTIAL STEPS

1. Establish laparoscopic access, place trocars, and explore the abdominal cavity.
2. Position the patient so as to obtain appropriate exposure.
3. Identify the ileocolic vessels by traction on the cecum. Incise the peritoneum overlying the junction of the ileocolic vessels with the SMA.
4. Dissect and control the ileocolic vessels and perform associated lymphadenectomy (for malignancy).
5. Dissect the plane anterior to the Toldt fascia. Identify and protect the duodenum and head of pancreas.
6. Identify and protect the ureter and gonadal vessels.

J.J. Hoballah and C.E.H. Scott-Conner (eds.), *Operative Dictations in General and Vascular Surgery*, DOI 10.1007/978-1-4614-0451-4_41,
© Springer Science+Business Media, LLC 2012

7. If indicated by extent of needed resection, dissect and divide the right colic and right branch of the middle colic vessels and complete mesenteric dissection of transverse colon.

8. Complete retroperitoneal dissection of all attachments of ascending colon.

9. Mobilize ascending colon and hepatic flexure.

10. *For an extracorporeal anastomosis:*
    - Create a midline periumbilical 5-cm incision and place a wound protector.
    - Deliver the specimen.
    - Complete the proximal and distal mesenteric and bowel dissection extracorporeally with GIA staplers.
    - Perform a standard side-to-side anastomosis extracorporeally, avoiding any twists, and close the mesenteric defect.
    - Reintroduce the bowel into abdominal cavity perform a final laparoscopic exploration after closure of the access site using number one PDS suture.
    - Close all 10-mm trocar sites at the level of the fascia and closure of all skin defects.

11. *For an intracorporeal anastomosis:*
    - Divide the mesentery of the small bowel followed by division of terminal ileum and transverse colon using Endo GIA.
    - Perform an intracorporeal side-to-side anastomosis using Endo GIA, followed by closure of common enterotomy and mesenteric defect.
    - Place the specimen into an extraction bag and deliver it via a properly placed small incision.
    - Close all 10-mm trocar sites at the level of the fascia and close all skin defects.

NOTE THESE VARIATIONS

- Intracorporeal versus extracorporeal anastomosis.
- A hand assist technique may be used. In the hand assist technique, a small incision is strategically placed at the beginning of the operation and a specific hand assist device is used to allow the introduction of the non-dominant hand of the surgeon into the abdominal cavity to assist with the operation. The site is typically chosen so as the non-dominant hand does not interfere with a camera the site can also be used for the extraction of the specimen and for the

performance of the extracorporeal anastomosis. In the hand assist technique, the access incision is usually placed either in the midline (periumbilically) or in the right upper quadrant. The surgeon's hand is used to retract the small bowel, elevate the colon, and facilitate laparoscopic dissection.

COMPLICATIONS

- Access related complications (bowel injury, vascular injury, and retroperitoneal injury).
- Vascular injury (bleeding).
- Anastomotic complications (leak, fistula, twist, obstruction, and edema).

TEMPLATE OPERATIVE DICTATION

Preoperative diagnosis: List specific pathology indicating surgery *(see indications above)*, e.g., *malignant neoplasm of ascending colon.*

Procedure: Laparoscopic right hemicolectomy.

Postoperative diagnosis: List specific intraoperative findings, e.g., *malignant neoplasm of ascending colon.*

Indications: This ___-year-old *male/female* patient presented with ____ and on workup was found to have_____. *If malignancy: staging workup was completed and showed_____.* He/she is now presenting for elective laparoscopic right hemicolectomy. The indications, alternatives and risks, and benefits of the surgery were discussed with the patient and informed consent was obtained.

Details of operation: The patient was brought to the operating room and placed on the operating table in the lithotomy position. The abdomen was clipped, prepped with 2% chlorhexidine solution, and draped in the standard fashion. A time-out was completed verifying correct patient, procedure, site, positioning, and implant(s) and/or special equipment prior to beginning this procedure. *A vertical 1 cm supraumbilical incision was used to access the peritoneal cavity/A Verres needle was introduced into the abdominal cavity* and pneumoperitoneum was achieved. An additional 12-mm trocar was then placed under direct vision in the midline in the supra-pubic taking care to avoid injury to the bladder. Two additional 5-mm trocars were placed, one in the left anterior axillary line and the other one at the level of the mid-clavicular of the line to the right of the abdominal cavity below the umbilicus. *An additional 5-mm trocar was placed in the sub-xiphoid area to allow for the assistant to retract the transverse colon upward.* The patient was then positioned in 30° reverse Trendelenburg position with the patient's right side up to allow for small bowel to drop clear of the operative field. The 10-mm scope was introduced from the suprapubic port at the initial part of the procedure. The cecum was grasped with the left hand of the operating surgeon and lifted up to tent the ileocolic artery. The dissection was then started at the base of the ileocolic artery where it joined the superior mesenteric artery. The peritoneum overlying the takeoff of the ileocolic artery was opened using *electrocautery/an appropriate energy device*. This opening of the peritoneum was carried all the way up to the base of the transverse mesocolon. With the ileocolic artery retracted by traction on the cecum, gentle dissection was used to identify its takeoff from the superior mesenteric artery. The ileocolic artery and vein were then dissected and divided using endo-GIA vascular load or Ligasure device. The divided vessels were then elevated and dissection proceeded in the retroperitoneal using a traction counter-traction technique with gentle sweeping and visualization of the ureter. This dissection is carried along the plane of the Toldt fascia to the duodenum. The Duodenum and its attachments were swept downward. The C loop of the duodenum as well as a head of the pancreas were fully visualized with dissected and preserved. This dissection was continued in the avascular plane until the liver or gallbladder were encountered. By creating a window in the avascualr plane of the mesentery of the transverse colon. Dissection then continued on the right side of the superior mesenteric artery leading to the identification of the right colic artery and vein which were then gently dissected and divided.

For extended right hemicolectomy: the middle colic vessels were also dissected by opening the peritoneum overlying them and dissecting them at the takeoff from the superior mesenteric artery. The middle colic vessels were then divided followed by complete division of the mesentery of the transverse colon to the right of the middle colic vessels.

The lateral attachments of the ascending colon were then divided including mobilization of the retroperitoneal attachments of the terminal ileum. This mobilization was carried out until the posterior plane of dissection that was started from the medial approach was encountered, completing the liberation of the ascending colon and its hepatic flexure.

The Omentum attached to resected portions of colon was divided and resected with the specimen.

If extracorporeal anastomosis: A grasper was placed on the ascending colon and an access incision made by enlarging the umbilical trocar site to a total length of about 4–5 cm. A wound protector was then placed into the peritoneal cavity to prevent port site implantation as well as minimize the risk of wound infection. The ascending and transverse colon were then delivered and extracted. The small bowel and colon were then divided extracorporeally using a GIA device. The mesenteric dissection was completed as needed on the small bowel and colonic sides and the specimen resection was thus completed. The specimen was removed. The two ends of the ileum and transvers colon were then aligned, ensuring that the mesentery was not twisted, and a stapled end-to-end anastomosis was created in the usual manner. The mesenteric defect was then closed with _____ sutures and the bowel reintroduced into the peritoneal cavity. The fascia was then closed with _____. The peritoneum was again insufflated and the anastomosis, alignment of the bowel, and hemostasis were checked.

***If intracorporeal anastomosis:** The specimen was placed on the right side of the abdominal cavity. The terminal ileum and the transverse colon were approximated with a single 3-0 PDS suture. Enterotomies were made and the 60-mm Endo GIA 3.8-mm stapler was used to construct a stapled side-to-side anastomosis. The common enterotomy was closed using 3-0 PDS suture. The rent in the mesentery was also approximated with 3-0 PDS suture. The specimen was then placed in and Endocatch bag and extracted from an appropriately placed incision (right lower quadrant muscle splitting or Pfannestiel). Following extraction of the specimen the fascia of the extraction site was closed would number one PDS suture.*

The trocars were removed under direct vision and any fascial defects larger than 10 mm closed with a number one PDS suture. The skin was closed with 4-0 PDS sutures in a running fashion and a dry sterile dressing was applied. The sponge and instrument count was correct, blood loss was minimal, and there were no complications. The patient tolerated the procedure well and was transferred to the post-anesthesia care unit in stable condition.

NOTES

Chapter 42
Left Hemicolectomy

Simon Roh, M.D. and John C. Byrn, M.D.

INDICATIONS
- Cancer.
- Diverticular disease.
- Sigmoid volvulus.

ESSENTIAL STEPS
1. Long midline incision.
2. *Explore the abdomen for metastatic disease (liver and peritoneum and ovaries in female).*
3. Incise the line of Toldt and mobilize the colon toward midline.
4. Identify and protect both ureters.
5. Mobilize the splenic flexure.
6. Divide the colon proximally and distally.
7. Ligate the mesenteric vessels.
8. Remove the specimen (tag proximal and distal ends).
9. Anastomose the colon.
10. Check the anastomosis for patency and integrity.
11. Close the abdomen.

NOTE THESE VARIATIONS
- Stapled or sutured anastomosis.
- Size/type of stapler and type of sutures.
- High ligation of inferior mesenteric artery.

J.J. Hoballah and C.E.H. Scott-Conner (eds.), *Operative Dictations in General and Vascular Surgery*, DOI 10.1007/978-1-4614-0451-4_42,
© Springer Science+Business Media, LLC 2012

- *Presence/extent of metastatic disease.*
- *Closure of mesenteric defect rarely possible.*

COMPLICATIONS
- Injury to the ureter.
- Injury to the spleen.
- Anastomotic leak.

TEMPLATE OPERATIVE DICTATION

Preoperative diagnosis: *Carcinoma of the descending colon/ diverticular disease.*

Procedure: Left hemicolectomy with mobilization of splenic flexure and primary anastomosis (coloproctostomy).

Postoperative diagnosis: Same *(enumerate any metastatic disease found).*

Indications: This ____-year-old *male/female* with *abdominal pain/ bleeding/obstructive symptoms/recurrent bouts of diverticulitis* was found to have *carcinoma of the descending colon/diverticular disease.* Elective resection was indicated.

Description of procedure: *An epidural catheter was placed by anesthesia prior to the start of the operation.* The patient was placed in the supine position and general endotracheal anesthesia was induced. Preoperative antibiotics were given. A Foley catheter, orogastric tube, and sequential pneumatic compression device were placed. The abdomen was prepped and draped in the usual sterile fashion. A time-out was completed verifying correct patient, procedure, site, positioning, and implant(s) and/or special equipment prior to beginning this procedure.

A vertical midline incision was made from xiphoid to just above the pubis. This was deepened through the subcutaneous tissues and hemostasis was achieved with electrocautery. The linea alba was identified and incised and the peritoneal cavity entered. Patient was repositioned in a slight Trendelenburg position. The abdomen was explored. *Adhesions were lysed sharply under direct vision with Metzenbaum scissors. A mass/diverticulum was palpated in the descending colon. The liver, omentum, peritoneum, and ovaries (if present) were inspected for the evidence of metastatic disease. Metastatic disease was noted ____/no metastatic disease was noted.*

The descending colon was inspected and retracted medially using a moist towel and self-retaining retractor. Using electrocautery/Metzenbaum scissors, the colon was freed from its peritoneal attachments along the line of Toldt proximally from the splenic flexure and distally to the rectosigmoid junction. Both ureters were identified and protected.

Attention was then turned to mobilizing the splenic flexure. The peritoneum covering the splenic flexure was dissected using electrocautery. The splenocolic ligament and the pancreaticocolic ligaments were divided. The distal transverse colon was dissected from the stomach by freeing the greater omentum.

Points of transection were selected proximally and distally *(specify locations)*. The bowel was divided with the linear cutting stapler. The peritoneum on the medial aspect of mesentery was then scored with electrocautery and the vessels were serially clamped, divided, and ligated individually with 2-0 silk sutures. The dissection proceeded to the inferior mesenteric artery which was identified and double ligated with 2-0 silk sutures. The location of the left ureter was confirmed prior to dividing the IMA. Dissection continued to the sigmoid artery which was divided and ligated with 2-0 silk. The rectosigmoid junction was mobilized and the loose tissues in the presacral space were sharply dissected with electrocautery down to the level of the sacral promontory. The rectosigmoid junction was identified by the splaying of the teniae at the level of the sacral promontory. The bowel was transected at the junction using a GIA-60/TA-55 stapler. The specimen was removed, proximal and distal ends tagged, and sent to pathology. Hemostasis was checked in the operative field. The two ends of the bowel were checked and found to be viable, with excellent blood supply.

[Choose one:]

If stapled anastomosis: Attention was turned to performing a coloproctostomy with the EEA stapler. The staple line from the distal colon was sharply excised and edges were grasped with Allis clamps. The diameter of EEA to be used was measured with EEA sizers. A purse-string suture was placed around the distal colon using 0 Prolene. The anvil was inserted into the distal colon and the purse-string was tied down. The EEA stapler was passed via the anus so that it abutted the proximal colon TA staple line at the top of the rectum. The spike was deployed through the rectum and the EEA stapler was mated with the anvil. The stapler was tightened down and fired. Once the stapler along with the anvil had been removed, two intact donut anastomoses were visualized. A leak test was performed and no leaks were found.

If sutured: The fat was gently cleared from the terminal 2–3 mm of the bowel ends. The two ends of the bowel were brought into apposition and found to lie comfortably without excessive tension.

A two-layer hand-sewn end-to-end anastomosis was then constructed using an outer layer of interrupted 3-0 silk Lembert sutures and an inner running layer of 3-0 Vicryl.

The anastomosis was checked and found to be intact and widely patent. *Mesenteric defect was checked for herniated bowel.* The abdominal cavity was then copiously irrigated and hemostasis was checked.

(Optional: 10 Fr JP drain was placed through a stab incision in the LLQ and left in pelvis near the anastomosis.)

(Optional: Multiple interrupted through-and-through retention sutures of ___were placed.) The fascia was closed with *a running suture of ___/a Smead-Jones closure of interrupted ___.* The skin was closed with *skin staples/subcuticular sutures of___/other.*

The patient tolerated the procedure well and was taken to the postanesthesia care unit in stable condition.

ACKNOWLEDGMENT

This chapter was contributed by Nate Thepjatri, MD in the first edition.

NOTES

Chapter 43

Laparoscopic Left Hemicolectomy

Faek R. Jamali, M.D.

INDICATIONS

- Left colon cancer or polyps.
- Resection of specific benign conditions of the descending and sigmoid colon (arteriovenous malformations, diverticular disease and ischemic strictures).
- Sigmoid volvulus.

ESSENTIAL STEPS

1. Establish laparoscopic access, place trocars, and perform laparoscopic exploration of abdominal cavity.
2. Position the patient to obtain appropriate exposure.
3. Place the sigmoid colon under traction and incise the peritoneum overlying the base of the left colon mesentery to identify the inferior mesenteric artery (IMA).
4. Dissect and control the IMA and perform lymphadenectomy.
5. Dissect the plane anterior to the Toldt fascia and identify and preserve the left ureter.
6. Complete the mesenteric dissection on the left up to ligament of Treitz and down to sacral promontory; identify and preserve the hypogastric nerve bundles.
7. Complete the lateral mobilization of left colon.
8. Take down the splenic flexure, if indicated by tumor location (medial to lateral or lateral to medial).
9. Dissect and divide the mesorectum at the level of the promontory with division of superior hemorrhoidal vessels.

J.J. Hoballah and C.E.H. Scott-Conner (eds.), *Operative Dictations in General and Vascular Surgery*, DOI 10.1007/978-1-4614-0451-4_43,
© Springer Science+Business Media, LLC 2012

10. Transect the left colon distally at the rectosigmoid junction level with Endo GIA 3.8-mm stapler.
11. Perform a Pfannestiel (or left lower quadrant) access incision and place a wound protector.
12. Deliver the specimen, transect the colon proximally and place and appropriate sized EEA anvil proximally into the descending colon while ensuring adequate length and blood supply of colon.
13. Reinsert the colon and anvil back into the peritoneal cavity. Close the access incision in layers.
14. Perform a stapled EEA anastomosis.
15. Check the donuts and perform the air leak test.
16. Remove trocars under direct vision and close all fascial defects >10 mm.

NOTE THIS VARIATION

■ A hand assist technique may be used. In the hand assist technique, a small incision is strategically placed at the beginning of the operation and a specific hand assist device is used to allow the introduction of the non-dominant hand of the surgeon into the abdominal cavity to assist with the operation. The site is typically chosen so as the non-dominant hand does not interfere with the camera. The site can also be used for the extraction of the specimen and for the performance of the extracorporeal anastomosis. In the hand assist technique, the access incision is usually placed either in the midline (periumbilically) or in the left lower quadrant. The surgeon's hand is used to retract the small bowel, elevate the colon, and facilitate laparoscopic dissection.

COMPLICATIONS

■ Access-related complications (bowel injury, vascular injury, and retroperitoneal injury).
■ Vascular injury (bleeding).
■ Anastomotic complications (leak, fistula, twist, obstruction, and edema).

TEMPLATE OPERATIVE DICTATION

Preoperative diagnosis: List specific pathology indicating surgery *(see indications above)*, e.g., *malignant neoplasm of descending colon.*

Procedure: Laparoscopic left hemicolectomy.

Postoperative diagnosis: List specific intraoperative findings, e.g., *malignant neoplasm of descending colon*.

Indications: This ___-year-old *male/female* patient was found to have list specific preoperative diagnosis. Staging workup was completed and showed ____. *He/she* is now presenting for elective laparoscopic left hemicolectomy. The indications, alternatives and risks, and benefits of the surgery were discussed with the patient and informed consent was obtained.

Details of operation: The patient was brought to the operating room and placed on the operating table in the lithotomy position. The abdomen was clipped, prepped with 2% Chlorhexidine solution, and draped in the standard fashion. A time-out was completed verifying correct patient, procedure, site, positioning, and implant(s) and/or special equipment prior to beginning this procedure.

[Choose one:]

A Verres needle was introduced into the abdominal cavity and penumoperitoenum was achieved and a 10 mm optical trocar was inserted.

An open approach was used to access the peritoneal cavity. Using the S retractors, the subcutaneous tissue was dissected all the way down to the fascia. The fascia was grasped between two Kocher clamp and opened using the 11 blade vertically. The peritoneum was then incised and the trocar placed under direct vision.

An additional 12-mm trocar was then placed under direct vision in the right lower quadrant and two additional 5-mm trocars one on the right anterior axillary line at the level of umbilicus and another on the left anterior axillary line at the level of the umbilicus. A 5-mm trocar was placed in the suprapubic area to allow the assistant to retract the sigmoid colon.

The patient was then positioned in 30° Trendelenburg and with the patient's left side up to allow for small bowel to drop out of the operative field. The sigmoid was grasped with the assistant's hand lifted up to tent the IMA. The dissection was then started at the base of the IMA, at its takeoff from the aorta. The peritoneum overlying the takeoff of the IMA was opened using ____. This incision in the peritoneum was carried all the way up to the base of the ligament of Treitz and inferiorly to the level of peritoneal reflection. The IMA was then dissected near its origin from the aorta. This was coupled with a retroperitoneal dissection (using a traction counter-traction technique and gentle sweeping) along the plane of the Toldt fascia to identify and preserve the left ureter at this level. Once the left ureter has been clearly identified, the IMA was divided using ____. The dissection was then continued in the avascular plane anterior to the Toldt fascia cephalad to the level of the ligament of Treitz and distally to the level of the peritoneal reflection taking care to preserve the left ureter throughout its course. At this stage, the hypogastric plexus of nerves was identified at the level of the pelvic brim and preserved. The lateral mobilization of the colon was then carried out by dividing any lateral attachments of the descending in sigmoid colon as well as dividing the white line of told. This dissection was carried on retroperitoneally until it met with the medial-to-lateral dissection that had already been done. The dissection was also carried out upward to the level of the splenic flexure.

If splenic flexure mobilized: *The mobilization of the splenic flexure was performed to allow sufficient length of colon to perform a tension-free anastomosis.* **Choose one:** *Dissection progressed along the white line of Toldt with subsequent division of omental attachments to distal transverse colon and the splenic felxure takedown was completed from lateral to medial. The mesenteric dissection was continued in a medial to lateral approach cephalad all the way up to the tail of the pancreas and the retroperitoneal attachments of the mesentery of the transverse colon were incised at the inferior border of the tail of the pancreas. Completing the splenic flexure mobilization.*

The dissection was continued distally to the level of the rectosigmoid junction at the level of the peritoneal reflection and the mesentery of the colon at that level was dissected with ____ including division of the superior hemorrhoidal vessels. The colon at that level was transected with an Endo GIA 60-mm stapling device with 3.8-mm staples. An access incision was then made in the *Pfannenstiel manner in the suprapubic area/left lower quadrant via a muscle splitting incision*. A wound protector was inserted and the specimen delivered through this access incision. Completion of the mesenteric transection proximately was done. Care was taken to ensure grossly negative margins and removal of all of the mesentery of the left colon for a proper lymphadenectomy. The colon was transected proximally. A running over and over 2-0 prolene suture was used to tighten the proximal colon onto the appropriate sized anvil.

The colon and the anvil were then reintroduced back into the peritoneal cavity. The access incision was closed in layers with 3-0 Vicryl for the peritoneal layer and number one PDS for the fascia. Reinsufflation of the abdominal cavity was carried out. The EEA stapler was then introduced into the anus following gentle dilatation and appropriate lubrication. It was guided under direct vision up to the level of the distal staple line on the rectal stump. The spike of the EEA device was then deployed to pierce the rectal stump, the anvil was then attached to this spike, and the EEA device is closed and fired to perform a stapled end-to-end anastomosis. The doughnuts produced by the EEA stapler were checked to ensure that they were complete. Furthermore, an air leak test was carried out by insufflating air gently into the rectum, while the anastomosis was bathed underwater. A clamp was placed on the proximal colon to prevent its distention. Once the anastomosis was properly tested, the patient was repositioned back in the normal anatomical position. The trocars were removed under direct vision and any fascial defects larger than 10 mm closed with a number one PDS suture. The skin was closed with 4-0 PDS sutures in a running fashion and a dry sterile dressing is applied. The sponge and instrument count were correct, blood loss was minimal, and there were no complications. The patient tolerated the procedure well and was transferred to the post-anesthesia care unit in stable condition.

NOTES

Chapter 44
Low Anterior Resection

Eanas S. Yassa, M.D. and John C. Byrn, M.D.

INDICATION
- Carcinoma of the rectosigmoid colon higher than 5 cm from the anal verge.

ESSENTIAL STEPS
1. *Combined lithotomy–supine position*.
2. Lower midline incision.
3. Explore the abdomen for metastatic disease (liver and peritoneum and ovaries in female).
4. Incise the line of Toldt to free the rectosigmoid colon from peritoneal attachment.
5. Identify and protect both ureters.
6. *Mobilize the splenic flexure*.
7. Transect the bowel proximally and distally.
8. Ligate the mesenteric vessels and remove the specimen (tag proximal and distal ends).
9. *Stapled/sutured* anastomosis.
10. Check the anastomosis for patency and integrity.
11. Place drains.
12. Close the abdomen.

NOTE THESE VARIATIONS
- Note and document any metastatic disease.
- *Stapled* vs. *sutured* anastomosis.

J.J. Hoballah and C.E.H. Scott-Conner (eds.), *Operative Dictations in General and Vascular Surgery*, DOI 10.1007/978-1-4614-0451-4_44,
© Springer Science+Business Media, LLC 2012

- *Size of stapler/type of suture.*
- *Add diverting loop ileostomy, if integrity of the anastomosis is in question or if anastomosis is at less than 7 cm from anal verge.*

COMPLICATIONS
- Injury to the ureters.
- Injury to the spleen.
- Anastomotic leak.

TEMPLATE OPERATIVE DICTATION

Preoperative diagnosis: Carcinoma of the rectosigmoid colon.

Procedure: Low anterior resection with primary anastomosis.

Postoperative diagnosis: Same *(enumerate any metastatic disease found)*.

Indications: This ____-year-old *male/female* with *abdominal pain/ bleeding/obstructive symptoms* was found to have carcinoma of the rectosigmoid colon located ____ cm from the anal verge. Workup with *computed tomography scan of the abdomen and pelvis and CXR* revealed *no evidence of metastatic disease/other*. Elective resection was indicated.

Description of procedure: *An epidural catheter was placed by anesthesia prior to the start of the operation.* The patient was placed in the *combined lithotomy–supine* position and general endotracheal anesthesia was induced. Preoperative antibiotics were given. A Foley catheter and orogastric tube were placed. The abdomen was prepped and draped in the usual sterile fashion. A time-out was completed verifying correct patient, procedure, site, positioning, and implant(s) and/or special equipment prior to beginning this procedure. A lower midline incision was made from just above the umbilicus to the pubic symphysis. This was deepened through the subcutaneous tissues and hemostasis was achieved with electrocautery. The linea alba was identified and incised and the peritoneal cavity entered sharply. The abdomen was explored. *Adhesions were lysed sharply under direct vision with Metzenbaum scissors. A mass was palpated in the descending colon.* The liver, omentum, peritoneum, *and ovaries (if present)* were inspected for the evidence of metastatic disease. *Metastatic disease was noted ____/no metastatic disease was noted.*

The small bowel was inspected and retracted to the right using a moist towel and self-retaining retractor. Using electrocautery, the colon was freed from its peritoneal attachments along the line of Toldt proximally from the splenic flexure and distally to the pelvic inlet. Left ureter was identified and protected. Omentum was freed from the transverse colon and the splenic flexure was mobilized.

With the descending colon and splenic flexure rotated medially, the plane anterior to the aorta was entered and colon, mesenteric fat were mobilized from the retroperitoneum overlying the sacral promontory and into the pelvis. The sympathetic plexus at the IMA origin was protected, as was the left ureter and gonadal vessel. The mesentery was scored and the inferior mesenteric artery identified and ligated at its origin with *2-0 silk/using a ligasure device*. A proximal point of division was selected, and the colon was divided using a linear cutting stapler.

The mesorectum was then mobilized posteriorly using sharp dissection. Care was taken not to enter the presacral venous plexus. The lateral rectal stalks were divided using medial traction and electrocautery. Anteriorly the plane between the *bladder and rectum/prostate and rectum* (Denonvilliers fascia) was incised and the mesorectal plane mobilized anteriorly. The lesion was palpable and the rectum was carefully elevated until an adequate distal margin was noted. This was confirmed with digital rectal exam or rigid sigmoidoscopy.

[Choose one:]

If stapled: A reticulating linear stapler was then used to divide the rectum at least __ cm distal to the palpable lesion. Proximal and distal ends of the bowel were tagged and the specimen removed and sent to pathology. The proximal colon was carefully inspected, noted to reach easily into the pelvis and to have an excellent blood supply. Mesenteric fat was cleared from the distal centimeter of bowel. The field was isolated with laparotomy pads and the bowel opened and sized. It was determined that a ____ mm circular stapler could be accommodated. A purse-string suture of 3-0 nylon/prolene was placed, the anvil was inserted, and the purse-string suture was tied. The circular stapler was introduced through the anus and guided under direct vision along the rectal stump. The "spike" was pierced through the midportion of the staple line/anterior taenia adjacent to the staple line. The proximal bowel with anvil in place was engaged with the circular stapler and the stapler was then fired. The anastomosis was tested for leaks with irrigation solution and air introduced through the rectum and was found to be patent and intact. Two complete donuts were obtained and submitted to pathology, after being marked as proximal and distal.

If sutured: The proximal bowel was brought down to the pelvis and made to lie comfortably in a end-to-end fashion. Using retractors to assist with exposure, an anastomosis was then constructed using interrupted 3-0 Vicryl ± an outer layer of interrupted 3-0 silk Lembert sutures. The anastomosis was checked and found to be patent and intact.

The pelvis was then copiously irrigated. Hemostasis was again checked. Closed suction drain was placed in the pelvis to lay posterior to the anastomosis and brought out through a separate stab incision.

***If a diverting loop ileostomy created:** A suitably mobile loop of ileum is selected and confirmed to reach to the anterior abdominal wall and the site of ostomy marking. A window is made in the mesentery and an umbilical tape passed. A marking stitch was placed/the serosa was scored with electrocautery to ensure distal and proximal orientation was maintained. Kocher clamps were used to maintain alignment of the dermis and fascia. An ellipse of skin was excised at the site of ostomy marking and the subcutaneous tissues divided vertically. Using hand held retractors, the anterior rectus fascia was exposed and vertically incised for a length of approximately 2–3 cm. Rectus fibers were spread in the direction of their travel and the posterior rectus fascia was incised with care taken to protect the underlying bowel. Ostomy hole admitted two fingers. The loop of bowel was passed through and orientation confirmed. Ostomy was checked to ensure no tension or torsion. Fascia and skin were closed as below and the ostomy was matured using 3-0 chromic/vicryl in an eccentric/brooke fashion to open and allow drainage from the proximal limb. Ostomy bag was applied.*

(Optional: Multiple interrupted through-and-through retention sutures of ____were placed.) The fascia was closed with *a running suture of ____/a Smead-Jones closure of interrupted ____*. The skin was closed with *skin staples/subcuticular sutures of____/other.*

The patient tolerated the procedure well was extubated in the operating room and was taken to the postanesthesia care unit in stable condition.

ACKNOWLEDGMENT

This chapter was contributed by Nate Thepjatri, MD in the first edition.

NOTES

Chapter 45

Laparoscopic Low Anterior Resection

Mohammad Khreiss, M.D. and Vassiliki Liana Tsikitis, M.D.

INDICATION

- Rectal adenocarcinoma.

ESSENTIAL STEPS

1. Place the patient in the lithotomy position, with both arms tucked and well padded. Secure the patient carefully to the table to avoid movement when the table is tilter. Place a Foley catheter and an orogastric tube.
2. Perform rigid proctosigmoidoscopy to identify and mark the distal margin from the anal verge.
3. We perform a diverting loop ileostomy for all anastomosis less than 5 cm from the anal verge.
4. Placement of four trocars: Three 5-mm trocars in the supraumbilical, left lower abdomen and one suprapubic, one 12-mm trocar in the right lower abdomen (use the site that was marked by the enterostomy nurse for this trocar; this will be the site of the future diverting ileostomy if needed).
5. Explore the abdomen for the evidence of metastatic disease.
6. Place the patient in steep Trendelenburg position.
7. Mobilize the left colon from medial to lateral and identify the vascular pedicle. Have the assistant elevate this pedicle at the level of the sacral promontory.
8. Create and enlarge an opening in the peritoneum. Sweep the retroperitoneum downwards while the mesentery

J.J. Hoballah and C.E.H. Scott-Conner (eds.), *Operative Dictations in General and Vascular Surgery*, DOI 10.1007/978-1-4614-0451-4_45,
© Springer Science+Business Media, LLC 2012

of the colon is lifted upwards and identify the left ureter and gonadal vessels. Sweep these back into the retroperitoneum.

9. Identify the superior rectal artery of the IMA and divide it with the surgeon's preferred energy source device. Alternatively, high ligation of the IMA at its origin can be performed, but has not been found to offer an oncologic benefit.

10. Mobilize the descending colon laterally along the white line of Toldt all the way up to the splenic flexure.

11. Lift the rectum and mesorectum anteriorly.

12. Start the dissection along the presacral fascia in the avascular plane (use sharp dissection with electrocautery).

13. Identify the hypogastric nerves and isolate them.

14. Continue the dissection all the way down to the levator muscles posteriorly (to the pelvic floor).

15. Proceed with the lateral dissection and take down the lateral stalks of the rectum protecting the ureters at all time.

16. In a female, a stitch may be placed in the uterus to fix the uterus to the anterior abdominal wall if the uterus obstructs the anterior plane of dissection.

17. The anterior dissection is done as the rectum is retracted posteriorly and the prostate/vagina retracted anteriorly. Continue the dissection down to the levator ani muscles.

18. Divide the rectum using a reticulated laparoscopic stapler at a point distal to the mass such that a negative margin is respected.

19. Create a Pfannenstiel's incision, apply the wound protector.

20. Exteriorize the sigmoid colon and the rectum through the incision.

21. Divide the mesentery of the sigmoid and divide the colon at the level of the sigmoid with a stapler or a thermal device of the operating surgeon's choice.

22. Send the specimen to pathology and check for adequacy of the distal margin (at least 1 cm distal margin).

23. Perform a rectal exam, dilate the anus, and measure the adequate diameter with sizers before choosing the size of the circular stapler.

24. Open the staple line of the proximal colon and insert the anvil, we prefer that the spike of the anvil comes out 1 cm at the side of the tenia coli. Close the defect either with a linear staple or in a hand sewn manner. Place a purse

string suture around the anvil (we prefer a side-to-end anastomosis).

25. Perform a side-to-end anastomosis using the CEEA. Make sure that the mesentery of the colon is in the proper alignment and that there is no tension at the anastomosis (mesentery of the colon should be medial).

26. Perform a rigid proctosigmoidoscopy and check the anastomotic line.

27. Test the anastomosis with air insufflation, with the pelvis filled with saline.

28. Identify the ileocecal valve at this time.

29. *If ileostomy is elected*:
    - Run the small bowel proximally and identify a point around 25–30 cm proximal to ileocecal valve.
    - Use the 12-mm trocar site to construct an ileostomy site and exteriorize the small bowel.
    - Mature the loop ileostomy in the regular fashion. Make sure that there is no twist in the mesentery of the small bowel.

30. Check for adequate hemostasis and suction all fluid in the pelvis.

31. Remove all trocars under vision.

32. Close the Pfannenstiel incision.

33. Close skin with a running subcuticular monocryl suture at all trocar sites and Pfannestiel incision.

34. *Apply a dressing and stoma appliance (connect the stoma bag to the stoma base before applying it to the skin)*.

35. Extubate patient and transfer to PACU.

NOTE THESE VARIATIONS

- The abdomen may be entered using an open Hassan's technique.
- A hand-assisted procedure may be employed. Hand port is placed at the site of the Pfannenstiel's incision at the beginning of the case.
- The IMA and IMV may be divided at the beginning of the procedure and the dissection can be carried medially up to the level of the splenic flexure.
- The IMA/IMV may be divided, if there is not enough length or if there is tension at the anastomosis. The transverse colon can also be further mobilized in this situation.
- The diverting loop ileostomy is optional.

COMPLICATIONS

- Injury to small bowel.
- Injury to both ureters (this could happen upon identifying the left ureter originally or during lateral dissection of the rectum).
- Injury to the spleen.
- Injury to the hypogastric nerves.
- Injury to the posterior wall of the vagina.
- Anastomotic leak.
- Bleeding from the presacral venous plexus.
- Injury to left common iliac vessels.
- Injury to the rectum itself.
- Sexual dysfunction.

TEMPLATE OPERATIVE DICTATION

Preoperative diagnosis: Rectal cancer s/p neoadjuvant chemoradiotherapy.

Procedure: Rigid sigmoidoscopy, laparoscopic low anterior resection with colorectal stapled anastomosis. *Diverting loop ileostomy*.

Postoperative diagnosis: Same.

Indications: The patient is ___-year-old *male/female* recently diagnosed with rectal cancer.

Description of procedure: After general anesthesia was established, the patient was placed in the lithotomy position using allen stirrups. The abdomen and perineal areas were prepped and draped in the regular manner. A time-out was completed verifying correct patient, procedure, site, positioning, and implant(s) and/or special equipment prior to beginning this procedure. Preoperative antibiotics and DVT prophylaxis were given. Insufflation of the abdominal cavity was done with a *Veress needle/Hassan cannula/optical trocar* after a *5-/10-mm* supraumbilical incision was made. Pneumoperitoneum was established. Exploration of the abdominal cavity took place to rule out any metastatic disease. The liver and peritoneum were examined and no metastasis was identified. Following that, two 5-mm trocars were inserted in the suprapubic area in the midline and in the left lower quadrant. A 12-mm trocar was inserted in the right lower quadrant. The sigmoid colon was then retracted anteriorly and the vascular pedicle was identified. An incision in the peritoneum was done at the level of the sacral promontory and dissection was carried out to bring up the mesentery of the sigmoid from the retroperitoneum. The left ureter and the gonadal vessels are identified and protected at all times. Dissection then was carried laterally along the white line of

Toldt until the splenic flexure was reached. All the splenic flexure attachments were taken down either with bovie electrocautery. *The sigmoidal branches and the superior rectal vessels of the IMA were then identified and divided with a thermal device/the IMA was identified and divided at its origin.* After that posterior dissection of the rectum was done in the presacral space using electrocautery till the levator ani muscles to complete the posterior portion of TME. Lateral dissection was performed. Care was taken to avoid injury to the ureters. The lateral attachments were taken down using bovie electrocautery. Anteriorly, the peritoneal reflection was opened up and the dissection was carried distally. The dissection was carried down till the levators. The mesentery of the rectum was taken down with thermal device about 2 cm inferior to the tumor height. The rectum was then divided using a laproscopic stapler. Following that a 6 cm Pfannenstiel incision was done. The specimen was exteriorized through the incision after applying the wound protector. The sigmoid was divided with the stapler. Sizers were used to measure the diameter of the rectum and a 29-mm CEEA stapler was used. A purse string suture was applied around the Tenia coli on the antimesenteric side of the colon. A small opening was done in the staple line and the anvil was inserted. The spike was inserted through the Tenia at a point 1 cm proximal to the staple line that was now closed with a new stapler. After that a side-to-end stapled anastomosis was performed using the 29-mm CEEA stapler. Donuts were inspected and found to be intact. St Mark's retractor was used to achieve adequate exposure of the pelvis. The anastomosis was checked for leak using air insufflation test. Rigid sigmoidoscopy was also performed carefully to check the staple line. There was no evidence of tension at the anastomosis.

If Diverting Loop Ileostomy: *The ileocecal valve was identified. The small bowel was run and at a point 25 cm from the ileocecal valve the small bowel was exteriorized through the right 12-mm trochar site. A loop ileostomy was fashioned in the regular manner.*

Hemostasis was secured. All trocars were removed under vision. There was no evidence of any trocar site bleeding. The abdomen was irrigated with saline. Closure of the Pfannenstiel's incision was done using number 1 vicryl interrupted sutures. The skin was closed using 4.0 monocryl subcuticular sutures. The same was done to the port sites. Dressing was applied. The stoma appliance was then applied. Patient was extubated and transferred to the PACU in good condition.

NOTES

Chapter 46
Abdominoperineal Resection

Eanas S. Yassa, M.D. and John C. Byrn, M.D.

INDICATION

- Carcinoma of the anus/rectum when sphincter sparing procedure not feasible.

ESSENTIAL STEPS

1. Combined lithotomy–supine position.
2. Lower midline incision.
3. Explore the abdomen for metastatic disease (liver and peritoneum and ovaries in female).
4. *Rigid sigmoidoscopy/digital rectal exam to confirm level of the lesion and sphincter involvement (can also be done prior to incision or at any point prior to division of colon).*
5. Incise the line of Toldt to free the rectosigmoid colon from the peritoneal attachment.
6. Identify and protect both ureters.
7. Transect the bowel proximally.
8. Ligate the mesenteric vessels.
9. Incise the peritoneum and elevate from the hollow of sacrum, circumferentially to levators.
10. Working from below, incise from skin around the anus.
11. Enter the peritoneal cavity in posterior midline; incise levators anteriorly.
12. Pass the specimen through posteriorly.
13. Complete anterior dissection.
14. *If male: Avoid injury to the urethra.*

J.J. Hoballah and C.E.H. Scott-Conner (eds.), *Operative Dictations in General and Vascular Surgery*, DOI 10.1007/978-1-4614-0451-4_46, © Springer Science+Business Media, LLC 2012

15. *If female: May excise back wall of the vagina with the specimen.*
16. Place drains.
17. Make an opening for the colostomy.
18. Deliver the colon, tack to the peritoneum.
19. Close the abdomen and perineum.
20. Mature colostomy.

NOTE THESE VARIATIONS
■ Note and document any metastatic disease.
■ *If female: Excision of part of back wall of the vagina.*

COMPLICATIONS
■ Injury to ureters.
■ Injury to the urethra (male).
■ Hemorrhage from the presacral venous plexus.
■ Non-healing perineal wound.
■ Sexual dysfunction.

TEMPLATE OPERATIVE DICTATION
Preoperative diagnosis: Carcinoma of the anus/rectum.
Procedure: Abdominoperineal resection of the anus and rectum.
Postoperative diagnosis: Same *(enumerate any metastatic disease found)*.
Indications: This ____-year-old *male/female* with *abdominal pain/ bleeding/obstructive symptoms* was found to have carcinoma of the rectum located *at/____ cm from* the anal verge or involving the sphincter complex. Workup with *computed tomography scan of the abdomen and pelvis and CXR for evaluation of metastatic disease, and MRI/endorectal ultrasound for the evaluation of locoregional spread* revealed ____. Elective resection was indicated. Because of *proximity to sphincter complex/concern for functional outcome with low anastomosis/other____* abdominoperineal resection was chosen.
Description of procedure: *An epidural catheter was placed by anesthesia prior to the start of the operation.* The patient was placed in the supine position and general endotracheal anesthesia was induced. Preoperative antibiotics were given. A Foley catheter and orogastric tube were placed. The patient was then positioned in *Lloyd-Davies/other* stirrups with care taken to pad all pressure points. The abdomen and perineum were prepped and draped in the usual sterile fashion. A time-out was completed verifying correct patient, procedure, site, positioning, and implant(s) and/

or special equipment prior to beginning this procedure. *Procedure was begun with digital rectal exam and/or rigid sigmoidoscopy to confirm the level of the lesion.* A lower midline incision was made from just above the umbilicus to the pubic symphysis. This was deepened through the subcutaneous tissues and hemostasis was achieved with electrocautery. The linea alba was identified and incised and the peritoneal cavity entered. The abdomen was explored. *Adhesions were lysed sharply under direct vision with Metzenbaum scissors. A mass was palpated in the descending colon.* The liver, omentum, peritoneum, *and ovaries (if present)* were inspected for the evidence of metastatic disease. *Metastatic disease was noted ____/no metastatic disease was noted.*

The small bowel was inspected and retracted to the right using a moist towel and self-retaining retractor. Using electrocautery, the colon was freed from its peritoneal attachments along the line of Toldt beginning distally at the pelvic inlet and proceeding proximally to the splenic flexure. Both ureters were identified and protected.

With the descending colon and splenic flexure rotated medially, the plane anterior to the aorta was entered and colon, mesenteric fat were mobilized from the retroperitoneum overlying the sacral promontory and into the pelvis. The sympathetic plexus at the IMA origin was protected, as was the left ureter and gonadal vessel. The mesentery was scored and the inferior mesenteric artery identified and ligated at its origin with *2-0 silk/using a ligasure device.* A proximal point of division was selected and the colon was divided using a linear cutting stapler.

The mesorectum was then mobilized posteriorly using sharp dissection. Care was taken not to enter the presacral venous plexus. The lateral rectal stalks were divided using medial traction and electrocautery. Anteriorly, the plane between the *bladder and rectum/prostate and rectum* (denonvilliers fascia) was incised and the mesorectal plane mobilized anteriorly.

The lesion was palpable and the rectum was carefully elevated until the level of the coccyx/coning of the mesentery was identified.

Attention was then turned to the perineal phase of the dissection. The bony prominences of the ischial tuberosities were marked bilaterally, the coccyx and the perineal body were marked. An elliptical incision was made connecting these points and encompassing the anus *(if female, optional) and extending up to include a portion of the back wall of the vagina.* Dissection then progressed through subcutaneous tissues circumferentially. Hemostasis was achieved with electrocautery. *If male: The transversus perinei muscle was identified and dissection was kept posterior to this anatomic landmark to avoid injury to the prostate and urethra.* The abdomen was entered posterior to the anus in the midline and anterior to the coccyx. The levators were then divided with electrocautery beginning posteriorly and progressing anteriorly. The specimen was delivered through this posterior incision into the perineal field. The remaining anterior attachments were then severed (*in the male: care was taken to palpate the foley catheter and avoid injury to the urethra*) and the specimen removed. Hemostasis was achieved in the pelvis and perineal wound.

The perineal skin was closed with *skin staples/subcuticular sutures of ____/vertical mattress sutures of 3-0 nylon/vicryl. The back wall of the vagina was carefully reapproximated and closed with a subcuticular suture of running 4-0 monocryl.*

The abdominal cavity was then copiously irrigated. Hemostasis was again checked. A closed suction drain was passed via a separate stab incision and placed in the pelvis. A tongue of omentum was brought to lay in the pelvis over the rectal fossa. *The pelvic peritoneum was closed with running 3-0 Vicryl.* A disk of skin was removed in the preselected site for the colostomy. This incision was deepened through subcutaneous tissues, fascial layers, and rectus muscle in a muscle splitting fashion until an opening sufficient for two fingers was created. The colon was then delivered through this opening without tension or torsion. *It was tacked circumferentially to the peritoneum with interrupted 3-0 silk and laterally to the peritoneum in such a manner as to eliminate the lateral trap.* Attention was then turned to abdominal closure.

(Optional: Multiple interrupted through-and-through retention sutures of ____ were placed.) The fascia was closed with *a running suture of ____/a Smead-Jones closure of interrupted ____.* The skin was closed with *skin staples/subcuticular sutures of ____/other.* A dressing was applied.

The colostomy was then matured with multiple interrupted sutures of 3-0 Vicryl placed in such a way as to tack the full thickness of the edge of the colon to a subcuticular layer of the skin. An ostomy appliance was placed.

The patient was repositioned in the supine position and a dressing of *kerlix fluffs/ABD pads/mesh shorts* was applied to the perineal wound. The patient was extubated in the operating room after tolerating the procedure well and was taken to the postanesthesia care unit in stable condition.

NOTES

Chapter 47

Laparoscopic Abdominoperineal Resection

Mohammad Khreiss, M.D. and Vassiliki Liana Tsikitis, M.D.

INDICATIONS

- Low rectal adenocarcinoma; location precludes adequate 1 cm distal margin for a sphincter preserving procedure.
- Melanoma of the anorectum involving the sphincters.
- Anal carcinoma recurrence after Nigro protocol.

ESSENTIAL STEPS

1. Place patient in the lithotomy position with both arms tucked and well padded. Secure the patient carefully to the operating table, to avoid movement when the table is steeply tilted. Place a Foley catheter and an orogastric tube. Close the anus with a purse string stitch.

2. Place four trocars: three 5-mm trocars are used; one supraumbilical, one in the left lower abdomen (in the site marked by the enterostomal nurse for the end colostomy), and one suprapubic. Place a 12-mm trocar in the right lower abdomen.

3. Explore the abdomen for the evidence of metastatic disease.

4. Place the patient in steep Trendelenburg position.

5. Mobilize the left colon from medial to lateral, identifying and elevating the inferior mesenteric artery (IMA) at the level of the sacral promontory so that the left ureter can be identified. Once the left ureter and the gonadal vessels are identified, sweep them back into the retroperitoneum.

J.J. Hoballah and C.E.H. Scott-Conner (eds.), *Operative Dictations in General and Vascular Surgery*, DOI 10.1007/978-1-4614-0451-4_47,

6. Identify the superior rectal artery of the IMA and divide it with the surgeon's energy source device. Alternatively, the IMA may be divided at its origin.

7. Mobilize the descending colon laterally along the white line of Toldt all the way up to the splenic flexure. The degree of mobilization depends on the colon length needed to create the end colostomy.

8. Life the rectum and mesorectum anteriorly.

9. Identify the hypogastric nerves posteriorly and isolate them.

10. Start the dissection along the presacral fascia in the avascular plane (use sharp dissection with electrocautery) and continue the dissection down to the levator muscles posteriorly (to the pelvic floor).

11. Then proceed with the lateral dissection and take down the lateral stalks of the rectum while protecting the ureters at all time.

12. In a female, elevate the uterus with a stitch to the anterior abdominal wall, if it obstructs the anterior plane of dissection.

13. Continue the anterior dissection to the levator ani muscles as the rectum is retracted posteriorly and the prostate/vagina is retracted anteriorly.

14. Divide the colon at the level of the sigmoid using the laparoscopic stapler and keep the orientation so the colon does not twist as it is exteriorized for the construction of the stoma. The colostomy is constructed at the end of the case.

15. Place one pelvic drain through the right lower quadrant trocar.

16. Proceed with the perineal portion of the resection (the specimen has been freed from all attachments and is at the pelvic floor).

17. Perform an elliptical incision around the anus involving the sphincteric complex and enter the peritoneal cavity after the anococcygeal ligament is incised.

18. Free the specimen circumferentially and pass it through the perineal incision. Care must be taken not to injure the vagina in a woman and the urethra in a man when the last part (anterior) of the specimen dissection from the levators takes place.

19. Close the pelvic incision in layers.

20. Close the fascia at the 12-mm trocar site.

21. Close the skin at the trocar sites in a subcuticular manner.
22. Mature the stoma with 3.0 vicryl stitches and apply an ostomy appliance.

NOTE THESE VARIATIONS

- The abdomen may be entered using an open Hassan's technique or using the optiview camera if a 5-mm camera is used.
- Level of division of vascular pedicle (high ligation of the IMA/IMV is optional and has not been shown to convey oncologic benefits).
- The skin of the perineal incision may be closed with interrupted sutures.

COMPLICATIONS

- Injury to small bowel.
- Injury to both ureters (this could happen upon identifying the left ureter originally or during lateral dissection of the rectum).
- Injury to the spleen.
- Injury to the sympathetic and parasympathetic nerves leading to sexual dysfunction.
- Injury to the posterior wall of the vagina in a female.
- Injury to the bladder.
- Bleeding from the pelvic venous plexus.
- Injury to left common iliac vessels.
- Injury to the rectum itself.
- Pelvic collection.
- Dehiscence of the perineal wound.

TEMPLATE OPERATIVE DICTATION

Preoperative diagnosis: *Low rectal cancer/anal carcinoma.*
Procedure: Laparoscopic Abdominoperineal Resection with end colostomy.
Postoperative diagnosis: Same.
Indications: The patient is _____-year-old *male/female* diagnosed with *low rectal cancer/anal carcinoma after failure of NIGRO protocol/other.*
Description of procedure: Under general anesthesia, the patient was placed in the lithotomy position using Allen stirrups. The anus was closed using a 2.0 silk suture. The abdomen and perineal areas were prepped and draped in the regular manner.

A time-out was completed verifying correct patient, procedure, site, positioning, and implant(s) and/or special equipment prior to beginning this procedure. Antibiotics were given. Insufflation of the abdominal cavity was done with the optiview camera after a 5-mm supraumbilical incision is made. Pneumoperitoneum was established. Exploration of the abdominal cavity took place to rule out any metastatic disease. The liver and peritoneum were examined and no metastasis was identified.

Next, two 5-mm trocars were inserted in the suprapubic area in the midline and in the left lower quadrant. A 12-mm trocar was inserted in the right lower quadrant. The sigmoid colon was then retracted anteriorly and the vascular pedicle was identified. An incision in the peritoneum was done and dissection was carried through the mesentery of the sigmoid. The left ureter was identified and isolated. Dissection was carried laterally along the white line of Toldt until the splenic flexure and then the flexure was taken down. *The sigmoidal branches and the superior rectal vessels of the IMA were then identified and divided with _____/the IMA was identified and divided at its origin with _____.* Posterior dissection of the rectum was performed in the presacral space using electrocautery until the levator ani muscles to complete the posterior portion of TME. Lateral dissection was performed. Care was taken to avoid injury to the ureters and the iliac vessels. The lateral attachments were taken down using *electrocautery/_____.* Anteriorly the peritoneal reflection was opened up and the dissection was carried distally. The dissection was carried down till the levators. The sigmoid colon was then divided using the laparoscopic stapler. We made certain that the proximal colon reached the abdominal wall freely. The completely dissected recturm was tucked into the pelvis to facilitate removal through the perineum. The colon was exteriorized through the left trocar site whose size was augmented and an end colostomy was fashioned in the regular manner. All trocars were removed under vision. There was no bleeding from the trocar sites. The fascial defect at the 12-mm trochar site was closed using number 1 vicryl suture. The skin was closed using 4.0 monocryl subcuticular sutures. Dressing was applied. The stoma appliance was applied.

We then proceeded with the perineal part of the procedure. An elliptical incision around the anus was done. The dissection was carried down through skin and subcutaneous tissue posteriorly. We enter the pelvis anterior to the coccyx, after sharp dissection of the anococcygeal ligament. The levator muscles were divided both laterally with bovie electrocautery. We address possible bleeding from the inferior hemorrhoidal vessels with electrocautery.

The whole specimen was delivered through the perineal posterior incision. We proceeded with the anterior dissection of the perineum last. The specimen was removed and excellent hemostasis of the perineum was achieved. The perineal incision was then closed in layers. 3.0 Vicryl sutures were used for closure of the pelvic peritoneum, and 4.0 monocryl sutures for the skin closure. A pelvic drain was placed through a separate stab wound before closure. Patient tolerated the procedure well and was extubated and then transferred to PACU in a good condition.

NOTES

Chapter 48
Subtotal Colectomy with Ileostomy and Hartmann's Pouch

Samy Maklad, M.D. and John W. Cromwell, M.D.

INDICATION

- Emergency resection for lower gastrointestinal bleeding, ischemia, or intractable colitis when primary anastomosis is unwise.

ESSENTIAL STEPS

1. Midline incision.
2. Explore the abdomen.
3. Mobilize the right colon:
   - Incise lateral peritoneal reflection from the cecum to hepatic flexure.
   - Sharply divide adhesions of the colon to retroperitoneum.
   - Identify and protect the right ureter and duodenum.
4. Mobilize the transverse colon by sharply dividing greater omentum from the colon.
5. Mobilize the splenic flexure and left colon:
   - Incise the peritoneum lateral to the left colon from the splenic flexure to the sigmoid colon.
   - Reflect the colon medially, sharply dividing adhesions to the retroperitoneum.
   - Identify and protect the left ureter.
6. Identify points of transection on the terminal ileum and rectosigmoid colon.
7. Divide the terminal ileum with a linear cutting stapler.

J.J. Hoballah and C.E.H. Scott-Conner (eds.), *Operative Dictations in General and Vascular Surgery*, DOI 10.1007/978-1-4614-0451-4_48,
© Springer Science+Business Media, LLC 2012

8. Score the peritoneum overlying the intended line of mesenteric division.
9. Divide the mesentery, securing vessels with 2-0 silk ties and suture ligatures.
10. Identify the point of division on the rectosigmoid colon (in general above the peritoneal reflection, at the point where taeniae converge to form a continuous longitudinal muscle layer of rectum).
11. Divide the rectosigmoid colon with a linear cutting stapler and remove the specimen.
12. Check hemostasis.
13. Create an opening in the left lower quadrant for ileostomy.
14. Pass the terminal ileum through opening.
15. Anchor the terminal ileum to the peritoneum circumferentially.
16. Close the lateral peritoneal defect.
17. Close the abdomen.
18. Mature ileostomy.

NOTE THESE VARIATIONS
- Level of distal transection varies depending upon pathology.
- Hartmann's pouch may be tacked to the presacral fascia or marked with long monofilament sutures.

COMPLICATIONS
- Necrosis of ileostomy.
- Small bowel obstruction.

TEMPLATE OPERATIVE DICTATION
Preoperative diagnosis: *Lower gastrointestinal bleeding/ischemia/ intractable colitis*.
Procedure: Subtotal colectomy with end ileostomy.
Postoperative diagnosis: Same.
Indications: This ____-year-old *male/female* had *lower gastrointestinal bleeding/mesenteric ischemia/other* and on workup was found to have ____. Resection was required.
Description of procedure: An epidural catheter was placed by anesthesia prior to the start of the operation. The patient was placed in the supine position and general endotracheal anesthesia was induced. Preoperative antibiotics were given. A Foley

catheter and nasogastric tube were placed. The abdomen was prepped and draped in the usual sterile fashion. A time-out was completed verifying correct patient, procedure, site, positioning, and implant(s) and/or special equipment prior to beginning this procedure. A vertical midline incision was made. This was deepened through the subcutaneous tissues and hemostasis was achieved with electrocautery. The linea alba was identified and incised and the peritoneal cavity entered. The abdomen was explored. *Adhesions were lysed sharply under direct vision with Metzenbaum scissors*.

The abdominal cavity was inspected for gross abnormalities. *(Detail appearance of the colon and extent of disease.)* The small bowel was also inspected for the evidence of disease and was found to be normal. With the exception of the region of the terminal ileum, no blood was found in the lumen of the small bowel and there were no other abnormalities noted.

Initially, the right colon was mobilized by incising the peritoneal attachment from the cecum to the hepatic flexure. The colon and terminal ileum was mobilized medially, taking care to protect the duodenum and right ureter. The greater omentum was then taken from the transverse colon up to the splenic flexure. The lateral peritoneal attachment of the left colon was then incised from the splenic flexure to the sigmoid colon. The left colon was mobilized medially. Care was taken to protect the left ureter.

Points of division on the terminal ileum and rectosigmoid colon were then chosen. The bowel was divided with a linear cutting stapler. The mesentery was scored and divided. Mesenteric vessels were secured with ties and suture ligatures of 2-0 silk. The specimen was removed.

Hemostasis was checked. Attention was then turned to the right lower quadrant, where a disk of skin was excised at the previously marked site. This was deepened through the subcutaneous tissues and the fascia was incised. An opening in the abdominal wall sufficient to pass *two/three fingers* through was created. The ileum was passed through this opening and determined to lie comfortably without tension. The terminal ileum was tacked to the peritoneum circumferentially with interrupted sutures of 3-0 silk and the lateral peritoneal defect was obliterated with a running suture of 3-0 Vicryl.

(Optional: Multiple interrupted through-and-through retention sutures of ____ were placed.) The fascia was closed with *a running suture of ____/a Smead-Jones closure of interrupted ____*. The skin was closed with *skin staples/subcuticular sutures of____/other*.

A dressing was placed over the incision and the ileostomy was matured with multiple interrupted sutures of 3-0 Vicryl placed full thickness through the edge of the ileum, catching a submucosal bite at the skin level and then suturing the ileum to the subcuticular level of the skin. A nicely everted ileostomy with good protrusion was thus produced. An ostomy bag was applied.

The patient tolerated the procedure well and was taken to the postanesthesia care unit in stable condition.

ACKNOWLEDGMENT

This chapter was contributed by Mazen M. Hashisho, MD in the first edition.

NOTES

Chapter 49

Laparoscopic Subtotal Colectomy with Ileostomy and Hartmann's Pouch

Maher A. Abbas, M.D.

INDICATIONS
- Fulminant colitis.
- Acute lower gastrointestinal hemorrhage.

ESSENTIAL STEPS
1. Lithotomy position, both arms are tucked.
2. Foley catheter and orogastric tube are introduced.
3. 15 mmHg pneumoperitoneum.
4. Place five trocars.
   - Three 5-mm trocars in the supraumbilical, the right and left mid-abdomen.
   - Two 12-mm trocars in the right and left lower abdomen.
5. Place the table in Trendelenburg position.
6. Retract the sigmoid colon anteriorly and identify the inferior mesenteric artery.
7. Open the peritoneum at a level anterior to the inferior mesenteric artery and isolate the sigmoid vessels. Identify and protect the left ureter.
8. Divide the sigmoid vessels using a vascular stapler, an energy source, or clips.
9. Dissect more superior to identify the left colic vessels which are divided in a similar fashion.
10. Lift the mesocolon off the retroperitoneum from a medial to lateral approach and dissect as far as possible.
11. Place the patient in the reverse Trendelenburg position.

J.J. Hoballah and C.E.H. Scott-Conner (eds.), *Operative Dictations in General and Vascular Surgery*, DOI 10.1007/978-1-4614-0451-4_49,
© Springer Science+Business Media, LLC 2012

12. Mobilize the left colon from the lateral to medial approach by incising the lateral attachments.
13. Takedown the splenic flexure by lifting the omentum off the distal transverse colon and joining the dissection with the medially mobilized descending colon.
14. Identify and divide the middle colic vessels.
15. Lift the ascending colon anteriorly and identify the ileocolic artery and vein. Open a mesenteric window on both sides of these vascular structures.
16. Identify the duodenum and keep down toward the spine and away from the ileocolic vessels.
17. Divide the ileocolic vessels using a vascular stapler, an energy source, or clips.
18. Lift the right mesocolon off the retroperitoneum and dissect bluntly in this medial-to-lateral plane toward the hepatic flexure.
19. Mobilize the ascending colon from a lateral-to-medial approach by incising the lateral attachments.
20. Make a 10-cm Pfannenstiel's incision.
21. Exteriorize the colon and divide the bowel at the terminal ileum and rectosigmoid junction.
22. Bring an end ileostomy through a right lower quadrant trephine site previously marked by the enterostomal nurse or at the right lower quadrant trocar.
23. Remove all trocars under direct camera visualization and close the fascia of the 12-mm left lower quadrant trocar.
24. Close the skin at the trocar sites.
25. Cover all wounds.
26. Fashion an end ileostomy.

NOTE THESE VARIATIONS

- Hand-assisted subtotal colectomy with a hand port established at the beginning of the operation through a Pfannenstiel's incision.
- All five trocars can be 5 mm if no stapling is necessary (energy source is used for vascular pedicle division).

COMPLICATIONS

- Transection of the ureter.
- Perforation of the duodenum or stomach.
- Laceration of the spleen.
- Small bowel enterotomy.
- Stomal-related complications.

TEMPLATE OPERATIVE DICTATION

Preoperative diagnosis: Fulminant colitis (or lower gastrointestinal bleeding).

Procedure: Laparoscopic subtotal colectomy with end ileostomy and Hartmann's pouch.

Postoperative diagnosis: Same.

Indications: The patient is _____-year-old *male/female* with a history of _____. Different treatment options were discussed with the patient. The procedure of laparoscopic (possible open) subtotal colectomy with end ileostomy and Hartmann's pouch was reviewed with the patient. The procedure, indication, alternatives, risks, and complications were reviewed with the patient. The patient verbalized understanding and wished to proceed. Informed consent was obtained.

Description of procedure: The patient was brought to the operating room and after instillation of general endotracheal anesthesia, he/she was placed in the lithotomy position with both arms tucked. A time-out was completed verifying correct patient, procedure, site, positioning, and implant(s) and/or special equipment prior to beginning this procedure. Intravenous antibiotic and subcutaneous heparin were administered. A Foley catheter and an orogastric tube were inserted. All extremities were well padded. The rectum was irrigated with betadine. The abdomen and perineum were shaved and prepped in the usual sterile fashion.

Using a 5-mm supraumbilical incision, the abdomen was insufflated with a Veress needle and a 5-mm trocar was established. Under direct visualization, a 12-mm trocar was placed in the right lower quadrant and one in the left lower quadrant followed by two additional 5-mm trocars in the right and left midabdomen. The patient was placed in the Trendelenburg position. The sigmoid colon was grabbed and retracted anteriorly. The inferior mesenteric artery pedicle was identified and a mesenteric window was opened anterior to it. The sigmoid vessels were isolated and divided after identifying the left ureter which was kept out of harm's way. Next the left colic vessels were identified, isolated, and divided in a similar fashion. The left mesocolon was then lifted off the retroperitoneum from a medial to lateral approach and blunt dissection was carried out toward the splenic flexure. The patient was placed in the reverse Trendelenburg position and the left colon was mobilized from a lateral to medial approach by incising the lateral attachments. The splenic flexure was taken down by lifting the omentum off the distal transverse colon and joining the dissection with the mobilized descending colon. The transverse colon was lifted anteriorly and the middle colic vessels were identified, isolated, and divided with the laparoscopic vascular stapler. The ascending colon was lifted anteriorly and the ileocolic vessels were isolated by creating mesenteric windows on each side and divided with the laparoscopic vascular stapler after identifying the duodenum and keeping it out of harm's way toward the spine. The right mesocolon was lifted off the retroperitoneum and blunt dissection was carried from a medial to lateral approach toward the hepatic flexure. The hepatic flexure was taken down and the ascending colon was mobilized medially by incising the lateral attachments. A 10-cm Pfannenstiel's incision was made and a wound protector was placed. The terminal ileum and rectosigmoid colon were divided sequentially using a GIA 80-mm stapler. The specimen was sent for histologic evaluation. The abdomen was irrigated. The transected end of the terminal ileum was identified and brought through the right lower quadrant trocar site which was enlarged as a stomal trephine. It was secured above the skin with a clamp. Care was taken not to twist the ileostomy. All trocars were removed under direct camera visualization and the left lower quadrant fascial site closed with 0 vicryl in a figure of eight fashion. The trocar site skin wounds were closed with 3.0 vicryl suture in a subcuticular fashion. An end Brooke ileostomy was finally matured using 3.0 chromic sutures. Appliance was placed. All instruments, needles, and sponges count was correct times two. The patient tolerated the procedure well and was taken to the recovery unit in stable condition.

NOTES

Chapter 50

Total Proctocolectomy with Ileoanal Reservoir and Ileoanal Anastomosis

Danny Liu, M.D. and John W. Cromwell, M.D.

INDICATIONS
- Ulcerative or Crohn's colitis refractory to medical management.
- Familial polyposis syndromes.

ESSENTIAL STEPS
1. Combined lithotomy–supine position.
2. Midline incision.
3. Explore the abdomen.
4. Mobilize the right colon:
   - Incise the lateral peritoneal reflection from the cecum to the hepatic flexure.
   - Sharply divide adhesions of the colon to the retroperitoneum.
   - Identify and protect the right ureter and duodenum.
5. Mobilize the transverse colon by dividing greater omentum from the colon.
6. Mobilize the splenic flexure and left colon:
   - Incise the peritoneum lateral to the left colon from the sigmoid colon to splenic flexure.
   - Reflect the colon medially, sharply dividing adhesions to the retroperitoneum.
   - Identify and protect the left ureter.
7. Identify the point of transection on the terminal ileum.
8. Divide the terminal ileum with a linear cutting stapler carefully preserving the terminal ileal vasculature.

J.J. Hoballah and C.E.H. Scott-Conner (eds.), *Operative Dictations in General and Vascular Surgery*, DOI 10.1007/978-1-4614-0451-4_50,
© Springer Science+Business Media, LLC 2012

9. Score the peritoneum overlying the intended line of mesenteric division.
10. Divide the mesentery, securing vessels with 2-0 Vicryl ties and suture ligatures, or using Ligasure.
11. Incise the peritoneum and elevate the rectum along the TME plane.
12. Continue dissection circumferentially to levators, staying close to the rectum to avoid autonomic nerves.
13. Divide the rectum and remove the specimen.
14. Construct an ileal reservoir.
15. Perform stapled/sutured anastomosis from below.
16. *Place drain (optional).*
17. *Temporary diverting loop ileostomy (optional).*
18. Close the abdomen.

NOTE THESE VARIATIONS
- Mucosectomy vs. simple anastomosis.
- J vs. S vs. W reservoir.
- Optional temporary diverting loop ileostomy.

COMPLICATIONS
- Injury to the ureters.
- Hemorrhage from the presacral venous plexus.
- Sexual dysfunction.
- Urinary retention.
- Anastomotic leak/stricture.
- Incontinence.
- Infertility.

TEMPLATE OPERATIVE DICTATION
Preoperative diagnosis: *Ulcerative colitis/Crohn's colitis refractory to medical management/familial polyposis for cancer prophylaxis.*
Procedure: Total proctocolectomy with ileal reservoir and ileoanal anastomosis.
Postoperative diagnosis: Same.
Indications: This ___-year-old *male/female* has *ulcerative colitis refractory to medical management/familial polyposis*. Total proctocolectomy with ileal reservoir and ileoanal anastomosis was chosen for definitive management and cancer prophylaxis.
Description of procedure: The patient was brought to the operating room and placed in the supine position. General endotracheal anesthesia was induced without complications. A Foley catheter and *oral/naso*gastric tube were placed. The patient was then

positioned in *Lloyd-Davies/Allen* stirrups with care taken to pad all pressure points. The abdomen and perineum were prepped and draped in the usual sterile fashion. A time-out was completed verifying correct patient, procedure, site, positioning, and implant(s) and/or special equipment prior to beginning this procedure.

[Choose one:]

If mucosal proctectomy: The anus was gently dilated. Gelpi retractors/Lone Star retractor were placed to expose the dentate line and evert the anus. A solution of dilute epinephrine was infiltrated in the submucosal plane. An incision was made at the dentate line and the mucosal excised in a sleeve-like fashion to a distance ___ cm above the dentate line. It was divided, excised, and submitted to pathology. Hemostasis was achieved with electrocautery.

A vertical midline incision was made sharply. This was deepened through the subcutaneous tissues and hemostasis was achieved with electrocautery. The linea alba was identified and incised and the peritoneal cavity entered. *Adhesions were lysed sharply under direct vision with Metzenbaum scissors.*

The abdominal cavity was inspected for gross abnormalities. *No abnormalities/the following abnormalities (enumerate) were found. No evidence of Crohn's disease was visualized in the small intestine.* The right colon was mobilized by incising the peritoneal attachment along the white line of Toldt from the cecum to the hepatic flexure. The colon and terminal ileum was mobilized medially, taking care to protect the duodenum and right ureter. The hepatocolic ligament was divided using electrocautery. The greater omentum was then taken from the transverse colon up to the splenic flexure. The lateral peritoneal attachment of the left colon was then incised from the splenic flexure to the sigmoid colon. The splenocolic ligament was divided using electrocautery. The left colon was mobilized medially. Care was taken to protect the left ureter.

A point of division was chosen on the terminal ileum close to the cecum. The bowel was divided with a linear cutting stapler. The mesentery was scored and divided, taking care to preserve the ileocolic artery and its branches. Mesenteric vessels were secured with ties and suture ligatures of 2-0 silk. The inferior mesenteric artery was then identified and divided near the root. Dissection was carried down on both sides of the rectosigmoid to the cul-de-sac, while staying close to the rectosigmoid colon to avoid injuring the pelvic nerves. Care was also taken not to damage the ureters and gonadal vessels.

The rectum was then mobilized along the total mesorectal excision (TME) plane into the hollow of the sacrum by using blunt and electrocautery dissection. The rectum was carefully elevated until the endopelvic fascia and levator sling were identified. The peritoneum anterolateral to the rectum was incised and the rectum is freed from adjacent structures by blunt and electrocautery dissection. The rectum was divided with *electrocautery/curved cutting stapler* close to the dentate line and the specimen was removed.

If rectal mucosectomy: *Total mucosectomy was confirmed.* The pelvis was inspected for hemostasis, irrigated, and packed.

Attention was turned to the terminal ileum, which was inspected for viability. A *J-pouch/S-pouch/W-pouch* was planned and it was confirmed that the apex of the pouch reached easily into the pelvis without tension. The antimesenteric borders of the limbs of the reservoir were aligned and secured with several sutures of 3-0 Vicryl. Enterotomies were made to admit the stapler. The linear cutting stapler was used to create the reservoir. *Stab wounds were closed with a linear stapler (if not placed at apex).*

Attention was then turned to the perineal field. The reservoir was passed down into the pelvis and aligned with the rectal remnant in such a way as to avoid torsion and tension. The apex of the reservoir was *brought through the muscular cuff and* then *stapled/sutured to the anus at the dentate line with multiple interrupted sutures of 4-0 PDS/__mm circular stapler.*

Closed suction drains were placed in the pelvis and brought out through separate stab wounds lateral to the abdominal incision. These were secured in place with 3-0 nylon.

If temporary loop ileostomy: *A proximal loop of ileum was identified and an opening was made in the abdominal wall in the left upper quadrant. The loop of ileum was passed through this opening without tension or torsion.*

The abdominal cavity was then copiously irrigated. Hemostasis was again checked.

The fascia was closed with *a running suture of 0 PDS.* The skin was closed with *skin staples/subcuticular sutures of ___/other.* A dressing was applied.

If temporary loop ileostomy: *The terminal ileum was opened on the inferior margin and matured in a Brooke's fashion with multiple interrupted sutures of 3-0 Vicryl. An ostomy appliance was placed.*

The patient tolerated the procedure well and was taken to the postanesthesia care unit in stable condition.

NOTES

Chapter 51

Laparoscopic Total Proctocolectomy with Ileal Pouch to Anal Canal Anastomosis with Diverting Loop Ileostomy

Maher A. Abbas, M.D.

INDICATIONS
- Mucosal ulcerative colitis.
- Familial polyposis.

ESSENTIAL STEPS
1. Lithotomy position, both arms are tucked.
2. Foley catheter and orogastric tube.
3. Place five trocars.
   - Three 5-mm trocars in the supraumbilical, and the right and left mid-abdomen.
   - Two 12-mm trocars in the right and left lower abdomen.
4. Place the table in Trendelenburg position.
5. Retract the sigmoid colon anteriorly and identify the inferior mesenteric artery.
6. Open the retroperitoneum at the level of the sacral promontory and dissect retrograde to the level of the inferior mesenteric artery. Identify and protect the left ureter from this angle.
7. Isolate the inferior mesenteric artery and divide using a vascular stapler, an energy source, or clips.
8. Dissect more lateral to identify the inferior mesenteric vein which is divided in a similar fashion.
9. Lift the mesocolon off the retroperitoneum from a medial to lateral approach and dissect as far as possible.

J.J. Hoballah and C.E.H. Scott-Conner (eds.), *Operative Dictations in General and Vascular Surgery*, DOI 10.1007/978-1-4614-0451-4_51,
© Springer Science+Business Media, LLC 2012

10. Place the patient in the reverse Trendelenburg position.

11. Mobilize the left colon from the lateral to medial approach by incising the lateral attachments.

12. Takedown the splenic flexure by lifting the omentum off the distal transverse colon and joining the dissection with the medially mobilized descending colon.

13. Identify and divide the middle colic vessels.

14. Lift the ascending colon anteriorly and identify the ileocolic artery and vein. Open a mesenteric window on both sides of these vascular structures.

15. Identify the duodenum and keep down toward the spine and away from the ileocolic vessels.

16. Divide the ileocolic vessels using a vascular stapler, an energy source, or clips.

17. Lift the right mesocolon off the retroperitoneum and dissect bluntly in this medial-to-lateral plane toward the hepatic flexure.

18. Mobilize the ascending colon from a lateral to medial approach by incising the lateral attachments.

19. Place the patient in the Trendelenburg position again.

20. Identify the hypogastric nerves at the sacral promontory in the previously opened window. Protect the nerves.

21. Use blunt dissection and electrocautery to carry the dissection in the avascular presacral plane all the way down to the levator muscles.

22. Take down the lateral attachments of the rectum and open the peritoneal reflection anteriorly staying behind Denonviellers' fascia [unless patient has rectal carcinoma then may need to open anterior to the fascia depending on the location of the tumor]. Carry the dissection down to the levator muscles.

23. Divide the rectum at the anorectal junction using the laparoscopic stapler.

24. Make an 8–10 cm Pfannenstiel's skin incision. Create subcutaneous flaps and divide the anterior fascia and peritoneum in a vertical fashion.

25. Place wound protector.

26. Extract the colorectum through the wound and divide the terminal ileum with a linear stapler.

27. Fashion a 15–20 cm ileal J pouch using a linear stapler.

28. Place purse-string suture at apex of J pouch and tie after introducing the anvil of an EEA circular stapler.

29. Expose the pelvis with a St. Mark's retractor and perform a stapled side -to-end ileoanal anastomosis. The orientation

of the mesentery is checked prior to the stapling to ensure that the pouch is properly oriented and not twisted.

30. Test the anastomosis by transanally insufflating the pouch with the pelvis submerged with saline solution.
31. Run the ileum in a retrograde fashion and identify a segment about 30–40 cm proximal to the pouch.
32. Exteriorize this segment through the right lower quadrant trocar site or an alternative site previously marked by the enterostomal nurse. Secure bowel over a rod at the skin level. Care is taken not to twist the bowel.
33. Remove all trocars under direct visualization through the Pfannenstiel's incision.
34. Close the Pfannenstiel's incision in three layers (peritoneum, fascia, and skin).
35. Close the anterior fascia of the 12-mm left lower quadrant trocar.
36. Close the skin at the trocar sites.
37. Cover all wounds.
38. Mature a diverting loop ileostomy.
39. Cover the ileostomy with the proper appliance.

NOTE THESE VARIATIONS

- Hand-assisted total proctocolectomy with a hand port established at the beginning of the operation through a Pfannenstiel's incision.
- All five trocars can be 5 mm if no stapling is necessary (energy source is used for vascular pedicle division and anorectum is extracted transanally following mucosectomy).
- Anal mucosectomy with handsewn ileoanal anastomosis.
- The proctectomy portion of the operation performed by dividing the mesorectum next to the rectal wall instead of the total mesorectal excision dissection which was described above.
- Omission of the ileostomy in a select group of patients.

COMPLICATIONS

- Transection of the ureter.
- Perforation of the duodenum or stomach.
- Laceration of the spleen.
- Small bowel enterotomy.
- Transection of the hypogastric nerve trunk.

- Anastomotic leak.
- Twisting of the pouch.

TEMPLATE OPERATIVE DICTATION

Preoperative diagnosis: *Mucosal ulcerative colitis refractory to medical management/familial polyposis.*

Procedure: Laparoscopic total proctocolectomy with ileal pouch to anal canal anastomosis, diverting loop ileostomy.

Postoperative diagnosis: Same.

Indications: The patient is _____-year-old *male/female* with a history of _____. Different treatment options were discussed with the patient. The procedure of laparoscopic (possible open) total proctocolectomy with ileal pouch to anal canal anastomosis with diverting loop ileostomy was reviewed with the patient. The procedure, indication, alternatives, risks, and complications were reviewed with the patient. The patient verbalized understanding and wished to proceed. Informed consent was obtained.

Description of procedure: The patient was brought to the operating room and after instillation of general endotracheal anesthesia; he/she was placed in the lithotomy position with both arms tucked. A time-out was completed verifying correct patient, procedure, site, positioning, and implant(s) and/or special equipment prior to beginning this procedure.

Intravenous antibiotic and subcutaneous heparin were administered. A Foley catheter and an orogastric tube were inserted. All extremities were well padded. The rectum was irrigated with betadine. The abdomen was shaved and prepped in the usual sterile fashion. Using a 5-mm supraumbilical incision, the abdomen was insufflated with a Veress needle and a 5-mm trocar was established. Under direct visualization, a 12-mm trocar was placed in the right lower quadrant and one in the left lower quadrant followed by two additional 5-mm trocars in the right and left midabdomen. The patient was placed in the Trendelenburg position. The sigmoid colon was grabbed and retracted anteriorly. The inferior mesenteric artery pedicle was identified and the retroperitoneum was opened posterior to the vessel just superior to the sacral promontory. Using retrograde dissection, a window was created between the artery and the retroperitoneum. The left ureter was identified and kept out of harm's way for the entirety of the operation. The inferior mesenteric artery was then isolated and divided using a laparoscopic vascular stapler. Next the inferior mesenteric vein was identified, isolated, and divided in a similar fashion. The left mesocolon was then lifted off the retroperitoneum from a medial to lateral approach and blunt dissection was carried out toward the splenic flexure. The patient was placed in the reverse Trendelenburg position and the left colon was mobilized from a lateral to medial approach by incising the lateral attachments. The splenic flexure was taken down by lifting the omentum off the distal transverse colon and joining the dissection with the mobilized descending colon. The transverse colon was lifted anteriorly and the middle colic vessels were identified, isolated, and divided with the laparoscopic vascular stapler. The ascending colon was lifted anteriorly and the ileocolic vessels were isolated by creating mesenteric windows on each side and divided with the laparoscopic vascular stapler after identifying the duodenum and keeping it out of harm's way toward the spine. The right mesocolon was lifted off the retroperitoneum and blunt dissection was carried from a medial to lateral approach toward the hepatic flexure. The hepatic flexure was taken down and the ascending colon was mobilized medially by incising the lateral attachments. The patient was placed in the Trendelenburg position again and the small bowel was retracted out of the pelvis. The sacral promontory was visualized and both hypogastric nerves were identified and protected. Using blunt dissection and electrocautery, the presacral avascular plane was developed. Dissection was carried down to the levator muscles. The lateral attachments of the rectum were divided. The peritoneal reflection was opened anteriorly and dissection was carried posterior to Denonviellers' fascia. Once the dissection was complete circumferentially at the level of the pelvic floor, the rectum was divided at the anorectal junction using the 45-mm laparoscopic endoGIA (3.5 mm) (alternative is the 4.8-mm staple height). A 10-cm Pfannenstiel's skin incision was made and subcutaneous flaps were raised superiorly and inferiorly. The anterior fascia and peritoneum were divided at the midline in a vertical fashion. A small wound protector was used to retract the wound. The colorectum was extracted through the wound and the terminal ileum was divided with a linear 80-mm stapler. A 20-cm ileal J pouch was created using the 80-mm linear stapler. A purse-string was placed at the apex of the pouch using a 2.0 prolene suture and the anvil of a circular stapler [size range from 25 to 34 mm, depending on bowel and anus size]. The pelvis was exposed with a St. Mark's retractor, the pouch was brought down to the pelvis taking care not to twist the mesentery and a side to end stapled anastomosis was performed with the EEA circular stapler. The anastomosis was insufflated transanally with air after submerging the pelvis with sterile saline and gently occluding the ileum proximal to the pouch. No evidence of airleak. A loop of small bowel was identified 30 cm proximal to the pouch and was exteriorized over a plastic rod through a stomal trephine created at the site of the right lower quadrant trocar. Care was taken not to twist the ileostomy. The remaining trocars were removed under direct visualization through the Pfannenstiel incision. The incision was then closed in three layers, approximating the peritoneum with 0 vicryl suture, the anterior fashion with 0 PDS suture, and the skin with metal staplers. The anterior fascia of the 12-mm left lower quadrant trocar was closed with 0 vicryl. The trocar site skin wounds were approximated with metal staples and all wounds were dressed. A diverting loop ileostomy was finally matured using 3.0 chromic sutures. Appliance was placed. All instruments, needles, and sponges count was correct times two. The patient tolerated the procedure well and was taken to the recovery unit in stable condition.

NOTES

Chapter 52

Total Proctocolectomy with Ileostomy

Danny Liu, M.D. and John W. Cromwell, M.D.

INDICATION
- Ulcerative or Crohn's colitis refractory to medical management, when sphincter preservation is not desired or feasible.

ESSENTIAL STEPS
1. Combined lithotomy–supine position.
2. Purse-string suture to close the anus (optional).
3. Midline incision.
4. Explore the abdomen.
5. Mobilize the right colon:
    - Incise the lateral peritoneal reflection from the cecum to the hepatic flexure.
    - Divide adhesions of the colon to the retroperitoneum.
    - Identify and protect the right ureter and duodenum.
6. Mobilize the transverse colon by dividing greater omentum from the colon.
7. Mobilize the splenic flexure and left colon:
    - Incise the peritoneum lateral to the left colon from the sigmoid colon to splenic flexure.
    - Reflect the colon medially, dividing adhesions to the retroperitoneum.
    - Identify and protect the left ureter.
8. Identify the point of transection on the terminal ileum.
9. Divide the terminal ileum with a linear cutting stapler.

J.J. Hoballah and C.E.H. Scott-Conner (eds.), *Operative Dictations in General and Vascular Surgery*, DOI 10.1007/978-1-4614-0451-4_52,
© Springer Science+Business Media, LLC 2012

10. Score the peritoneum overlying the intended line of mesenteric division.
11. Divide the mesentery, securing vessels with 2-0 silk ties and suture ligatures, or using Ligasure.
12. Incise the pelvic peritoneum and elevate the rectum along the TME plane.
13. Continue dissection circumferentially to the levators, staying close to the rectum to avoid autonomic nerves.
14. Switch to perineal approach, incise skin around the anus.
15. Enter the peritoneal cavity in posterior midline; incise levators anteriorly.
16. Complete anterior dissection.
17. *If male: Avoid injury to the urethra. If female: carefully dissect along the rectovaginal plane.*
18. Pass the specimen through.
19. Place drain(s).
20. *Close the pelvic peritoneum.*
21. Make an opening for the ileostomy.
22. Deliver the terminal ileum, tack to the peritoneum, and obliterate lateral recess.
23. Close the abdomen and perineum.
24. Mature ileostomy in Brooke's fashion.

COMPLICATIONS

- Injury to the ureters.
- Injury to the urethra (male).
- Hemorrhage from the presacral venous plexus.
- Sexual dysfunction.
- Urinary retention.

TEMPLATE OPERATIVE DICTATION

Preoperative diagnosis: *Ulcerative colitis/Crohn's colitis* refractory to medical management.
Procedure: Total proctocolectomy with ileostomy.
Postoperative diagnosis: Same.
Indications: This ___-year-old *male/female* has *ulcerative colitis/Crohn's colitis with extensive rectal involvement* refractory to medical management. Sphincter preservation is not desired or feasible. Total proctocolectomy with ileostomy was chosen for definitive management.
Description of procedure: The patient was brought to the operating room and placed in the supine position. General

endotracheal anesthesia was induced without complications. A Foley catheter and *oral/naso*gastric tube were placed. The patient was then positioned in *Lloyd-Davies/Allen* stirrups with care taken to pad all pressure points. A time-out was completed verifying correct patient, procedure, site, positioning, and implant(s) and/ or special equipment prior to beginning this procedure. *The anus was closed with a purse-string suture of 2-0 silk.* The abdomen and perineum were prepped and draped in the usual sterile fashion. A multidisciplinary time-out was performed confirming the correct patient, procedure, and preoperative antibiotics were given. A vertical midline incision was made sharply. This was deepened through the subcutaneous tissues and hemostasis was achieved with electrocautery. The linea alba was identified and incised and the peritoneal cavity entered. *Adhesions were lysed sharply under direct vision with Metzenbaum scissors.*

The abdominal cavity was inspected for gross abnormalities. *No abnormalities/the following abnormalities (enumerate) were found.* The right colon was mobilized by incising the peritoneal attachment along the white line of Toldt from the cecum to the hepatic flexure. The colon and terminal ileum was mobilized medially, taking care to protect the duodenum and right ureter. The hepatocolic ligament was divided using electrocautery. The greater omentum was then taken from the transverse colon up to the splenic flexure. The lateral peritoneal attachment of the left colon was then incised from the splenic flexure to the sigmoid colon. The splenocolic ligament was divided using electrocautery. The left colon was mobilized medially. Care was taken to protect the left ureter.

A point of division was chosen on the terminal ileum. The bowel was divided with a linear cutting stapler. *The mesentery was scored and divided/using the Ligasure. Mesenteric vessels were secured with ties and suture ligatures of 2-0 silk.* The inferior mesenteric artery was then identified and divided near the root. Dissection was carried down on both sides of the rectosigmoid to the cul-de-sac, while staying close to the rectosigmoid colon to avoid injuring the pelvic nerves. Care was also taken not to damage the ureters and gonadal vessels.

The rectum was then mobilized along the total mesorectal excision (TME) plane into the hollow of the sacrum by using blunt and electrocautery dissection. The rectum was carefully elevated until the endopelvic fascia and levator sling were identified. The peritoneum anterolateral to the rectum was incised and the rectum is freed from adjacent structures by blunt and electrocautery dissection. *If male: The dissection carried down behind the prostate.*

The pelvic dissection is continued to the lowest level possible to facilitate the perineal excision.

Attention was then turned to the perineal phase of the dissection. A narrow elliptical incision was made encompassing the anus. Dissection then progressed through subcutaneous tissues circumferentially. Hemostasis was achieved with electrocautery. The posterior portion of the incision is extended over the coccyx, entering the abdomen. The levators were then divided with electrocautery beginning posteriorly and progressing anteriorly. *If male: The prostate and the urethral catheter is palpated and protected from accidental injury. If female: Dissection through the rectovaginal plane was carefully completed.* The remaining anterior attachments were then severed and the specimen removed. Hemostasis was achieved in the pelvis and perineal wound.

Closed suction drains were placed in the pelvis and brought out through separate stab wounds. The drains were secured in place with 3-0 nylon. The perineal wound was closed in layers with interrupted 2-0 Vicryl and the skin was closed with vertical mattress sutures of 3-0 Nylon.

The abdominal cavity was then copiously irrigated. Hemostasis was again checked. *The pelvic peritoneum was closed with running 3-0 Vicryl.* A disk of skin was removed in the preselected site for the ileostomy. This incision was deepened through subcutaneous tissues and muscular and fascial layers until an opening sufficient for two fingers was created. The ileum was then delivered through this opening without tension or torsion. *It was tacked circumferentially to the peritoneum with interrupted 3-0 Vicryl and laterally to the peritoneum in such a manner as to eliminate the lateral trap.*

The fascia was closed with *a running suture of 0 looped PDS.* The skin was closed with *skin staples/subcuticular sutures of ___/ other.* A dressing was applied.

The ileostomy was then matured in a Brooke's fashion with multiple interrupted sutures of 3-0 Vicryl. An ostomy appliance was placed.

The patient tolerated the procedure well and was taken to the postanesthesia care unit in stable condition.

NOTES

Chapter 53

Laparoscopic Total Proctocolectomy with End Ileostomy

Maher A. Abbas, M.D.

INDICATIONS

- Mucosal ulcerative colitis.
- Crohn's disease.
- Familial polyposis.

ESSENTIAL STEPS

1. Lithotomy position, both arms are tucked.
2. Foley catheter and orogastric tube.
3. Pneumoperitoneum to 15 mmHg.
4. Place five trocars:
    - Three 5-mm trocars in the supraumbilical, and the right and left mid-abdomen sites.
    - Two 12-mm trocars in the right and left lower abdomen.
5. Place the table in Trendelenburg position.
6. Retract the sigmoid colon anteriorly and identify the inferior mesenteric artery.
7. Open the retroperitoneum at the level of the sacral promontory and dissect retrograde to the level of the inferior mesenteric artery. Identify and protect the left ureter from this angle.
8. Isolate the inferior mesenteric artery and divide using a vascular stapler, an energy source, or clips.
9. Dissect more lateral to identify the inferior mesenteric vein which is divided in a similar fashion.

J.J. Hoballah and C.E.H. Scott-Conner (eds.), *Operative Dictations in General and Vascular Surgery*, DOI 10.1007/978-1-4614-0451-4_53,
© Springer Science+Business Media, LLC 2012

10. Lift the mesocolon off the retroperitoneum from a medial to lateral approach and dissect as far as possible.
11. Place the patient in the reverse Trendelenburg position.
12. Mobilize the left colon from the lateral to medial approach by incising the lateral attachments.
13. Takedown the splenic flexure by lifting the omentum off the distal transverse colon and joining the dissection with the medially mobilized descending colon.
14. Identify and divide the middle colic vessels.
15. Lift the ascending colon anteriorly and identify the ile-ocolic artery and vein. Open a mesenteric window on both sides of these vascular structures.
16. Identify the duodenum and keep down toward the spine and away from the ileocolic vessels.
17. Divide the ileocolic vessels using a vascular stapler, an energy source, or clips.
18. Lift the right mesocolon off the retroperitoneum and dissect bluntly in this medial to lateral plane toward the hepatic flexure.
19. Mobilize the ascending colon from a lateral to medial approach by incising the lateral attachments.
20. Divide the terminal ileum just proximal to the ileocecal valve using a laparoscopic endoGIA.
21. Place the patient in the Trendelenburg position again.
22. Identify the hypogastric nerves at the sacral promontory in the previously opened window. Protect the nerves.
23. Use blunt dissection and electocautery to carry the dissec-tion in the avascular presacral plane, all the way down to the levator muscles.
24. Take down the lateral attachments of the rectum and open the peritoneal reflection anteriorly staying behind Denonviellers' fascia *(unless patient has rectal carcinoma then may need to open anterior to the fascia depending on the location of the tumor)*. Carry the dissection down to the levator muscles.
25. Switch to the perineal portion of the operation.
26. Close the anus with a purse-string suture.
27. Perform circumferential subcutaneous dissection around the anus.
28. Retract the wound with a Lone Star retractor.
29. Carry the dissection deeper and incise the levator and connect with the peritoneal cavity.
30. Extract the entire colorectum through the perineal wound.

31. Irrigate the perineal wound and close in multiple layers.
32. Reestablish the pneumoperitoneum.
33. Identify the transected end of the terminal ileum and bring out through a stomal trephine at the level of the right lower quadrant trocar site or an alternative site previously marked by the enterostomal nurse. Secure bowel at the level of the skin using a clamp.
34. Remove all trocars under direct camera visualization and close the fascia of the 12-mm left lower quadrant trocar.
35. Close the skin at the trocar sites.
36. Cover all wounds.
37. Mature an end ileostomy.
38. Cover the ileostomy with the proper appliance.

NOTE THESE VARIATIONS

- Hand-assisted total proctocolectomy with a hand port established at the beginning of the operation through a Pfannenstiel's incision.
- All five trocars can be 5 mm, if no stapling is necessary (if an energy source is used for vascular pedicle division and anorectum is extracted transanally following the perineal dissection).
- An intersphincteric proctectomy can be performed preserving the external anal sphincter muscle to minimize the morbidity of the perineal wound.
- The proctectomy portion of the operation may be performed by dividing the mesorectum next to the rectal wall instead of the total mesorectal excision dissection which was described above.

COMPLICATIONS

- Transection of the ureter.
- Perforation of the duodenum or stomach.
- Laceration of the spleen.
- Small bowel enterotomy.
- Transection of the hypogastric nerve trunk.
- Stomal-related complications.

TEMPLATE OPERATIVE DICTATION

Preoperative diagnosis: Mucosal ulcerative colitis (Crohn's disease or familial polyposis).
Procedure: Laparoscopic total proctocolectomy with end ileostomy.

Postoperative diagnosis: Same.

Indications: The patient is _____-year-old *male/female* with a history of _____. Different treatment options were discussed with the patient. The procedure of laparoscopic (possible open) total proctocolectomy with permanent end ileostomy was reviewed with the patient. The procedure, indication, alternatives, risks, and complications were reviewed with the patient. The patient verbalized understanding and wished to proceed. Informed consent was obtained.

Description of procedure: The patient was brought to the operating room and after instillation of general endotracheal anesthesia; he/she was placed in the lithotomy position with both arms tucked. A time-out was completed verifying correct patient, procedure, site, positioning, and implant(s) and/or special equipment prior to beginning this procedure.

Intravenous antibiotic and subcutaneous heparin were administered. A Foley catheter and an orogastric tube were inserted. All extremities were well padded. The rectum was irrigated with betadine. The abdomen and perineum were shaved and prepped in the usual sterile fashion. Using a 5-mm supraumbilical incision, the abdomen was insufflated with a Veress needle and a 5-mm trocar was established. Under direct visualization, a 12-mm trocar was placed in the right lower quadrant and one in the left lower quadrant followed by two additional 5-mm trocars in the right and left mid-abdomen. The patient was placed in the Trendelenburg position. The sigmoid colon was grabbed and retracted anteriorly. The inferior mesenteric artery pedicle was identified and the retroperitoneum was opened posterior to the vessel just superior to the sacral promontory. Using retrograde dissection, a window was created between the artery and the retroperitoneum. The left ureter was identified and kept out of harm's way for the entirety of the operation. The inferior mesenteric artery was then isolated and divided using a laparoscopic vascular stapler. Next the inferior mesenteric vein was identified, isolated, and divided in a similar fashion. The left mesocolon was then lifted off the retroperitoneum from a medial to lateral approach and blunt dissection was carried out toward the splenic flexure. The patient was placed in the reverse Trendelenburg position and the left colon was mobilized from a lateral to medial approach by incising the lateral attachments. The splenic flexure was taken down by lifting the omentum off the distal transverse colon and joining the dissection with the mobilized descending colon. The transverse colon was lifted anteriorly and the middle colic vessels were identified, isolated, and divided with the laparoscopic vascular stapler. The ascending colon was lifted anteriorly and the ileocolic vessels were isolated by creating mesenteric windows on each side and divided with the laparoscopic vascular stapler after identifying the duodenum and keeping it out of harm's way toward the spine. The right mesocolon was lifted off the retroperitoneum and blunt dissection was carried from a medial to lateral approach toward the hepatic flexure. The hepatic flexure was taken down and the ascending colon was mobilized medially by incising the lateral attachments. The terminal ileum was transected just proximal to the ileocecal valve using a laparoscopic endoGIA. The patient was placed in the Trendelenburg position again and the small bowel was retracted out of the pelvis. The sacral promontory was visualized and both hypogastric nerves were identified and protected. Using blunt dissection and electrocautery, the presacral avascular plane was developed. Dissection was carried down to the levator muscles. The lateral attachments of the rectum were divided. The peritoneal reflection was opened anteriorly and dissection was carried posterior to Denonviellers' fascia. Once the dissection was complete circumferentially at the level of the pelvic floor, the pelvis was irrigated. Attention was then directed to the perineal portion of the operation. The anus was closed using a 0 Vicryl purse-string. Electrocautery was used to perform a perianal subcutaneous circumferential dissection all the way to the level of the pelvic floors which were divided. The perineal dissection was connected with the peritoneal cavity and the colorectum was exteriorized through the perineal wound. The wound was irrigated and closed in three layers using 0 Vicryl for the pelvic floor muscles and subcutaneous tissue and 3-0 Vicryl for the subcuticular skin closure. The wound was covered antibiotic ointment followed by a dry dressing. The pneumoperitoneum was reestablished. The transected end of the terminal ileum was identified and brought through the right lower quadrant trocar site which was enlarged as a stomal trephine. It was secured above the skin with a clamp. Care was taken not to twist the ileostomy. All trocars were removed under direct camera visualization and the left lower quadrant fascial site closed with 0 Vicryl in a figure of eight fashion. The trocar site skin wounds were closed with 3.0 Vicryl suture in a subcuticular fashion. An end Brooke ileostomy was finally matured using 3.0 chromic sutures. Appliance was placed. All instruments, needles, and sponges count was correct times two. The patient tolerated the procedure well and was taken to the recovery unit in stable condition.

NOTES

Chapter 54
End Ileostomy

Emily Steinhagen, M.D. and Celia M. Divino, M.D.

INDICATIONS

- Colon cancer.
  - ○ Perforation.
  - ○ Obstruction.
- Colitis (ulcerative colitis, Crohn's colitis, infectious colitis, ischemic colitis).
  - ○ Fulminant colitis requiring emergent colectomy.
  - ○ Defunctioning of bowel.
  - ○ Unsafe to perform anastomosis at time of surgery.
- Trauma.
  - ○ Perforation.

ESSENTIAL STEPS

1. Mark the stoma site with patient awake and upright/sitting.
2. Midline incision.
3. Terminal ileum and right colon mobilization.
4. *Resection.*
5. Select site of diversion if not clear from resection; divide bowel and mesentery.
6. Create stoma site.
   - Excise skin.
   - Divide anterior sheath/rectus/posterior sheath and peritoneum.
7. Bring terminal ileum through stoma site.

J.J. Hoballah and C.E.H. Scott-Conner (eds.), *Operative Dictations in General and Vascular Surgery*, DOI 10.1007/978-1-4614-0451-4_54,
© Springer Science+Business Media, LLC 2012

8. Confirm length and orientation.
9. Check hemostasis.
10. Close abdominal incision.
11. Excise stapled end of ileum.
12. Evert ileostomy and mature.

NOTE THESE VARIATIONS
- Usually performed as part of a larger procedure.
- Options for distal end of the bowel: mucous fistula or Hartmann's pouch.
- Can be performed as part of laparoscopic procedure.

COMPLICATIONS
- Necrosis.
- Internal hernia.
- Obstruction/ileus.
- Stoma retraction.
- Stoma prolapse.
- Parastomal hernia.

TEMPLATE OPERATIVE DICTATION
Preoperative diagnosis: *Ischemia/infection/perforation/obstruction* of the colon.
Procedure: *(Specify type)* Resection and end ileostomy *with mucous fistula or Hartman's pouch.*
Postoperative diagnosis: Same.
Indications: The patient is a ___ -year-old *male/female* who presented with _____ and required *(resection performed)* and end ileostomy.
Description of the procedure: Informed consent was obtained including a discussion of risks, benefits, and alternatives. The need for possible stoma was discussed with the patient. The patient's abdomen was marked for stoma while the patient was in the upright and seated positions. The patient was brought to the operating room and placed on the operating table in the supine position. General anesthesia was induced. A time-out was completed verifying correct patient, procedure, site, positioning, and implant(s) and/or special equipment prior to beginning this procedure. Perioperative antibiotics were given. A Foley catheter was placed. The abdomen was prepped and draped in the usual sterile fashion.

A midline incision was made in the skin and carried down through the subcutaneous tissues to the fascia. The fascia was divided and the peritoneal cavity was entered. Careful exploration of the abdomen was performed and adhesions were carefully lysed.

The right colon and terminal ileum were mobilized. The ureter was identified during the dissection and was protected throughout the procedure.

(Include details of the resection if performed)

The terminal ileum was inspected and the location of transection was determined. The avascular plane in the mesentery was identified and a window was created adjacent to the bowel. The bowel was divided using(the harmonic scalpel electrocautary clams and ties with a liner stapler. *The mesentery was also divided and mesenteric vessels were secured with nonabsorbable ties* . The proximal end of the ileum easily reached the intended right lower quadrant stoma site.

A small circular disc of skin was excised at the pre-selected site in the right lower quadrant. The subcutaneous fat was retracted and held out of the field. The anterior rectus sheath was incised *(vertically/horizontally/with a cruciate incision)*. The rectus fibers were dissected bluntly with clamps. The posterior rectus sheath and peritoneum were then entered with a *(vertical/horizontal/cruciate)* incision. The area was checked for hemostasis; the inferior epigastric artery was identified and also found to be intact. A large *(babcock)* clamp was passed through the hole. The proximal edge of the ileum was grasped and carefully delivered through the stoma, along with the supporting mesentery. Care was taken to keep the ileum in its correct orientation and to avoid torsion. There was no tension on the ileum and adequate length was present.

The cut edge of the mesentery was secured to the peritoneum of the anterior abdominal wall.

The distal end of the bowel was matured to form a mucous fistula/carefully placed in an anatomic position in the abdomen as a Hartmann's pouch.

The midline incision was then closed. The fascia was closed with _____ and the skin was closed with staples. A sterile towel was placed over the incision to protect while the stoma was matured.

The stapled edge of the ileum was excised to produce a fresh bleeding edge. The ileostomy was then everted and matured. An orienting suture were placed in each quadrant that went through the full thickness of the bowel at the cut edge, then through the seromuscular layer 3–5 cm proximally, just adjacent the skin, and finally to the dermis. All orienting sutures were tied. Additional interrupted sutures were placed between the orienting sutures from the cut edge of the bowel to the dermis until the stoma was securely formed. An stoma appliance was placed and a sterile dressing was placed over the midline incision.

The patient tolerated the procedure well. All counts were correct. Anesthesia was reversed and the patient was extubated. The patient was taken to the postoperative care unit in stable condition.

ACKNOWLEDGMENT

This chapter was contributed by Kareem A. Hamdy, MD, in the first edition.

NOTES

Chapter 55

Loop Ileostomy

Laura Doyon, M.D. and Kaare Weber, M.D.

INDICATIONS

- Any situation that requires complete, temporary diversion of fecal stream.
- Allows for relative ease and less invasive approach for reversal.

ESSENTIAL STEPS

1. For ease in the patient's access, mark the site with the patient awake and sitting upright.
2. Create a lower midline incision.
3. Identify the terminal ileum by using the cecum as a guide.
4. Choose a freely mobile loop of distal ileum (or more proximally as needed for small bowel anastomoses.) Consider placing marking stitches at the proximal and distal ends of the apex of the loop in order not to confuse orientation.
5. At the marked site, excise an appropriately sized disc of skin and subcutaneous tissue. Carry incision down to the fascia, and make an adequately sized incision in the fascia and peritoneum.
6. Carry intended loop through the ostomy site, taking care not to rotate the distal/proximal orientation. A penrose drain threaded under the loop can facilitate this.
7. Confirm that the loop is tension-free.
8. Confirm hemostasis, then close the lower midline abdominal incision. Protect wound.

J.J. Hoballah and C.E.H. Scott-Conner (eds.), *Operative Dictations in General and Vascular Surgery*, DOI 10.1007/978-1-4614-0451-4_55,
© Springer Science+Business Media, LLC 2012

9. Make a four-fifths circumferential incision toward the proximal side of the apex of the loop.
10. Evert the cut edges of ileum and suture in place to the cut edge of the skin.
11. Exchange the penrose for a short plastic rod, to minimize chance of retraction. A piece of cut foley catheter can bridge each end of the rod to create a ring and prevent rod from being dislodged.
12. Place appliance.

NOTE THIS VARIATION

■ Instead of carrying out a complete loop and then cutting, everting, and maturing the ileostomy, one can staple across the apex of the loop using a mechanical stapler, without violating the mesentery. The complete proximal limb and one corner of the distal limb are delivered through the ostomy site. The proximal staple line is excised, and then matured as with an end ileostomy. Only the exposed portion of the distal limb's staple line is excised, to allow for decompression; this cut end is then matured as above.

COMPLICATIONS

■ Ostomy ischemia, necrosis.
■ Parastomal hernia, internal hernia.
■ Retraction, prolapse.
■ Paraileostomy abscess.
■ Skin excoriation.

TEMPLATE OPERATIVE DICTATION

Preoperative diagnosis: *Obstruction/perforation* of the colon.
Procedure: *(Resection with primary anastomosis)* and diverting loop ileostomy.
Postoperative diagnosis: Same.
Indications: This ___-year-old *male/female* presented with *colonic obstruction/perforation* requiring temporary fecal diversion, for which loop ileostomy was performed.
Description of procedure: After explaining the risks and benefits of the procedure and obtaining informed consent, the patient was brought to the operating room and placed in a supine position. General anesthesia was induced. A time-out was completed verifying correct patient, procedure, site, positioning, and implant(s) and/or special equipment prior to beginning this procedure. Venous

compression devices and a Foley catheter placed, and the abdomen was prepped and draped in the usual sterile fashion. A lower midline incision was made and then carried down through the subcutaneous tissue with electrocautery dissection, ensuring excellent hemostasis. The exposed linea alba was incised, taking care not to injure underlying bowel, and the fascia and peritoneum were opened.

Attention was turned to the cecum, in order to identify the terminal ileum. An appropriate segment of distal ileum with adequate mesenteric length was selected. Next, a Kelly clamp was used to carefully dissect a small hole in the associated mesentery just below the apex of the loop, in order to thread a Penrose drain to hold the loop. Marking stitches were placed in order to identify the proximal and distal ends of the ostomy.

A circular disc of skin and subcutaneous tissue was excised from the previously determined ostomy site. Hemostasis was achieved, and the underlying fascia was incised in order to allow two fingerbreadths of space. With the guidance of the penrose, and care not to disturb the correct orientation of the ends of the ileostomy, the loop was delivered through the ostomy site.

After checking that the mesentery was not under tension, and that hemostasis was achieved, the midline abdominal incision was closed. First, the fascia was reapproximated with 2-0 running PDS, followed by 3-0 interrupted subcutaneous sutures, and finally a 4-0 monocryl running subcuticular suture. The wound was protected with towels to prevent contamination.

The Penrose drain was exchanged for a plastic rod to support the ostomy. A four-fifths circumferential incision was made toward the proximal aspect of the ileal loop, leaving at least one centimeter of space from the incision to the skin edge. After removing the marking stitches, the cut edges were everted to create a spigot shape of the ostomy. The bowel edges were sutured to the surrounding skin by taking full-thickness bites of the edges of the ileum, then to a seromuscular bite at the base of the ostomy, and then to the dermis of the skin. This was carried out around the complete circumference of the ostomy.

The ostomy appliance was placed, and the midline wound was dressed with a sterile bandage. The patient was awoken from anesthesia and taken to the recovery room in stable condition. All instruments, needles, and towels had been accounted for, and the attending surgeon was present through the entirety of the procedure.

ACKNOWLEDGMENT

This chapter was contributed by Kareem A. Hamdy, MD, in the first edition.

NOTES

Chapter 56
Closure of Loop Ileostomy

Walid Faraj, M.D., F.R.C.S. and Ahmad Zaghal, M.D.

INDICATION
- Healed distal anastomosis confirmed by endoscopic or contrast studies.

ESSENTIAL STEPS
1. Verify anal sphincter competency by physical exam or manometric study if the index procedure involved the anal sphincter mechanism.
2. Confirm adequate healing of distal anastomosis.
3. Make an incision around the stoma.
4. Dissect circumferentially until the fascia is reached and peritoneal cavity entered.
5. Clearly identify proximal and distal limbs.
6. Debride the edges of the enterotomy.
7. Determine if primary closure is feasible or if limited resection is needed.
8. Close the enterotomy/perform primary resection and anastomosis
   - Hand sewn or
   - Double-stapled technique
   - Rarely, segmental resection and anastomosis is needed.
9. Close the wound, or
   - Pack wound open for delayed closure.

J.J. Hoballah and C.E.H. Scott-Conner (eds.), *Operative Dictations in General and Vascular Surgery*, DOI 10.1007/978-1-4614-0451-4_56,
© Springer Science+Business Media, LLC 2012

NOTE THESE VARIATIONS
- Stoma may be closed with sutures or staples.
- Sometimes, a limited ileal resection is required if the stoma site is in poor condition.
- Packing the wound open for delayed closure is often a prudent alternative to primary closure.

COMPLICATIONS
- Infection.
- Bleeding.
- Anastomotic leak.
- Incisional hernia.

TEMPLATE OPERATIVE DICTATION
Preoperative diagnosis: ___months status post low anterior resection with protective loop ileostomy for colon/rectal cancer.
Procedure: Closure of loop ileostomy.
Postoperative diagnosis: Same.
Indications: This is a ___-year-old *male/female* who underwent ____ with proximal diverting loop ileostomy ___ months ago. *Contrast studies revealed a securely healed distal anastomosis/physical exam and manometric studies revealed an acceptable anal tone.*
Description of procedure: The patient was placed in a supine position. The procedure was performed under *local/general* anesthesia. The ileostomy bag was removed, the ileostomy site cleaned, then the *abdomen was* prepped and draped in a sterile manner. A time-out was completed verifying correct patient, procedure, site, positioning, and implant(s) and/or special equipment prior to beginning this procedure. An elliptical skin incision about 2 mm from mucocutaneous junction, around the ileostomy was performed. The incision was deepened in the subcutaneous tissue until the serosa of the emerging bowel appeared. Sharp dissection was continued circumferentially in this plane, dividing the fine adhesions between the bowel and its mesentery and the subcutaneous fat until the fascia was reached, and the peritoneal cavity entered, after which it was feasible to bring the emerging ileal loop through the wound, the mucocutaneous junction and the rim of skin were excised, the everted proximal end of the stoma was unfolded, and the edge of enterotomy freshened. The stoma was inspected and found to be *suitable for primary closure without resection/unsuitable for primary closure, and therefore a limited resection of the stoma site was performed to permit safe closure.*

[Choose one:]

If hand-sewn anastomosis: then a formal hand-sewn end-to-end anastomosis using seromuscular interrupted absorbable sutures was done to restore the intestinal continuity.

If stapled closure: then a transverse stapled closure of the ileal loop was done.

The site was checked for hemostasis, which was adequate, the loop of ileum was returned back to the abdominal cavity.

Hemostasis was secured, fascial defect was closed using continuous nonabsorbable suture, and skin *closed using interrupted nonabsorbable sutures/packed open for delayed primary closure.*

The patient tolerated the procedure well and was transferred to the postanesthesia care unit in stable condition.

NOTES

Chapter 57
Transverse Loop Colostomy

Gary William Swain, Jr., M.D. and Scott Q. Nguyen, M.D.

INDICATIONS
- For fecal diversion proximal to the splenic flexure:
  - Obstruction.
  - Perforation.

ESSENTIAL STEPS
1. Mark the location (preferably with patient awake).
2. Make transverse incision through planned colostomy site.
3. *Decompress colon if necessary.*
4. Bring the transverse colon through incision.
5. *Mobilize the hepatic flexure if necessary to add length.*
6. Create a mesenteric window.
7. *Pass plastic rod through the window.*
8. *Close fascia & skin medially/laterally around the colon if necessary to assure snugness.*
9. Mature colostomy and place ostomy appliance.

NOTE THESE VARIATIONS
- *For a markedly distended colon it may be necessary to make a controlled colostomy in the free tenia to aspirate the colonic contents. The colostomy is then closed with a pursestring suture of 3-0 silk.*

J.J. Hoballah and C.E.H. Scott-Conner (eds.), *Operative Dictations in General and Vascular Surgery*, DOI 10.1007/978-1-4614-0451-4_57,
© Springer Science+Business Media, LLC 2012

- *A fascial bridge may be created by suturing the fascia together under the mesenteric window with interrupted sutures instead of placing the plastic rod.*
- *To ensure total diversion, a stapler may be applied across the distal segment without cutting.*

COMPLICATIONS
- Ischemia, necrosis.
- Parastomal hernia.
- Prolapse.

TEMPLATE OPERATIVE DICTATION

Preoperative diagnosis: Left colon obstruction.

Procedure: Transverse loop colostomy.

Postoperative diagnosis: Same.

Indications: This ___-year-old *male/female* with colonic obstruction required fecal diversion and loop colostomy was elected.

Description of procedure: The patient was taken to the operating room and placed supine on the table and general endotracheal anesthesia was induced. A time-out was completed verifying correct patient, procedure, site, positioning, and implant(s) and/or special equipment prior to beginning this procedure. A Foley catheter and nasogastric tube were inserted, and the abdomen was prepped and draped in the usual sterile fashion. Intravenous antibiotics were given prior to incision. A short transverse incision was made in the right upper quadrant. This incision was carried down deep through the subcutaneous tissues with electrocautery. The muscular and aponeurotic layers were incised with cruciate incisions and spread with retractors. The peritoneum was sharply entered. The transverse colon was immediately encountered and noted to be markedly distended.

In order to deliver the colon through the incision it was necessary to decompress it. The greater omentum was swept cephalad. A pursestring suture of 3-0 silk was made at a free tenia. A large bore needle attached to suction was obliquely inserted into the colon wall and allowing gas and liquid stool to escape. The pursestring was then tied down to prevent any further leakage of enteric contents. A loop of transverse colon was then brought through the incision. *Additional length was obtained by lysing the peritoneal attachments and mobilizing the hepatic flexure.* The greater omentum over the proposed colostomy area was then dissected free from the colon and ligated.

A mesenteric window was created under the colon by incising the mesentery adjacent to the colon wall. A plastic rod was inserted under the colon through the mesenteric window in order to hold the exteriorized segment of transverse colon above the skin and fascia. The colon was then allowed to rest on the rod. The size of the fascial defect was assessed. Interrupted sutures of 0 vicryl were placed medial/lateral to the colon to close the fascia so that it was tight enough to allow only the loop of colon plus and one index finger, thus ensuring that the defect was snug but not overly constricting. The skin was closed around the colon with interrupted subcuticular absorbable suture using the same principle. Towels were placed to protect the field and the colon was incised and opened transversely. The colonic contents were suctioned out. The double barrel colostomy was matured with multiple interrupted mucoserous cutaneous sutures of 3-0 Vicryl circumferentially in Brooke fashion. After maturation, the colostomy was noted to be pink and viable. A 32-French urinary catheter was cut and secured to either end of the rod forming a small loop. This acted to prevent the colostomy from falling into the abdominal wound. A colostomy appliance was then placed.

The patient tolerated the procedure well and was taken to the postanesthesia care unit in stable condition.

ACKNOWLEDGMENT

This chapter was contributed by Kareem A. Hamdy, MD, in the first edition.

NOTES

Chapter 58

Closure of Transverse Loop Colostomy

Catherine Madorin, M.D. and Scott Q. Nguyen, M.D.

INDICATION
- Colostomy/fecal diversion no longer required.

ESSENTIAL STEPS
1. Incise mucocutaneous border of colostomy.
2. Mobilize transverse colon past level of fascia.
3. If necessary, lyse adhesions to the abdominal wall.
4. Assess viability of the colon.
5. Freshen edges of bowel.
6. Close transversely in two layers.
7. Close fascia.
8. Place packing in the wound.

NOTE THIS VARIATION
- Stapled closure with side to side anastomosis.

COMPLICATION
- Anastomotic leak.
- Stricture.

TEMPLATE OPERATIVE DICTATION
Preoperative diagnosis: Transverse loop colostomy.
Procedure: Closure of transverse loop colostomy.
Postoperative diagnosis: Same.

J.J. Hoballah and C.E.H. Scott-Conner (eds.), *Operative Dictations in General and Vascular Surgery*, DOI 10.1007/978-1-4614-0451-4_58,
© Springer Science+Business Media, LLC 2012

Indications: This ___-year-old *male/female* had previously underwent transverse loop colostomy for *obstruction/perforation* secondary to _____. He/*she* now returns for elective colostomy reversal.

Description of procedure: The patient was taken to the operating room and placed supine on the table. A time-out was completed verifying correct patient, procedure, site, positioning, and implant(s) and/or special equipment prior to beginning this procedure. Following induction of general endotracheal anesthesia, a Foley catheter was placed and preoperative intravenous antibiotics given. The abdomen was prepped and draped in standard sterile fashion. An incision was made circumferentially around the colostomy at the mucocutaneous border. The subcutaneous tissues were dissected off the colonic wall down to the level of the fascia. The colon was circumferentially dissected off the fascia and peritoneal attachments were divided with the help of a finger inserted into the peritoneal cavity, bluntly dissecting the colon from the anterior abdominal wall. Care was taken to not injure the serosal layer of the colon wall.

The colon was inspected and found to be in excellent condition.

For primary closure: The mucocutaneous border of the ostomy was excised to obtain healthy clean edges of colon. The colon was closed transversely in two layers, an inner running layer of adsorbable suture and an outer layer of interrupted Lembert sutures of 3-0 silk. The colon lumen was widely patent. Hemostasis was assured and the colon was then returned to the peritoneal cavity.

For stapled closure: An adequate length of transverse colon was freed and pulled out of the abdominal wound. A linear GIA 80 cm stapler was inserted into either barrel of the colostomy and fired along the antimesenteric border to form a side to side anastomosis. The common colotomy of the anastomosis was closed using a TA 90 cm stapler, removing the mucocutaneous border of the colostomy. A 3-0 silk suture was placed at the "crotch" of the anastomosis. 3-0 silk was used to reinforce the staple lines in Lembert fashion. The colon was then returned to the peritoneal cavity. The abdomen was irrigated, aspirated, and assured to be hemostatic.

The fascia was closed with *interrupted figure of eight sutures of 0-vicryl*. The wound was thoroughly irrigated. The skin was packed open and left to heal by secondary intention.

The patient tolerated the procedure well and was taken to the postanesthesia care unit in stable condition.

ACKNOWLEDGMENT

This chapter was contributed by Kareem A. Hamdy, MD, in the first edition.

NOTES

Chapter 59
Subtotal Colectomy for Lower GI Bleeding

Brian A. Coakley, M.D. and Celia M. Divino, M.D.

INDICATIONS
- Bleeding from the lower gastrointestinal tract, for which the location within the colon cannot be determined.
- Bleeding from the lower gastrointestinal tract that is refractory to nonoperative treatment measures.
- Bleeding from the lower gastrointestinal tract due to diffuse diverticular disease.

ESSENTIAL STEPS
1. Make a vertical incision in the midline.
2. Explore all the four quadrants of the abdominal cavity.
3. The right colon should be mobilized:
   - Make a division in the lateral peritoneal reflection and extend this opening from the cecum to the hepatic flexure. Take down any adhesions between the retroperitoneum and colon. Identify and preserve the duodenum and right ureter against any injury.
4. The transverse colon should be mobilized by dividing the greater omentum near the colon.
5. The splenic flexure and left colon should be mobilized:
   - Make a division in the lateral peritoneal reflection and extend this opening from the splenic flexure to the sigmoid colon. The left colon should be reflected medially by taking down any adhesions between it and the retroperitoneum.

J.J. Hoballah and C.E.H. Scott-Conner (eds.), *Operative Dictations in General and Vascular Surgery*, DOI 10.1007/978-1-4614-0451-4_59,
© Springer Science+Business Media, LLC 2012

- Identify points of transection on the terminal ileum and rectosigmoid colon.
6. Identify the point of intended transaction of both the rectosigmoid colon and the terminal ileum.
7. Use a linear-cutting stapler to divide the terminal ileum.
8. Use electrocautery to score the peritoneum overlying the intended line of mesenteric resection.
9. Use 2-0 ties and suture ligatures or, alternatively, an electronic vessel-sealing system, to divide the mesentery.
10. Plan the site of intended division of the rectosigmoid colon (usually above the peritoneal reflection, at the point where the taenia fuse to form a single longitudinal muscular layer on the rectum).
11. Divide the rectosigmoid junction with a linear-cutting stapler and remove the specimen.
12. Obtain hemostasis.
13. *If using staplers to create the anastomosis*:
    - *Bring together the stapled ends of the terminal ileum and rectosigmoid colon.*
    - *Place two stay sutures with 3-0 silk.*
    - *Use electrocautery to make enterotomies.*
    - *Place a linear-cutting stapler across the common wall and fire (take care to ensure that no mesentery protrudes into the intended staple line).*
    - *Inspect the staple line for hemostasis. Use gentle electrocautery along the staple line, as needed.*
    - *Use either a linear-cutting stapler or two-layer suture closure to close the remaining enterotomies.*
14. *If using sutures to create the anastomosis*:
    - *Bring together the end of the rectosigmoid colon and the antimesenteric border of the terminal ileum.*
    - *Create a two-layered anastomosis between the rectosigmoid stump and the antimesenteric border of the terminal ileum. For the inner layer, use running or interrupted 3-0 Vicryl and for the outer layer use interrupted 3-0 silk.*
15. Check the luminal size and integrity of the anastomosis. Ensure there is no tension on the anastomosis.
16. Obtain hemostasis.
17. Irrigate abdomen.
18. Place drains, if desired.
19. Close the midline wound in layers.

NOTE THESE VARIATIONS

- Primary anastomosis vs. diverting ileostomy with Hartmann's pouch or mucus fistula.
- Stapled vs. sutured anastomosis.

COMPLICATIONS

- Ureteral or duodenal injury.
- Recurrent bleeding.
- Anastomotic leak.
- Abscess.

TEMPLATE OPERATIVE DICTATION

Preoperative diagnosis: Lower gastrointestinal bleed.
Procedure: Subtotal colectomy with ileoproctostomy.
Postoperative diagnosis: Same.
Indications: This ___-year-old *male/female* developed bright red blood from the rectum, and on workup with *tagged red blood cell scan/sigmoidoscopy/colonoscopy/angiography* was found to have *angiodysplasia/diverticular disease/indeterminate colonic source* refractory to blood transfusion and conservative management. After a full discussion was held with the patient regarding the potential risks, potential benefits and alternative treatment options to surgery, *he/she* ultimately decided to undergo subtotal colectomy with ileocolonic anastomosis for definitive management.
Description of procedure: The patient was properly identified in the holding area and taken to the operating room. *Epidural catheter was placed for postoperative pain relief.* The patient was placed in the supine on the operating room table and sequential compression stocking were placed bilaterally. An IV line was inserted, general anesthesia was induced and the patient was successfully intubated. A time-out was completed verifying correct patient, procedure, site, positioning, and implant(s) and/or special equipment prior to beginning this procedure. Preoperative antibiotics were given. A Foley catheter and *orogastric/nasogastric* tube were inserted. The abdomen was prepped and draped in the usual sterile fashion. A vertical midline incision was made. This was deepened through the subcutaneous layer and hemostasis was achieved with electrocautery. The linea alba was incised and the peritoneal cavity entered. The abdomen was explored. *Given that the patient had undergone previous abdominal surgery, adhesions were sharply taken down under direct vision with the Metzenbaum scissors.*

The abdominal cavity was inspected for gross abnormalities. The colon appeared to be full of blood *with an extensive amount of diverticula throughout the colon, starting somewhat above the sacral promontory at the peritoneal reflection all the way to the cecum/ other.* The small bowel was also inspected for evidence of bleeding. With the exception of the region of the terminal ileum, no blood was found in the lumen of the small bowel and there were no abnormalities noted.

Initially the right colon was mobilized by dividing the peritoneal attachment from the cecum to the hepatic flexure. The colon and terminal ileum were mobilized medially, ensuring preservation of the duodenum and right ureter. We then sharply took down attachments of the greater omentum from the transverse colon extending up to the splenic flexure. At this point, we divided the lateral peritoneal reflection of the left colon, from the splenic flexure to the sigmoid colon. The left colon was reflected medially. Care was taken at all times to protect the left ureter.

Points of division on the terminal ileum and rectosigmoid colon were then selected. The bowel was divided in both locations with a linear-cutting stapler. The mesentery was scored and divided. The mesenteric vasculature was secured *ties and suture ligatures/an electronic vessel-sealing system.* The specimen was removed and sent to pathology.

Hemostasis was ensured along the staple line.

[Choose one:]

If **stapled anastomosis:** *The end of the rectosigmoid colon was brought together with the antimesenteric border of the terminal ileum and two3-0 silk were placed. Enterotomies were made. The linear-cutting stapler was inserted and fired along the common wall. The staple line was inspected for hemostasis. The linear-cutting stapler/a two-layer suture closure technique was used to close the enterotomies. The staple lines were imbricated with ___ suture.*

If **sutured anastomosis:** *The rectosigmoid colon was then sutured to the antimesenteric border of the terminal ileum in two layers: An inner layer of interrupted/running 3-0 Vicryl with an outer layer of interrupted 3-0 silk.*

The luminal size and strength of the anastomosis was verified. Hemostasis was ensured. A *drain was placed near the anastomosis.*

(Optional: Multiple interrupted through-and-through retention sutures of ____ were placed.) The fascia was closed with *interrupted _____/a running suture of ____.* The skin was closed with *skin staples/subcuticular sutures of ___/other.*

A sterile dressing was applied. The patient was successfully extubated at the end of the procedure. All needle, sponge, and instrument counts were correct at the end of the case. The patient tolerated the procedure well and was taken to the postanesthesia care unit in stable condition.

ACKNOWLEDGMENT
This chapter was contributed by Mazen M. Hashisho, MD, in the first edition.

NOTES

Chapter 60
Hartmann's Procedure

Carol E.H. Scott-Conner, M.D.

INDICATIONS

- Diverticular disease with perforation.
- Other situations in which conditions are not favorable for anastomosis.

ESSENTIAL STEPS

1. Long midline incision.
2. Explore the abdomen.
3. Culture any pus.
4. Incise the line of Toldt to free the colon from peritoneal attachment.
5. Identify and protect the ureters.
6. *Mobilize the splenic flexure.*
7. Divide the colon proximally and distally.
8. Ligate the mesenteric vessels.
9. Remove the specimen (tag proximal and distal ends).
10. Create ostomy site and deliver the colon.
11. Close the abdomen.
12. Mature colostomy.

NOTE THESE VARIATIONS

- Mobilization of the splenic flexure optional.
- Primary anastomosis with diverting loop ileostomy is an alternative in some situations.

J.J. Hoballah and C.E.H. Scott-Conner (eds.), *Operative Dictations in General and Vascular Surgery*, DOI 10.1007/978-1-4614-0451-4_60,
© Springer Science+Business Media, LLC 2012

COMPLICATIONS

- Injury to the ureter.
- Injury to the spleen.

TEMPLATE OPERATIVE DICTATION

Preoperative diagnosis: *Diverticular disease/other* with perforation.

Procedure: Left colon resection with colostomy (Hartmann's procedure).

Postoperative diagnosis: Same.

Indications: This ___-year-old *male/female* with *abdominal pain/ fever/obstructive symptoms/recurrent bouts of diverticulitis* was found to have *an acute perforation of the sigmoid colon/other.* Elective resection was indicated.

Description of procedure: *An epidural catheter was placed by anesthesia prior to the start of the operation.* The patient was placed in the supine position and general endotracheal anesthesia was induced. A time-out was completed verifying correct patient, procedure, site, positioning, and implant(s) and/or special equipment prior to beginning this procedure. Preoperative antibiotics were given. A Foley catheter and nasogastric tube were placed. The abdomen was prepped and draped in the usual sterile fashion. A vertical midline incision was made from xiphoid to just above the pubis. This was deepened through the subcutaneous tissues and hemostasis was achieved with electrocautery. The linea alba was identified and incised and the peritoneal cavity entered. The abdomen was explored. *Adhesions were lysed sharply under direct vision with Metzenbaum scissors. Generalized peritonitis/an abscess in the left lower quadrant/a mass in the sigmoid colon/other* was found.

The small bowel was inspected and retracted to the right using a moist towel and self-retaining retractor. Using electrocautery, the colon was freed from its peritoneal attachments along the line of Toldt proximally from the splenic flexure and distally to the pelvic inlet. Both ureters were identified and protected. Omentum was freed from the transverse colon and the splenic flexure was mobilized.

Points of transection were selected proximally and distally *(specify locations).* The bowel was divided with the linear cutting stapler. The peritoneum overlying the mesentery was then scored with electrocautery and the left colic artery was identified, double ligated with 2-0 silk sutures, and transected. The peritoneum overlying the mesentery was scored and remaining mesentery divided and ligated with 2-0 silk. *The inferior mesenteric artery was ligated near its origin from the aorta and all associated nodal tissue swept down with the specimen (if cancer).* The specimen was removed, proximal and distal ends tagged, and sent to pathology. The abdominal cavity was then copiously irrigated and hemostasis was checked.

The proximal colon reached easily to the proposed colostomy site without tension. A disk of skin was removed from the colostomy site in the left lower quadrant. The incision was deepened through all layers of the abdominal wall and dilated to admit *two/three* fingers. The colon was passed out through the ostomy site without torsion or tension. It was tacked to the peritoneum with several interrupted sutures of 3-0 silk. The lateral gutter was obliterated with a running suture of 3-0 Vicryl.

(Optional: The Hartmann's pouch was tacked to the presacral fascia/tagged with two long sutures of 2-0 prolene and allowed to fall into the pelvis.)

Two closed suction drains were placed in the pelvis and brought out through separate stab wounds lateral to the incision. These were secured with 3-0 nylon.

(Optional: Multiple interrupted through-and-through retention sutures of ____ were placed.) The fascia was closed with *a running suture of ____/a Smead-Jones closure of interrupted ____.* The skin was closed with *skin staples/subcuticular sutures of ___/other.*

The colostomy was matured with multiple interrupted sutures of 3-0 Vicryl. An ostomy bag was applied.

The patient tolerated the procedure well and was taken to the postanesthesia care unit in stable condition.

NOTES

Chapter 61

Closure of Hartmann's Procedure (Open)

Samy Maklad, M.D. and John W. Cromwell, M.D.

INDICATION

- Restoring continuity following diverting end colostomy and Hartmann's pouch procedure.

ESSENTIAL STEPS

1. Barium enema or colonoscopy preoperatively to confirm patency and rule out distal obstruction of colon.
2. Position patient in dorsal lithotomy position.
3. Close ostomy site with 0-vicryl pursestring suture and cover with Tegaderm to prevent contamination of surgical field.
4. Enter abdominal cavity via low midline incision through previous incisional scar.
5. Identify the Hartman's pouch and free from surrounding adhesions.
6. Reduce colostomy into abdomen via circumferential elliptical incision.
7. Mobilize splenic flexure as needed to create enough length for a tension-free anastomosis.
8. Assess both ends of bowel for perfusion/viability and freshen ends of bowel by stapling off the distal 2 cm.
9. Create tension-free anastomosis via one of several techniques: (a) End-to-end anastomotic stapler (EEA stapler) or (b) hand-sewn end-to-end.
10. Test anastomosis for leak by insufflating the rectum while submerging anastomosis in saline.

J.J. Hoballah and C.E.H. Scott-Conner (eds.), *Operative Dictations in General and Vascular Surgery*, DOI 10.1007/978-1-4614-0451-4_61,
© Springer Science+Business Media, LLC 2012

11. Check for hemostasis.
12. Close midline incision.

NOTE THESE VARIATIONS

■ Type of anastomosis: EEA stapler or end-to-end hand-sewn anastomosis.
■ Temporary diverting loop ileostomy.

COMPLICATIONS

■ Anastomotic stricture.
■ Anastomotic leak.
■ Wound infection.
■ Ureteral injury.

TEMPLATE OPERATIVE DICTATION

Preoperative diagnosis: *Diverting end colostomy and Hartmann's pouch.*

Procedure: *Closure of Hartmann's pouch.*

Postoperative diagnosis: Same.

Indications: This is ___-year-old *male/female* that underwent diverting end colostomy and Hartman's pouch for ____. He presents today for take down of his Hartmann's pouch. He/she was informed of all possible risks of surgery including but not limited to the risk of leak, PE, DVT, death, anesthetic complications, infection, bleeding requiring transfusions, bowel and vascular injury, decubitus ulceration, and nerve palsies. He was also made aware of the possibilities of developing small bowel obstruction and internal hernia as long-term complications of this operation. The patient understands and is willing to proceed with our recommendations.

Description of procedure: The patient was taken to the operating room and placed in the supine position. General endotracheal anesthesia was induced without any difficulty. A time-out was completed verifying correct patient, procedure, site, positioning, and implant(s) and/or special equipment prior to beginning this procedure. Both upper extremities were placed in the extended position on arm boards. A Foley catheter and an orogastric tube were placed. Preoperative antibiotics were given. The patient was re-positioned in the dorsal lithotomy position with stirrups and care was taken to pad all pressure points. The colostomy was *closed with a 0-vicryl pursestring stitch or the colostomy was covered* *with a Tegaderm* to prevent fecal contamination of the surgical field. The patient's abdomen and perineum were then prepped and draped in the usual sterile fashion.

Using a #10 blade a vertical low midline incision was made overlying the previous midline incisional scar. This was depended through the subcutaneous tissues using electrocautery. Hemostasis was achieved and maintained throughout the case using electrocautery. The fascia was identified and incised and the peritoneal cavity was entered.

The abdomen was explored. *Adhesions were lysed sharply under direct vision with Metzenbaum scissors.* The bowel was inspected for gross abnormities. *No abnormalities/the following abnormalities* were found. A self-retaining abdominal wall retractor was placed and the small bowel was carefully retracted into the right upper quadrant. The Hartmann's pouch was identified by a marker proline stitch noted on the end to the pouch which appeared healthy. The distal colon was mobilized and freed from any adjacent adhesions during which time the left ureter was identified and protected within the retroperitoneum.

Attention was turned toward taking down the colostomy. An elliptical incision encompassing the colostomy was made using a #15 blade and deepened through the subcutaneous and surrounding fascia using electrocautery. Once the proximal colon was freed from the fascia and reduced into the abdomen, the two ends were freshened by stapling the distal 2 cm with a gastrointestinal anastomosis (GIA) stapler. *The proximal colon was found to lie adjacent to the pouch without tension/The left colon was mobilized by incising the white line of toldt up to the splenic flexure allowing the proximal colon to lie adjacent to the pouch without tension.* A tension-free anastomosis was created between the proximal and distal colon in the following manner.

If using an EEA stapler: *A purse string stitch using a 2-0 Prolene was placed in the proximal end of the colon and fastened around the anvil. EEA sizer was used to dilate the rectum to 33, 29, or 25 Fr and to assure the absence of any stricture. A 33, 29, or 25 Fr EEA stapler was advanced carefully by an assistant from below and a second purse string stitch was placed on the rectal stump and fastened around EEA stapler. The antimesenteric boarders were aligned. The EEA stapler was attached to the anvil and fired. The stapler was removed and the rings of tissue retained in the stapler were inspected and found to be complete and intact rings. The staple line was found to be a complete 360° with an intact staple line/was not complete and a reinforcing layer of interrupted 3-0 silk or Vicryl Lembert suture were placed.*

If using hand-sewn anastomotic technique: The antime-senteric boarders were aligned in an end-to-end fashion and approximated in two layers, an outer layer of interrupted 3-0 silk Lembert stitches and an inner layer of running 3-0 Vicryl.

If temporary loop ileostomy: An opening in the abdominal wall to the right of midline, opposite the colostomy site was made. The fascial opening was widened to allow two fingers to pass through easily. A proximal loop of ileum was passed through and tacked to the peritoneum in several areas with interrupted 3-0 Vicryl.

The anastomosis was tested for patency and integrity by filling the abdomen with saline and insufflating the rectum with air while occluding the colon proximal to the anastomosis. No bubbles were noted and air was seen to pass across the anastomosis proximally. The abdomen was copiously irrigated with normal saline and the self-retaining retractor was removed. Hemostasis was checked and omentum was brought down to lie over the anastomosis. The fascia was close with a running suture of looped 0-PDS. The skin was closed with *skin staples/running subcuticular stitch using 4-0 Monocryl suture*. The midline incision was dressed with 4×4 gauze and Tegaderm.

If temporary loop ileostomy: The proximal loop of ileum was opened on the inferior margin and matured in a brook fashion using multiple interrupted 3-0 Vicryl stitches. This was done by inverting the ileum and taking full thickness bites of the edge of the ileum to a sero-muscular bite of ileum and then a subcuticular layer of skin. An ostomy appliance was then placed.

The patient tolerated the procedure well and was extubated and taken to the postoperative care unit in stable condition accompanied by the surgical and anesthesia teams.

NOTES

Chapter 62
Laparoscopic Closure of Hartmann's Procedure

Maher A. Abbas, M.D.

INDICATIONS

- Prior sigmoidectomy for perforated diverticulitis, carcinoma, penetrating trauma, bleeding, inflammatory bowel disease, ischemia, or infection.
- Anastomotic leak following prior left hemicolectomy, sigmoidectomy, or anterior resection requiring conversion to Hartmann's procedure.

ESSENTIAL STEPS

1. Lithotomy position, both arms are tucked.
2. Foley catheter and orogastric tube.
3. If short rectal stump on preoperative evaluation, multiple prior abdominopelvic operations, and then stent both ureters.
4. Close the colostomy with a purse-string and disconnect it at the mucocutaneous junction.
5. Dissect around the colostomy in the subcutaneous plane until the fascia is reached.
6. Dissect the bowel circumferentially and free it from the abdominal wall.
7. Perform a limited lysis of adhesions through this stomal wound and begin to mobilize the descending colon.
8. Inspect the visualized portion of the colon and trim the distal aspect of the bowel to good quality edges.
9. Establish purse-string and place anvil of circular EEA stapler.

J.J. Hoballah and C.E.H. Scott-Conner (eds.), *Operative Dictations in General and Vascular Surgery*, DOI 10.1007/978-1-4614-0451-4_62,
© Springer Science+Business Media, LLC 2012

10. Reduce descending colon back inside abdominal cavity.
11. Approximate the fascia with a purse-string suture around a 12-mm trocar. Tie the purse-string.
12. Establish pneumoperitoneum.
13. Under direct visualization, place three trocars in the right lower quadrant (12 mm), supraumbilical area (5 mm), and right mid abdomen (5 mm).
14. Lyse adhesions.
    • Additional trocars may be needed depending on the extent of intra-abdominal adhesions.
15. Mobilize the splenic flexure to ensure a tension-free anastomosis (needed in some cases).
    • Place the patient in the reverse Trendelenburg position again.
    • Mobilize the left colon from the lateral to medial approach by incising the lateral attachments.
    • Take down the splenic flexure by lifting the omentum off the distal transverse colon and joining the dissection with the medially mobilized descending colon.
16. Identify rectal stump by bringing a rectal dilator transanally and advance to the top of the rectal stump.
17. If the apex of the rectal stump is soft and pliable then remove dilator and advance circular EEA stapler transanally and perform an end-to-end stapled colorectal anastomosis.
18. If the apex of the rectal stump is fibrotic then can either perform an end-to-side stapled colorectal anastomosis (anterior rectum) or alternatively dissect and resect the upper/mid aspect of the rectum and perform a high or low anterior resection type anastomosis. In such case, identify the left ureter and keep out of harm's way prior to transecting the rectum.
19. Test the anastomosis by insufflating the rectum transanally with the pelvis submerged in saline solution.
20. Irrigate and suction the pelvis.
21. Consider a pelvic drain if extensive pelvic dissection or prior radiation.
22. Remove all trocars and close the fascia of the 12-mm trocars.
23. Close the skin wounds with metal staples except for the prior stoma site which is partially approximated leaving its central portion open to drain.
24. Dress all wounds.

NOTE THESE VARIATIONS

- In a minority of patients, a completion proctectomy of the rectal stump is necessary with a coloanal anastomosis (i.e., in the case of multiple prior pelvic operations, extensive pelvic fibrosis).
- Splenic flexure mobilization is commonly, but not always, needed for tension-free anastomosis.

COMPLICATIONS

- Transection of the ureter.
- Laceration of the spleen.
- Small bowel enterotomy.
- Transection of the hypogastric nerve trunk.
- Anastomotic leak.
- Severe bleeding.
- Need for conversion to open procedure if extensive intrabdominal adhesions and fibrosis are encountered.

TEMPLATE OPERATIVE DICTATION

Preoperative diagnosis: Prior sigmoidectomy with Hartmann's procedure for _____.

Procedure: Laparoscopic closure of Hartmann's pouch.

Postoperative diagnosis: Same.

Indications: The patient is _____-year-old *male/female* with a history of _____. Different treatment options were discussed with the patient. The procedure of laparoscopic possible open closure of Hartmann's procedure was reviewed with the patient. The procedure, indication, alternatives, risks, and complications were reviewed with the patient. The patient verbalized understanding and wished to proceed. Informed consent was obtained.

Description of procedure: The patient was brought to the operating room and after instillation of general endotracheal anesthesia, he/she was placed in the lithotomy position with both arms tucked. A time-out was completed verifying correct patient, procedure, site, positioning, and/or special equipment prior to beginning this procedure. Intravenous antibiotic and subcutaneous heparin were administered. A Foley catheter and an orogastric tube were inserted. *(If ureteral stents are needed then cystoscopy and bilateral ureteral stents performed at this stage.)* All extremities were well padded. The rectum was irrigated with betadine. The abdomen was shaved and prepped in the usual sterile fashion.

The colostomy was closed with a purse-string suture using 2.0 Vicryl. Electrocautery was used to disconnect the mucocutaneous junction and dissection was carried in the subcutaneous plane until the fascia was reached and the bowel is dissected circumferentially and freed from the abdominal wall. Limited adhesiolysis was performed through the stomal wound and a short segment of the descending colon was mobilized. It was visually inspected and the colostomy portion of the bowel was trimmed. A 2.0 prolene suture was used as a purse-string and the anvil of a (25–34 mm range) circular EEA stapler was placed and the purse-string was tied. The descending colon was reduced inside the abdominal cavity. The fascia was approximated with a 0 Vicryl purse-string suture and a 12-mm trocar was placed and the suture was tied. The pneumoperitoneum was established. Under direct visualization, three trocars were placed in the right lower quadrant (12 mm), supraumbilical area (5 mm), and right mid abdomen (5 mm). Adhesiolysis was performed (if additional trocars are needed, they are placed as dictated by the location of the adhesions). Splenic flexure mobilization was performed to ensure a tension-free anastomosis. The patient was placed in the reverse Trendelenburg position and the left colon was mobilized from a lateral to medial approach by incising the lateral attachments. The splenic flexure was taken down by lifting the omentum off the distal transverse colon and joining the dissection with the mobilized descending colon. The patient was positioned in the Trendelenburg position again. A rectal dilator was introduced transanally and advanced to the apex of the rectal stump. The stump was mobilized off the pelvic side wall (*if significant fibrosis then need to mobilize the pelvic portion of the rectum and resect as needed*). The dilator was then exchanged for a circular EEA stapler and a stapled *end-to-end/end-to-anterior rectal side* anastomosis was performed under direct visualization. The anastomosis was tested by insufflating the rectum transanally after submerging the pelvis with saline solution and gently occluding the proximal descending colon. No air leak was noted. The pelvis was irrigated and suction. *A 19 French closed suction drain was placed in the pelvis through the right lower quadrant trocar site and secured to the skin with 2.0 nylon suture*. Under direct visualization with the camera through the 12-mm prior stoma site, all trocars were removed. The skin was closed with metal staples. The purse-string at the stoma site was removed and the anterior fascia was closed with single interrupted 0 PDS sutures and the skin was partially approximated with metal staples. The central portion of the wound was left open to drain. All wounds were dressed. All instruments, needles, and sponges count was correct times two. The patient tolerated the procedure well and was taken to the recovery unit in stable condition.

NOTES

Chapter 63

Sigmoidectomy and Rectopexy (Frykman-Goldberg Procedure)

Sergy Khaitov, M.D.

INDICATION

- Full-thickness rectal prolapse with constipation.

ESSENTIAL STEPS

1. Modified lithotomy position.
2. Lower midline laparotomy, *optional – Phannenstiel incision*.
3. Incise peritoneal attachments of the sigmoid colon and rectum.
4. Identify ureters.
5. Identify, isolate, and divide superior hemorrhoidal artery.
6. Identify and dissect presacral avascular space.
   - Preserve hypogastric nerves.
7. Continue mobilization of rectum down to the pelvic floor with preservation of the lateral stalks.
8. Reduce the rectum from the pelvis with upward traction, defining distal resection margin to plan the anastomosis at the level of sacral promontory – upper rectum.
9. Define proximal resection margin at the sigmoid colon to plan the anastomosis at the level of the sacral promontory.
   - Avoid mobilizing sigmoid colon proximally into the descending colon.
10. Transect the mesorectum and sigmoid colon mesentery with clamps and ties or energy device.

J.J. Hoballah and C.E.H. Scott-Conner (eds.), *Operative Dictations in General and Vascular Surgery*, DOI 10.1007/978-1-4614-0451-4_63,
© Springer Science+Business Media, LLC 2012

11. Divide of upper rectum with the GIA or TA stapler.
12. Divide proximal sigmoid colon with purse-string device and placement of EEA stapler anvil.
13. Create EEA anastomosis at the level of the sacral promontory.
14. Air leak test the anastomosis.
15. Rectopexy to presacral fascia with nonabsorbable sutures (avoid presacral plexus bleeding).
16. Irrigate the pelvis and check for hemostasis.
17. Close the abdomen.

VARIATIONS

- Optional use of preoperative bowel prep.
- No resection for patients with diarrhea, rectopexy only.
- Optional use of drains.
- Laparoscopic procedure.

COMPLICATIONS

- Recurrence.
- Anastomotic leak.
- Infection.
- Bleeding.
- Inadvertent injuries to ureters, hypogastric nerves.

TEMPLATE OPERATIVE DICTATION

Preoperative diagnosis: Full-thickness rectal prolapse with constipation.
Procedure: Sigmoid Resection and rectopexy.
Postoperative: Same.
Indications: This ___-year-old male/female presented with full-thickness rectal prolapse and constipation. Preoperative colonoscopy was negative for malignancy. Sigmoid resection and rectopexy was chosen for management.
Description of the procedure: Epidural catheter placement was performed by anesthesia team at preoperative holding area and subcutaneous heparin injection was given as well. Patient was brought to the operating room and positioned on the operating table supine, sequential compression stockings were applied. Preoperative antibiotic prophylaxis was administered. After induction of general endotracheal anesthesia patient was repositioned into modified lithotomy position using Allen stirrups. A time-out was completed verifying correct patient, procedure, site, position-

ing, and implant(s) and/or special equipment prior to beginning this procedure. All bony prominences were well-padded and protected. Foley catheter was placed into the urinary bladder under sterile technique. Orogastric tube was placed by anesthesiologist. Operating field was prepped and draped in standard surgical fashion. *Lower midline laparotomy/Phannenstiel* incision was performed with a knife and Bovie electrocautery. Peritoneal cavity was entered sharply without difficulties. Exploration of peritoneal cavity revealed: list findings. Small bowel was packed off to the upper abdomen was moist lap pads.

Lateral attachments of the junction between the descending colon and sigmoid were opened with Bovie electrocautery and incision of the pelvic peritoneum was continued to the pelvic floor on both sides. Both ureters were clearly identified and preserved. Redundant sigmoid colon was retracted out of the pelvis and base of the rectosigmoid mesentery was palpated and avascular behind it was sharply dissected with preservation of hypogastric nerves. At this point, superior hemorrhoidal artery was clearly identified and isolated. Position of both ureters was confirmed and they were preserved. Superior hemorrhoidal artery was clamped and ligated with 0 Vicryl ligatures/divided with LigaSure device. Dissection was continued in avascular presacral plane in the distal direction down to the pelvic floor until levators plate was identified. Limited mobilization lateral attachments of the rectum were performed with preservation of lateral stalks. The mesorectum was divided with clamps and ties and the level of the upper rectum to plan the anastomosis at the level of the sacral promontory. Rectal wall was cleared off the mesenteric fat and it was transected with *TA-60/GIA* stapler and transected. The mesentery of the sigmoid colon was divided with clamps and ties to the level of proximal sigmoid colon to accomplish tension-free anastomosis to the upper rectum. The wall of sigmoid colon was cleared of mesenteric fat and was transected after the application of purse-string device. The specimen was handled off the field.

Sigmoid lumen was measured with EEA sizers and 31/28 mm EEA anvil was placed into sigmoid colon and purse-string stitch was tied. Stapled EEA anastomosis was created between the upper rectum and proximal sigmoid colon at the level of the sacral promontory. The air leak test was performed and was negative.

Rectopexy was accomplished with the application of 2/3 interrupted 2/0 Prolene sutures between presacral fascia and upper rectum distal to the anastomosis. Hemostasis was confirmed and pelvis was irrigated and dried. Operative instruments, suture materials, and laparotomy pack counts were reported to be correct.

Laparotomy was closed with running looped #1PDS suture and the level of the fascia. Incision was irrigated and dried. Final counts of operative instruments, suture materials, and pads were reported to be correct. Skin was closed with staples. Sterile dressing was applied. Patient was repositioned into the supine position, successfully extubated in the operating room and transferred to the postanesthesia care unit in stable and alert condition.

NOTES

Section V

Anus, Rectum, and Pilonidal Region

Chapter 64
Rubber Band Ligation of Hemorrhoids

Shauna Lorenzo-Rivero, M.D.

INDICATION
- Internal hemorrhoids with prolapse or bleeding, refractory to medical management.

ESSENTIAL STEPS
1. Rectal exam.
2. Anoscopy.
3. Identification of internal hemorrhoids.
4. For each of three pedicles:
   - Clamp applied to the proximal redundant mucosa.
   - Rubber band applied.
   - Mucosa inspected.
5. Anoscope withdrawn.

NOTE THESE VARIATIONS
- Number of pedicles varies but in general, three can be defined at the left lateral, right posterior, and right anterior locations.
- A pair of bands, rather than a single band, may be used.

COMPLICATIONS
- Pain due to rubber band application too close to dentate line.
- Bleeding.

J.J. Hoballah and C.E.H. Scott-Conner (eds.), *Operative Dictations in General and Vascular Surgery*, DOI 10.1007/978-1-4614-0451-4_64,
© Springer Science+Business Media, LLC 2012

- Sepsis.
- Recurrence.
- Urinary retention.

TEMPLATE OPERATIVE DICTATION

Preoperative diagnosis: First- to second-degree hemorrhoids.
Procedure: Anoscopy, rubber band ligation of hemorrhoids.
Postoperative diagnosis: Same.
Indications: This___-year-old *male/female* was found to have internal hemorrhoids that did not respond to bulk-forming agents.
Description of procedure: The patient was placed in the prone jackknife position *and given sedation*. A time-out was completed verifying correct patient, procedure, site, positioning, and implant(s) and/or special equipment prior to beginning this procedure. Digital rectal exam was performed. A generously lubricated anoscope was inserted into the anal canal. The three hemorrhoidal pedicles were identified and the redundant rectal mucosa just above the largest internal hemorrhoid grasped with a clamp. The patient did not complain of excessive pain. Using the applicator, *a rubber band was/two rubber bands were* placed around this tissue and the clamp was released. The *band was/bands were* noted to be in good position. This procedure was repeated on the other two pedicles. The mucosa was inspected for bleeding prior to withdrawal of the anoscope.

The patient tolerated the procedure well *and was taken to the postanesthesia care unit in stable condition (if sedation used)*.

NOTES

Chapter 65

Hemorrhoidectomy

Shauna Lorenzo-Rivero, M.D.

INDICATIONS

- Second-degree hemorrhoids resistant to medical management or band ligation.
- Third- and fourth-degree hemorrhoids.
- Hemorrhoids complicated by ulceration, fissures, fistulae, large hypertrophied anal papillae, or excessive skin tags.
- Strangulated hemorrhoids.
- Acute bleeding when suture ligation fails.

ESSENTIAL STEPS

1. Rectal exam.
2. Inject local anesthetic.
3. Dilate the anus and place anoscope.
4. Identify three hemorrhoidal pedicles.
5. Clamp pedicles at the base.
6. Retract the anal tissue externally.
7. Excise the skin and mucosa with elliptical incision.
8. Dissect the hemorrhoidal tissue free of surrounding structures taking care not to injury the sphincter muscles.
9. Clamp and ligate the pedicle at the apex.
10. Secure hemostasis.
11. Close incisions.
12. Repeat for other pedicles.

J.J. Hoballah and C.E.H. Scott-Conner (eds.), *Operative Dictations in General and Vascular Surgery*, DOI 10.1007/978-1-4614-0451-4_65,
© Springer Science+Business Media, LLC 2012

NOTE THESE VARIATIONS
- Prone jackknife position vs. lithotomy position.
- Number of hemorrhoids varies but is in general, three: left lateral, right posterior, and right anterior locations.

COMPLICATIONS
- Bleeding/hematoma.
- Anal incontinence.
- Sphincter spasm.
- Sepsis.
- Urinary retention.
- Recurrence.

TEMPLATE OPERATIVE DICTATION

Preoperative diagnosis: *Second/third/fourth-degree* hemorrhoids.
Procedure: Anoscopy, hemorrhoidectomy.
Postoperative diagnosis: Same.
Indications: This ___-year-old *male/female* was found to have symptomatic hemorrhoids *refractory to medical management/complicated by (specify)*.
Description of procedure: The patient was brought to the operating room and *general/spinal/caudal* anesthesia was induced. *He/she* was placed in the *prone jackknife lithotomy* position. A time-out was completed verifying correct patient, procedure, site, positioning, and implant(s) and/or special equipment prior to beginning this procedure. The buttocks were taped apart.

The perineum was prepped and draped in standard sterile fashion. Local anesthetic was injected *as a perianal/pudendal nerve block*. The anus was carefully dilated until three fingers could be introduced. An anoscope was introduced and the three hemorrhoidal pedicles were identified. A Kelly clamp/perforated towel clip was placed near the base of each pedicle near the dentate line and retracted externally to exteriorize the hemorrhoidal pedicles.

Each pedicle was excised in turn in the following fashion. An elliptical incision was made extending from perianal skin to anorectal ring including both internal and external hemorrhoids and excising a minimum amount of anoderm. Flaps were developed on both aspects of the incision, taking care to elevate only skin and mucosa. The dilated venous mass was dissected using Metzenbaum scissors from the underlying sphincter muscle. The base was secured with a Kelly clamp. The pedicle was amputated from the base and secured with a 2-0 Vicryl suture ligature. Hemostasis was achieved using electrocautery.

Following hemostasis, the skin and mucosal incisions were closed with a running lock stitch of 2-0 Vicryl on the mucosal aspect and converted to subcuticular once skin was encountered. The anal canal was then injected with local anesthetic. A gauze pad was tucked between the gluteal folds.

The patient tolerated the procedure well and was *extubated and* taken to the postanesthesia care unit in stable condition.

NOTES

Chapter 66

Procedure for Prolapsed Hemorrhoids (Stapled Hemorrhoidectomy)

Susan Skaff Hagen, M.D., M.S.P.H.

INDICATIONS

- Second degree hemorrhoids after multiple failures with rubber band treatment.
- Third or fourth degree hemorrhoids.
- Rectal mucosal prolapse.

ESSENTIAL STEPS

1. General anesthesia.
2. Lithotomy position.
3. Examine rectum.
4. Place dilator in anal canal and secure to perineum.
5. Place pursestring.
6. Open circular stapler and position head proximal to pursestring and tie.
7. With traction on pursestring, tighten device and hold for 30 s.
8. Fire stapler and keep closed for 20 s.
9. Remove stapler.
10. Examine staple line.
11. Secure hemostasis.

NOTE THESE VARIATIONS

- Suture over staple line.
- Packing with Surgicel or Xylocaine post procedure.

J.J. Hoballah and C.E.H. Scott-Conner (eds.), *Operative Dictations in General and Vascular Surgery*, DOI 10.1007/978-1-4614-0451-4_66,

COMPLICATIONS

- Damage to rectal wall.
- Short or long term dysfunction.
- Pelvic Sepsis.

TEMPLATE OPERATIVE DICTATION

Preoperative diagnosis: *Hemorrhoids/Rectal mucosal prolapse.*
Procedure: PPH Hemorrhoidal Stapling.
Postoperative diagnosis: Same.
Indications: Patient is a ___-year old *male/female* with ___ hemorrhoids that are *painful/bleeding/prolapsing. He/she* presents for a PPH hemorrhoidal stapling.
Description of procedure: Patient was brought into the operating room and general endotracheal anesthesia was administered. The patient was then placed in the *lithotomy/prone jack knife* position. A time-out was completed verifying correct patient, procedure, site, positioning, and implant(s)and/or special equipment prior to beginning this procedure. The patient was prepped with *Betadine/Chlorhexidine* and draped in the usual sterile fashion.

The perineal and rectal areas were examined. The patient was found to have *prolapsing internal hemorrhoids and external hemorrhoids*. The hemorrhoidal stapling kit was opened and the dilator was placed in the anal canal. The obturator was removed. The dilator kit was secured to the perineum using 3-0 silk suture. The dentate line was identified. The purse-string suture anoscope was placed through the dilator. Approximately 1.5 cm above the dentate line, a 2-0 Prolene purse-string suture was placed. Next the stapling gun was fully opened and the anvil was placed above the purse-string suture. The purse-string suture was tied down. The two ends of the suture were brought through the opening in the stapler device. With traction on the pursestring, the stapling gun was closed until the green indicator was present within the window. The stapling gun was kept in the closed position for 30 s. The stapler gun was fired and kept in position for 20 s. The device was then was removed. The staple line was examined. *There was one bleeding point at ___o'clock that was sutured using 4-0 Vicryl suture*. After hemostasis, *a piece of Surgicel and Xylocaine lubricant* were placed in the rectum. Mesh undergarments with ABD were applied. The patient tolerated the procedure well and was brought to the PACU in stable condition.

NOTES

Chapter 67
Drainage of Perirectal Abscess

Shauna Lorenzo-Rivero, M.D.

INDICATION
- Perirectal or perianal abscess.

ESSENTIAL STEPS
1. Rectal exam.
2. Inject local anesthetic.
3. Proctoscopy.
4. Aspirate the abscess.
5. Incise and drain.
6. Break loculations *digitally/with hemostat*.
7. Irrigate.
8. Pack open.

NOTE THESE VARIATIONS
- Submucosal or supralevator abscess requires internal drainage.
- In extremely favorable circumstances, fistulotomy may be done simultaneously.

COMPLICATIONS
- Bleeding/hematoma formation.
- Recurrent abscess.
- Fistula formation.
- Urinary retention.

J.J. Hoballah and C.E.H. Scott-Conner (eds.), *Operative Dictations in General and Vascular Surgery*, DOI 10.1007/978-1-4614-0451-4_67,

TEMPLATE OPERATIVE DICTATION

Preoperative diagnosis: *Perirectal/perianal/submucosal* abscess.

Procedure: Anoscopy, drainage of perirectal/perianal abscess.

Postoperative diagnosis: *Perirectal/perianal/submucosal* abscess.

Indications: This ___-year-old *male/female* was found to have *palpable/suspected perirectal/perianal/submucosal* abscess.

Description of procedure: The patient was brought to the operating room and *general/spinal/monitored care* anesthesia was induced. The patient was then repositioned in *lithotomy/left lateral decubitus position*. A time-out was completed verifying correct patient, procedure, site, positioning, and implant(s) and/or special equipment prior to beginning this procedure. A rectal examination was performed and the abscess/mass identified and confirmed to be *infralevator/submucosal* . The patient was prepped and draped in the usual sterile fashion. Local anesthetic was injected *as a perianal/pudendal nerve block*. Proctoscopy was performed. The area of swelling was aspirated using an 18-gauge needle and the presence of pus confirmed.

[Choose one:]

If infralevator perirectal or perianal: An incision was made through the skin over the abscess as close as possible to the anal verge. The surrounding structures were dissected using a hemostat until the abscess cavity was encountered. The hemostat was then used to break up loculations, pus was suctioned from the cavity, and a finger introduced to confirm the absence of remaining loculations. The abscess was irrigated. Hemostasis was achieved with electrocautery and the cavity packed open with gauze.

If submucosal : The overlying mucosa was incised and pus allowed to drain into the rectum. Loculations were broken with a hemostat. The cavity was irrigated and left open (or a Penrose drain was placed in the cavity).

The patient tolerated the procedure well and was *extubated and* taken to the postanesthesia care unit in stable condition.

NOTES

Chapter 68
Anorectal Fistulotomy

Shauna Lorenzo-Rivero, M.D.

INDICATION
- Fistulo-in-ano.

ESSENTIAL STEPS
1. Rectal exam.
2. Identify the external opening.
3. Inject local anesthetic.
4. *Anoscopy/anal retraction*.
5. Identify the internal opening.
6. Pass the probe from the external to internal opening.
7. Unroof the fistula.
8. Identify any side-tracks and unroof.
9. Biopsy the tract and send to pathology.
10. Hemostasis.

NOTE THESE VARIATIONS
- Penrose drain or seton for:
  - Complex fistulae.
  - Multiple tracts.
  - Crohn's disease.

COMPLICATIONS
- Recurrent abscess/fistula.
- Incontinence.

J.J. Hoballah and C.E.H. Scott-Conner (eds.), *Operative Dictations in General and Vascular Surgery*, DOI 10.1007/978-1-4614-0451-4_68,
© Springer Science+Business Media, LLC 2012

- Bleeding.
- Urinary retention.

TEMPLATE OPERATIVE DICTATION

Preoperative diagnosis: Fistula-in-ano.
Procedure: Anoscopy, fistulotomy.
Postoperative diagnosis: Same.
Indications: This ___-year-old *male/female* developed fistulo-in-ano *after previous incision and drainage of perirectal abscess.*
Description of procedure: The patient was brought to the operating room and *general/spinal/monitored care* anesthesia was induced. The patient was then positioned in the *prone jackknife/lithotomy/ left lateral decubitus* position. A time-out was completed verifying correct patient, procedure, site, positioning, and implant(s) and/or special equipment prior to beginning this procedure. The perineum was prepped and draped in the usual sterile fashion. The external opening(s) of the fistula(e) *was/were* identified. Local anesthetic was injected *as a perianal/pudendal nerve block.* The anus was gently dilated and a Hill-Ferguson retractor was inserted, exposing the anal crypts. These were explored using a crypt hook until the internal opening of the fistula was identified. The tract was cannulated from the external opening and the flexible probe passed through to the internal opening with care and without resistance. Electrocautery was used to divide the overlying soft tissues. This was accomplished in stages. A portion of the margin was resected as a biopsy and sent to pathology. *All tracts were unroofed/a Penrose drain/seton was placed in the defect and sutured to the perianal skin using a 3-0 silk interrupted suture.*

Hemostasis was achieved using electrocautery. A gauze pad was tucked between the buttocks.

The patient tolerated the procedure well and was *extubated and* taken to the postanesthesia care unit in stable condition.

NOTES

Chapter 69

Anal Fistula Plug

Shauna Lorenzo-Rivero, M.D.

INDICATION
- Fistula-in-Ano.

ESSENTIAL STEPS
1. Rectal exam.
2. Identify the external opening.
3. Inject local anesthetic.
4. *Anoscopy/anal retraction.*
5. Inject the external opening. Identify the internal opening.
6. Pass the probe from the external to internal opening.
7. Prepare the fistula plug and attach to the fistula probe.
8. Withdraw the probe and insert the plug.
9. Trim internal portion of plug and close opening.
10. Leave external opening open and apply 5% Flagyl topical ointment.

NOTE THIS VARIATION
- None currently recommended for best results.

COMPLICATIONS
- Recurrence.
- Pain.
- Infection.
- Dislodgement of plug.

J.J. Hoballah and C.E.H. Scott-Conner (eds.), *Operative Dictations in General and Vascular Surgery*, DOI 10.1007/978-1-4614-0451-4_69,
© Springer Science+Business Media, LLC 2012

- Bleeding.
- Urinary retention.

TEMPLATE OPERATIVE DICTATION

Preoperative diagnosis: Fistula-in-Ano.
Postoperative diagnosis: Same.
Indications: This ___-year-old *male/female* developed fistulo-in-ano *after previous incision and drainage of perirectal abscess.* A Seton has been in place for 6–8 weeks and all sepsis controlled.
Description of Procedure: The patient was brought to the operating room and *general/spinal/monitored care* anesthesia was induced. The patient was then positioned in the *prone jackknife/lithotomy/left lateral decubitus* position. A time-out was completed verifying correct patient, procedure, site, positioning, and implant(s) and/or special equipment prior to beginning this procedure. The perineum was prepped and draped in the usual sterile fashion. The external opening(s) of the fistula(e) *was/were* identified. Local anesthetic was injected *as a perianal/pudendal nerve block.* The anus was gently dilated and a Hill-Ferguson retractor was inserted, exposing the anal crypts.

A 1:1 mixture of hydrogen peroxide and saline was injected from the external opening to both identify the internal opening and flush the tract. The tract was cannulated from the external opening and the flexible probe passed through to the internal opening with care and without resistance. The fistula plug which had already been soaking in saline was then prepared by suturing with a 2-0 Vicryl through the apex of the plug and tying it to the internal end of the fistula probe. It was brought out through the external opening until the plug fit snuggly but without excessive resistance. The probe was removed from the stitch. The plug was removed from the internal opening to cut the base (large end) so that it lies just beneath the mucosa. A 2-0 Vicryl suture was placed through the base of the plug and the external suture was pulled to secure the plug in place. The internal stitch that was still attached to the base was used to perform a figure of eight stitch to cover the base with mucosa. Any visible plug at the external opening was trimmed.

Hemostasis was achieved using electrocautery. The patient was cleaned and dried. 5% Flagyl topical ointment was applied to the external opening followed by a gauze pad tucked between the buttocks.

The patient tolerated the procedure well and was *extubated and* taken to the postanesthesia care unit in stable condition.

NOTES

Chapter 70

Lateral Internal Sphincterotomy for Chronic Anal Fissure

Shauna Lorenzo-Rivero, M.D.

INDICATION

- Chronic anal fissure.

ESSENTIAL STEPS

1. Rectal exam.
2. Inject local anesthetic.
3. Anoscopy.
4. Identify the fissure and curet the base.
5. Identify the intersphincteric groove and make an incision.
6. Elevate and divide fibers of the internal sphincter.
7. Achieve hemostasis.
8. Close the wound.

NOTE THESE VARIATIONS

- Prone jackknife vs. lithotomy position vs. left lateral decubitus.
- Longitudinal incision into the anal canal (open technique) on occasion used.

COMPLICATIONS

- Bleeding/hematoma formation.
- Incontinence.
- Recurrence.
- Urinary retention.

J.J. Hoballah and C.E.H. Scott-Conner (eds.), *Operative Dictations in General and Vascular Surgery*, DOI 10.1007/978-1-4614-0451-4_70,
© Springer Science+Business Media, LLC 2012

TEMPLATE OPERATIVE DICTATION

Preoperative diagnosis: Chronic anal fissure.
Procedure: Lateral internal sphincterotomy.
Postoperative diagnosis: Same.
Indications: This ___-year-old *male/female* had anal fissure of duration refractory to medical management. Lateral internal sphincterotomy was elected for management.
Description of procedure: The patient was brought to the operating room and *general/spinal/monitored care* anesthesia was induced. The patient was placed in the *prone jackknife/lithotomy/ left lateral decubitus* position. A time-out was completed verifying correct patient, procedure, site, positioning, and implant(s) and/ or special equipment prior to beginning this procedure. The perineum was prepped and draped in the usual sterile fashion. Local anesthetic was injected *as a perianal/pudendal nerve block*. The anus was gently dilated and anoscopy performed to identify the fissure. The anoscope was replaced with a Hill-Ferguson retractor and the base of the fissure scraped with a curet.

The intersphincteric groove was identified. A short, 4- to 5-mm incision was made directly over the intersphincteric groove on the *right/left* side. A hemostat was used to dissect the internal sphincter free of anoderm and external sphincter. Fibers were then elevated into the wound using a right-angle clamp and divided with *electrocautery/sharp dissection* until the hypertrophic sphincter felt relaxed on digital exam. Hemostasis was achieved by holding pressure. The incision was left open to drain.

The patient tolerated the procedure well and was *extubated and* taken to the postanesthesia care unit in stable condition.

Chapter 71
Anoplasty for Anal Stenosis

Carol E.H. Scott-Conner, M.D.

INDICATION
- Fibrotic stricture of the anal canal.

ESSENTIAL STEPS
1. Rectal exam.
2. Gently dilate the anus.
3. Hill-Ferguson retractor.
4. Incision from the dentate line upward into rectum 1.5 cm.
5. Y-extension through the anoderm.
6. Elevate the flaps.
7. *Internal sphincterotomy (if necessary)*.
8. Perform Y-V advancement and suture.

NOTE THIS VARIATION
- Internal sphincterotomy.

COMPLICATIONS
- Recurrence.
- Anal ulcer.
- Urinary retention.

TEMPLATE OPERATIVE DICTATION
Preoperative diagnosis: Anal stricture.
Procedure: Anoplasty *with lateral internal sphincterotomy*.

J.J. Hoballah and C.E.H. Scott-Conner (eds.), *Operative Dictations in General and Vascular Surgery*, DOI 10.1007/978-1-4614-0451-4_71,
© Springer Science+Business Media, LLC 2012

Postoperative diagnosis: Same.

Indications: This ___-year-old *male/female* developed anal stricture *after previous hemorrhoidectomy/other*.

Description of procedure: The patient was brought to the operating room and *general/spinal* anesthesia was induced. The patient was then positioned in the *prone jackknife/lithotomy* position. A time-out was completed verifying correct patient, procedure, site, positioning, and implant(s) and/or special equipment prior to beginning this procedure. The perineum was prepped and draped in the usual sterile fashion. The anus was gently dilated and a Hill-Ferguson retractor was inserted, exposing the dentate line. An incision was made commencing at the dentate line and extending upward onto rectal mucosa for 1.5 cm. It was then extended through the anoderm in a Y-fashion. Flaps were elevated by sharp dissection. Hemostasis was achieved by electrocautery.

If internal sphincterotomy: It was noted that incising the anoderm and associated fibrosis did not completely release the stricture; therefore, an internal sphincterotomy was performed in such a manner as to completely release the stricture.

The Y-flap was advanced in a V fashion and sutured in place with a running suture of 4-0 PDS/PG.

Hemostasis was rechecked. A gauze pad was tucked between the buttocks.

The patient tolerated the procedure well and was *extubated and* taken to the postoperative care unit in stable condition.

NOTES

Chapter 72
Marsupialization of Pilonidal Sinus

Daniel Calva-Cerqueira, M.D.

INDICATIONS
- Recurrent infected pilonidal cyst.
- Pilonidal sinus with secondary tracts encountered.

ESSENTIAL STEPS
1. Prone jackknife position.
2. Identify and cannulate tracts.
3. *Inject with methylene blue and hydrogen peroxide (optional).*
4. Incise the skin overlying the probe with electrocautery.
5. Remove a narrow wedge of adjacent skin.
6. Curet base.
7. Suture skin to the base of the tract with interrupted sutures of 3-0 Vicryl.
8. Pack.

NOTE THESE VARIATIONS
- Injection with methylene blue/hydrogen peroxide optional.
- All tracts must be identified and laid open; number and location varies.

COMPLICATIONS
- Delayed healing.
- Recurrence.

J.J. Hoballah and C.E.H. Scott-Conner (eds.), *Operative Dictations in General and Vascular Surgery*, DOI 10.1007/978-1-4614-0451-4_72,
© Springer Science+Business Media, LLC 2012

TEMPLATE OPERATIVE DICTATION

Preoperative diagnosis: Chronic infections of pilonidal *cyst/ sinus*.

Procedure: Marsupialization of pilonidal *cyst/sinus*.

Postoperative diagnosis: Same.

Indications: This is a ___-year-old *male/female* who has *chronic infections/secondary sinus tracts* of a pilonidal *cyst*, which is chronic of ___ duration *requiring incision and drainage*. Marsupialization was indicated for definitive management.

Description of procedure: The patient was brought to the operating room and underwent general anesthesia and endotracheal intubation. All appropriate monitoring devices were in place. The patient was then placed in the prone jackknife position, and the buttocks were gently spread with tape. All pressure points were padded, and then the presacral region was prepped and draped in the usual sterile fashion. A time-out was completed verifying correct patient, procedure, site, positioning, and implant(s) and/or special equipment prior to beginning this procedure.

Optional variation: *An opening was/several openings were evident on the midline. The largest was cannulated with a small plastic intravenous cannula and injected with a mixture of methylene blue and hydrogen peroxide. This bubbled from the secondary openings, but all staining remained midline.*

A probe was inserted and the main tract along the midline readily identified. Electrocautery was used to open the skin overlying the probe. Secondary tracts were identified and opened in a similar fashion. The skin edges were grasped with Allis clamps and a narrow band of skin was excised from the lateral aspect of *each/the* incision using electrocautery. *All blue-stained tissue was exposed.* The base of the tracts was curetted.

The skin edges were then brought down and sutured to the tract margin with interrupted 2-0 Vicryl. Hemostasis was checked. The wound was irrigated copiously with saline and packed.

The patient tolerated the procedure well was extubated and reversed from general anesthesia. *He/She* was taken to the postanesthesia care unit in stable condition.

ACKNOWLEDGMENT

This chapter was contributed by Mohamad Allam, MD in the first edition.

NOTES

Chapter 73

Excision and Primary Closure of Pilonidal Sinus

Daniel Calva-Cerqueira, M.D.

INDICATIONS
- Pilonidal *cyst/sinus* without infection or secondary tracts.

ESSENTIAL STEPS
1. Prone jackknife position.
2. Identify and cannulate the tract.
3. *Inject with methylene blue and hydrogen peroxide (optional).*
4. Excise ellipse of skin overlying the tract and including all midline openings.
5. Deepen the incision to *the fascia, well below probe.*
6. Completely excise the pilonidal sinus with adequate margins.
7. Achieve hemostasis.
8. Develop flaps.
9. Close the wound.

NOTE THESE VARIATIONS
- Injection with methylene blue/hydrogen peroxide is optional.
- All tracts must be identified; if secondary tracts are encountered, convert to marsupialization.

COMPLICATIONS
- Wound breakdown.
- Recurrence.

J.J. Hoballah and C.E.H. Scott-Conner (eds.), *Operative Dictations in General and Vascular Surgery*, DOI 10.1007/978-1-4614-0451-4_73,
© Springer Science+Business Media, LLC 2012

TEMPLATE OPERATIVE DICTATION

Preoperative diagnosis: Chronic pilonidal *cyst/sinus.*

Procedure: Excision and primary closure of pilonidal *cyst/sinus.*

Postoperative diagnosis: Same.

Indications: This is a ___-year-old *male/female* who has chronic pilonidal *cyst/sinus* of ___ duration *requiring incision and drainage* limited to the midline and currently without evidence of infection. Excision and primary closure was elected for management.

Description of procedure: The patient was brought to the operating room and underwent general anesthesia and endotracheal intubation. All appropriate monitoring devices were in place. The patient was then placed in the prone jackknife position, and the buttocks were gently spread with tape. All pressure points were padded, and then the presacral region was prepped and draped in the usual sterile fashion. A time-out was completed verifying correct patient, procedure, site, positioning, and implant(s) and/or special equipment prior to beginning this procedure.

Optional variation: *An opening was/several openings were evident on the midline. The largest was cannulated with a small plastic intravenous cannula and injected with a mixture of methylene blue and hydrogen peroxide. This bubbled from the secondary openings, but all staining remained midline.*

A probe was inserted and the midline tract readily identified. An elliptical incision was made around the *opening/openings* and the entire tract. This was deepened through subcutaneous tissue using electrocautery. The incision was continued until *fascia/ normal tissue* deep to the tract was encountered. The pilonidal sinus tract *and all blue-stained tissue* was thus excised cleanly in its entirety.

Hemostasis was achieved with electrocautery. After ensuring that there is no infection and that the wound was clean, flaps were developed until the skin and subcutaneous tissues could be approximated in the midline without tension. The incision was then closed with interrupted vertical mattress sutures of 3-0 nylon, placed in such a fashion as to completely close the dead space by incorporating a bite of *fascia/deep tissue.* The wound was dressed.

The patient tolerated the procedure well, was extubated and reversed from general anesthesia. *He/she* was taken to the postanesthesia care unit in stable condition.

ACKNOWLEDGMENT

This chapter was contributed by Mohamad Allam, MD in the first edition.

NOTES

Section VI

Hepatobiliary Tract

Chapter 74
Cholecystectomy

Jennifer E. Hrabe, M.D.

INDICATIONS

- Symptomatic cholelithiasis.
- Acute or chronic cholecystitis.
- Choledocholithiasis (resolved).
- Biliary pancreatitis (resolved).
- Carcinoma of the gallbladder.
- Trauma.
- Conversion from laparoscopic cholecystectomy.
- Inability of patient to tolerate pneumoperitoneum.
- Incidental to other procedures, when abnormalities noted.

ESSENTIAL STEPS

1. Right subcostal incision.
2. Divide the falciform ligament.
3. Inspect the abdomen.
4. *Decompress the gallbladder.*
5. Identify and encircle the cystic duct and cystic artery.
6. Remove the gallbladder from the fundus down.
7. *Perform cholangiogram.*
8. Ligate and divide the cystic duct and cystic artery.
9. Check hemostasis.
10. *Place closed-suction drain.*
11. Close the abdomen.

J.J. Hoballah and C.E.H. Scott-Conner (eds.), *Operative Dictations in General and Vascular Surgery*, DOI 10.1007/978-1-4614-0451-4_74,
© Springer Science+Business Media, LLC 2012

NOTE THESE VARIATIONS

- Back wall of the gallbladder may be left in situ if severe inflammation.
- Antegrade dissection is feasible alternative.
- Cholangiogram is optional.
- Drain placement is optional.
- Wedge excision of the liver and regional lymphadenectomy may be added for carcinoma of the gallbladder.

COMPLICATIONS

- Injury to the common bile duct or right hepatic duct.
- Bile leak.
- Subhepatic abscess.
- Retained common bile duct stones.

TEMPLATE OPERATIVE DICTATION

Preoperative diagnosis: *Symptomatic cholelithiasis/acute or chronic cholecystitis/choledocholithiasis/biliary pancreatitis/trauma/ cancer of the gallbladder.*

Procedure: Cholecystectomy *with operative cholangiogram.*

Postoperative diagnosis: Same.

Indications: This ___-year-old *male/female* with *right upper quadrant pain/nausea/vomiting/fever/leukocytosis/other* was found on workup to have *cholelithiasis with a normal common duct/cholecystitis/choledocholithiasis/biliary pancreatitis/possible early cancer of gallbladder/other* on workup. *Laparoscopic cholecystectomy was attempted but was unable to be completed due to ___. The patient was not a candidate for laparoscopic cholecystectomy due to ___.* Open cholecystectomy was indicated.

Description of procedure: The patient was placed on the operating table in the supine position. General anesthesia was induced. A time-out was completed verifying correct patient, procedure, site, positioning, and implant(s)and/or special equipment prior to beginning this procedure. Preoperative antibiotics were administered. A Foley catheter and nasogastric/orogastric tube were placed. The abdomen was prepped and draped in the usual sterile fashion. A right subcostal incision was made two finger breadths below the costal margin, extending from just to the right of the xiphoid to the anterior axillary line. This was deepened through the subcutaneous tissues and hemostasis was achieved with electrocautery. The fascial and aponeurotic layers of the abdominal wall were divided with electrocautery and the peritoneal cavity entered.

The falciform ligament was doubly ligated with 2-0 silk and divided. The abdomen was inspected.

If gallbladder inflamed: An extensive number of adhesions of omentum and bowel to the region of the gallbladder were noted. The gallbladder appeared inflamed. Adhesions were lysed sharply under direct vision with Metzenbaum scissors.

If trocar decompression: The gallbladder was noted to be tensely distended. A pursestring suture of 3-0 silk was placed in the fundus and a biliary trocar used to suction bile and stones. The trocar was removed and bile was cultured.

Traction was placed on the fundus of the gallbladder. The cystic duct and cystic artery were identified. Starting at the fundus and continuing downward to the cystic duct and cystic artery, the peritoneum overlying was incised and the gallbladder was dissected off the liver bed.

If cholangiogram: A clip was placed on the cystic duct close to the neck of the gallbladder. A nick was made in the cystic duct and a cholangiogram catheter threaded. A cholangiogram was obtained and showed good flow of bile into the duodenum, an intact biliary tree, and absence of any filling defects/other.

The cystic duct and cystic artery were ligated with 3-0 silk and divided and the gallbladder was removed. Hemostasis was checked and the hepatoduodenal ligament inspected and found to be intact, without palpable abnormalities. *A closed-suction drain was placed in the gallbladder fossa and secured to the skin with 3-0 nylon.* Omentum was laid in the operative field.

The incision was closed in layers with *running/interrupted ___.* The skin was *closed with skin staples/subcuticular sutures of ___/ packed open.*

The patient tolerated the procedure well and was taken to the postanesthesia care unit in stable condition.

ACKNOWLEDGMENT

This chapter was contributed by Mazen M. Hashisho, MD, in the first edition.

NOTES

Chapter 75

Laparoscopic Cholecystectomy

Jennifer E. Hrabe, M.D.

INDICATIONS

- Symptomatic cholelithiasis.
- Acute or chronic cholecystitis.
- Choledocholithiasis (resolved).
- Biliary pancreatitis (resolved).

ESSENTIAL STEPS

1. Induce the pneumoperitoneum.
2. Place a laparoscope through the infraumbilical port.
3. Inspect the abdomen.
4. Reverse Trendelenburg position.
5. Additional trocars in the epigastrium, right midclavicular line, and right anterior axillary line.
6. Grasp and elevate the fundus of the gallbladder.
7. Gently dissect any adhesions to the omentum, colon, and duodenum.
8. Incise the peritoneum over the infundibulum.
9. Define the cystic duct and cystic artery close to the gallbladder.
10. *Perform cholangiogram.*
11. Doubly clip and divide the cystic artery and cystic duct.
12. Dissect the gallbladder from the liver with electrocautery.
13. Check hemostasis.
14. Remove the gallbladder.
15. *Place a closed suction drain.*

J.J. Hoballah and C.E.H. Scott-Conner (eds.), *Operative Dictations in General and Vascular Surgery*, DOI 10.1007/978-1-4614-0451-4_75,
© Springer Science+Business Media, LLC 2012

16. Remove trocars.
17. Close large trocar sites.

NOTE THESE VARIATIONS
- Cholangiogram is optional.
- Drain placement is optional.
- Fundus-down dissection is a feasible alternative.

COMPLICATIONS
- Injury to the common bile duct or right hepatic duct.
- Bile leak.
- Subhepatic abscess.
- Retained common bile duct stones.
- Need for conversion to open cholecystectomy (**note:** this is not a complication but rather a sign of sound judgment when conditions are not favorable).

TEMPLATE OPERATIVE DICTATION
Preoperative diagnosis: *Symptomatic cholelithiasis/cholecystitis/ choledocholithiasis/biliary pancreatitis.*

Procedure: Laparoscopic cholecystectomy *with operative cholangiogram.*

Postoperative diagnosis: Same.

Indications: This ___-year-old *male/female* developed *right upper quadrant pain/nausea/vomiting/fever/leukocytosis* and on workup was found to have *cholelithiasis with a normal common duct/ cholecystitis/choledocholithiasis/biliary pancreatitis.* Laparoscopic cholecystectomy was elected.

Description of procedure: The patient was placed on the operating table in the supine position. General anesthesia was induced. A time-out was completed verifying correct patient, procedure, site, positioning, and implant(s) and/or special equipment prior to beginning this procedure. *A nasogastric/orogastric tube was placed.* The abdomen was prepped and draped in the usual sterile fashion.

An incision was made in a natural skin line below the umbilicus.

[Choose one:]

For Veress needle: The fascia was elevated and the Veress needle inserted. Proper position was confirmed by aspiration and saline meniscus test.

For Hassan cannula: The fascia was elevated and incised. The peritoneum was elevated and incised. Entry into the peritoneum was confirmed visually and no bowel was noted in the vicinity of the incision. Two anchoring sutures of 2-0 Vicryl were placed and the Hassan cannula inserted under direct vision. The sutures were anchored around the cannula.

The abdomen was insufflated with carbon dioxide to a pressure of 12–15 mmHg. The patient tolerated insufflation well. *A 10/12-mm trocar was then inserted.*

The laparoscope was inserted and the abdomen inspected. No injuries from initial trocar placement were noted. Additional trocars were then inserted in the following locations: a 10/12-mm trocar in the right epigastrium and two 5-mm trocars along the right costal margin. The abdomen was inspected and *no abnormalities/ the following abnormalities* were found. The table was placed in the reverse Trendelenburg position with the right side up.

Filmy adhesions between the gallbladder and omentum/duodenum/transverse colon were lysed sharply. The dome of the gallbladder was grasped with an atraumatic grasper passed through the lateral port and retracted over the dome of the liver. The infundibulum was also grasped with an atraumatic grasper through the midclavicular port and retracted toward the right lower quadrant. This maneuver exposed Calot's triangle. The peritoneum overlying the gallbladder infundibulum was then incised and the cystic duct and cystic artery identified and circumferentially dissected. *If cholangiogram: A clip was placed on the cystic duct close to the neck of the gallbladder. A nick was made in the cystic duct and a cholangiogram catheter threaded. A cholangiogram was obtained and showed good flow of bile into the duodenum, an intact biliary tree, and absence of any filling defects/other.* The cystic duct and cystic artery were then doubly clipped and divided close to the gallbladder.

The gallbladder was then dissected from its peritoneal attachments by electrocautery. Hemostasis was checked and the gallbladder and contained stones were removed *using an endoscopic retrieval bag placed* through the subxiphoid port. The gallbladder was passed off the table as a specimen. The gallbladder fossa was copiously irrigated with saline and hemostasis was obtained. There was no evidence of bleeding from the gallbladder fossa or cystic artery or leakage of the bile from the cystic duct stump. *A closed suction drain was placed in the gallbladder fossa and brought out through the lateral port site.*

Secondary trocars were removed under direct vision. *No bleeding was noted/trocar site bleeding was controlled by electrocautery/suture placement.* The laparoscope was withdrawn and the umbilical trocar removed. The abdomen was allowed to collapse. The fascia of the 10/12 trocar sites was closed with simple/figure-of-eight 0 vicryl sutures. The skin was closed with subcuticular sutures of 4-0 monocryl and steristrips/topical skin adhesive. *The nasogastric/orogastric tube was removed.*

The patient tolerated the procedure well and was taken to the postanesthesia care unit in stable condition.

ACKNOWLEDGMENT

This chapter was contributed by Mazen M. Hashisho, MD, in the first edition.

NOTES

Chapter 76

Open Common Bile Duct Exploration

Christopher Bunch, M.D.

INDICATIONS

- Choledocholithiasis.
- Acute suppurative cholangitis due to choledocholithiasis.
- Common duct stones found during open biliary tract surgery.
- On occasion done as adjunct to complex biliary tract surgery.

ESSENTIAL STEPS

1. *Correct coagulopathy, if present.*
2. Right upper quadrant incision.
3. *Cholecystectomy and cholangiogram, if not previously performed.*
4. Kocher maneuver.
5. Place two stay sutures in the common bile duct.
6. Longitudinal incision.
7. Aspirate bile and culture.
8. Explore the duct with *scoops, biliary Fogarty catheters, baskets, and/or choledochoscope.*
9. Number of stones retrieved should equal number identified on pre-exploration study.
10. Close the bile duct in watertight fashion around T-tube.
11. Perform completion cholangiogram.
12. Place closed suction drain in the subhepatic space.
13. Check hemostasis.
14. Place omentum in the field.
15. Close the abdomen.

J.J. Hoballah and C.E.H. Scott-Conner (eds.), *Operative Dictations in General and Vascular Surgery*, DOI 10.1007/978-1-4614-0451-4_76,
© Springer Science+Business Media, LLC 2012

NOTE THESE VARIATIONS
- *Cholecystectomy if not already done.*
- *Instruments used to clear common bile duct.*
- *Use of choledochoscope: Fiberoptic/rigid.*
- *Size of T-tube.*

COMPLICATIONS
- Retained common bile duct stones.
- Bile leak.
- Stricture of the common bile duct.
- Pancreatitis.

TEMPLATE OPERATIVE DICTATION

Preoperative diagnosis: *Choledocholithiasis/suppurative cholangitis/other.*

Procedure: *Cholecystectomy with* common bile duct exploration with cholangiogram.

Postoperative diagnosis: Same.

Indications: This ____-year-old *male/female* developed *right upper quadrant pain/jaundice/fever/leukocytosis* and on workup was found to have choledocholithiasis. Endoscopic clearance was *unsuccessful/not available* and open common bile duct exploration was elected.

Description of procedure: An epidural catheter was placed by anesthesia prior to the start of the operation. The patient was placed in the supine position and general endotracheal anesthesia was induced. Preoperative antibiotics were given. A Foley catheter and nasogastric tube were placed. The abdomen was prepped and draped in the usual sterile fashion. A time-out was completed verifying correct patient, procedure, site, positioning, and implant(s) and/or special equipment prior to beginning this procedure. A right subcostal incision was made two finger breadths below the costal margin and extending from just to the right of the xiphoid to the anterior axillary line. This was deepened through the subcutaneous tissues and hemostasis was achieved with electrocautery. The fascial and aponeurotic layers of the abdominal wall were divided with electrocautery and the peritoneal cavity entered.

The falciform ligament was doubly ligated with 2-0 silk and divided. The abdomen was explored.

[Choose one:]

If cholecystectomy: The gallbladder was elevated and the peritoneum overlying Calot's triangle incised. The cystic duct and cystic artery were identified and encircled with silk ties. The cystic duct was cannulated with a ____ catheter and cholangiograms obtained that demonstrated a dilated common bile duct containing ____ stones. Cholecystectomy was completed in the usual fashion and the gall-bladder removed.

If cholecystectomy had been performed previously: *The common bile duct was identified and palpated. A ____ gauge butterfly needle was used to cannulate the duct and obtain cholangiograms. These demonstrated a dilated common bile duct containing ____ stones.*

A Kocher maneuver was performed by incising the peritoneal attachments lateral to the duodenum and gently rotating the duodenum and head of pancreas medially. The common duct and head of pancreas were palpated and *found to be normal/a stone was palpated in the common duct.* The peritoneum overlying the common duct was then incised to expose the anterior wall of the common bile duct 2 cm proximal to the pancreas. Two stay sutures of 4-0 silk were placed on the anteromedial wall and the common bile duct was then incised between these sutures for a length of 1.5 cm. Bile was sampled for cultures and gram stain and aspirated.

Common bile duct stones were gently milked from the distal duct and emerged from the choledochotomy, where they were retrieved. *Scoops/stone forceps/biliary Fogarty catheter* were passed proximally and distally and stones retrieved. The common bile duct was irrigated proximally and distally until no debris was obtained.

Attempt was then made to pass a ____ French *coude catheter/ Bakes dilator* through the ampulla. This *was/was not successful. A flexible fiberoptic/rigid choledochoscope was introduced into the choledochotomy and stone(s) retrieved front the distal duct under direct vision with a stone basket/biliary Fogarty catheter.*

When all stones had been retrieved and the duct appeared clear, completion choledochoscopy was then performed and *no additional stones or debris were noted/additional calculus material was retrieved.* Patency of the ampulla was confirmed by noting the ampulla to dilate when irrigated with saline.

A ____ French T-tube was then placed in the common duct, and the choledochotomy was closed using 4-0 Prolene suture in a continuous fashion *below/above* the T-tube. The closure was tested with saline and a single figure-of-eight 4-0 Prolene used to completely approximate the choledochotomy edges *inferior to/ superior to* the T-tube. Air was then expelled from the long limb of the T-tube by placing a smaller diameter tubing into the T-tube and instilling saline while removing the inner tubing.

A completion cholangiogram was obtained using under ____ fluoroscopic guidance. *The contrast did not initially enter the duodenum. However, after administration of ____ intravenously, a subsequent infusion of dye revealed free passage into the duodenum.* No stones were noted.

The T-tube was brought along the inferior border of the liver medially and out through a separate incision inferior to the subcostal incision. A closed suction drain was placed in the subhepatic space and brought out through a separate skin incision lateral to the T-tube exit site. The T-tube was sewn to the skin with considerable slack in the tubing. Both drains were affixed to the abdominal skin using 3-0 nylon suture. Hemostasis was checked, the field was irrigated, and omentum was placed over the choledochotomy.

The incision was closed in layers with *running/interrupted* ____. The skin was *closed with skin staples/subcuticular sutures of ___/ packed open.* The T-tube drain was placed to gravity drainage. The JP drain was placed to closed bulb suction.

The patient tolerated the procedure well and was taken to the postanesthesia care unit in stable condition.

NOTES

Chapter 77

Laparoscopic Exploration of Common Bile Duct

Walid Faraj, M.D., F.R.C.S. and Ahmad Zaghal, M.D.

INDICATIONS

- Symptomatic common bile duct stone(s).
- Dilated common bile duct.
- Common bile duct stones found during laparoscopic cholecystectomy.
- Common bile duct injury.

ESSENTIAL STEPS

1. Check the availability of a digital C-arm unit with real-time fluoroscopy in the operating room.
2. Skin incisions and trocars placement as for laparoscopic cholecystectomy.
3. Calot's triangle dissection, identification of cystic duct and artery.
4. Cholangiography.
5. IV glucagon.
6. Flush of cholangiogram catheter with saline.
7. *Transcystic exploration: choledochoscope, basket retrieval.*
8. *Laparoscopic choledochotomy.*
9. Completion cholangiography.
10. Cholecystectomy, if not previously performed.
11. Secure hemostasis.
12. *Close the cystic duct stump/Place T-tube, close choledochotomy, place closed-suction drains.*
13. Wound closure.

J.J. Hoballah and C.E.H. Scott-Conner (eds.), *Operative Dictations in General and Vascular Surgery*, DOI 10.1007/978-1-4614-0451-4_77,
© Springer Science+Business Media, LLC 2012

NOTE THESE VARIATIONS

- Laparoscopic transcystic exploration (most common method).
- Laparoscopic choledochotomy.
- Cholecystectomy, if not previously performed.
- Use of Fogarty catheter instead of basket.
- Retrieval may be guided by fluoroscopy or by choledochoscope.

COMPLICATIONS

- Transient hyperamylasemia/pancreatitis.
- Retained common bile duct stones.
- Bleeding.
- Bile leak.
- Duodenal injury.

TEMPLATE OPERATIVE DICTATION

Preoperative diagnosis: *Choledocholithiasis/CBD injury.*

Procedure: *Laparoscopic cholecystectomy, with* intraoperative cholangiogram, and laparoscopic common bile duct exploration.

Postoperative diagnosis: Same.

Indications: This is a ___-year-old *male/female* who presented with a history of right upper quadrant pain, fever, jaundice, and leukocyosis, workup revealed elevated serum liver function test, and choledocholithiasis, ERCP failed to clear the biliary tract, so the decision was to perform *laparoscopic cholecystectomy, with* intraoperative cholangiogram, and CBD exploration.

Description of procedure: Under general anesthesia, with the patient placed in the supine position, the whole abdomen was prepped and draped in the usual sterile fashion. A time-out was completed verifying correct patient, procedure, site, positioning, and implant(s) and/or special equipment prior to beginning this procedure.

A Veress needle was placed and the abdomen insufflated to 15 mmHg. A 10-mm trocar was placed in the supraumbilical location and the abdomen inspected. A second 10-mm trocar was placed in an epigastric location under direct vision. Two additional 5-mm trocars were then placed in the right upper quadrant.

[Choose one:]

The gall bladder was retracted cephalad using a ratcheted grasper, exposing the peritoneum overlying the Calot's triangle, that was incised using electrocautery, then cystic artery and cystic duct were identified, then the cystic duct was skeletonized at the gallbladder–cystic duct junction after which a hemoclip was applied proximally, then a small cystic duct ductotomy was made.

If cholecystectomy previously performed: *Adhesions were carefully lysed and a cystic duct remnant identified and grasped.*

A cholangiogram catheter was then introduced *into the abdomen percutaneously and fed into the cystic duct/through the right lateral trocar using a cholangiogram clamp.* A cholangiogram was the obtained that showed a dilated CBD containing ___ filling defects.

The patient was then given 10 mg of glucagon intravenously (to relax the sphincter of Oddi), and 10 ml of NSS were vigorously flushed through the cholangiogram catheter under fluoroscopic guidance, then cholangiography was repeated to evaluate whether the stone has passed.

[Choose one:]

If the filling defect in the CBD disappeared: *The procedure was concluded at this stage, and attention was then drawn toward completion of the cholecystectomy in the usual fashion, after withdrawing the cholangiography catheter.*

If the filling defect persisted: *The decision was to proceed with a choledochoscopy: (trans-cystic exploration):*

Choledochoscopy was performed by dissecting the cystic duct within 1 cm of the junction with the CBD, a cystic duct ductotomy was then performed, and a guide wire was advanced into the cystic duct through a 3-mm introducer in the right subcostal trocar. (Alternatively, if the cholangiogram catheter was placed percutaneously: the site was dilated and a cystic duct introducer that was placed to pass the choledochoscope). The choledochoscope was then advanced over the guide wire into the dilated duct, after it was dilated using balloon dilator.

Continuous saline irrigation through the choledochoscope under pressure no greater than 50–100 mmHg was used to facilitate visualization as the choledochoscope was being advanced.

A stone was visualized, a stone basket was passed through the working channel of the choledochoscope, the basket was then opened so that the middle of the basket was aligned with the middle of the stone, careful manipulation of the basket in an in-and-out manner aided in the stone capture, then the stone was brought within the basket wires, the basket was closed around the stone, and the stone was pulled to the tip of the scope, both the scope and basket were then withdrawn as one unit.

The maneuver was repeated ___ times to retrieve all the stones from the CBD. The stones were placed in a plastic collection sac for retrieval at the completion of bile duct exploration.

After the duct was cleared of stones, the scope passed easily into the duodenum.

Completion cholangiography was then performed, showing no filling defects in the CBD, and dye was able to reach the duodenum, then the cystic duct was closed with a pretied ligature, and cholecystectomy was completed in the usual fashion, and *gall bladder removed*, hemostasis secured.

If the stone was inaccessible, transcystic exploration was abandoned in favor of laparoscopic choledochotomy/postoperative ERCP.

Laparoscopic choledochotomy: *The gallbladder was retracted cephalad, the CBD was dissected till approximately 1–2 cm distal to the junction of the cystic duct, then Two stay sutures were placed in the CBD, an additional 5-mm trocar was placed in the right lower quadrant for insertion of an additional needle driver, a vertical choledochotomy was then made using curved microscissors, on the anterior aspect of the duct while the stay sutures were elevated, the duct was then flushed with saline to remove any loose stones, the choledochoscope was then introduced directly into the CBD through the choledochotomy, and stones were removed with a basket retrieval technique similar to transcystic choledochoscopy. After clearing the duct of stones, a (12/14)F T-tube was inserted into the choledochotomy and the ductal defect was closed with interrupted absorbable sutures, the T-tube was brought out through the subcostal port, and a __F closed-suction drain was brought out through the most lateral port.*

Cholecystectomy was completed as the usual fashion, and gall bladder removed, hemostasis secured.

The skin incisions were closed in layers, O/PDS interrupted sutures for the fascia, and 4-0 monocryl subcuticular sutures for the approximation of the skin.

The T-tube drain was connected to gravity drainage, the closed-suction drain was connected to closed bulb suction, and both were fixed to the skin using 3/O nylon sutures.

The patient tolerated the operation very well, and was transferred to the postanesthesia care unit in a stable condition.

NOTES

Chapter 78

Roux-en-Y Hepaticojejunostomy or Choledochojejunostomy

Susan Skaff Hagen, M.D., M.S.P.H.

INDICATIONS

- Biliary stricture.
- Biliary injury.
- Bile duct tumor.
- Bypass of nonresectable pancreatic or periampullary malignancy.

ESSENTIAL STEPS

1. Right subcostal incision.
2. Mobilization.
3. Identify hepatic artery/replaced right hepatic artery.
4. *Perform cholecystectomy (if not already done).*
5. Identify bile duct.
6. *Cholangiogram.*
7. Dissect the hepatoduodenal ligament
8. Identify the ligament of Treitz.
9. Create Roux limb.
10. Divide the transverse mesocolon.
11. Jejunojejunostomy *stapled or hand sewn.*
12. Bring jejunal limb *through transverse mesocolon* in close apposition to biliary tree.
13. Create antimesenteric jejunostomy.
14. Construct posterior layer of *end-to-side/side-to-side* anastomosis.
15. Place *T-tube/stent.*

J.J. Hoballah and C.E.H. Scott-Conner (eds.), *Operative Dictations in General and Vascular Surgery*, DOI 10.1007/978-1-4614-0451-4_78,
© Springer Science+Business Media, LLC 2012

16. Construct anterior closure.
17. Place closed suction drain.
18. Close abdomen.

NOTE THESE VARIATIONS
- Epidural catheter.
- Level of anastomosis (common duct – choledocho vs. hepatic duct – hepatico).
- Cholecystectomy (if not previously done).
- Retrocolic vs. antecolic.
- T-tube/stent.

COMPLICATIONS
- Leak.
- Stricture.

TEMPLATE OPERATIVE DICTATION
Preoperative diagnosis: Biliary stricture/injury/tumor/other.
Procedure: Roux-en-Y hepaticojejunostomy/choledochojejunostomy.
Postoperative diagnosis: Same.
Indications: Patient is a ___-year-old *male/female* who developed obstructive jaundice with subsequent workup showing a *biliary stricture/injury/tumor/other* which was not amenable to endoscopic treatment. Biliary enteric anastomosis was elected for definitive management.
Description of procedure: *An epidural catheter was placed by anesthesia prior to the start of the operation.* Patient was brought into the operating room and placed on the table in the supine position. General endotracheal anesthesia was administered. A time-out was completed verifying correct patient, procedure, site, positioning, and implant(s) and/or special equipment prior to beginning this procedure. Preoperative antibiotics were administered. A Foley catheter and nasogastric tube were placed. All bony prominences were padded. The patient was prepped with *Betadine/Chlorhexidine* and draped in the usual sterile fashion. *A right subcostal incision was made two finger breadths below the costal margin from the right of the xiphoid to the anterior axillary line. The previously made incision in the right subcostal area was re-incised with a scalpel.* This was deepened through the subcutaneous tissues and hemostasis was achieved with electrocautery. *Dense adhesions were taken down.* The fascial and aponeurotic layers of the abdominal wall were divided with electrocautery

and the peritoneal cavity entered. The abdomen was explored and (*detail findings*). The falciform ligament was doubly ligated with 2-0 silk and divided.

The *Thompson/Omni* retractor was placed for exposure of the porta hepatis. Approximately __ h of dissection was required to safely identify structures. The location of the hepatic artery was identified first to prevent injury. The main artery was located by palpation and Doppler ultrasound on the left side of the hepatoduodenal ligament. The artery then looped anteriorly in the porta hepatis. No replaced right hepatic artery was palpable.

If cholecystectomy:

The gallbladder was elevated and the peritoneum overlying Calot's triangle was incised. The cystic duct and cystic artery were identified and encircled with silk ties. *The cystic duct was cannulated with a ___ catheter and a cholangiogram was obtained that demonstrated a dilated common bile duct with distal stricture/ tumor.* Cholecystectomy was completed in the usual fashion and the gallbladder was removed.

Or

The gallbladder was freed from the liver bed, starting from the fundus. The cystic duct and cystic artery were ligated and divided. A cholangiogram was performed to delineate the anatomy.

If cholecystectomy already performed:

If intact common bile duct: The common bile duct stent was palpable in the usual anterolateral portion of the hepatoduodenal ligament. There was no discreet mass. The distal common bile duct was identified and was of normal caliber just above the duodenum.

If unusual location of common bile duct: The common bile duct was not found in the usual anterolateral portion of the hepatoduodenal ligament. Upon further exploration, it appeared the common bile duct was clipped multiple times and likely transected. The area of injury was identified at (describe findings). The distal common bile duct was identified and was of normal caliber just above the duodenum.

If cholangiogram:

The anterior wall of the bile duct was incised superiorly to approximately 2 cm from the liver capsule. An intraoperative cholangiogram was performed under surgeon directed fluoroscopy via the common hepatic duct and confirmed the presence (describe findings).

The hepatic plate was then dropped by incising the peritoneal layer between the liver capsule and the hepatoduodenal ligament just above the hepatic duct. This exposed the proximal common hepatic duct at its bifurcation which was mildly dilated to __ mm.

The duct was entered just below the bifurcation and a probe was easily passed into all three major ducts *(or describe findings and if intraoperative cholangiogram performed under surgeon directed fluoroscopy via the previously placed PTC)*. The open edge of the duct was trimmed slightly and healthy bleeding was seen around the duct. The duct opening was then extended to the left along the anterior surface of the left hepatic duct until the opening was 15 mm in length. Again patency of both the left and right hepatic arteries was confirmed by *palpation/Doppler interrogation. The distal common bile duct was ligated with 4-0 Prolene suture.*

Attention was then turned to creation of the roux limb. The ligament of Treitz was located and the jejunum was divided with a GIA stapler ___ cm from the ligament where a loop of jejunum easily approximated to the liver. The distal staple line was imbricated with 4-0 silk sutures. The divided distal end of jejunum was then brought through an aperture in the transverse mesocolon.

If stapled: The jejunojejunostomy anastomosis we performed approximately 40 cm distal to the roux limb. This anastomosis was performed in side-to-side functional end-to-end fashion. Two limbs of jejunum were approximated with 3-0 silk sutures. Enterotomies were made and the GIA stapler was introduced and fired. The staple line was checked for hemostasis and the enterotomy closed with *a linear stapler/two layers of sutures.* The staple line was inspected for hemostasis. *The staple line was inverted using interrupted 4-0 silk Lembert sutures.* The defect in the mesentery was then closed using *running 3-0 Vicryl suture/interrupted 3-0 silk sutures.*

If sutured: A hand sewn two layer end-to-side enteroenterostomy was then performed between the proximal jejunal limb and the jejunum 40 cm distal to the roux limb using 3-0 Vicryl and 3-0 silk. The anastomosis was checked for integrity and noted to be widely patent. The mesenteric defect was re-approximated with *running 3-0 Vicryl suture/interrupted 3-0 silk sutures.* The roux limb was also fixed to the mesocolon with interrupted silks.

Next, attention was turned to the biliary tract. *The distal end of the bile duct was then freshened to the point where there was clean tissue.* Interrupted 5-0 PDS sutures were placed at 3 and 9 o'clock in the bile duct. An enterotomy was made in the roux limb ___ cm from the distal end on the antimesenteric border. The back wall of the end-to-side *hepaticojejunostomy/choledochojejunostomy* was completed with interrupted 5-0 PDS. If stent: *A stent was fashioned from a 5 French pediatric feeding tube and placed across the anastomosis and into the left hepatic duct. The stent was fixed to the roux limb with a chromic stitch/not sutured in place.* If t-tube: *A T-tube was placed across the anastomosis. The vertical limb was brought out of the duct 1 cm proximal to the anastomosis. This was then brought out of through the abdominal wall through a stab incision.* The anastomosis was then completed with interrupted 5-0 PDS on the anterior wall.

The abdomen was copiously irrigated with *warm saline/GU irrigation fluid*. The hepatic artery was again interrogated with Doppler and found to have normal triphasic signal. The liver had normal color and was soft. No further bilious drainage was evident. Attention was turned to closure.

A *19 round Blake/Jackson-Pratt* drain was placed posterior to the biliary anastomosis and brought through a separate skin incision. *An additional drain was placed anterior to the biliary anastomosis.* The *drain(s) was/*were sutured to the skin with 3-0 Nylon and connected to closed bulb suction. The subcostal fascia was closed in a single layer with running #1 *PDS/Prolene*. The wound was irrigated and the skin re-approximated with staples. A dry sterile dressing was applied. The patient tolerated the procedure well. There were no intraoperative complications. All instrument and sponge counts were correct at the end of the case. The patient was extubated and transferred to the recovery room in stable condition.

ACKNOWLEDGMENT

This chapter was contributed by Natisha Busick, MD, in the first edition.

NOTES

Chapter 79

Carcinoma of Hepatic Duct Bifurcation

Rajesh Shetty, M.D. and Thomas E. Collins, M.D.

INDICATION

- Cholangiocarcinoma (Klatskin tumor).

ESSENTIAL STEPS

1. Preoperative assessment and planning includes the following:
   - Imaging including cholangiogram and axial imaging (MRI or CT) to determine resectability and the type of liver resection required (right or left trisegmentectomy).
   - Preoperative placement of percutaneous transhepatic cholangiocatheters may be considered if surgery is not scheduled within 1–2 weeks.
   - Preoperative assessment of liver function by history and laboratory studies.
2. B/L subcostal (roof top) incision.
3. Completely mobilize the liver.
4. Carefully evaluate for evidence of metastatic disease by palpation and intraoperative ultrasound of liver including the caudate lobe, subhilar and retroduodenal area.
5. Examine all peritoneal surfaces.
6. Perform cholecystectomy by top-down technique.
7. Perform a complete Kocher maneuver.
8. Dissect the porta hepatis including the following:
   - Circumferential dissection of the portal vein and hepatic artery.

J.J. Hoballah and C.E.H. Scott-Conner (eds.), *Operative Dictations in General and Vascular Surgery*, DOI 10.1007/978-1-4614-0451-4_79,
© Springer Science+Business Media, LLC 2012

- Dissection of the segmental branches of the portal vein and hepatic artery (right or left) depending on planned liver resection.
- Division of the common bile duct at the level of the duodenum.
- Inclusion of all hepatoduodenal lymph nodes and tissue with the liver specimen to be resected.

9. Transect the liver parenchyma to complete either a right or left trisegmentectomy utilizing cautery, and obliterate the parenchyma by ultrasound or waterjet. (CVP maintained at five or below during transaction.)
10. Place or reposition transhepatic stent.
11. Complete biliary reconstruction utilizing retrocolic Roux-en-Y hepaticojejunostomy.
12. Place drain(s) and close.

NOTE THESE VARIATIONS
- Use of preoperative biliary decompression.
- Extent of liver resection.
- Stapled vs. sutured jejunojejunostomy.
- Running vs. interrupted biliary anastomosis.
- Use of fibrin glue on cut surface of liver.

COMPLICATIONS
- Hemorrhage.
- Bile leak.
- Cholangitis.
- Subhepatic abscess.
- Recurrence.

TEMPLATE OPERATIVE DICTATION
Preoperative diagnosis: Carcinoma of the hepatic duct bifurcation.
Procedure:
1. Exploratory laparotomy with intraoperative ultrasound.
2. Liver resection (right or left trisegmentectomy).
3. Roux-en-Y hepaticojejunostomy to intrahepatic bile duct.
4. Percutaneous transhepatic cholangiocatheter placement.
Postoperative diagnosis: Same.
Indications: This ___-year-old *male/female* developed obstructive jaundice and workup revealed Klatskin tumor. Resection with biliary enteric anastomosis was elected for definitive management.

Preoperative imaging indicated the tumor would best be resected with a (right/left) trisegmentectomy.

Description of procedure: The patient was placed in the supine position and general endotracheal anesthesia was induced. Appropriate arterial and venous access was obtained for monitoring and resuscitation. Preoperative antibiotics were given prior to incision. Foley catheter and nasogastric tubes were placed. The abdomen was prepped and draped in the usual sterile fashion. A time-out was completed verifying correct patient, procedure, site, positioning, and implant(s) and/or special equipment prior to beginning this procedure.

A bilateral subcostal incision (roof top) was made two finger breadths below the costal margins with superior xiphoid extension if necessary. This was deepened through the subcutaneous tissues, fascial and muscular layers of the abdominal wall with electrocautery. The peritoneal cavity was entered and a self-retaining retractor was placed for exposure. The falciform ligament was divided and ligated with 2-0 silk. Exploration was begun with careful bimanual palpation of the liver for any unsuspecting masses. The gastrohepatic ligament was incised taking care not to injure an accessory or replaced left hepatic artery if present. The caudate lobe was examined and palpated. A Kocher maneuver was performed to access the retroduodenal lymph nodes. The liver was completely mobilized by taking down both right and left triangular ligaments and dividing the inferior right lobe retroperitoneal attachments. The entire liver was examined with intraoperative ultrasound to ensure no tumor was present in the planned residual liver. No evidence of metastatic disease was found and resection was therefore elected. If present, the gallbladder was removed in top-down fashion with cautery. Care was taken to preserve the posterior right-sided portal structures. The cystic artery and duct were divided and ligated.

Next the portal dissection was carried out to evaluate for vascular involvement of the vessels supplying the planned residual liver segments. The hepatic artery and portal vein were identified and circumferentially dissected. The remaining lymph tissue in the porta hepatis was kept in continuity with the bile duct to be resected en bloc with the planned liver specimen. Next the segmental vascular structures were dissected into the liver in preparation for parenchymal transection.

[Choose one:]

Left trisegmentectomy: The right posterior hepatic artery and portal vein were dissected circumferentially.

Right trisegmentectomy: The left hepatic artery and vein were dissected to the umbilical fissure. Once the vascular dissection revealed no evidence of vascular invasion precluding resection, the common bile duct was transected at the superior aspect of the duodenum. The distal bile duct margin was then excised and sent for frozen section *which returned negative/which revealed the presence of tumor. Additional bile duct was/was not resected (if not, give reason).* The distal common bile duct stump was suture ligated.

Next attention was turned to transection of the liver. The central venous pressure was monitored and was 5 or less throughout the resection.

[Choose one:]

If left trisegmentectomy: The liver was further mobilized by ligating the venous branches draining into the vena cava. The right anterior and left portal vein and hepatic arteries were ligated and divided. The resulting demarcation on the surface of the liver was then scored with cautery to a depth of 1 cm. The (waterjet/ultrasound) dissector was then used to transect the parenchyma in the sectoral plane between the anterior (segments 5 and 8) and posterior (segments 6 and 7) sectors. Visible bile ducts and vessels were ligated or clipped. Once the dissection reached the bile duct it was sharply transected and the distal margin sent for frozen section. The caudate lobe was included in the specimen. The GIA stapler was used to transect the posterior aspect containing large venous branches.

If right trisegmentectomy: The liver was further mobilized by ligating the venous branches draining into the vena cava. The right portal vein and hepatic arteries were ligated and divided. Early portal and arterial branches to segment 4 were also divided and ligated. The surface of the liver was then scored with cautery to a depth of 1 cm approximately, about 1 cm. to the right of the falciform ligament. The junction between the caudate and the left lateral segment was scored with cautery to facilitate removal of the caudate lobe. The (waterjet/ultrasound) dissector was then used to transect the parenchyma. Visible bile ducts and vessels were ligated or clipped. The caudate lobe was included in the specimen. Once the dissection reached the bile duct it was sharply transected and the distal margin sent for frozen section. The GIA stapler was used to transect the posterior aspect of the specimen.

Next hemostasis was obtained on the cut surface of the liver with cautery and suture ligature. Additionally, bile leaks on the cut surface were identified and suture ligated.

Unless already present from preoperative placement, a transhepatic stent was brought through the abdominal wall above the incision. A Bakes dilator was used to probe the open bile duct into the liver. The dilator was then pushed though the surface of the liver and the stent was tied to the dilator to be brought through the liver and out the cut bile duct. The side holes on the stent were placed in the liver and an absorbable purse string suture was placed around the tube to secure it to the liver surface and prevent bile leakage.

Next attention was turned to biliary reconstruction. The jejunum was divided 30–40 cm distal to the ligament of Treitz with a GIA stapler. The distal staple line was oversewn with interrupted 3-0 silk sutures. The transverse mesocolon was incised to the left of the middle colic vessels and the distal staple line was brought through the mesocolon and in proximity to the open hepatic duct. The roux limb was secured to the mesocolon with interrupted 3-0 silk sutures. An antimesenteric enterotomy was performed 5 cm. proximal to the end of the distal Roux limb about one half of the length of the bile duct and an end to side, single layer, interrupted, anastomosis was performed using 5-0 PDS suture. The initial step being approximating the posterior wall of the duct to the posterior wall of the jejunum with positioning the stent into the roux limb and then completing the anterior wall. Bowel continuity was restored by a jejunojejunostomy 30–40 cm distal on the Roux limb using a stapling device or a two-layer hand-sewn closure. The resulting mesenteric defect was reapproximated with interrupted 3-0 silk sutures.

The abdomen was copiously irrigated with saline. The cut surface of the liver was again examined and treated for bleeding or bile leak. Closed suction drains were placed under the biliary anastomosis and proximate to the cut liver surface and brought through separate stab incisions below the subcostal incision. The drains and transhepatic stent were fixed to the abdomen with suture. The fascia was closed in two layers with monofilament absorbable suture. The subcutaneous tissues were irrigated and hemostasis ensured. The skin was closed with staples and a dry sterile dressing applied.

The patient tolerated the procedure well and was taken to the postanesthesia care unit in stable condition.

ACKNOWLEDGMENT

This chapter was contributed by Natisha Busick, MD, in the first edition.

NOTES

Chapter 80
Hepatic Wedge Resection

Georgios Tsoulfas, M.D.

INDICATION
- Metastatic disease peripheral in the liver.

ESSENTIAL STEPS
1. Right subcostal incision, with extension if needed.
2. Explore the abdomen and identify the lesion.
3. Mobilize the liver by dividing its ligamentous attachments.
4. Establish margins of resection around the lesion by cauterizing the hepatic capsule.
5. Transect the parenchyma using *cautery, finger fracture, or ultrasonic aspirator.*
6. Obtain hemostasis and bile stasis by *clipping or ligating* vessels and bile ducts >2 mm encountered.
7. Irrigate.
8. *Place drain (optional).*
9. Place omentum in the operative field.
10. Close the abdomen.

NOTE THESE VARIATIONS
- Method of parenchymal transection.
- Use of drain.
- Several lesions may be resected if necessary.

J.J. Hoballah and C.E.H. Scott-Conner (eds.), *Operative Dictations in General and Vascular Surgery*, DOI 10.1007/978-1-4614-0451-4_80,
© Springer Science+Business Media, LLC 2012

COMPLICATIONS

- Recurrence.
- Bile leak.
- Bleeding.

TEMPLATE OPERATIVE DICTATION

Preoperative diagnosis: Metastatic ____ cancer of the ____ segment of the liver.

Procedure: Wedge resection in ____ segment of the liver.

Postoperative diagnosis: Same.

Indications: This ___-year-old *male/female* had undergone resection of ____ primary ___ *month/years* ago. On evaluation with computed tomography *and positron emission tomography scan* a lesion was noted in the ____ segment of the liver. Fine needle aspiration of the lesion revealed ____ consistent with ____ primary. This led to the decision to proceed with a wedge resection of the lesion.

Description of procedure: An epidural catheter was placed by anesthesia prior to the start of the operation. The patient was placed in the supine position and general endotracheal anesthesia was induced. A time-out was completed verifying correct patient, procedure, site, positioning, and implant(s) and/or special equipment prior to beginning this procedure. Preoperative antibiotics were given. A Foley catheter and nasogastric tube were placed. The abdomen was prepped and draped in the usual sterile fashion. A long right subcostal incision was made from the midline to the anterior axillary line, two finger breadths below the costal margin. This was deepened through the subcutaneous tissues and hemostasis was achieved with electrocautery. Muscles and aponeurotic layers were divided with electrocautery. The abdomen was explored. *Adhesions were lysed sharply under direct vision with Metzenbaum scissors.*

Inspection revealed the mass in the ____ segment of the ____ lobe without evidence of other metastatic disease. Perihepatic adhesions were divided and the ligamentous attachments of the liver were divided to fully mobilize it. The planned margin of resection was estimated by palpation and the liver capsule was scored using cautery to outline at least a 1-cm margin from the lesion.

The parenchyma was transected using *cautery/finger fracture/ ultrasonic aspirator.* Bile ducts and vessels were identified and secured with *clips/ligatures. Hemostasis of the liver edge was performed with figure-of-eight 2-0 silk sutures in an interrupted fashion along the length of the resection.* The area was copiously irrigated with saline and reinspected for hemostasis. There was no evidence of active bleeding or bile leakage.

The omentum was placed in the operative field. *A closed suction drain was placed and brought out through a separate stab wound.*

(Optional: Multiple interrupted through-and-through retention sutures of ____ were placed.) The fascia was closed with *a running suture of ____/a Smead-Jones closure of interrupted ____.* The skin was closed with *skin staples/subcuticular sutures of ____/other.*

The patient tolerated the procedure well and was taken to the postanesthesia care unit in stable condition.

NOTES

Chapter 81
Right Hepatic Lobectomy

Georgios Tsoulfas, M.D.

INDICATIONS
- Tumor metastatic to the right lobe of the liver.
- Hepatocellular carcinoma confined to the right lobe.

ESSENTIAL STEPS
1. Bilateral subcostal incision with vertical midline extension.
2. Explore the abdomen and identify the lesion.
3. Mobilize the liver by dividing its ligamentous attachments.
4. Perform cholecystectomy to enhance exposure of the hilar vasculature.
5. Identify and ligate the right hepatic artery, right portal vein, and right hepatic bile duct (in that order).
6. After controlling the afferent vessels, turn attention to and ligate the short hepatic veins between the right lobe and inferior vena cava.
7. Identify and transect the right hepatic vein.
8. Transect the liver parenchyma along line of vascular demarcation between the lobes using *cautery, finger fracture, or ultrasonic aspirator.*
9. Obtain hemostasis and bile stasis by *clipping or ligating* small vessels and bile ducts encountered.
10. Irrigate the wound.
11. Place omentum *and closed suction drain* adjacent to the transected liver surface.

J.J. Hoballah and C.E.H. Scott-Conner (eds.), *Operative Dictations in General and Vascular Surgery*, DOI 10.1007/978-1-4614-0451-4_81,
© Springer Science+Business Media, LLC 2012

12. Reapproximate the falciform ligament to prevent postoperative torsion and vascular compromise.
13. Close the abdomen.

NOTE THESE VARIATIONS
- Technique of parenchymal transection.
- Division of hepatic veins sometimes performed later in procedure, which is the decision can be made to obtain control at the hilum, transect the parenchyma, and THEN divide the right hepatic vein.
- Use of drain optional.

COMPLICATIONS
- Major bleeding.
- Injury to the hilar structures of the remaining liver.
- Bile collection.

TEMPLATE OPERATIVE DICTATION
Preoperative diagnosis: Metastatic ___ cancer of the liver.
Procedure: Right hepatic lobectomy.
Postoperative diagnosis: Same.
Indications: This ___ -year-old *male/female* with a history of stage ___ carcinoma of ___ resected in ___ now has a mass in the right lobe of the liver. Computed tomography *and positron emission tomography scan* revealed metastatic lesions limited to the right lobe of the liver. This led to the decision to proceed with a right hepatic lobectomy.
Description of procedure: An epidural catheter was placed by anesthesia prior to the start of the operation. The patient was placed in the supine position and general endotracheal anesthesia was induced. A time-out was completed verifying correct patient, procedure, site, positioning, and implant(s) and/or special equipment prior to beginning this procedure. Preoperative antibiotics were given. A Foley catheter and nasogastric tube were placed. The abdomen was prepped and draped in the usual sterile fashion. A bilateral subcostal incision was made two finger breadths below the costal margin with a vertical midline extension up toward the xiphoid process. Further dissection through the muscular and aponeurotic layers of the abdominal wall was performed with a combination of sharp dissection and electrocautery. The peritoneum was entered and the abdominal cavity inspected. Palpation of the liver revealed ___ lesions *(specify number, size, and location)*.

The left lobe appeared to be clean of disease. No other metastatic disease was identified.

The Omni retractor system was employed to retract the chest wall. The falciform ligament was divided between Pean clamps and tied with 2-0 silk sutures. The triangular ligament was divided with electrocautery up to the inferior vena cava at the diaphragm. *Adhesions from previous surgery were taken down sharply.*

An umbilical tape was placed around the hilar structures to be able to perform a Pringle maneuver, if vascular control is needed. The right lobe was completely mobilized to the level of the cava and rotated anteriorly and medially and the attachments to the posterior structures divided with electrocautery. The gallbladder was removed in the usual fashion by grasping the fundus and performing the dissection from the top down to the level of the cystic duct, which was cleared and tied with 2-0 silk sutures. The cystic artery was identified and ligated with 2-0 silk sutures and the gallbladder removed from the field and sent to pathology. The suture around the cystic duct was used to provide traction medially, so as to uncover the right hepatic artery and portal vein.

Attention was turned to the hilum of the liver. The right lateral aspect of the hepatoduodenal ligament was incised and the hepatic arteries were found lateral to the common hepatic duct. Surrounding lymphatic vessels were ligated with 3-0 silk ties, and the right hepatic artery was temporarily occluded while palpating the artery to the opposite liver lobe to ensure patency to the arterial supply to the liver remnant. Having done this the right hepatic artery was identified and double ligated with 2-0 silk sutures and divided. The common bile duct was retracted anteriorly with a vein retractor and the portal vein bifurcation was identified. The right portal vein branch was freed from surrounding lymphoareolar tissue and ligated with a vascular stapler. The right hepatic bile duct was divided at this point. A clear line of vascular demarcation along the principal plane between the lobes was identified.

After controlling the afferent vessels, the hepatic veins were approached. Multiple short hepatic veins between the inferior vena cava and the liver were ligated using 3-0 silk ties, as the liver was retracted anteriorly and to the left, starting infrahepatically and proceeding cephalad. The main right hepatic vein was exposed after dividing the retrocaval ligament bridging segments 1 and 7 and a vascular stapler was used to transect it and the parenchymal side was ligated using a running 5-0 prolene.

The parenchyma was transected on the line of vascular demarcation along the principal plane using *finger fracture/ electrocautery/ultrasonic aspirator/combination of these.* Bile ducts and small vessels on the resection side were clipped and ligated using 3-0 silk ties on the remnant side. The parenchyma of the caudate lobe was transected to expose the anterior surface of the vena cava.

Hemostasis and bile stasis were obtained with a combination of cautery, clips, and 2-0 silk sutures. A *closed suction drain was inserted from a separate skin incision and placed adjacent to the transected liver surface and brought out dependently through the abdominal wall. The falciform ligament was reapproximated to prevent torsion of the liver remnant mid-postoperative vascular compromise.* Omentum was brought up to the operative field. After confirming hemostasis, the wound was irrigated with warm saline.

(Optional: Multiple interrupted through-and-through retention sutures of __ were placed.) The fascial layers were closed with *running sutures of __/a Smead-Jones closure of interrupted __.* The skin was closed with *skin staples/subcuticular sutures of __/ other.* The drain was secured with a suture of 3-0 nylon.

The patient tolerated the procedure well and was taken to the postanesthesia care unit in stable condition.

NOTES

Chapter 82
Left Hepatic Lobectomy

Georgios Tsoulfas, M.D.

INDICATIONS

- Tumor metastatic to the medial segments of the left lobe of the liver.
- Hepatocellular carcinoma confined to the left lobe.

ESSENTIAL STEPS

1. Bilateral subcostal incision with vertical midline extension.
2. Explore the abdomen and identify the lesion.
3. Mobilize the liver by dividing its ligamentous attachments.
4. Identify and ligate the left hepatic artery, left portal vein, and left hepatic bile duct (in that order).
5. After controlling the afferent vessels, turn attention to and ligate the short hepatic veins between the caudate lobe and inferior vena cava.
6. Transect the liver parenchyma along the line of vascular demarcation between the lobes using *cautery, finger fracture, or ultrasonic aspirator.*
7. Identify and transect the left hepatic vein.
8. Obtain hemostasis and bile stasis by *clipping or ligating* small vessels and bile ducts encountered.
9. Irrigate the wound.
10. Place omentum *and closed suction drain* adjacent to the transected liver surface.
11. Close the abdomen.

J.J. Hoballah and C.E.H. Scott-Conner (eds.), *Operative Dictations in General and Vascular Surgery*, DOI 10.1007/978-1-4614-0451-4_82,
© Springer Science+Business Media, LLC 2012

NOTE THESE VARIATIONS

- Technique of parenchymal transection.
- Division of hepatic veins sometimes performed later in procedure, if the decision is made to control the afferent vessels in the hilum, transect the parenchyma and then divide the hepatic vein.
- Removal of the gallbladder is optional as one may wish not to perform any unnecessary dissection close to the right lobe.
- Use of drain optional.

COMPLICATIONS

- Major bleeding.
- Injury to the hilar structures of the remaining liver.
- Bile collection.

TEMPLATE OPERATIVE DICTATION

Preoperative diagnosis: Metastatic cancer of the liver.

Procedure: Left hepatic lobectomy.

Postoperative diagnosis: Same.

Indications: This ___-year-old *male/female* with a history of stage carcinoma of resected in now has mass in medial segments of the left lobe of the liver. Computed tomography *and positron emission tomography scan* revealed metastatic lesions limited to the left lobe of the liver. This led to the decision to proceed with a left hepatic lobectomy.

Description of procedure: An epidural catheter was placed by anesthesia prior to the start of the operation. The patient was placed in the supine position and general endotracheal anesthesia was induced. A time-out was completed verifying correct patient, procedure, site, positioning, and implant(s) and/or special equipment prior to beginning this procedure. Preoperative antibiotics were given. A Foley catheter and a nasogastric tube were placed. The abdomen was prepped and draped in the usual sterile fashion. A bilateral subcostal incision was made two finger breadths below the costal margin with a vertical midline extension up toward the xiphoid process. Further dissection through the muscular and aponeurotic layers of the abdominal wall was performed with a combination of sharp dissection and electrocautery. The peritoneum was entered and the abdominal cavity inspected. Palpation of the liver revealed *lesions (specify number, size, and location)*. The right lobe appeared to be clean of disease. No other metastatic disease was identified.

The Omni retractor system was employed to retract the chest wall. The falciform ligament was divided between Pean clamps and tied with 2-0 silk sutures. The triangular ligament was divided with electrocautery up to the inferior vena cava at the diaphragm. *Adhesions from previous surgery were taken down sharply.*

An umbilical tape was placed around the hilar structures to be able to perform a Pringle maneuver, if vascular control is needed. The left lobe was completely mobilized to the level of the cava and the attachments to the posterior structures divided with electrocautery. The gallbladder was removed in the usual fashion by grasping the fundus and performing the dissection from the top clown to the level of the cystic duct, which was cleared and tied with 2-0 silk sutures. The cystic artery was identified and ligated with 2-0 silk sutures and the gallbladder removed from the field and sent to pathology.

Attention was turned to the hilum. The gastrohepatic omentum was divided and the left hepatic artery was approached through the lesser sac. Surrounding lymphatic vessels were ligated with 3-0 silk ties, and the left hepatic artery was temporarily occluded while palpating the artery to the opposite liver lobe to ensure patency to the arterial supply to the liver remnant. Having done this the left hepatic artery was identified and double-ligated with 2-0 silk sutures and divided. The common bile duct was retracted anteriorly with a vein retractor and the portal vein bifurcation was identified. The left portal vein branch was freed from surrounding lymphoareolar tissue and ligated with a vascular stapler. The left hepatic bile duct was divided at this point by double-clamping, transaction, and ligation. A clear line of vascular demarcation along the principal plane between the lobes was identified.

After controlling the afferent vessels, the hepatic veins were approached. Multiple short hepatic veins between the inferior vena cava and the caudate lobe of the liver were ligated using 3-0 silk ties to mobilize segment 1 inferiorly. As the veins are ligated and divided, segment 1 was retracted anteriorly, and the remainder of the hepatic veins between the inferior vena cava and the caudate lobe were divided. Division of the retrocaval ligament from the left side of the inferior vena cava allowed complete mobilization of segment 1.

The parenchyma was transected on the line of vascular demarcation along the principal plane using *finger fracture/electrocautery/ ultrasonic aspirator/a combination of these.* Bile ducts and small vessels on the resection side were clipped and ligated using 3-0 silk ties on the remnant side.

The main left hepatic vein was exposed where it joins the middle hepatic vein and a vascular stapler was used to transect it and the parenchymal side was ligated using running 5-0 prolene. The specimen was removed from the operative field.

Hemostasis and bile stasis were obtained with a combination of cautery and 2-0 silk sutures. *A closed suction drain was inserted from a separate skin incision and placed adjacent to the transected liver surface and brought out dependently through the abdominal wall.* Omentum was brought up to the operative field. After confirming hemostasis, the wound was irrigated with warm saline.

(Optional: Multiple interrupted through-and-through retention sutures of ___ were placed.) The fascial layers were closed with *running sutures of ___/a Smead-Jones closure of interrupted ___*. The skin was closed with *skin staples/subcuticular sutures of ___/other.* The drain was secured with a suture of 3-0 nylon.

The patient tolerated the procedure well and was taken to the postanesthesia care unit in stable condition.

NOTES

Chapter 83

Packing of Liver Injury with Damage Control Laparotomy

Mohammad Khreiss, M.D. and Bellal A. Joseph, M.D.

INDICATIONS

- Penetrating abdominal injury
- Blunt abdominal injury with hemodynamic Instability

ESSENTIAL STEPS

1. Supine position with both arms abducted
2. Prep the chest, abdomen, and both lower extremities table to table
3. Establish Central Venous catheter access through neck, insert foley, IV antibiotics
4. Activate massive transfusion protocol
5. Perform trauma laparotomy; midline incision from xiphoid to above pubic tubercle
6. Evacuate heamoperitoneum and bowel contents (if present)
7. Pack all four quadrants with laparotomy pads (RUQ, LUQ, LLQ, and RLQ)
8. Apply direct pressure to sources of bleeding, bimanual compression of liver
9. Allow anesthesia to catch up through transfusion of warm blood and blood products (use level one transfuser)
10. Remove packs and inspect for sources of bleeding, control spillage from bowel injury if present (when removing packs, start with lower quadrants then LUQ then RUQ, if spillage from bowel is not present then an auto transfusion device is used)

J.J. Hoballah and C.E.H. Scott-Conner (eds.), *Operative Dictations in General and Vascular Surgery*, DOI 10.1007/978-1-4614-0451-4_83,

11. Remove RUQ packing and inspect for liver injury (visual and tactile)
12. Mobilize liver and identify injury (divide falciform, round, coronary and triangular ligaments, mobilization only on side of injury)
13. If bleeding is not controlled with manual compression, perform a Pringle maneuver by encircling the portal triad between thumb and index fingers (may use vascular clamp).
14. Inspect the injury site and perform hepatotomy to expose bleeding vessels (may use finger fracture technique ,Kelly fracture technique, or stapler device)
15. Suture ligate bleeding vessels using 3.0 prolene sutures
16. Use hemostatic adjuncts such as thrombin soaked gel foam, Tisseel, etc.
17. Release Pringle maneuver and reinspect
18. Damage control packing of the liver if bleeding continues and pt develops acidosis, coagulopathy, and hypothermia
19. Apply packs between the liver and kidney, the liver and diaphragm in a clockwise fashion making a sandwich (avoid applying pack over IVC or portal vein to prevent compression of either one)
20. Temporary closure of the abdomen (may use towel clips, skin closure only, use of Bogota bag, application of wound VAC; we prefer us of wound VAC closure...)
21. Transfer patient to ICU for further resuscitation

NOTE THESE VARIATIONS

- Carefully document findings and management of any additional injuries.
- The incision may be extended to the right subcostal area for further exposure and an abdominal wall retractor may be applied (we prefer the Thompson retractor)
- Cholecystectomy may be needed if gallbladder is damaged or ischemic – not recommended routinely
- The right hepatic artery may arise from the SMA
- Failure of the Pringle maneuver to control bleeding may indicate hepatic veins or supra hepatic IVC injury
- Adequate packing of the liver should not need more than seven laparotomy pads if done correctly
- A steri drape may be applied against the liver parenchyma before applying the packs (this will prevent rebleeding upon removal of the packs in direct contact with raw liver surface)

- Avoid inserting the packs into the laceration. This will increase the degree of injury
- Always keep count of the number of pads used and document in the chart and in the operative dictation

COMPLICATIONS
- Injury to the CBD upon performing Pringle maneuver
- Iatrogenic injury to the spleen upon inspection
- Hepatic necrosis and abscess formation
- Biloma formation
- Acidosis, hypothermia, and coagulopathy
- Abdominal compartment syndrome may develop in the ICU
- Death

TEMPLATE OPERATIVE DICTATION

Preoperative diagnosis: Penetrating abdominal injury with hemodynamic instability

Procedure: Damage control laparotomy, packing of segment ___ stellate liver injury *(list any additional procedures)*, temporary abdominal closure with wound VAC

Postoperative diagnosis: Stellate Liver injury to segment ___ *(list any additional injuries)*.

Indications: The patient is ___ -year-old *male/female* sustained injury due to ___. Patient was brought to the ED by EMS. He/she underwent intubation and resuscitation in the emergency department according to ATLS protocols; however, the patient was a transient responder and was rushed to the operating room for exploration. Type and cross match was drawn.

Description of procedure: Under general anesthesia and with the patient in the supine position with both upper extremities abducted, the chest abdomen and both lower extremities were prepped and draped in the usual sterile manner. A time-out was completed verifying correct patient, procedure, site, positioning, and implant(s) and/or special equipment prior to beginning this procedure. Foley catheter was inserted and IV antibiotics were infused. At the same time, an arterial line and large bore central venous access were accomplished by the anesthesia team. Massive transfusion protocol was activated.

A midline skin incision extending from the xiphoid to above the pubic tubercle was performed. Dissection was carried through skin and subcutaneous tissue, until the peritoneal cavity was entered. ___ liters of hemoperitoneum were evacuated. There was *evidence of/no evidence of bowel contents and the auto-transfusion device was applied.* Laparotomy pads were carefully applied to pack the right upper quadrant, left upper quadrant, left lower quadrant, and right lower quadrant, respectively. Packs were placed deep behind the spleen and liver. Bimanual compression to the liver was applied due to profuse bleeding. The anesthesia team was allowed to catch-up by transfusion of blood and blood products. After restoring hemodynamic stability, the lower abdominal packs were removed. The ligament of trietz was identified and a complete small bowel inspection was performed. There *was/ was no* evidence of injury to the small bowel *(detail injuries and management)*. The colon was then inspected and *was found to be injured in ___/no evidence of injury was present (detail injuries and management)*. There was no evidence of any mesenteric hematomas. No central or lateral retroperitoneal hematomas were identified. The left upper quadrant packing was removed. The spleen appeared *intact/was injured (detail management)*. There *was no/ was* evidence of left perinephric hematomas *(detail management)*. The right upper quadrant packs were removed. There was a evidence of profuse bleeding from the dome of the liver secondary to a stellate lesion of segments ___. Packs were reapplied. The incision was extended to the right subcostal margin. The round and falciform ligaments were divided along with the right triangular and coronary ligaments. The liver was mobilized and delivered into the midline. *The porta-hepatis was isolated and a Pringle maneuver was performed using a vascular clamp.* The packing was removed. It was noticed that the bleeding decreased markedly yet was still present. Hepatotomy was performed using finger fracture technique and several bleeding vessels were identified and suture ligated using 3.0 prolene sutures. The Pringle maneuver was released and it was noticed that bleeding resumed. The anesthesia team reported that the patient has received ___ units of blood, his temperature was ___, and his INR was ___. Decision was taken at this time to perform damage control and packing of the liver and transfer the patient to the ICU for further resuscitation and management. A folded steri drape was applied against the surface of the liver. Laparotomy pads were applied between the liver and the kidney laterally and between the liver and the diaphragm superiorly to control the bleeding between 7 O'clock and 5 O'clock in a clockwise fashion. No pads were applied above the IVC or portal vein to avoid compression of these structures. A total of seven pads were used. After that temporary closure of the abdominal cavity was done using a Wound Vac. Patient was transferred to the ICU in fair condition. The gravity of the situation was communicated to the family.

NOTES

Section VII

Pancreas

Chapter 84

Partial Pancreaticoduodenectomy (Whipple Procedure)

Prashant Khullar, M.D.

INDICATIONS

- Malignancy of the head of the pancreas, proximal duodenum, or distal bile duct.
- Chronic pancreatitis with failed nonoperative management.
- Cystadenoma of the head of the pancreas.
- Rarely, massive destruction of the pancreatic head–duodenum complex secondary to trauma

ESSENTIAL STEPS

1. *Upper midline/chevron* incision.
2. Explore for disease outside resection field (liver metastasis, peritoneal nodules, or lymph nodes, ascites).
3. Place appropriate mechanical retraction device, e.g., Bookwalter's, Fowlers, Omni-Tract, etc.
4. Extensive Kocher maneuver to allow visualization of the superior mesenteric artery.
5. Mobilize gall bladder from the gall bladder fossa, divide the cystic artery, and mobilize the cystic duct till the junction with the common bile duct.
6. Divide the common hepatic duct close to the level of the cystic duct entry site and retract it caudally to identify the portal vein
7. Assess for a replaced/accessory right or common hepatic artery

J.J. Hoballah and C.E.H. Scott-Conner (eds.), *Operative Dictations in General and Vascular Surgery*, DOI 10.1007/978-1-4614-0451-4_84,
© Springer Science+Business Media, LLC 2012

8. Identify, dissect, clamp, ligate, and divide the gastroduodenal artery.
9. Identify and dissect the superior mesenteric vein caudal to the neck of the pancreas, and develop a plane superior to the vein and posterior to the neck of the pancreas. Loop the neck of the pancreas with a Penrose drain.
10. Circumferentially dissect the first and second parts of the duodenum and divide it 3 cm distal to the pylorus using a linear stapling device.
11. Divide the neck of the pancreas after placing stay sutures cranially and caudally on the pancreatic remnant to control bleeding.
12. Divide the proximal jejunum about 10 cm distal to the ligament of Trietz and deliver it dorsal to the superior mesenteric vessels from left to right into the supracolic compartment.
13. Separate the uncinate process from the portal vein, superior mesenteric vein, and artery gently by serially clamping, dividing, and ligating the vascular branches off the SMV, SMA, and PV.
14. Remove and send marked specimen to pathology for analysis of the common hepatic duct, pancreatic duct, and uncinate process margins.
15. *Place piece of pediatric feeding tube into the pancreatic duct as stent.*
16. Pass the distal end of the jejunum into the supracolic compartment through an opening created in the transverse mesocolon.
17. Create a retrocolic pancreaticojejunostomy with either a duct-to-mucosal anastomosis or with an invagination technique; 4-0 or 5'0 PDS full thickness sutures between the pancreatic duct and the jejunum and 3'0 silk interrupted stitches incorporating the pancreatic capsule and the seromuscular layer of the jejunum.
18. For the invagination technique, use 4'0 PDS interrupted sutures to anastomose the full thickness jejunum and the pancreatic capsule with underlying parenchyma in an end-to-end fashion. This inner layer should incorporate the pancreatic duct for several bites to splay it open. The outer layer consists of 3'0 interrupted silk sutures approximating the pancreatic capsule and the underlying pancreatic parenchyma to the seromuscular layer of the jejunum in such a manner so as to 'dunk' the pancreatic remnant into the lumen of the jejunum.

19. End-to-side biliary-enteric anastomosis of the common bile duct to proximal ascending loop, 7–10 cm distal to the pancreaticojejunostomy in a single layer using interrupted/continuous absorbable sutures, e.g., 5′0 PDS.
20. Antecolic duodenojejunostomy in case of pyloric preserving pancreatoduodenectomy is done 10–15 cm distal to the biliary-enteric anastomosis in a single interrupted/continuous layer with absorbable suture.
21. Place nasogastric tube in efferent limb of duodenojejunostomy (*18 French gastrostomy drainage tube brought out through the abdomen is an alternative*).
22. Check hemostasis.
23. Place omentum and closed suction drains in proximity to anastomoses.
24. Secure drains with 3-0 nylon.
25. *(Optional) place feeding jejunostomy.*
26. Close the abdomen.

NOTE THESE VARIATIONS

- Hepatic artery arising from the superior mesenteric artery may be encountered and should be preserved.
- Classical pancreatoduodenectomy versus pylorus preserving may be done. A two layer gastrojejunostomy is done instead of a duodenojejunostomy.
- Anastomotic technique, use of stents.

COMPLICATIONS

- Pancreatitis or leak from pancreaticojejunostomy.
- Bile leak.
- Inadvertent ligation of an anomalous hepatic artery leading to hepatic hypoperfusion.
- Injury to the portal vein, superior mesenteric vein.
- Delayed gastric emptying, commonly secondary to pancreaticojejunostomy anastomotic leak.
- Leak from gastrojejunostomy.
- Intra-abdominal abscess.

TEMPLATE FOR OPERATIVE DICTATION

Preoperative diagnosis: *Carcinoma of head of pancreas/distal bile duct/duodenum/other.*

Procedure: Partial pancreaticoduodenectomy (Whipple procedure).

Postoperative diagnosis: Same.

Indications: This ___-year-old *male/female* developed *progressive jaundice/weight loss/diabetes/abdominal pain* and was found to have a ___. Evaluation with *computed tomography scan/ERCP/ endoscopic ultrasound* demonstrated no obvious metastatic disease and a high probability of resectability. Exploration for partial pancreaticoduodenectomy was indicated.

Description of the procedure: An epidural catheter was placed by anesthesia prior to the start of the operation. The patient was placed in the supine position and general endotracheal anesthesia was induced. A time-out was completed verifying correct patient, procedure, site, positioning, and implant(s) and/or special equipment prior to beginning this procedure. Preoperative antibiotics were given. A Foley catheter and a nasogastric tube were placed. The abdomen was prepped and draped in the usual sterile fashion. *A vertical midline incision was made from xiphoid to just below the umbilicus/a bilateral subcostal incision was made two finger breadths below the costal margin.* This was deepened through the subcutaneous tissues and hemostasis was achieved with electrocautery. Fascial layers were divided with electrocautery and the peritoneal cavity entered. The abdomen was explored. *Adhesions were lysed sharply under direct vision with Metzenbaum scissors.* There was no evidence of spread outside the planned resection field; specifically, no liver or peritoneal nodules, obvious local extension, ascites, or lymphadenopathy. Mechanical retractors were placed.

An extensive Kocher maneuver was performed to identify the superior mesenteric vessels. The head of the pancreas and superior mesenteric vessels were palpated to assure resectability. The mass appeared to be localized to the head of the pancreas and did not appear to involve the mesenteric vessels. The decision was made to proceed with resection.

The gastrohepatic ligament was dissected and the common bile duct was freed circumferentially.

The gall bladder was separated from the underlying gall bladder fossa, and the cystic artery was identified, ligated, and divided. The common hepatic duct was divided close to the level of the cystic duct entry site and retracted caudally to identify the portal vein. Absence/presence of a replaced/accessory right or common hepatic artery was confirmed. The artery was carefully preserved. The gastroduodenal artery was identified, dissected, clamped, divided, and ligated.

The superior mesenteric vein caudal to the neck of the pancreas was identified, dissected and a plane superior to the vein and posterior to the neck of the pancreas was identified. The neck of the pancreas was looped with a Penrose drain.

[Choose one:]

If standard Whipple: Identify, ligate, and divide the right gastric artery, and the terminal branches of the left gastric artery at the junction of the antrum and the body of the stomach. The antrum of the stomach was stapled and transected at the junction of the antrum and the body of the stomach just below the visible branches of the vagus nerve. The antrum was reflected superiorly and to the right laterally.

If pylorus-preserving Whipple: The first and second parts of the duodenum were circumferentially dissected and divided 3 cm distal to the pylorus using a linear stapling device.

The neck of the pancreas was divided with electrocautery/knife after placing stay sutures cranially and caudally on the pancreatic remnant to control potential bleeding.

The proximal jejunum about 10 cm distal to the ligament of Trietz was divided using a linear stapling device and delivered dorsal to the superior mesenteric vessels from left to right into the supracolic compartment. The uncinate process was dissected free from the portal vein, superior mesenteric vein, and artery gently by serially clamping, dividing, and ligating the vascular branches off the SMV, SMA, and PV. The specimen was removed, marked, and sent to pathology for analysis of the common hepatic duct, pancreatic duct, and uncinate process margins.

The distal end of the jejunum was passed into the supracolic compartment through an opening created in the transverse mesocolon.

Choose one:

A retrocolic pancreaticojejunostomy was performed with a duct-to-mucosal anastomosis. 4-0 or 5'0 PDS full thickness sutures were taken between the pancreatic duct and the jejunum and 3'0 silk interrupted stitches incorporating the pancreatic capsule and the seromuscular layer of the jejunum were used for the outer layer.

For the invagination technique, 4'0 PDS interrupted sutures were used to anastomose the full thickness jejunum and the pancreatic capsule with underlying parenchyma in an end-to-end fashion. This inner layer incorporated the pancreatic duct for several bites to splay it open. The outer layer was done with 3'0 interrupted silk sutures approximating the pancreatic capsule and the underlying pancreatic parenchyma to the seromuscular layer of the jejunum in such a manner so as to 'dunk' the pancreatic remnant into the lumen of the jejunum.

End-to-side biliary-enteric anastomosis of the common bile duct to proximal ascending loop was performed 7–10 cm distal to the pancreaticojejunostomy in a single layer using interrupted/continuous 5'0 PDS.

Choose one:

An antecolic duodenojejunostomy in case of pyloric preserving pancreatoduodenectomy was done 10–15 cm distal to the biliary-enteric anastomosis in a single interrupted/continuous layer with absorbable suture.

A gastrojejunostomy was performed as a two-layered sutured anastomosis between the gastric remnant and the jejunum. This was constructed with an inner running layer of 4-0 PDS and an outer layer of interrupted 3-0 silk Lembert sutures. A three-corner stitch was placed at the angle of sorrow.

All anastomoses were checked and found to be patent and intact. *The nasogastric tube was positioned in the desired location/a Stamm gastrostomy was created in the usual fashion and the nasogastric tube removed. A Witzel feeding/needle catheter jejunostomy was then constructed in the usual fashion.* Mesenteric defects were closed. Hemostasis was checked. Closed suction drains were placed in close proximity to the anastomoses and brought out *(detail locations).* All tubes, stents, and drains were brought out through the anterior abdominal wall and secured to the skin with 3-0 nylon sutures.

(Optional: Multiple interrupted through-and-through retention sutures of ___ were placed.) The fascia was closed with *a running suture of ___/a Smead-Jones closure of interrupted ___.* The skin was closed with *skin staples/subcuticular suture of ___/other.*

The patient tolerated the procedure well and was taken to the postanesthesia care unit in stable condition.

ACKNOWLEDGMENT

This chapter was contributed by Natisha Busick, MD in the first edition.

NOTES

Chapter 85

Total Pancreaticoduodenectomy

Prashant Khullar, M.D.

INDICATIONS

- Multicentricity of tumor as identified on imaging or operative exploration
- Rare giant tumors, for example, cystadenocarcinomas or sarcomas involving the entire pancreas
- Diffuse intraductal papillary mucinous neoplasm
- Positive margins after a Whipple's operation as documented on frozen section

ESSENTIAL STEPS

1. *Upper midline/chevron* incision.
2. Explore for disease outside resection field (liver metastasis, peritoneal nodules, ascites, or lymph nodes).
3. Place appropriate mechanical retraction device, e.g., Bookwalter's, Fowlers, Omni-Tract, etc.
4. Mobilize the right colon and hepatic flexure to access the duodenum and the head of the pancreas.
5. Assess for a replaced/accessory right or common hepatic artery
6. Retract the colon medially and inferiorly to visualize the third and fourth portions of the duodenum.
7. Extensive Kocher maneuver to expose the superior mesenteric vessels.
8. Palpate the head of the pancreas and superior mesenteric vessels to determine resectability.

J.J. Hoballah and C.E.H. Scott-Conner (eds.), *Operative Dictations in General and Vascular Surgery*, DOI 10.1007/978-1-4614-0451-4_85,
© Springer Science+Business Media, LLC 2012

9. Widely open the gastrocolic omentum to expose the body of the pancreas.

10. Detach the greater omentum from the left transverse colon.

11. Divide the proximal jejunum about 10 cm distal to the ligament of Trietz and deliver it dorsal to the superior mesenteric vessels from left to right into the supracolic compartment.

12. Mobilize gall bladder from the gall bladder fossa, divide the cystic artery, and mobilize the cystic duct till the junction with the common bile duct.

13. Divide the common hepatic duct close to the level of the cystic duct entry site and retract it caudally to identify the portal vein.

14. Identify, dissect, clamp, ligate, and divide the gastroduodenal artery to open the plane anterior to the portal vein behind the neck of the pancreas.

15. Identify, ligate, and divide the right gastric artery, and the terminal branches of the left gastric artery at the junction of the antrum and the body of the stomach.

16. Transect the stomach at the junction of the antrum and the body of the stomach with a linear stapling device and retract the stomach laterally.

17. Gently apply traction on the spleen medially and divide the lienorenal ligament.

18. Divide the splenocolic ligament to free the left colon inferiorly.

19. Ligate the short gastric arteries.

20. Retract the stomach superiorly and medially.

21. Mobilize the spleen and pancreas from retroperitoneal attachments.

22. Divide the inferior mesenteric vein.

23. Dissect the spleen and pancreas medially to identify origin of the splenic artery and vein at the superior mesenteric vein-splenic vein junction.

24. Ligate and divide the splenic artery and splenic vein.

25. Ligate veins from the duodenum and pancreas as they come into the portal vein and superior mesenteric vein.

26. Separate the uncinate process from the portal vein, superior mesenteric vein, and artery gently by serially clamping, dividing, and ligating the vascular branches off the SMV, SMA, and PV.

27. Remove the specimen.

28. Pass the distal end of the jejunum into the supracolic compartment through an opening created in the transverse mesocolon.
29. An end-to-side biliary-enteric anastomosis of the common bile duct to proximal ascending loop, in a single layer using interrupted/continuous absorbable sutures, for e.g., 5'0 PDS is created
30. Antecolic gastrojejunostomy in case of classical total pancreatoduodenectomy is done 10–15 cm distal to the biliary-enteric anastomosis in two layers with absorbable suture for the inner layer and interrupted silk sutures for the seromuscular outer layer.
31. Place nasogastric tube in efferent limb of gastrojejunostomy *(18 French gastrostomy drainage tube brought out the abdomen is an alternative).*
32. Check hemostasis.
33. Replace omentum and closed suction drains in proximity to anastomoses.
34. Secure drains with 3-0 nylon.
35. *(Optional) place feeding jejunostomy.*
36. Close the abdomen.

NOTE THESE VARIATIONS

- Anomalous replaced/accessory/common hepatic artery arising from the superior mesenteric artery may be encountered and should be preserved.
- Exact order of dissection varies.
- Pylorus preserving versus classical pancreatoduodenectomy may be done. A duodenojejunostomy is done instead of a gastrojejunostomy 10–15 cm distal to the biliary-enteric anastomosis in a single interrupted/continuous layer with absorbable suture.
- *Gastrostomy, feeding jejunostomy optional.*

COMPLICATIONS

- Brittle diabetes.
- Bleeding.
- Bile leak.
- Recurrence of cancer.
- Intra-abdominal abscess.

TEMPLATE FOR OPERATIVE DICTATION

Preoperative diagnosis: *Carcinoma/cystadenoma/other of pancreas.*

Procedure: Total pancreaticoduodenectomy.

Postoperative diagnosis: Same.

Indications: This ___-year-old *male/female* developed progressive *jaundice/weight loss/diabetes/abdominal pain* and was found to have a ___. Evaluation with *computed tomography scan/ERCP/ endoscopic ultrasound* demonstrated no obvious metastatic disease and a high probability of resectability with total pancreatectomy. Exploration for total pancreaticoduodenectomy was indicated.

Description of the procedure: An epidural catheter was placed by anesthesia prior to the start of the operation. The patient was placed in the supine position and general endotracheal anesthesia was induced. A time-out was completed verifying correct patient, procedure, site, positioning, and implant(s) and/or special equipment prior to beginning this procedure. Preoperative antibiotics were given. A Foley catheter and nasogastric tube were placed. The abdomen was prepped and draped in the usual sterile fashion. *A vertical midline incision was made from xiphoid to just below the umbilicus/a bilateral subcostal incision was made two finger breadths below the costal margin.* This was deepened through the subcutaneous tissues and hemostasis was achieved with electrocautery. Fascial layers were divided with electrocautery and the peritoneal cavity entered. The abdomen was explored. *Adhesions were lysed sharply under direct vision with Metzenbaum scissors.* There was no evidence of spread outside the planned resection field; specifically, no liver or peritoneal nodules, ascites, obvious local extension, or lymphadenopathy. Mechanical retractors were placed.

The right colon and hepatic flexure were mobilized and retracted medially and inferiorly. The gastrocolic omentum was widely divided to expose the pancreas. An extensive Kocher maneuver was performed. The head of the pancreas and superior mesenteric vessels were palpated to assure resectability. The mass appeared to be localized to the pancreas and did not appear to involve the mesenteric vessels. The decision was made to proceed with resection.

The gastrohepatic ligament was dissected and the common bile duct was freed circumferentially.

The gall bladder was separated from the underlying gall bladder fossa, and the cystic artery was identified, ligated, and divided. The common hepatic duct was divided close to the level of the cystic duct entry site and retracted caudally to identify the portal vein. Absence/presence of a replaced/accessory right or common hepatic artery was confirmed. The artery was carefully preserved.

The gastroduodenal artery was identified, dissected, clamped, divided, and ligated.

The superior mesenteric vein caudal to the neck of the pancreas was identified, dissected and a plane superior to the vein and posterior to the neck of the pancreas was identified.

[Choose one:]

If standard total pancreatoduodenectomy: The right gastric artery, and the terminal branches of the left gastric artery at the junction of the antrum and the body of the stomach were identified, ligated, and divided. The antrum of the stomach was stapled and transected just below the visible branches of the vagus nerve. The antrum was reflected superiorly and to the right laterally.

If pylorus-preserving Whipple: The first and second parts of the duodenum were circumferentially dissected and divided 3 cm distal to the pylorus using a linear stapling device.

Using electrocautery, the greater omentum was separated from the transverse colon. The splenic flexure was mobilized. Gentle traction on the spleen was applied medially to divide the lienorenal and splenocolic ligaments to free the left colon inferiorly. The short gastric arteries were ligated, and the stomach was retracted superiorly and medially. The spleen and pancreas were mobilized from their retroperitoneal attachments and the inferior mesenteric vein was divided and ligated.

The spleen and pancreas were dissected free medially to identify origin of the splenic artery and vein at the superior mesenteric vein–splenic vein junction. The splenic artery and splenic vein were divided and ligated at the origin of the splenic artery. The veins from the duodenum and pancreas as they entered into the portal vein and superior mesenteric vein were identified, ligated, and divided. The uncinate process was separated from the portal vein, superior mesenteric vein, and artery gently by serially clamping, dividing, and ligating the vascular branches off the SMV, SMA, and PV. The specimen was sent off to pathology for histopathological assessment. The distal end of the jejunum was passed into the supracolic compartment through an opening created in the transverse mesocolon. End-to-side biliary-enteric anastomosis of the common bile duct to proximal ascending loop was performed in a single layer using interrupted/continuous 5'0 PDS.

[Choose one:]

An antecolic duodenojejunostomy in case of pyloric preserving total pancreatoduodenectomy was done 10–15 cm distal to the biliary-enteric anastomosis in a single interrupted/continuous layer with absorbable suture.

A gastrojejunostomy was performed as a two-layered sutured anastomosis between the gastric remnant and the jejunum. This was constructed with an inner running layer of 4-0 PDS and an outer layer of interrupted 3-0 silk Lembert sutures. A three-corner stitch was placed at the angle of sorrow.

All anastomoses were checked and found to be patent and intact. *The nasogastric tube was positioned in the desired location/a Stamm gastrostomy was created in the usual fashion and the nasogastric tube removed. A Witzel feeding/needle catheter jejunostomy was then constructed in the usual fashion.* Hemostasis was checked. Mesenteric defects were closed. Closed suction drains were placed in close proximity to the anastomoses and brought out *(detail locations).* All tubes, stents, and drains were brought out through the anterior abdominal wall and secured to the skin with 3-0 nylon sutures.

(Optional: Multiple interrupted through-and-through retention sutures of ___ were placed.) The fascia was closed with *a running suture of ___/a Smead-Jones closure of interrupted ___.* The skin was closed with *skin staples/subcuticular suture of ___/other.*

The patient tolerated the procedure well and was taken to the postanesthesia care unit in stable condition.

ACKNOWLEDGMENT

This chapter was contributed by Natisha Busick, MD in the first edition.

NOTES

Chapter 86
Distal Pancreatectomy

Prashant Khullar, M.D.

INDICATIONS
- Trauma.
- Tumor of the pancreatic body or tail.
- Pseudocyst of the tail of the pancreas.

ESSENTIAL STEPS
1. *Diagnostic laparoscopy may be indicated since the risk of occult metastatic disease is higher in pancreatic cancer involving the body and tail.*
2. Midline or left subcostal/chevron incision.
3. Explore for disease outside resection field (liver metastasis, peritoneal nodules, ascites, or lymph nodes).
4. Place appropriate mechanical retraction device, e.g., Bookwalter's, Fowlers, Omni-Tract, etc.
5. Widely divide the gastrocolic omentum and gastrosplenic ligament to enter the lesser sac.
6. Confirm pathology and resectability. Kocherise the duodenum to palpate head and uncinate process of pancreas.
7. *In case of splenic vein thrombosis and resulting portal hypertension, it is beneficial to dissect and isolate the splenic artery origin with a vessel loop early in the operation. The splenic artery can be ligated, if excessive bleeding occurs during subsequent dissection.*
8. *If splenectomy:*
   - Gently apply traction on the spleen medially and divide the lienorenal ligament.

418

J.J. Hoballah and C.E.H. Scott-Conner (eds.), *Operative Dictations in General and Vascular Surgery*, DOI 10.1007/978-1-4614-0451-4_86,
© Springer Science+Business Media, LLC 2012

- Divide the splenocolic ligament to free the left colon inferiorly.
- Ligate the short gastric arteries.
- Retract the stomach superiorly and medially.
- Mobilize the spleen and pancreas from retroperitoneal attachments.
- Ligate and divide the inferior mesenteric vein, if it drains into the splenic vein.
- Dissect the spleen and pancreas medially to identify origin of the splenic artery and vein at the superior mesenteric vein–splenic vein junction.
- Ligate and divide the splenic artery and splenic vein.
- *If splenic preservation: Develop plane deep to the pancreas but superficial to the splenic vessels.*
- *Clip and divide multiple tributaries linking the tail and body of the pancreas with the splenic vessels until the distal pancreas is completely free.*

9. Divide the neck of the pancreas after placing stay sutures cranially and caudally on the pancreatic remnant to control bleeding.
10. Send off specimen for frozen sections of margins in case of malignant etiology. Mark resection bed with metallic clips as a guide to postoperative radiation therapy if needed.
11. Proximal stump of the pancreatic duct can be secured with figure of eight silk suture.
12. Check hemostasis.
13. Close the abdomen and secure drains.

NOTE THESE VARIATIONS
- Choice of incision.
- Preservation of the spleen.

COMPLICATIONS
- Bleeding.
- Pancreatitis or pancreatic leak.
- Subphrenic abscess.

TEMPLATE FOR OPERATIVE DICTATION
Preoperative diagnosis: *Tumor of/trauma to the body/tail* of the pancreas.
Procedure: Distal pancreatectomy with *splenectomy/splenic preservation.*

Postoperative diagnosis: Same.

Indications: This ___-year-old *male/female* had *tumor/trauma* isolated to *the body/tail* of the pancreas. Distal pancreatectomy with *splenectomy/splenic preservation* was elected.

Description of procedure: An epidural catheter was placed by anesthesia prior to the start of the operation. The patient was placed in the supine position and general endotracheal anesthesia was induced. A time-out was completed verifying correct patient, procedure, site, positioning, and implant(s) and/or special equipment prior to beginning this procedure. Preoperative antibiotics were given. A Foley catheter and a nasogastric tube were placed. The abdomen was prepped and draped in the usual sterile fashion. *A vertical midline incision was made from xiphoid to just below the umbilicus/left subcostal/chevron incision was made two finger breadths below the left costal margin.* This was deepened through the subcutaneous tissues and hemostasis was achieved with electrocautery. The fascia was identified and incised and the peritoneal cavity entered. The abdomen was explored and the pathology confirmed *(enumerate findings, specifically absence of metastatic disease for tumor, and extent of exploration for trauma). Adhesions were lysed sharply under direct vision with Metzenbaum scissors.* Mechanical retractors were placed. The colon was mobilized and the splenic flexure was reflected downward. The gastrocolic ligament was divided widely to open the lesser sac and expose the pancreas.

[Choose one:]

If splenectomy: The spleen was mobilized by incising the splenocolic ligament. The splenic flexure was mobilized. Gentle traction on the spleen was applied medially to divide the lienorenal and splenocolic ligaments to free the left colon inferiorly. The short gastric arteries were ligated and the stomach was retracted superiorly and medially. The spleen and pancreas were mobilized from their retroperitoneal attachments and the inferior mesenteric vein was divided and ligated. The spleen and pancreas were dissected free medially to identify origin of the splenic artery and vein at the superior mesenteric vein–splenic vein junction. The splenic artery and splenic vein were divided and ligated at the origin of the splenic artery. The pancreas was transected with a TA 55 stapler after placing stay sutures cranially and caudally on the pancreatic remnant to control bleeding.

If splenic preservation: The spleen was reflected anteromedially and the posterior surface of the spleen and pancreas were freed. A point of transection was chosen ___ cm distal to the superior mesenteric vein. The pancreas was gently elevated from the retroperitoneum. The pancreas was transected with a TA 55 stapler after placing stay sutures cranially and caudally on the pancreatic remnant to control bleeding. The end of the pancreatic duct was oversewn with figure-of-eight 3-0 silk sutures. The distal pancreas was elevated and multiple small tributaries linking the splenic vessels and pancreas were clipped and divided until the pancreas was free.

The specimen was removed and sent for frozen section to assess margin status. The field was checked for hemostasis. Closed suction drains were placed in the operative field. The colon and stomach were placed in the correct anatomic position. Drains were brought out on the left side of the abdomen and secured with 3-0 nylon.

(Optional: Multiple interrupted through-and-through retention sutures of ___ were placed.) The fascia was closed with *a running suture of ___/a Smead-Jones closure of interrupted ___*. The skin was closed with *skin staples/subcuticular sutures of ___/other.*

The patient tolerated the procedure well and was taken to the postanesthesia care unit in stable condition.

ACKNOWLEDGMENT

This chapter was contributed by Natisha Busick, MD in the first edition.

NOTES

Chapter 87
Laparoscopic Distal Pancreatectomy

Prashant Khullar, M.D.

INDICATIONS
- Benign/malignant tumor of the pancreatic body or tail.
- Pseudocyst of the tail of the pancreas.

ESSENTIAL STEPS
1. Supine or a right semilateral position, depending on the location of the lesion.
   - Lesions closer to the tail of the pancreas are best approached in the right semilateral decubitus position. The operating surgeon stands to the right of the patient.
   - Alternatively, the patient can be in a lithotomy position with the surgeon stationed between the legs of the patient.
2. Create pneumoperitoneum with camera port at or above the umbilicus
3. Introduce the laparoscope and perform a peritoneal exploration for disease outside resection field (liver metastasis, peritoneal nodules, ascites, or lymph nodes).
4. Place three 5 mm ports along the right subcostal margin, right abdomen, and along the left mid-clavicular line, 5 cm below the costal margin. The third port can be upsized to a 15 mm port to allow the placement of Endo-GIA staplers. Additional 10 mm port can be placed in the sub-xiphoid region.

J.J. Hoballah and C.E.H. Scott-Conner (eds.), *Operative Dictations in General and Vascular Surgery*, DOI 10.1007/978-1-4614-0451-4_87,
© Springer Science+Business Media, LLC 2012

5. Enter the lesser sac through gastrocolic omentum.
6. Mobilize the splenic flexure and divide the gastrocolic omentum along the greater curvature of the stomach using a laparoscopic Harmonic™ scalpel or a LigaSure™.
7. Introduce a fan blade retractor through the sub-xiphoid port and retract the stomach anterosuperiorly.
8. *If desired, use laparoscopic ultrasound to identify the tumor and the blood vessels to determine the line of transection and preservation of blood vessels.*
9. Mobilize inferior margin of pancreas by developing a plane between the root of the transverse colon and the anterior fascia of the pancreas.
10. Identify and isolate the splenic vessels at the level of transection, approximately 1 cm proximal to the tumor.
11. Transect the pancreas with an Endo-GIA™ stapler (4.8 mm). *Use of ePTFE-buttressed stapler to transect the pancreas may be associated with a lower rate of postoperative pancreatic fistula.*
12. The splenic vessels can be transected separately with a vascular load of the Endo-GIA stapler.
13. Oversew the pancreatic staple line and secure hemostasis with endoscopic clip application as needed.
14. Dissect the pancreatic tail (specimen) from the retroperitoneum in a medial-to-lateral direction.
15. Divide the splenic vessels again as far from the splenic hilum as possible, taking care to preserve short gastric vessels and potential collaterals, (Warshaw technique).
    If splenectomy:
    • Gently apply traction on the spleen medially and divide the lienorenal ligament.
    • Divide the splenocolic ligament to free the left colon inferiorly.
    • Ligate the short gastric arteries.
    • Retract the stomach superiorly and medially using a fan blade retractor introduced through the sub-xiphoid port.
    • Mobilize the spleen and pancreas from retroperitoneal attachments.
    • Ligate and divide the inferior mesenteric vein, if it drains into the splenic vein.
    • Dissect the spleen and pancreas medially to identify the splenic artery and vein at the level of the line of transection.
    • Transect the pancreas as above.

16. Retrieve specimen in a retrieval bag.
17. Pancreas staple line can be reinforced with fibrin glue as needed.
18. Secure a Blake drain and close port sites in a standard fashion.

NOTE THIS VARIATION
- Preservation of the spleen.

COMPLICATIONS
- Bleeding.
- Pancreatitis or pancreatic leak.
- Subphrenic abscess.

TEMPLATE FOR OPERATIVE DICTATION

Preoperative diagnosis: *Tumor of the body/tail* of the pancreas.

Procedure: Laparoscopic distal pancreatectomy with *splenectomy/splenic preservation*.

Postoperative diagnosis: Same.

Indications: This ___-year-old *male/female* had *tumor* isolated to *the body/tail* of the pancreas. Laparoscopic distal pancreatectomy with *splenectomy/splenic preservation* was elected.

Description of procedure: An epidural catheter was placed by anesthesia prior to the start of the operation. The patient was placed in the *supine/right semilateral decubitus position* and general endotracheal anesthesia was induced. Preoperative antibiotics were given. A Foley catheter and a nasogastric tube were placed. A time-out was completed verifying correct patient, procedure, site, positioning, and implant(s) and/or special equipment prior to beginning this procedure. The abdomen was prepped and draped in the usual sterile fashion. A *12–15 mm Hasson port/Veress needle* was placed above the umbilicus and carbon dioxide pneumoperitoneum was induced up to a pressure of 15 mmHg. The laparoscope was introduced and a general peritoneal exploration was done for disease outside resection field and *none was noted/(detail location and biopsy if performed, procedure generally terminated at this point)*. Three 5 mm ports were introduced along the right subcostal margin, right abdomen, and along the left anterior axillary line, 3–4 cm below the costal margin. A 15 mm epigastric port was introduced.

The lesser sac was entered via the gastrocolic omentum. The splenic flexure was mobilized and the gastrocolic omentum was divided along the greater curvature of the stomach. Stomach is retracted away using a fan blade retractor introduced through the epigastric port. *Laparoscopic ultrasound was used to identify the tumor and the blood vessels to determine the line of transection and preservation of blood vessels.*

Choose one: If splenectomy: *The spleen was mobilized by incising the splenocolic ligament. The splenic flexure was mobilized. Gentle traction on the spleen was applied medially to divide the lienorenal and splenocolic ligaments to free the left colon inferiorly. The short gastric arteries were ligated and the stomach was retracted superiorly and medially. The spleen and pancreas were mobilized from their retroperitoneal attachments and the inferior mesenteric vein was divided and ligated. The spleen and pancreas were dissected free medially to the junction of the splenic vein and the SMV. The splenic artery and splenic vein were transected with vascular Endo-GIA staplers at the level of the pancreatic transection. The pancreas was transected with an Endo-GIA stapler (4.8 mm).*

If splenic preservation: *The inferior margin of pancreas was mobilized by developing a plane between the root of the transverse colon and the anterior fascia of the pancreas. Splenic vessels were identified and isolated at the level of transection, approximately 1 cm proximal to the tumor. The Endo-GIA stapler (4.8 mm) was used to transect the pancreas. The splenic vessels were transected separately with a vascular load of the Endo-GIA stapler. The pancreas specimen was dissected from the retroperitoneum in a medial to lateral direction. The splenic vessels were transected again as far from the splenic hilum as possible using a vascular load of the Endo-GIA stapler, taking care to preserve short gastric vessels and potential collaterals (Warshaw technique).*

Pancreatic staple line was oversewn and hemostasis was secured with endoscopic clip application as needed. The specimen was retrieved in an endocatch bag. The pancreatic staple line was reinforced with fibrin glue. A Blake drain was secured and port sites were closed in a standard fashion.

The patient tolerated the procedure well and was taken to the postanesthesia care unit in stable condition.

NOTES

Chapter 88

Pancreatic Cystogastrostomy

Prashant Khullar, M.D.

INDICATIONS

- Persistent clinical symptoms for example, abdominal pain, nausea, vomiting, and biliary obstruction.
- Failure of interventional/endoscopic drainage.
- Cyst enlargement on serial imaging or size more than 6 cm.
- Increasing risk of complications, for example, bleeding, rupture, infection, and obstruction.

ESSENTIAL STEPS

1. *Upper midline/left subcostal/chevron incision* over the palpable mass.
2. Palpate and confirm the isolated pseudocyst adherent to the back wall of the stomach.
3. Place mechanical retractors, for example, Fowler's, Bookwalter's, or Omni-Tract.
4. *Roux-en-Y jejunal loop is an option if these conditions are not met.*
5. Place 2-0 silk stay sutures in the anterior wall of the stomach, distant from the pylorus.
6. Longitudinal/transverse gastrotomy, approximately 5–8 cm.
7. Place retractors to expose the back wall of the stomach.
8. Palpate the pseudocyst and aspirate through the back wall of the stomach (to confirm location and absence of blood and send for culture if turbid. Fluid is also sent for biochemistry and tumor markers).

J.J. Hoballah and C.E.H. Scott-Conner (eds.), *Operative Dictations in General and Vascular Surgery*, DOI 10.1007/978-1-4614-0451-4_88,
© Springer Science+Business Media, LLC 2012

9. Place stay sutures in the posterior gastric wall.
10. Enter the cyst with electrocautery or sharp hemostat.
11. Decompress with suction.
12. Enlarge hole in the posterior gastric wall to approximately 3 cm.
13. Send wedge of the cyst wall to frozen section pathology to exclude cystic neoplasm.
14. Debride the necrotic material and address any underlying ductal abnormalities.
15. Palpate retroperitoneum to assure no other masses.
16. Assure hemostasis at edges.
17. Place running lock-stitch of 2-0 PDS around cystogastrostomy in such a fashion as to incorporate full thickness of the gastric and cyst wall.
18. Position nasogastric tube in the stomach.
19. Close the anterior gastrotomy *two-layer sutured/stapled.*
20. Place omentum over the gastrotomy.
21. *Address any biliary abnormalities. A Roux-en-Y hepaticojejunostomy or a choledochoduodenostomy may be required to relieve biliary obstruction.*
22. Recheck hemostasis.
23. Close the abdomen without drainage.

NOTE THESE VARIATIONS

- Stapled vs. sutured closure of anterior gastrotomy.
- Cystojejunostomy (with Roux-en-Y limb) if not adherent to the stomach.
- Biliary abnormalities (gallstones, stricture of distal common duct from chronic pancreatitis) may need to be addressed as described above.

COMPLICATIONS

- Recurrence.
- Suture line (upper gastrointestinal) bleeding.
- Gastric leak.

TEMPLATE FOR OPERATIVE DICTATION

Preoperative diagnosis: Pancreatic pseudocyst.
Procedure: Cystogastrostomy.
Postoperative diagnosis: Same.
Indications: This ___-year-old *male/female* developed chronic pseudocyst ___ weeks after acute pancreatitis. The cyst *failed to*

resolve/was enlarging/was associated with abdominal pain and cystogastrostomy was elected.

Description of procedure: An epidural catheter was placed by anesthesia prior to the start of the operation. The patient was placed in the supine position and general endotracheal anesthesia was induced. A time-out was completed verifying correct patient, procedure, site, positioning, and implant(s) and/or special equipment prior to beginning this procedure. Preoperative antibiotics were given. A Foley catheter and a nasogastric tube were placed. The abdomen was prepped and draped in the usual sterile fashion. *A vertical midline incision was made from xiphoid to just below the umbilicus/a left subcostal/a chevron incision two finger breadths below the costal margin was made.* This was deepened through the subcutaneous tissues and hemostasis was achieved with electrocautery. The fascia was incised and the peritoneal cavity entered. The abdomen was explored. Mechanical retractors were placed. *Adhesions were lysed sharply under direct vision with Metzenbaum scissors.* The retrogastric pseudocyst, adherent to the back wall of the stomach, was noted. *No other abnormalities were noted/(detail abnormalities).* The decision was made to proceed with cystogastrostomy.

The stomach was visualized and two interrupted 2-0 silk stay sutures were placed in the anterior wall, away from the pylorus. Electrocautery was then used to incise the gastric wall and the stomach was entered. Retractors were placed to expose the back wall of the stomach overlying the pseudocyst. An 18-gauge needle was then passed through the posterior gastric wall into the pseudocyst. Fluid was aspirated and found to be nonbloody. A fluid sample was sent to microbiology for stat gram stain, culture, biochemistry, and tumor markers.

Two interrupted 2-0 silk stay sutures were then placed in the posterior gastric wall. The pseudocyst was entered with *electrocautery/a sharp hemostat.* The cyst was decompressed using suction. The incision was extended to approximately 3–5 cm and a section of the edge submitted for frozen section pathology. The cyst was debrided of all necrotic tissue. Hemostasis was assured at the edges. The cystogastrostomy anastomosis was then oversewn with a running lock-stitch of 2-0 PDS placed through the full thickness of the posterior gastric wall and the pseudocyst.

The retroperitoneum was palpated and no other masses were identified. Hemostasis was again assured and a nasogastric tube was passed into the stomach. The anterior wall gastrostomy was then closed.

[Choose one:]

If sutured: The inner layer was sutured with a running 3-0 PDS Connell suture and the outer layer with interrupted 3-0 silk Lembert sutures.

If stapled: The gastrotomy was closed with the linear stapler. Omentum was then placed over the gastric closure.

The patient had *no underlying/the following underlying* biliary abnormalities requiring further intervention (*detail cholecystectomy, ductal drainage procedures, or any other biliary procedure done*).

(Optional: Multiple interrupted through-and-through retention sutures of ___ were placed.) The fascia was closed with *a running suture of ___/a Smead-Jones closure of interrupted ___*. The skin was closed with *skin staples/subcuticular sutures of ___/other.*

The patient tolerated the procedure well and was taken to the postanesthesia care unit in stable condition.

ACKNOWLEDGMENT

This chapter was contributed by Natisha Busick, MD in the first edition.

NOTES

Chapter 89

Pancreaticojejunostomy (Puestow Procedure)

Kevin A. Bridge, M.D., M.S.P.H

INDICATION

- Symptomatic chronic pancreatitis with pancreatic ductal obstruction and/or dilated pancreatic duct (^{3}5 mm).

ESSENTIAL STEPS

1. Upper midline or left subcostal/chevron incision.
2. Widely open the gastrocolic omentum to expose the pancreas.
3. Separate peritoneal attachments between the posterior walls of the stomach and pancreas.
4. Identify the pancreatic duct *(aspirate with 22-gauge needle if difficulty locating)*.
5. *Perform ductogram using Hypaque (if no preoperative study)*.
6. *Perform cholangiogram if the common bile duct obstructed.*
7. Open the pancreatic duct from head to tail.
8. Identify the ligament of Treitz and create 3-cm opening in the mesocolon adjacent to the ligament.
9. Transect the jejunum in mobile portion 12–15 cm distal to the ligament of Treitz.
10. Pass the stapled distal limb up through the defect in the transverse mesocolon.
11. Approximate the antimesenteric border of the jejunum to the pancreas with stapled end toward the tail, and then make a longitudinal enterotomy.

J.J. Hoballah and C.E.H. Scott-Conner (eds.), *Operative Dictations in General and Vascular Surgery*, DOI 10.1007/978-1-4614-0451-4_89,
© Springer Science+Business Media, LLC 2012

12. Suture the pancreatic duct to the jejunum with a *single layer of 4-0 Vicryl interrupted sutures/double layer of running 3-0 Vicryl and interrupted 3-0 silk Lembert sutures.*
13. Close the mesocolon defect with continuous running Vicryl suture.
14. Construct the end-to-side jejunojejunostomy 60 cm distal to the pancreaticojejunostomy.
15. Place one or two closed suction drain(s) in close proximity to the pancreaticojejunostomy.
16. Check hemostasis.
17. Place omentum in the operative site.
18. Close the abdomen.

NOTE THESE VARIATIONS
May be combined with distal pancreatectomy with or without splenectomy.

COMPLICATIONS
- Pancreatic fistula.
- Leak from jejunojejunostomy.
- Abdominal abscess.
- Recurrent symptoms.

TEMPLATE OPERATIVE DICTATION
Preoperative diagnosis: Symptomatic chronic pancreatitis.
Procedure: Pancreaticojejunostomy.
Postoperative diagnosis: Same.
Indications: This ___-year-old *male/female* with symptomatic chronic pancreatitis. Workup with *endoscopic retrograde cholangiopancreatography/computed tomography/magnetic resonance imaging* demonstrated a pancreatic duct obstruction and/or a dilated pancreatic duct. Longitudinal pancreaticojejunostomy was indicated.
Description of procedure: *An epidural catheter was placed by anesthesia prior to the start of the operation.* The patient was placed in the supine position and general endotracheal anesthesia was induced. A time-out was completed verifying correct patient, procedure, site, positioning, and implant(s) and/or special equipment prior to beginning this procedure.

Preoperative antibiotics were given. A Foley catheter and a nasogastric tube were placed. The abdomen was prepped and draped in the usual sterile fashion.

A vertical midline incision was made from xiphoid to just below the umbilicus/left subcostal/chevron incision was made two finger breadths below the left costal margin. This was deepened through the subcutaneous tissues and hemostasis was achieved with electrocautery. The fascia was identified and incised and the peritoneal cavity entered. The abdomen was explored and the pathology confirmed (*enumerate findings, specifically presence or absence of pseudocysts, biliary tract disease*).

The gastrocolic omentum was opened widely and the pancreas fully exposed by lysing adhesions to the posterior wall of the stomach. The pancreas was palpated and found to be consistent with chronic pancreatitis. The dilated pancreatic duct *was/was not* palpable along the upper one-third of the pancreas. The lesser sac was entered through the greater omentum with occasional ligation of the larger omental vessels. The *location of the pancreatic duct was determined by aspiration with a 22-gauge needle and the* duct was opened with a scalpel first and the duct was filleted open using *Pott's scissors/electrocautery over a probe.* It was widely opened for a length of ___ cm. *Stones were retrieved from the proximal duct. Biopsy of the pancreas was submitted for pathology/frozen section.*

Attention was turned toward the jejunum. The ligament of Treitz was identified and a proximal mobile loop of jejunum was identified approximately 15 cm distal to the ligament of Treitz. The bowel was divided with a linear cutting stapler. A window was then created in an avascular portion of the transverse mesocolon adjacent to the ligament of Treitz. The distal limb of jejunum passed easily through this window and was brought adjacent to the pancreas. The limb was arranged so that the blind stapled end was aligned with the tail and the antimesenteric border of the loop lay along the dilated duct toward the head.

A side-to-side anastomosis was then performed with *4-0 interrupted Vicryl sutures/two layers, an inner layer of running 3-0 Vicryl and an outer layer of 3-0 silk Lembert sutures.* Mucosa of duct was approximated to mucosa of jejunum and the capsule of the pancreas apposed to the serosa of the jejunum. At the conclusion, the anastomosis appeared intact and the loop lay comfortably without torsion or tension.

The jejunojejunostomy was then performed at a point 60 cm distal to the anastomosis.

[Choose one:]

If stapled: The two limbs of jejunum were approximated with 3-0 silk sutures. Enterotomies were then made and the stapler was introduced and fired. This anastomosis was performed in side-to-side fashion using the GIA 55 and TA 55 staplers. The staple line was checked for hemostasis and the enterotomy closed with a linear stapler/two layers of sutures. The anastomosis was checked for integrity and noted to be widely patent in all three directions.

***If sutured:** A hand-sewn two-layer anastomosis was then made between the end of one limb of jejunum and the side of the jejunum using running 3-0 Vicryl and interrupted 3-0 silk.*

The patient had *no underlying/the following underlying* biliary abnormalities requiring further intervention *(detail cholecystectomy, ductal drainage procedures, or any other biliary procedure done).*

Closed suction drain(s) *was/were* placed in vicinity to the pancreaticojejunostomy and brought out through a separate stab wound. Hemostasis was checked and the abdomen was irrigated. Omentum was brought up and made to lie in the operative field.

The fascia was closed with *a running suture of ___/a Smead-Jones closure of interrupted ___.* The skin was closed with *skin staples/subcuticular sutures of ___/other.*

The patient tolerated the procedure well and was taken to the postanesthesia care unit in stable condition.

ACKNOWLEDGMENT

This chapter was contributed by Andrew A. Fedder, MD in the first edition.

NOTES

Section VIII

Spleen

Chapter 90

Splenectomy (Open) for Disease

Charles H. Mosher, M.D.

INDICATIONS

- Idiopathic immune thrombocytopenic purpura.
- Hereditary spherocytosis/elliptocytosis.
- Autoimmune hemolytic anemia.
- Primary splenic lymphoma.
- Myelofibrosis.
- (Other)

ESSENTIAL STEPS

1. Midline or left subcostal incision.
2. Pack/retract the colon downward.
3. Retract the stomach medially.
4. Incise the gastrosplenic ligament.
5. Palpate and expose the splenic artery.
6. Ligate the splenic artery.
7. Completely clamp and cut the gastrosplenic ligament.
8. Mobilize the spleen medially.
9. Incise the splenorenal ligament.
10. Ligate and cut the splenic artery and vein.
11. Remove the spleen.
12. Obtain hemostasis.
13. Search for accessory spleens; remove any that are found.
14. Close the abdomen.

J.J. Hoballah and C.E.H. Scott-Conner (eds.), *Operative Dictations in General and Vascular Surgery*, DOI 10.1007/978-1-4614-0451-4_90,
© Springer Science+Business Media, LLC 2012

NOTE THESE VARIATIONS

- Left subcostal incision vs. upper midline incision.
- Optional preliminary ligation of the splenic artery in the lesser sac.

COMPLICATIONS

- Portal vein thrombosis.
- Bleeding.
- Overwhelming postsplenectomy sepsis.
- Subphrenic abscess.
- Splenosis.
- Pancreatic injury.
- Gastric injury.
- Colon injury.
- Missed accessory spleen with recurrence of hematologic disorder.

TEMPLATE OPERATIVE DICTATION

Preoperative diagnosis: *Hematologic condition (list).*
Procedure: Splenectomy.
Postoperative diagnosis: Same.
Indications: This ___-year-old *male/female* was found to have *idiopathic thrombocytopenic purpura/hereditary spherocytosis/ autoimmune hemolytic anemia/other* ___ refractory to medical management. Splenectomy was indicated for the management of *thrombocytopenia/anemia/neutropenia/pancytopenia/other.*

Description of procedure: An epidural catheter was placed by anesthesia prior to the start of the operation. The patient was placed in the supine position and general endotracheal anesthesia was induced. A time-out was completed verifying correct patient, procedure, site, positioning, and implant(s) and/or special equipment prior to beginning this procedure. Preoperative antibiotics were given. A Foley catheter and a nasogastric tube were placed. The abdomen was prepped and draped in the usual sterile fashion.

A vertical midline incision was made from xiphoid to just below the umbilicus. This was deepened through the subcutaneous tissues and hemostasis was achieved with electrocautery. The linea alba was identified and incised and the peritoneal cavity entered/a left subcostal incision was made from the midline to the anterior axillary line, approximately two finger breadths below and parallel to the costal margin. It was deepened through the muscular and aponeurotic layers of the abdominal wall with electrocautery. Hemostasis was achieved with electrocautery and the peritoneal cavity entered.

The abdomen was explored. The spleen was found to be *normal in size/enlarged. (List any other abnormalities found.) Adhesions were lysed sharply under direct vision with Metzenbaum scissors.* The colon was packed inferiorly. Packs were placed superiorly to bring the spleen toward midline. The gastrocolic omentum was incised in an avascular area so as to open the lesser sac and expose the splenic artery. The splenic artery was palpated and carefully exposed and ligated close to the spleen. The gastrosplenic and splenocolic ligaments were then serially clamped, cut, and tied with 2-0 silk. The spleen was carefully mobilized medially to expose the splenorenal ligament, which was carefully incised with electrocautery. The spleen was elevated from the retroperitoneum, taking care not to injure the hilar vessels or pancreas.

The splenic artery and vein were next identified and then separately clamped and divided close to the spleen. The spleen was removed intact and the splenic artery and vein were then tied and suture ligated with 2-0 silk.

The left upper quadrant was inspected for hemostasis. Accessory splenic tissue was sought in the splenic hilum, tail of the pancreas, omentum, vicinity of the splenic artery, mesentery, and gonads. *An accessory spleen was identified in the ___. It was dissected free of surrounding tissues, the hilum was ligated with 2-0 silk, and the accessory spleen was removed intact.*

The *midline/subcostal* incision was then closed in the following manner. *(Optional: Multiple interrupted through-and-through retention sutures of ___ were placed.)* The fascia was closed *(in layers, if subcostal) with a running suture of ___/a Smead-Jones closure of interrupted ___.* The skin was closed with *skin staples/subcuticular sutures of ___/other.*

The patient tolerated the procedure well and was taken to the postanesthesia care unit in stable condition.

NOTES

Chapter 91
Laparoscopic Splenectomy

Carol E.H. Scott-Conner, M.D.

INDICATIONS
- Idiopathic immune thrombocytopenic purpura.
- Hereditary spherocytosis/elliptocytosis.
- Autoimmune hemolytic anemia.
- Myelofibrosis.
- (Other.)

ESSENTIAL STEPS
1. Lateral position, left side up.
2. Induce the pneumoperitoneum.
3. Place first trocar, insert 30 or 45° laparoscope, and inspect the abdomen.
4. Place additional trocars.
5. Detach the splenic flexure and mobilize the colon inferiorly and medially.
6. Divide the anterior peritoneal folds and short gastric vessels.
7. Mobilize the stomach medially.
8. Identify and divide the splenic artery and splenic vein.
9. Protect the pancreas.
10. Incise the lateral peritoneal attachments of the spleen.
11. Place the spleen in a bag.
12. Morcellate and remove.
13. Check hemostasis.
14. Inspect for accessory spleens.

J.J. Hoballah and C.E.H. Scott-Conner (eds.), *Operative Dictations in General and Vascular Surgery*, DOI 10.1007/978-1-4614-0451-4_91,
© Springer Science+Business Media, LLC 2012

15. Desufflate the abdomen.
16. Close trocar sites.

NOTE THESE VARIATIONS
- May be performed with patient supine.
- Splenic vessels may be ligated or secured with vascular stapler.

COMPLICATIONS
- Bleeding.
- Missed accessory spleens.
- Spillage of splenic tissue; splenosis.

TEMPLATE OPERATIVE DICTATION
Preoperative diagnosis: *Hematologic condition (list).*
Procedure: Laparoscopic splenectomy.
Postoperative diagnosis: Same.
Indications: This ___-year-old *male/female* was found to have *idiopathic thrombocytopenic purpura/hereditary spherocytosis/ autoimmune hemolytic anemia/other* ___ refractory to medical management. Splenectomy was indicated for the management of *thrombocytopenia/anemia/neutropenia/pancytopenia/other* and the laparoscopic approach was elected.
Description of procedure: The patient was brought to the operating room and general anesthesia was induced. An orogastric tube and Foley catheter were placed. The patient was positioned in the full lateral position with the left side up. A time-out was completed verifying correct patient, procedure, site, positioning, and implant(s) and/or special equipment prior to beginning this procedure. All pressure points were carefully padded.

An incision was made in a natural skin line at the left costal margin.

[Choose one:]
*If **Veress needle:** The fascia was elevated and the Veress needle inserted. Proper position was confirmed by aspiration and saline meniscus test.*

*If **Hassan cannula:** The fascia was elevated and incised. Entry into the peritoneum was confirmed visually and no bowel was noted in the vicinity of the incision. Two figure-of-eight sutures of 2-0 Vicryl were placed and the Hassan cannula inserted under direct vision. The sutures were anchored around the cannula.*

The abdomen was insufflated with carbon dioxide to a pressure of 12–15 mmHg. The patient tolerated insufflation well. *A 10/11-mm trocar was then inserted.*

The laparoscope was inserted and the abdomen inspected. No injuries from initial trocar placement were noted. Additional trocars were then inserted *along the left costal margin and in the left supraumbilical region/other.*

The splenic flexure of the colon was gently displaced inferiorly and the splenocolic ligament was incised with the ultrasonic shears. The colon was mobilized medially and inferiorly. Next, the peritoneal folds overlying the short gastric vessels and then the short gastric vessels were divided in a similar fashion. The stomach was mobilized medially to expose the hilum of the spleen and tail of the pancreas.

Peritoneum overlying the splenic artery and splenic vein was incised. The splenic artery and splenic vein were *divided with the endoscopic vascular stapler/doubly ligated and divided.* The tail of the pancreas was identified and protected.

The lateral peritoneal attachments and splenophrenic ligament were then divided. The spleen was completely mobilized and placed within a retrieval bag. The bag was drawn into an enlarged trocar site and the contained spleen morcellated and removed piecemeal. The bag was withdrawn and the trocar reinserted. Temporary closure of the trocar site was obtained with a towel clip.

The surgical field was inspected for hemostasis. Accessory spleens were sought and *none were found/one was identified in the following location ___. It was removed by sharp and blunt dissection.*

Hemostasis was again checked and the field irrigated. The abdomen was desufflated and secondary trocars were removed under direct vision. *No bleeding was noted/trocar site bleeding was controlled by electrocautery/suture placement.* The laparoscope was withdrawn and the viewing trocar removed. The abdomen was allowed to collapse. All trocar sites >5 mm were closed with ___. The skin was closed with subcuticular sutures of ___ and steristrips.

The patient tolerated the procedure well and was taken to the postanesthesia care unit in stable condition.

NOTES

Chapter 92

Splenectomy for Trauma

Charles H. Mosher, M.D.

INDICATION

- Splenic injury with significant damage to the hilum or unstable patient or multiple other injuries or failed splenic salvage.

ESSENTIAL STEPS

1. Long midline incision.
2. Pack the left upper quadrant for temporary hemostasis.
3. Evacuate blood and clots *(autotransfusion apparatus optional)*.
4. Thorough exploration for other injuries.
5. Pack/retract the colon downward.
6. Retract the stomach medially.
7. Compress the spleen manually and rotate medially.
8. Incise the lateral splenic attachments with electrocautery.
9. Mobilize the spleen from the retroperitoneum, taking care not to injure the pancreas.
10. Divide the short gastric vessels.
11. Clamp and divide the splenorenal and splenocolic ligaments.
12. Ligate and divide the splenic artery and vein.
13. Remove the spleen.
14. Obtain hemostasis.
15. Pack the left upper quadrant and reassess for other injuries.

J.J. Hoballah and C.E.H. Scott-Conner (eds.), *Operative Dictations in General and Vascular Surgery*, DOI 10.1007/978-1-4614-0451-4_92,
© Springer Science+Business Media, LLC 2012

16. Recheck hemostasis.
17. Close the abdomen.

NOTE THESE VARIATIONS
- Other injuries will require additional brief paragraphs that must be individualized.
- Autotransfusion apparatus.

COMPLICATIONS
- Bleeding.
- Overwhelming postsplenectomy sepsis.
- Subphrenic abscess.
- Splenosis.
- Pancreatic injury.
- Gastric injury.
- Colon injury.
- Missed injuries.
- Portal vein thrombosis.

TEMPLATE OPERATIVE DICTATION
Preoperative diagnosis: *Blunt/penetrating abdominal trauma with hemodynamic instability*.

Procedure: Splenectomy *(list any additional procedures)*.

Postoperative diagnosis: Splenic injury not amenable to splenic preservation due to *severity of injury/hemodynamic instability/other injuries (list any additional intra-abdominal injuries)*.

Indications: This ___-year-old *male/female* was found to have *blunt trauma to the abdomen, positive computed tomography scan/FAST (Focused Abdominal Sonography for Trauma), and hemodynamic instability/stab wound/gunshot wound to the abdomen*.

Description of procedure: The patient was placed in the supine position and general endotracheal anesthesia was induced. A time-out was completed verifying correct patient, procedure, site, positioning, and implant(s) and/or special equipment prior to beginning this procedure. Preoperative antibiotics were given. A Foley catheter and a nasogastric tube were placed. The abdomen was prepped and draped in the usual sterile fashion.

A vertical midline incision was made from xiphoid to pubis. This was deepened through the subcutaneous tissues and hemostasis was achieved with electrocautery. The linea alba was identified and incised and the peritoneal cavity entered.

The abdomen was explored. A large amount of blood and clot was suctioned and removed from the abdomen. The spleen was found to be ruptured. The left upper quadrant was packed to obtain temporary hemostasis and the remainder of the abdomen was explored. *No other injuries/the following additional injuries (list)* were found. *Adhesions were lysed sharply under direct vision with Metzenbaum scissors.*

Attention was returned to the left upper quadrant. The colon was packed inferiorly. The spleen was grasped and compressed with a pack so as to mobilize it medially and achieve temporary hemostasis. It was rapidly mobilized into the midline by incising the lateral peritoneal attachments with electrocautery. The short gastric vessels were clamped and divided with 2-0 silk ties. Packs were placed behind the spleen and the spleen was inspected. The decision was made to proceed with splenectomy rather than attempt splenorrhaphy *(for failed splenorrhaphy, commence dictation here)*. The gastrosplenic and splenocolic ligaments were then serially clamped, cut, and tied with 2-0 silk.

The splenic artery and vein were next identified and then separately clamped and divided close to the spleen. The spleen was removed and the splenic artery and vein were then tied and suture ligated with 2-0 silk.

The left upper quadrant was inspected for hemostasis. Packs were placed and the remainder of the abdomen inspected *(detail additional injuries found and managed)*.

The incision was then closed in the following manner. *(Optional: Multiple interrupted through-and-through retention sutures of ____ were placed.)* The fascia was closed with *a running suture of ____/a Smead-Jones closure of interrupted ____*. The skin was closed with *skin staples/subcuticular sutures of ___/other*.

The patient tolerated the procedure well and was taken to the postanesthesia care unit in stable but critical condition.

NOTES

Chapter 93

Partial Splenectomy

Charles H. Mosher, M.D.

INDICATIONS
- Splenic cysts.
- Injury to the upper or lower pole of the spleen (iatrogenic or traumatic).

ESSENTIAL STEPS
1. Upper midline or left subcostal incision.
2. Explore the abdomen.
3. Pack/retract the colon downward.
4. Retract the stomach medially.
5. Incise the gastrosplenic ligament.
6. Palpate and expose the splenic artery.
7. Place a Bulldog clamp on the splenic artery.
8. Incise the retroperitoneum and mobilize the spleen medially.
9. Identify the area involved.
10. Incise the gastrosplenic ligament to improve mobility and access to the segmental vasculature.
11. Identify major vessels to the upper or lower pole at the hilum.
12. Ligate blood supply to the area of planned resection *(if upper pole, also ligate short gastrics)*.
13. Remove Bulldog clamp.
14. Observe for line of demarcation.

J.J. Hoballah and C.E.H. Scott-Conner (eds.), *Operative Dictations in General and Vascular Surgery*, DOI 10.1007/978-1-4614-0451-4_93,
© Springer Science+Business Media, LLC 2012

15. Remove the demarcated area with cautery or stapling device.
16. Close the raw surface.

NOTE THESE VARIATIONS

- Closure of the splenic remnant (type of suture, use of stapler, and pledgets).
- Upper or lower pole resected.

COMPLICATIONS

- Infarction of the remnant.
- Bleeding.
- Injury to the stomach, colon, or tail of the pancreas.
- Subphrenic abscess.
- Splenosis.

TEMPLATE OPERATIVE DICTATION

Preoperative diagnosis: *Traumatic rupture of the spleen/splenic cyst/iatrogenic injury* limited to the *upper/lower* pole of the spleen.
Procedure: Partial splenectomy with preservation of the *lower/upper* pole with intact blood supply.
Postoperative diagnosis: Same.
Indications: This ___-year-old *male/female* was found to have *traumatic rupture of the spleen/iatrogenic injury/splenic cyst*.
Description of procedure: *An epidural catheter was placed by anesthesia prior to the start of the operation.* The patient was placed in the supine position and general endotracheal anesthesia was induced. A time-out was completed verifying correct patient, procedure, site, positioning, and implant(s) and/or special equipment prior to beginning this procedure. Preoperative antibiotics were given. A Foley catheter and a nasogastric tube were placed. The abdomen was prepped and draped in the usual sterile fashion.

A vertical midline incision was made from xiphoid to just below the umbilicus. This was deepened through the subcutaneous tissues and hemostasis was achieved with electrocautery. The linea alba was identified and incised and the peritoneal cavity entered/a left subcostal incision was made from the midline to the anterior axillary line, approximately two finger breadths below and parallel to the costal margin. It was deepened through the muscular and aponeurotic layers of the abdominal wall with electrocautery. Hemostasis was achieved with electrocautery and the peritoneal cavity entered.

The abdomen was explored. The spleen was found to be *normal in size/enlarged. (List any other abnormalities found.) Injury/pathology* was found to be limited to the *upper/lower* pole and therefore amenable to partial splenectomy. *Adhesions were lysed sharply under direct vision with Metzenbaum scissors.* The colon was packed inferiorly. The lateral peritoneal attachments were divided with electrocautery and the spleen mobilized into the midline. Care was taken to avoid injury to the pancreas or splenic hilum. Packs were placed behind the spleen.

The gastrosplenic ligament was identified and incised in an avascular area so as to open the lesser sac and expose the splenic hilum. The remaining gastrosplenic ligament was then clamped, divided, and ligated with 2-0 silk. A Bulldog clamp was placed on the splenic artery to provide temporary vascular control. The vessels supplying the *area/pole* were ligated. The Bulldog clamp was removed. A line of demarcation was observed to form and the spleen was divided along this line with *electrocautery/a linear stapling device with a ____ cartridge. The cut edge of the splenic remnant was closed with 2-0 running chromic/2-0 chromic inter-locking horizontal mattresses with pledgets of ____/omental buttress.* The remnant was inspected and found to be viable, with an intact blood supply from the splenic artery. Hemostasis was achieved. The splenic remnant was replaced in the left upper quadrant.

(Optional: Multiple interrupted through-and-through retention sutures of ____ were placed.) The fascia was closed with *a running suture of ____/a Smead-Jones closure of interrupted ____.* The skin was closed with *skin staples/subcuticular sutures of ___/other.*

The patient tolerated the procedure well and was taken to the postanesthesia care unit in stable condition.

NOTES

Chapter 94

Splenorrhaphy

Charles H. Mosher, M.D.

INDICATION

- Splenic injury with desire for splenic preservation.

ESSENTIAL STEPS

1. Upper midline incision.
2. Explore the abdomen.
3. Pack/retract the colon downward.
4. Retract the stomach medially.
5. Incise the gastrosplenic ligament.
6. Incise the peritoneum lateral to the spleen.
7. Mobilize the spleen atraumatically.
8. Divide the short gastric vessels.
9. Palpate and expose the splenic artery.
10. Place a Bulldog clamp on the splenic artery.
11. Identify the injured area.
12. *Apply hemostatic agents/omental fixation/placement of absorbable mesh wrap/suture placement with pledgets.*
13. Remove Bulldog clamp.
14. Observe for hemostasis.
15. If hemostasis is inadequate or the patient becomes critically unstable, proceed to splenectomy.

NOTE THESE VARIATIONS

- Hemostatic agent (type and result).
- Suture (type).

J.J. Hoballah and C.E.H. Scott-Conner (eds.), *Operative Dictations in General and Vascular Surgery*, DOI 10.1007/978-1-4614-0451-4_94,
© Springer Science+Business Media, LLC 2012

- Pledgets (use and type).
- Mesh (use and type).
- Failure requires partial or complete splenectomy (see Chaps. 92 and 93).

COMPLICATIONS

- Bleeding.
- Infarction of partial or entire spleen.
- Injury to the stomach, colon, or pancreas.
- Splenosis.

TEMPLATE OPERATIVE DICTATION

Preoperative diagnosis: *Traumatic rupture/laceration of the spleen/ iatrogenic injury.*

Procedure: Splenorrhaphy.

Postoperative diagnosis: Same.

Indications: This ___-year-old *male/female* was found to have *traumatic rupture/laceration of the spleen/iatrogenic injury and a desire for splenic preservation.*

Description of procedure: *An epidural catheter was placed by anesthesia prior to the start of the operation.* The patient was placed in the supine position and general endotracheal anesthesia was induced. A time-out was completed verifying correct patient, procedure, site, positioning, and implant(s) and/or special equipment prior to beginning this procedure. Preoperative antibiotics were given. A Foley catheter and a nasogastric tube were placed. The abdomen was prepped and draped in the usual sterile fashion.

A vertical midline incision was made from xiphoid to just below the umbilicus. This was deepened through the subcutaneous tissues and hemostasis was achieved with electrocautery. The linea alba was identified and incised and the peritoneal cavity entered. Hemostasis was achieved with electrocautery and the peritoneal cavity entered.

The abdomen was explored. A large amount of blood and clot was suctioned and removed from the abdomen. The spleen was found to be ruptured. The left upper quadrant was packed to obtain temporary hemostasis and the remainder of the abdomen was explored. *No other injuries/the following additional injuries (list) were found. Adhesions were lysed sharply under direct vision with Metzenbaum scissors.*

Attention was returned to the left upper quadrant. The colon was packed inferiorly. The spleen was grasped and compressed with a pack so as to mobilize it medially and achieve temporary hemostasis. It was rapidly and atraumatically mobilized into the midline by incising the lateral peritoneal attachments with electrocautery. The short gastric vessels were clamped, divided, and ligated with 2-0 silk ties. Packs were placed behind the spleen and the spleen was inspected. Injury was found to consist of a *capsular avulsion of ____ pole/stellate laceration with intact hilar vessels/complex laceration/simple laceration*. The patient was hemodynamically stable and the decision was made to proceed with splenorrhaphy. The gastrosplenic and splenocolic ligaments were then serially clamped, cut, and tied with 2-0 silk.

The colon was packed inferiorly. *A Bulldog clamp was placed on the splenic artery/direct pressure was applied to the spleen with a laparotomy pad* to control bleeding. *Hemostatic agents (detail type) were applied with direct pressure to stop bleeding/a capsular tear was repaired with a running 4-0 chromic suture/the fracture was repaired with horizontal mattresses and gelfoam pledgets using 2-0 chromic/a portion of the omentum was placed in the splenic fracture and fixed with horizontal mattresses/absorbable mesh was placed over the spleen and with a purse string at the hilum to tamponade the spleen, with care taken not to compress the splenic vein*. The Bulldog clamp was removed.

The spleen was inspected for hemostasis and then placed into the left upper quadrant. The remainder of the abdomen was again checked for other injuries. Hemostasis in the left upper quadrant was again inspected and found to be adequate.

(Optional: Multiple interrupted through-and-through retention sutures of ____ were placed.) The fascia was closed with *a running suture of ____/a Smead-Jones closure of interrupted ____*. The skin was closed with *skin staples/subcuticular sutures of ___/other*.

The patient tolerated the procedure well and was taken to the postanesthesia care unit in stable condition.

NOTES

Hernia Repairs and Surgery for Necrotizing Fasciitis

Chapter 95
Bassini Repair of Inguinal Hernia

Jessemae L. Welsh, M.D.

INDICATION

- Inguinal hernia, in particular, if simple indirect hernia in young patient or female patient.

ESSENTIAL STEPS

1. Verify and mark side of surgery!
2. *Local anesthesia and ilioinguinal nerve block.*
3. Groin incision.
4. Expose the external oblique aponeurosis and external ring.
5. Incise the external oblique aponeurosis in direction of fibers.
6. Identify and protect the ilioinguinal nerve.
7. Mobilize flaps of the external oblique.
8. Gently encircle the spermatic cord *(or round ligament, if female)* at the external ring with Penrose drain.
9. Seek the indirect hernia sac on the anteromedial surface of the cord *or round ligament*.
10. Dissect free of surrounding structures and open.
11. Reduce contents.
12. Suture ligate and reduce the sac.
13. *Suture ligate and divide the round ligament with the sac in female.*
14. Assess the floor of the canal.
15. Identify the conjoint tendon and assess mobility to the shelving edge of the inguinal ligament.

J.J. Hoballah and C.E.H. Scott-Conner (eds.), *Operative Dictations in General and Vascular Surgery*, DOI 10.1007/978-1-4614-0451-4_95,
© Springer Science+Business Media, LLC 2012

16. *Relaxing incision if any tension.*
17. Suture the conjoint tendon to the shelving edge of the inguinal ligament with interrupted sutures.
18. *In male: Leave enough room to pass Kelly clamp through the internal ring next to the cord.*
19. *In female: Completely close the internal ring.*
20. *A single stitch lateral to the internal ring is sometimes needed in males.*
21. Check hemostasis.
22. Close aponeurosis of the external oblique with running 3-0 Vicryl.
23. Close Scarpa's fascia with interrupted 3-0 Vicryl.
24. Close the skin.
25. After applying dressing, pull the testis down into normal position in the scrotum.

NOTE THESE VARIATIONS
- Type of suture material varies.
- Completely close the canal in females.
- In males, a dilated internal ring may require an additional stitch lateral to the cord.
- Relaxing incision commonly employed.
- Type of anesthesia, including local anesthesia, varies.
- If done for incarceration, note findings, including viability of the bowel.
- Cord lipoma may be present.

COMPLICATIONS
- Hematoma, including scrotal hematoma.
- Recurrence.
- Neuropraxia.
- Femoral vein injury.
- Bowel injury.

TEMPLATE OPERATIVE DICTATION
Preoperative diagnosis: *Left/right* indirect inguinal hernia.
Procedure: Bassini repair of *left/right* inguinal hernia *with local anesthesia by surgeon.*
Postoperative diagnosis: Same.
Indications: This ___-year-old *male/female* developed a symptomatic *left/right reducible/incarcerated* inguinal hernia *with/without* symptoms of obstruction. Repair was indicated, and because of the *patient's age/sex/nature of the hernia* a Bassini repair was elected.

Description of procedure: The patient was taken to the operating room. A time-out was completed verifying correct patient, procedure, site, positioning, and implant(s) and/or special equipment prior to beginning this procedure.

[Choose one:]

If not local anesthesia: *General/epidural/spinal anesthesia was induced.* The *left/right* groin was prepped and draped in the usual sterile fashion. An incision was marked in a natural skin crease parallel to the inguinal ligament and planned to end near the pubic tubercle.

If local anesthesia: *A field block was produced by raising skin wheals along the proposed skin incision, along a vertical line lateral to it, and along a horizontal line superior to it. A skin wheal was raised 1 cm lateral and superior to the anterior superior iliac spine and a fascial injection of lidocaine was made to block the ilioinguinal nerve. Additional local anesthesia was injected during the procedure under the external oblique aponeurosis, at the internal ring, and as needed. A total of ___ mL of 0.5/1% lidocaine was used.*

The skin crease incision was made with a knife and deepened through Camper's and Scarpa's fascia with electrocautery until the aponeurosis of the external oblique was encountered. This was cleaned and the external ring was exposed. Hemostasis was achieved in the wound. An incision was made in the midportion of the external oblique aponeurosis in the direction of its fibers. The ilioinguinal nerve was identified and protected throughout the dissection. Flaps of external oblique were developed cephalad and inferiorly.

The cord was identified. It was gently dissected free at the pubic tubercle and encircled with a Penrose drain. Attention was directed to the anteromedial aspect of the cord, where an indirect hernia sac was identified.

If male: *The sac was carefully dissected free of the cord down to the level of the internal ring. The vas deferens and testicular vessels were identified and protected from harm.*

If female: *The round ligament was doubly ligated and divided at a convenient point near the sac.*

The sac was opened and contents were inspected for viability and then reduced. A finger was passed into the peritoneal cavity and the floor of the inguinal canal assessed and found to be strong. The femoral canal was palpated and no hernia identified.

If male: *The sac was twisted and suture ligated with 2-0 silk.*

If female: *The round ligament and sac were twisted and suture ligated with 2-0 silk.*

Redundant sac was excised and submitted to pathology. The stump of the sac was checked for hemostasis and allowed to retract into the abdomen.

Attention was then turned to the floor of the canal, which appeared to be intact with the exception of a dilated internal ring. Conjoint tendon was identified and grasped with Allis clamps. It *reached/did not reach* easily to the shelving edge of the ligament without tension.

If tension: Accordingly, the decision was made to do a relaxing incision. The anterior rectus sheath was incised with electrocautery medial and well superior to the conjoint tendon. Hemostasis was checked. The conjoint tendon then reached easily to the inguinal ligament with no tension whatsoever.

The conjoint tendon was then sutured to the shelving edge of the inguinal ligament with multiple simple sutures of ___. This suture line began at the pubic tubercle and commenced laterally to the internal ring. Care was taken not to take deep bites and endanger the femoral vessels.

If male: At the conclusion of this, the internal inguinal ring accommodated the tip of a Kelly hemostat. (Optional: A single suture was placed lateral to the cord to additionally tighten it.)

If female: The internal ring was completely obliterated at the conclusion of this procedure.

Hemostasis was again checked. The Penrose drain was removed. The external oblique aponeurosis was closed with a running suture of 3-0 Vicryl, taking care not to catch the ilioinguinal nerve in the suture line. Scarpa's fascia was closed with interrupted 3-0 Vicryl. The skin was closed with a subcuticular *stitch of ___/skin clips/other*. A sterile dressing was applied.

If male: The testis was gently pulled down into its anatomic position in the scrotum.

The patient tolerated the procedure well and was taken to the postanesthesia care unit in stable condition.

ACKNOWLEDGMENT

This chapter was contributed by Mohamad Allam, MD in the first edition.

NOTES

Chapter 96
Shouldice Repair of Inguinal Hernia

Evgeny V. Arshava, M.D.

INDICATIONS
- Direct inguinal hernia.
- Indirect inguinal hernia in adults.
- Coexisting inguinal and femoral hernias.

ESSENTIAL STEPS
1. Verify side of surgery!
2. *Local anesthesia.*
3. Groin incision.
4. Expose the external oblique aponeurosis and external ring.
5. *Define the inguinal ligament and incise thigh fascia (if suspicious of femoral component).*
6. Incise the external oblique aponeurosis in direction of fibers.
7. Identify and protect the ilioinguinal *and iliohypogastric* nerves.
8. Mobilize flaps of the external oblique.
9. Incise and divide cremaster muscle to expose the spermatic cord *(or round ligament, if female).*
10. Seek the indirect hernia sac or any peritoneal protrusion on the anteromedial surface of the cord *or round ligament* and dissect free off surrounding structure.
11. Reduce indirect sac or peritoneal protrusion into preperitoneal space. *Suture ligate if neck is narrow.*

J.J. Hoballah and C.E.H. Scott-Conner (eds.), *Operative Dictations in General and Vascular Surgery*, DOI 10.1007/978-1-4614-0451-4_96,
© Springer Science+Business Media, LLC 2012

12. Assess inguinal floor for the presence of direct hernia.
13. Incise the transversalis fascia *and trim excess if needed*.
14. Assess for femoral hernia. *Reduce if present and perform complete groin repair.*
15. Identify the transversus aponeurotic arch and lateral border of rectus abdominis muscle.
16. Perform inguinal repair with four continuous lines *and tie free sutures to close femoral canal if complete groin repair was performed*.
17. Check hemostasis.
18. Close the external oblique aponeurosis.
19. Close Scarpa's fascia and skin.
20. After applying dressing, pull the testis down into normal position in the scrotum.

NOTE THESE VARIATIONS

- Type of anesthesia, including local anesthesia, varies.
- Complete groin repair required if femoral hernia present.

COMPLICATIONS

- Recurrence.
- Infection.
- Postherniorrhaphy groin pain syndromes.
- Retroperitoneal hematoma due to unrecognized injury to the epigastric vessels. Scrotal hematoma.
- Ischemic orchitis and testicular atrophy.

TEMPLATE OPERATIVE DICTATION

Preoperative diagnosis: *Left/right* inguinal hernia.
Procedure: Shouldice repair *(or complete groin repair)* of *left/right* inguinal hernia *with local anesthesia by surgeon*.
Postoperative diagnosis: Same.
Indications: Patient is a ___-year-old *male/female* with symptomatic *left/right* inguinal hernia for which repair is indicated.
Description of procedure: The patient was taken to the operating room. A time-out was completed verifying correct patient, procedure, site, positioning, and implant(s) and/or special equipment prior to beginning this procedure.

If not local anesthesia: General/epidural/spinal anesthesia was induced. The *left/right* groin was prepped and draped in the usual sterile fashion.

If local anesthesia: A skin wheal was raised 2 cm medial and superior to the anterior superior iliac spine and sequential subcutaneous injections of local anesthetic were performed to block the distribution of ilioinguinal and iliohypogastric nerves. Additional local anesthesia was administered during the procedure under the external oblique aponeurosis, cremaster muscle, transversalis fascia, and at the internal ring. A total of ___ mL of 0.25%, 0.5% lidocaine were used.

Patient was placed in slight Trendelenburg position to facilitate operation.

An incision was made two fingerbreadths above and parallel to inguinal crease/*1 cm above and parallel to inguinal ligament*, starting midway between anterior superior iliac spine and internal inguinal ring and extending medial to the pubic tubercle.

The incision was deepened through Camper's and Scarpa's fascia until the aponeurosis of the external oblique was encountered. This was cleaned and the external ring was exposed. Hemostasis was achieved in the wound. An incision was made in the midportion of the external oblique aponeurosis in the direction of its fibers. The ilioinguinal *and iliohypogastric* nerves were identified and protected throughout the dissection. Flaps of external oblique were developed cephalad and inferiorly.

Lower edge of inguinal ligament was defined. Thigh fascia medial to the femoral vein was identified and incised to rule out presence of femoral hernia and to relax inguinal ligament for subsequent repair. Femoral hernia was found/not found.

The cord was identified. The cremasteric muscle was split longitudinally and divided in two portions. The medial portion was excised and its stumps, ligated. The lateral portion, containing cremasteric vessels and genital branch of genitofemoral nerve, was ligated with 2-0 Vicryl and divided. Testicular vessels and vas were identified, encircled with Penrose drain, and protected throughout the operation.

Attention was directed to the anteromedial aspect of the cord, where a *small/medium/large indirect hernia sac/peritoneal protrusion* was identified. The sac *or peritoneal protrusion* was carefully dissected free of the cord down to the level of the internal ring. Sac was reduced into preperitoneal space.

The sac was opened and contents were reduced. Narrow neck was twisted and suture ligated with 2-0 silk and redundant sac excised and submitted to pathology. The stump of the sac was checked for hemostasis and allowed to retract into the abdomen.

Small/medium/large cord lipoma was identified. It was freed from the spermatic cord, excised and the stump ligated with 3-0 Vicryl.

If female: The round ligament was divided and ligated with 2-0 Vicryl and the level of internal ring and pubic tubercle.

Attention then turned to the floor of the canal, which appeared to be weakened without a well-defined direct hernia. *Small/medium/large direct hernia was identified.*

An incision of the transversalis fascia was made beginning at the internal inguinal ring and extending medially to the pubic tubercle along the border of inguinal arch. Inferolateral flap of transversalis fascia was developed *and its excess was trimmed*. The inferior epigastric vessels were identified and protected. Femoral space was examined and found to contain no hernia.

Small/medium/large femoral hernia was found and reduced. Complete hernia repair was performed. 2-0 Prolene suture was passed initially through the femoral defect from below the inguinal ligament. Then the bites were taken in such fashion to first incorporate the Cooper's ligament, then transversalis fascia and then the inguinal ligament in wide loops. Three sutures were placed in such fashion from pubic tubercle to the femoral vein to completely close the femoral canal. This was left untied extending inferiorly toward the thigh, but clamped together with hemostats. The ties were subsequently incorporated in the second, third, and fourth lines of inguinal repair and tied.

The inguinal floor was reconstructed with four continuous lines of 32 or 34 gauge stainless steel *or 0 Prolene*. First line was started at the pubic tubercle and brought the inferolateral flap of the transversalis fascia first beneath the lateral border of the rectus abdominal muscle medially and beneath the transversus aponeurotic arch laterally. The proximal stump of cremasteric was incorporated into the end of first line during formation of the new internal ring. The suture was reversed and the second line brought full-thickness layer of internal oblique, transversus abdominis muscles, and transversalis fascia to the shelving edge of the inguinal ligament. The tails of the first and second lines were tied at the pubic tubercle. The third line was started at the internal inguinal ring and incorporated the layer of internal oblique muscle and of inferolateral flap of external oblique aponeurosis. The suture was reversed at pubic tubercle and the forth line imbricated the same structures over the third line.

Interrupted Prolene sutures incorporated in the second, third, and fourth lines of inguinal repair were tied to complete groin repair.

No venous hypertension or congestion was appreciated in the cord after completion of the repair. Curved Kelly forceps was inserted through the internal ring to confirm adequate laxity and rule out preperitoneal bleeding.

The spermatic cord was replaced in the normal anatomic position under external oblique. Wound was irrigated and hemostasis assured. The external oblique was then closed over it with a running 3-0 Vicryl, taking care not to catch the ilioinguinal nerve in the suture line. The distal stump of cremaster muscles was included in the reconstruction of the external ring. Scarpa's fascia was closed with running *interrupted* 3-0 Vicryl. Skin was closed with running 4-0 Monocryl. Dressing was applied.

If male: *Testicle was gently pulled down into the scrotum to assure its appropriate position.*

The patient tolerated the procedure well and was taken to the postanesthesia care unit in stable condition.

ACKNOWLEDGMENT

With deep acknowledgment to Michael A.J. Alexander, M.B., B.S., Surgeon-in-Chief, Shouldice Hospital.

NOTES

Chapter 97
McVay Repair of Inguinal Hernia

Peter C. Fretz, M.D.

INDICATIONS
- Inguinal hernia.
- Femoral hernia.

ESSENTIAL STEPS
1. Verify side of surgery!
2. *Local anesthesia.*
3. Groin incision.
4. Expose the external oblique aponeurosis and external ring.
5. Incise the external oblique aponeurosis in the direction of the fibers.
6. Identify and protect the ilioinguinal nerve.
7. Mobilize flaps of the external oblique.
8. Gently encircle the spermatic cord *(or round ligament, if female)* at the external ring with Penrose drain.
9. Seek the indirect hernia sac on the anteromedial surface of the cord *or round ligament*.
10. Dissect free the surrounding structures and open.
11. Reduce contents.
12. Suture ligate and reduce the sac.
13. *Suture ligate and divide the round ligament with the sac in female.*
14. Assess the floor of the canal.

J.J. Hoballah and C.E.H. Scott-Conner (eds.), *Operative Dictations in General and Vascular Surgery*, DOI 10.1007/978-1-4614-0451-4_97,
© Springer Science+Business Media, LLC 2012

15. Expose Cooper's ligament by sharp and blunt dissection.
16. Identify the conjoint tendon and assess quality and mobility to Cooper's ligament.
17. Make relaxing incision in the anterior rectus sheath.
18. Suture the conjoint tendon to Cooper's ligament with interrupted sutures; begin at the pubic tubercle and progress laterally.
19. At the femoral canal, place transition stitch that incorporates the conjoint tendon, Cooper's ligament, and anterior femoral sheath.
20. Remaining sutures are placed to the anterior femoral sheath.
21. *In male: Leave enough room to pass Kelly clamp through the internal ring next to the cord.*
22. *In female: Completely close the internal ring.*
23. *A single stitch lateral to the internal ring is sometimes needed in males.*
24. Check hemostasis.
25. Close the aponeurosis of external oblique with running 3-0 Vicryl.
26. Close Scarpa's fascia with interrupted 3-0 Vicryl.
27. Close the skin.
28. After applying dressing, pull the testis down into normal position in the scrotum.

NOTE THESE VARIATIONS

- Type of suture material varies.
- Completely close the inguinal canal in females.
- In males, a dilated internal ring may require an additional stitch lateral to the cord.
- Type of anesthesia, including local anesthesia, varies.
- If done for acute incarceration, note findings, including viability of the bowel.

COMPLICATIONS

- Hematoma, including scrotal hematoma.
- Femoral vein injury.
- Recurrence.
- Neuropraxia.
- Hydrocele.
- Obstruction of the vas referens.
- Testicular artery injury, testicular atropay.

TEMPLATE OPERATIVE DICTATION

Preoperative diagnosis: *Left/right indirect/direct inguinal/femoral* hernia.

Procedure: McVay repair of *left/right inguinal/femoral* hernia *with local anesthesia by surgeon*.

Postoperative diagnosis: Same.

Indications: This ___-year-old *male/female* developed a symptomatic *left/right inguinal/femoral* hernia. Repair was indicated.

Description of procedure: The patient was taken to the operating room. A time-out was completed verifying correct patient, procedure, site, positioning, and implant(s) and/or special equipment prior to beginning this procedure.

[Choose one:]

If not local anesthesia: General/epidural/spinal anesthesia was induced. The *left/right* groin was prepped and draped in the usual sterile fashion. An incision was marked in a natural skin crease and planned to end near the pubic tubercle.

If local anesthesia: A field block was produced by raising skin wheals along the proposed skin incision, along a vertical line lateral to it, and along a horizontal line superior to it. A skin wheal was raised 1 cm lateral and superior to the anterior superior iliac spine and a fascial injection of lidocaine was made to block the ilioinguinal nerve. Additional local anesthesia was injected during the procedure under the external oblique aponeurosis, at the internal ring, and as needed. A total of ___mL of 0.5/1% lidocaine was used.

The skin crease incision was made with a knife and deepened through Scarpa's and Camper's fascia with electrocautery until the aponeurosis of the external oblique was encountered. This was cleaned and the external ring was exposed. Hemostasis was achieved in the wound. An incision was made in the midportion of the external oblique aponeurosis in the direction of its fibers. The ilioinguinal nerve was identified and protected throughout the dissection. Flaps of external oblique were developed cephalad and inferiorly.

The cord was identified. It was gently dissected free at the pubic tubercle and encircled with a Penrose drain. Attention was directed to the anteromedial aspect of the cord, where an indirect hernia sac was identified.

If male: The sac was carefully dissected free of the cord down to the level of the internal ring. The vas and testicular vessels were identified and protected from harm.

If female: The round ligament was doubly ligated and divided at a convenient point near the sac.

The sac was opened and contents were reduced. A finger was passed into the peritoneal cavity and the floor of the inguinal canal assessed and found to be strong. The femoral canal was palpated *and a hernia identified/no hernia identified.*

If male: *The sac was twisted and suture ligated with 2-0 silk.*

If female: *The round ligament and sac were twisted and suture ligated with 2-0 silk.*

Redundant sac was excised and submitted to pathology. The stump of the sac was checked for hemostasis and allowed to retract into the abdomen.

Attention then turned to the floor of the canal, which appeared to be *intact with the exception of dilated internal ring/weak.* The conjoint tendon was identified and grasped with Allis clamps, and a relaxing incision made in the following fashion. The anterior rectus sheath was incised with electrocautery medial and well superior to the conjoint tendon. Hemostasis was checked. The conjoint tendon then reached easily to Cooper's ligament with no tension whatsoever.

The conjoint tendon was then sutured to the shelving edge of the inguinal ligament with multiple simple sutures of ___. This suture line began at the pubic tubercle and commenced laterally to the femoral vessels. A transition stitch was placed incorporating both Cooper's ligament and the anterior femoral sheath. Remaining sutures were placed between the conjoint tendon and anterior femoral sheath. Care was taken not to take deep bites and endanger the femoral vessels.

If male: *At the conclusion of this, the internal inguinal ring accommodated the tip of a Kelly hemostat. (Optional: A single suture was placed lateral to the cord to additionally tighten it.).*

If female: *The internal ring was completely obliterated at the conclusion of this procedure.*

Hemostasis was again checked. The Penrose drain was removed. The external oblique aponeurosis was closed with a running suture of 3-0 Vicryl, taking care not to catch the ilioinguinal nerve in the suture line. Scarpa's fascia was closed with interrupted 3-0 Vicryl. The skin was closed with a *subcuticular stitch of ___/skin clips/other.* A dressing was applied.

If male: *The testis was gently pulled down into its anatomic position in the scrotum.*

The patient tolerated the procedure well and was taken to the postanesthesia care unit in stable condition.

NOTES

Chapter 98
Mesh Repair of Inguinal Hernia

Carol E.H. Scott-Conner, M.D.

INDICATION

- Inguinal hernia, in particular, if poor quality of fascia precludes autogenous repair, hernia is recurrent, repair with autogenous tissue would require excess tension, or patient or surgeon preference.

ESSENTIAL STEPS

1. Verify side of surgery!
2. Prophylactic antibiotics.
3. *Local anesthesia.*
4. Groin incision.
5. Expose the external oblique aponeurosis and external ring.
6. Incise the external oblique aponeurosis in the direction of fibers.
7. Identify and protect the ilioinguinal nerve.
8. Mobilize flaps of the external oblique.
9. Gently encircle the spermatic cord *(or round ligament, if female)* at the external ring with Penrose drain.
10. Seek the indirect hernia sac on the anteromedial surface of the cord *or round ligament*.
11. *Dissect free of surrounding structures and open.*
12. *Reduce contents.*
13. *Suture ligate and reduce the sac.*
14. Assess the floor of the canal.

J.J. Hoballah and C.E.H. Scott-Conner (eds.), *Operative Dictations in General and Vascular Surgery*, DOI 10.1007/978-1-4614-0451-4_98,
© Springer Science+Business Media, LLC 2012

15. Place mesh and suture, beginning at the pubic tubercle.
16. Avoid narrowing the internal ring too much or catching nerves in repair.
17. Check hemostasis.
18. Close the external oblique aponeurosis.
19. Close Scarpa's fascia.
20. Close the skin.
21. After applying dressing, pull the testis down into normal position in the scrotum.

NOTE THESE VARIATIONS
- Type of suture material and mesh varies.
- Type of anesthesia, including local anesthesia, varies.

COMPLICATIONS
- Hematoma, including scrotal hematoma.
- Recurrence.
- Neuropraxia.
- Injury to the cord structures.
- Mesh migration.
- Mesh infection.

TEMPLATE OPERATIVE DICTATION
Preoperative diagnosis: *Left/right* inguinal hernia.
Procedure: Bassini repair of *left/right* inguinal hernia *with local anesthesia by surgeon.*
Postoperative diagnosis: Same.
Indications: This ___-year-old *male/female* developed a symptomatic *left/right* inguinal hernia. Repair was indicated, and because of the *patient's age/nature of the hernia/preference* a prosthetic mesh repair was elected.
Description of procedure: The patient was taken to the operating room. A time-out was completed verifying correct patient, procedure, site, positioning, and implant(s) and/or special equipment prior to beginning this procedure.

[Choose one:]
If not local anesthesia: General/epidural/spinal anesthesia was induced. The *left/right* groin was prepped and draped in the usual sterile fashion. An incision was marked in a natural skin crease and planned to end near the pubic tubercle.
If local anesthesia: A field block was produced by raising skin wheals along the proposed skin incision, along a vertical line lateral

to it, and along a horizontal line superior to it. A skin wheal was raised 1 cm lateral and superior to the anterior superior iliac spine and a fascial injection of lidocaine was made to block the ilioinguinal nerve. Additional local anesthesia was injected during the procedure under the external oblique aponeurosis, at the internal ring, and as needed. A total of ___ mL of 0.5/1% lidocaine was used.

The skin crease incision was made with a knife and deepened through Scarpa's and Camper's fascia with electrocautery until the aponeurosis of the external oblique was encountered. This was cleaned and the external ring was exposed. Hemostasis was achieved in the wound. An incision was made in the midportion of the external oblique aponeurosis in the direction of its fibers. The ilioinguinal nerve was identified and protected throughout the dissection. Flaps of the external oblique were developed cephalad and inferiorly.

The cord was identified. It was gently dissected free at the pubic tubercle and encircled with a Penrose drain. Attention was directed to the anteromedial aspect of the cord, where an indirect hernia sac was identified. The sac was carefully dissected free of the cord down to the level of the internal ring. The vas and testicular vessels were identified and protected from harm. The sac was opened and contents were reduced. A finger was passed into the peritoneal cavity and the floor of the inguinal canal assessed and found to be strong. The femoral canal was palpated and no hernia identified. The sac was twisted and suture ligated with 2-0 silk. Redundant sac was excised and submitted to pathology. The stump of the sac was checked for hemostasis and allowed to retract into the abdomen.

Attention then turned to the floor of the canal, which appeared to be grossly weakened without a well-defined defect or sac. The *polypropylene/other* mesh was cut to the appropriate size with an oval medial portion and a longitudinal lateral opening. Beginning at the pubic tubercle, the mesh was sutured to the inguinal ligament inferiorly and the conjoint tendon superiorly using two continuous running 2-0 nonabsorbable sutures. Care was taken to assure that the mesh was placed in a relaxed fashion to avoid excessive tension and that no neurovascular structures were caught in the repair. Laterally, the tails of the mesh were crossed and the internal ring recreated, allowing for passage of the surgeon's fifth fingertip.

Hemostasis was again checked. The Penrose drain was removed. The external oblique aponeurosis was closed with a running suture of 3-0 Vicryl, taking care not to catch the ilioinguinal nerve in the suture line. Scarpa's fascia was closed with interrupted 3-0 Vicryl.

The skin was closed with a *subcuticular stitch of* ___/*skin clips/ other*. A dressing was applied.

If male: The testis was gently pulled down into its anatomic position in the scrotum.

The patient tolerated the procedure well and was taken to the postanesthesia care unit in stable condition.

ACKNOWLEDGMENT

This chapter was contributed by Benjamin E. Schneider, MD and Peter Fretz, MD in the first edition.

NOTES

Chapter 99

Laparoscopic Inguinal Hernia Repair: Transabdominal Preperitoneal (TAPP)

Jessica K. Smith, M.D.

INDICATIONS

- Recurrent hernia.
- Bilateral hernias.
- Incidental herniorrhaphy during another laparoscopic procedure.

ESSENTIAL STEPS

1. Verify side of surgery!
2. General anesthesia.
3. Patient supine with arms tucked.
4. Trendelenburg position, surgeon on opposite side of table from the hernia, single video monitor at foot of operating table.
5. First trocar (10–12 mm) placed at the umbilicus.
6. Two additional trocars (5 mm) lateral to the rectus sheath on either side just below the level of the umbilicus.
7. Angled laparoscope provides best visualization.
8. Inspect both inguinal regions; identify:
   - The median umbilical ligament.
   - The medial umbilical ligament.
   - The lateral umbilical fold.
9. *Divide the median umbilical ligament if necessary to improve exposure.*
10. Incise the peritoneum along a line superior to the hernia defect, extending from the anterior superior iliac spine to the median umbilical ligament.

J.J. Hoballah and C.E.H. Scott-Conner (eds.), *Operative Dictations in General and Vascular Surgery*, DOI 10.1007/978-1-4614-0451-4_99,
© Springer Science+Business Media, LLC 2012

11. Mobilize the peritoneal flap superiorly for several centimeters along the umbilical ligament.
12. Create the preperitoneal space beginning laterally and extending medially to the inferior epigastric vessels.
13. Cooper's ligament is identified and exposed medially to its junction with the femoral vein.
14. Identify the iliopubic tract.
15. Parietalize the cord structures and reduce any indirect or direct hernia contents.
16. *Direct hernia: Reduce the sac and preperitoneal fat from the hernia orifice by gentle traction.*
17. *Indirect hernia: Reduce with gentle traction. For a large sac: Divide the sac distal to the internal ring, leaving the distal sac in situ and dissect the proximal sac away from the cord structures.*
18. Ensure hemostasis.
19. Place mesh (at least 11×6 cm) over the myopectineal orifice and parietalized spermatic cord to completely cover the direct, indirect, and femoral spaces.
20. Fix mesh superiorly to abdominal wall inferiorly to Cooper's ligament and medially to the pectineal ligament avoiding the inferolateral edges to stay away from the triangle of pain(nerves) and the triangle of doom(vessels).
21. Excise redundant mesh.
22. Close the peritoneal flap over the mesh securing with tacks in similar positions of safety.
23. *Bilateral hernias can be repaired using one long transverse peritoneal incision extending from one anterior superior iliac spine to the other or, alternatively, with two separate peritoneal incisions preserving the peritoneum between the medial umbilical ligaments.*

NOTE THESE VARIATIONS
- Direct vs. indirect hernia.
- Sac of indirect hernia reduced or divided and left in situ.
- Bilateral hernia; repaired with single large sheet of mesh or through two incisions.
- In women, the round ligament is usually divided to complete the peritoneal flap.

COMPLICATIONS
- Vascular injuries, especially the inferior epigastric artery or spermatic vessels.

- Nerve injury, especially the branches of genitofemoral nerve, lateral femoral cutaneous nerve, and femoral nerve.
- Vas deferens and testicular complications.
- Recurrence of hernia.
- Bowel injury or obstruction.
- Osteitis pubis.

TEMPLATE OPERATIVE DICTATION

Preoperative diagnosis: *Left/right/bilateral* inguinal hernia.

Procedure: Transabdominal preperitoneal laparoscopic (TAPP) repair of *left/right/bilateral* inguinal hernia.

Postoperative diagnosis: Same.

Indications: This ___-year-old *male/female* developed a *symptomatic/recurrent left/right/bilateral* inguinal hernia. Repair was indicated, and because of the *patient's age/sex/nature of the hernia/patient preference* laparoscopic repair was elected.

Description of procedure: The patient was taken to the operating room and the correct side of surgery was verified. The patient was placed supine with arms tucked at the sides. After obtaining adequate anesthesia, the patient's abdomen was prepped and draped in standard sterile fashion. The patient was placed in the Trendelenburg position. A time-out was completed verifying correct patient, procedure, site, positioning, and implant(s) and/or special equipment prior to beginning this procedure. A Veress needle was placed at the umbilicus and pneumoperitoneum created with insufflation of carbon dioxide to 15 mmHg. After the Veress needle was removed, a 10-mm trocar was placed infraumbilically and the 45° angled laparoscope inserted. Two 5-mm trocars were then placed lateral to the rectus sheath under direct visualization. Both inguinal regions were inspected and the median umbilical ligament, medial umbilical ligament, and lateral umbilical fold were identified. The median umbilical ligament was divided sharply with electrocautery to achieve optimal exposure. The peritoneum was incised with endoscopic scissors along a line 2 cm above the superior edge of the hernia defect, extending from the median umbilical ligament to the anterior superior iliac spine. The peritoneal flap was mobilized inferiorly using blunt and sharp dissection. The inferior epigastric vessels were exposed and the pubic symphysis was identified. Cooper's ligament was dissected to its junction with the iliac vein. The dissection was continued inferiorly to the iliopubic tract, with care taken to avoid injury to the femoral branch of the genitofemoral nerve and the lateral femoral cutaneous nerve. The cord structures were parietalized. The direct hernia sac was identified and reduced by gentle traction.

Indirect hernia: The indirect hernia sac was noted to be small and was easily mobilized from the cord structures and reduced into the peritoneal cavity/the indirect hernia sac was noted to be large and was therefore divided just distal to the internal ring, leaving the distal sac in situ while the proximal sac was dissected away from the cord structures.

A large piece of mesh was rolled longitudinally into a compact cylinder and passed through a trocar. The cylinder was placed along the inferior aspect of the working space and unrolled into place to completely cover the direct, indirect, and femoral spaces. The mesh was secured into place superiorly to the anterior abdominal wall and inferiorly and medially to Cooper's/pectineal ligaments with absorbable/titanium tacks. Care was taken to avoid the inferolateral triangles containing the iliac vessels and genital nerves. The peritoneal flap was closed over the mesh and secured with tacks in similar positions of safety. After ensuring adequate hemostasis, the trocars were removed and the pneumoperitoneum allowed to escape. The trocar incisions were closed using ___ and dry dressing/skin adhesive dressings applied.

The patient tolerated the procedure well and was taken to the postanesthesia care unit in stable condition.

ACKNOWLEDGMENT

This chapter was contributed by Alvina Won, MD in the first edition.

NOTES

Chapter 100

Laparoscopic Inguinal Hernia Repair: Totally Extraperitoneal (TEP)

Jessica K. Smith, M.D.

INDICATIONS

- Recurrent hernia.
- Bilateral hernias.
- Surgeon or patient preference.

ESSENTIAL STEPS

1. Verify side of surgery!
2. Supine position, general anesthesia, arms tucked, and Foley catheter.
3. Trendelenburg position.
4. Make skin incision for the first trocar (10–12 mm) at the umbilicus. If the patient is tall, adjust you incision inferiorly so that you will clear the posterior sheath.
5. Open the anterior rectus sheath on the ipsilateral side and retract the muscle laterally to expose the posterior rectus sheath.
6. Insert finger over the posterior rectus sheath and develop space.
7. Insert a transparent balloon-tipped trocar or other device into this space directed toward the pubic symphysis.
8. Place laparoscope in the trocar and inflate the balloon under direct vision to create the extraperitoneal space. Deflate balloon and start CO_2 insufflation of the preperitoneal space. Alternatively, start CO_2 insufflation and create the space with the laparoscope itself using blunt dissection.

J.J. Hoballah and C.E.H. Scott-Conner (eds.), *Operative Dictations in General and Vascular Surgery*, DOI 10.1007/978-1-4614-0451-4_100,
© Springer Science+Business Media, LLC 2012

9. Place two additional trocars in the midline or bilateral lower quadrants under direct vision. For midline ports place:
    - The second (5 mm) 1 cm above the pubic symphysis.
    - The third (5 mm) midway between the first and second trocars. For lateral lower quadrant ports, place laterally and superiorly with respect to the bilateral anterior superior iliac spines (ASIS).
10. Use a 30 or 45° angled laparoscope for best visualization.
11. Identify the inferior epigastric vessels keeping them always anterior to the plane of dissection in their investing fat.
12. Beginning at the pubis dissect Cooper's ligament to its junction with the iliac vein.
13. Inspect the direct space medial to the inferior epigastric vessels and reduce any sac or preperitoneal fat with gentle traction.
14. *Direct hernias: Reduce the sac to the level of the ileopubic tract with gentle traction.*
15. Skeletonize the spermatic cord laterally to the inferior epigastric vessels to expose the ileopubic tract. Do not go lateral or posterior to this to avoid nerve injury.
16. *Indirect hernias: If an indirect hernia sac is identified mobilize the sac from the cord structures and reduce into the peritoneum. Reduce any lipomas of the spermatic cord. If the sac is exceptionally large and will not reduce with gentle traction it can be suture ligated.*
17. *Bilateral hernias: Repeat dissection on the contralateral side.*
18. Place mesh behind the spermatic cord structures (at least 10×12 cm) over the myopectineal orifice to completely cover the direct, indirect, and femoral spaces. A keyhole can be cut in the mesh but there must be overlap of the mash encircling the cord.
19. *Bilateral hernias: Either two separate pieces or one large piece of mesh may be used.*
20. A minimum number of absorbable vicryl or titanium tacks are used to secure the mesh. One tack is placed in the anterolateral abdominal fascia to secure the mesh as it is unfurled.
21. A second tack is placed to Cooper's ligament to secure the medial side of the mesh.
22. Additional tacks, if needed, can be placed in Coopers or the lateral anterior abdominal wall while palpating the end of the tacking device to avoid intraperitoneal injury.

23. Avoid placing staples directly into either pubic tubercle.
24. Ensure hemostasis.
25. Allow insufflation to escape while gently holding mesh in position.
26. Withdraw trocars.
27. Close anterior sheath and skin incisions.

NOTE THESE VARIATIONS

- Type of mesh, balloon dissector, tracking device, and number of tacks used varies.
- Midline or lateral operating port placement.
- Bilateral hernias can be repaired with the use of either a single large prosthesis or two separate pieces.
- A keyhole can be pre-cut in the mesh to accommodate the cord structures or the mesh can be left whole.

COMPLICATIONS

- Bladder injury.
- Vascular injuries, especially the inferior epigastric artery or spermatic vessels.
- Nerve injury, especially the branches of the genitofemoral nerve, lateral femoral cutaneous nerve, and femoral nerve.
- Vas deferens and testicular complications.
- Recurrence of hernia.
- Osteitis pubis.

TEMPLATE OPERATIVE DICTATION

Preoperative diagnosis: *Left/right/bilateral* inguinal hernia.
Procedure: Totally extraperitoneal laparoscopic (TEP) repair of *left/right/bilateral* inguinal hernia.
Postoperative diagnosis: Same.
Indications: This ___-year-old *male/female* developed a *symptomatic/recurrent left/right/bilateral* inguinal hernia. Repair was indicated, and because of the *patient's age/sex/nature of the hernia/ patient preference* laparoscopic repair was elected.
Description of procedure: The patient was taken to the operating room and the side of surgery was verified. The patient was placed supine with arms tucked at the sides. A time-out was completed verifying correct patient, procedure, site, positioning, and implant(s) and/or special equipment prior to beginning this procedure. After induction of general anesthesia, the patient's abdomen was prepped and draped in standard sterile fashion.

The patient was placed in the Trendelenburg position. The skin incision for the first trocar was made just below the umbilicus. The anterior rectus sheath on the ipsilateral side of the hernia was opened and the muscle retracted laterally to expose the posterior rectus sheath. This extraperitoneal space was gently developed with blunt dissection and a balloon-tipped 10-mm trocar placed into the space, directed toward the pubic symphysis. An angled laparoscope was placed into the trocar and the balloon inflated under direct vision to create the extraperitoneal space. A 5-mm trocar was placed at the pubic symphysis and the final 5-mm trocar placed midline between the first and second trocars. *Alternatively, two additional 5-mm trocars were placed under direct visualization in the bilateral lower quadrants.*

The preperitoneal space was further developed by exposing the inferior epigastric vessels and keeping them anterior to the dissection plane. Cooper's ligament was dissected laterally to its junction with the iliac vein. The dissection was continued inferiorly to the iliopubic tract, with care taken to avoid injury to the femoral branch of the genitofemoral nerve and the lateral femoral cutaneous nerve. The cord structures were skeletonized. The direct hernia sac was identified and reduced by gentle traction.

[Choose one:]

If indirect hernias: The indirect hernia sac was noted to be small and was easily mobilized from the cord structures and reduced into the peritoneal cavity/the indirect hernia sac was noted to be large and was therefore suture ligated and divided just distal to the internal ring leaving the distal sac in situ while the proximal sac was dissected away from the cord structure.

If bilateral hernias: The procedure was repeated on the contralateral side.

A 10×12 cm piece of mesh was marked for orientation and rolled longitudinally into a compact cylinder and passed through the camera trocar. The mesh was placed along the inferior aspect of the working space and unrolled into place to completely cover the direct, indirect, and femoral spaces. The mesh was tacked into place laterally and superiorly to the ileopubic tract and inferior and medially to Cooper's ligament. Excess mesh was trimmed and removed.

After ensuring adequate hemostasis using electrocautery, the insufflation was stopped and allowed to escape while the mesh was held gently in position. The trocars were removed and the balloon deflated. The anterior rectus sheath was closed using ____.

The trocar incisions were closed using ___ and dry dressings/skin adhesive were applied.

The patient tolerated the procedure well and was taken to the postanesthesia care unit in stable condition.

ACKNOWLEDGMENT

This chapter was contributed by Alvina Won, MD in the first edition.

NOTES

Chapter 101

Repair of Femoral Hernia

Jessemae L. Welsh, M.D.

INDICATION
- Femoral hernia.

ESSENTIAL STEPS
1. Verify and mark side of surgery!
2. Skin line incision *above the inguinal ligament/directly over the hernia.*
3. Develop flaps to expose the sac.
4. Reduce the hernia and open the sac if possible.
5. *If not reducible:*
   - *Divide the inguinal ligament cephalad to the sac, protecting the underlying cord structures.*
   - *Enlarge the femoral orifice.*
   - *Open the sac and inspect contents.*
   - *If viable, replace contents in the abdomen.*
   - *If nonviable, perform segmental bowel resection.*
6. Close the sac with 2-0 silk suture ligature.
7. Excise the redundant sac and allow to retract into the abdomen.
8. Close the femoral canal with mesh plug.
9. *Close defect in the inguinal ligament.*
10. Attain hemostasis.
11. Close the wound.

J.J. Hoballah and C.E.H. Scott-Conner (eds.), *Operative Dictations in General and Vascular Surgery*, DOI 10.1007/978-1-4614-0451-4_101,
© Springer Science+Business Media, LLC 2012

NOTE THESE VARIATIONS
- Femoral hernia may also be repaired through the inguinal canal (see McVay repair, Chap. 97) or via a laparoscopic (Chaps. 99 and 100) or preperitoneal approach.
- Incision directly over the hernia for small, easily reduced herniae.
- Incision over the inguinal canal allows better access and exposure.
- Type of mesh, suture, and local anesthesia used.
- Repair with autogenous tissue rather than mesh is possible.
- Local anesthesia is sometimes used in frail or elderly patients.
- Aberrant obturator artery may be encountered deep to the inguinal ligament.

COMPLICATIONS
- Injury to the bowel.
- Reduction of compromised/strangulated bowel into the abdomen.
- Injury to the femoral vessels.
- If the inguinal ligament divided: Injury to the cord or ilioinguinal nerve or bleeding from the aberrant obturator artery.
- Recurrence.

TEMPLATE OPERATIVE DICTATION
Preoperative diagnosis: *Left/right incarcerated* femoral hernia.
Procedure: Bassini repair of *left/right* femoral hernia *with local anesthesia by surgeon.*
Postoperative diagnosis: Same.
Indications: This ___-year-old *male/female* developed a *symptomatic/incarcerated left/right* femoral hernia *with/without* symptoms of obstruction. Repair was indicated.
Description of procedure: The patient was taken to the operating room and the side of surgery was verified.

[Choose one:]
   If not local anesthesia: *General/epidural/spinal anesthesia was induced.*

   If local anesthesia: *The area of the planned surgery was infiltrated with lidocaine. A total of ___ mL of 0.5%/1% lidocaine was used.*

A time-out was completed verifying correct patient, procedure, site, positioning, and implant(s) and/or special equipment prior to beginning this procedure. The *left/right* groin was prepped and draped in the usual sterile fashion. An incision was made in a natural skin crease parallel to the inguinal ligament *over the hernia bulge/over the inguinal canal.* The incision was deepened through the subcutaneous tissue. Hemostasis was achieved with electrocautery. *A flap was developed inferiorly to expose the hernia sac/the hernia sac was exposed.* The sac was gently dissected free of surrounding tissues. It was found to be *reducible/irreducible.*

If hernia reducible: *The hernial orifice was inspected after reduction of the hernial contents. The sac was opened and the opening suture ligated with 2-0 silk. Redundant sac was excised and the sac allowed to retract into the peritoneal cavity.*

If hernia not reducible: *The inguinal ligament cephalad to the femoral canal was divided with care to avoid injury to the underlying cord structures and ilioinguinal nerve. With this divided, the hernia sac was opened and the contents inspected and found to be viable/ nonviable (dictate bowel resection if done). The hernia was then reduced and the redundant sac amputated and ligated with 2-0 silk.*

A plug of ___ mesh was fashioned in such a way as to completely fill the defect without encroaching upon the femoral vein. It was placed in the femoral canal and sutured in place with multiple interrupted sutures of ___. Care was taken to protect the femoral vessels from harm. *The inguinal ligament was then reconstructed with multiple interrupted sutures of ___, with care taken to protect the underlying cord structures and ilioinguinal nerve.*

The wound was irrigated and closed with interrupted 3-0 Vicryl *and skin staples/a subcuticular closure of ___/other.*

The patient tolerated the procedure well and was taken to the postanesthesia care unit in stable condition.

ACKNOWLEDGMENT

This chapter was contributed by Kareem A. Hamdy, MD in the first edition.

NOTES

Chapter 102

Ventral Hernia Repair

Peter C. Fretz, M.D.

INDICATION

- Ventral (incisional) hernia.

ESSENTIAL STEPS

1. *Excise the old scar if necessary.*
2. Mobilize flaps at fascial level.
3. Define and dissect the hernia sacs.
4. *Enter the peritoneal cavity and lyse adhesions/mobilize the small bowel if necessary.*
5. Identify all defects and convert into single defect.
6. Tailor mesh.
7. Suture to fascial edges.
8. *Place closed suction drains.*
9. Check hemostasis.
10. Close the subcutaneous tissues and skin.

NOTE THESE VARIATIONS

- Excision of scar.
- Location and number of defects.
- Type of mesh and method of fixation.
- Drain placement is optional.
- Incarcerated hernias require individualized management.

J.J. Hoballah and C.E.H. Scott-Conner (eds.), *Operative Dictations in General and Vascular Surgery*, DOI 10.1007/978-1-4614-0451-4_102,
© Springer Science+Business Media, LLC 2012

COMPLICATIONS

- Infection.
- Recurrence.
- Enterocutaneous fistula.

TEMPLATE OPERATIVE DICTATION

Preoperative diagnosis: Ventral (incisional) hernia.
Procedure: *Mesh* repair of ventral hernia.
Postoperative diagnosis: Same.
Indications: This ___-year-old *male/female* developed a ventral hernia in the site of a previous ___ incision. This was *symptomatic/incarcerated* and repair was indicated.
Description of procedure: The patient was brought to the operating room and general anesthesia was induced. A time-out was completed verifying correct patient, procedure, site, positioning, and implant(s) and/or special equipment prior to beginning this procedure. Antibiotics were administered prior to making the incision. The anterior abdominal wall was prepped and draped in the standard sterile fashion. A *vertical midline incision/other* incorporating the old incision was made. *The old scar was completely excised.* The incision was deepened to the fascia. The hernia sac was then identified and dissected free. The peritoneum of the sac was entered and the contents were reduced *(detail findings if incarcerated).* The fascia was carefully palpated and *no additional defects/additional defects (detail location)* were identified. *Intervening fascial bridges were cut to create a single defect (if multiple).*

Adhesions to the underside of the abdominal wall were lysed and the fascia was assessed. A piece of ___ mesh was tailored to fit the defect and sutured to the fascial edges with *running/interrupted* sutures of ___. Hemostasis was checked. *Closed suction drains were placed.* Subcutaneous tissues were closed with 3-0 Vicryl and the skin was closed with *skin staples/subcuticular sutures of ___/other.*

The patient tolerated the procedure well and was brought to the postanesthesia care unit in stable condition.

NOTES

Chapter 103
Laparoscopic Ventral Hernia Repair

Susan Skaff Hagen, M.D., M.S.P.H.

INDICATION
- Ventral hernia.

ESSENTIAL STEPS
1. General Anesthesia.
2. Foley.
3. Insufflate abdomen either using Veress needle or Hassan cannula.
4. Place initial trocar.
5. Insert laparoscope and inspect abdomen.
6. Place additional trocars.
7. Decide primary or mesh repair.
8. If mesh repair, orient mesh with Ethibond suture outside abdomen then insert via a 12-mm trocar.
9. Nonadherent side of mesh toward bowel.
10. Place trans-facial sutures to anchor mesh with 5 cm overlap on all sides of the hernia.
11. Tack mesh to abdominal wall.
12. Place additional trans-facial sutures.
13. Collapse abdomen to pressure of 8 mmHg.
14. Tie sutures.
15. Check hemostasis.
16. Close.

J.J. Hoballah and C.E.H. Scott-Conner (eds.), *Operative Dictations in General and Vascular Surgery*, DOI 10.1007/978-1-4614-0451-4_103,
© Springer Science+Business Media, LLC 2012

NOTE THESE VARIATIONS

- Orogastric tube.
- Veress needle or Hassan cannula.
- Cutting or splitting trocars.
- Primary repair.
- Repair with mesh.
- Closing trocar sites.
- Local infiltration.
- Abdominal binder.

COMPLICATIONS

- Injury to bowel, bladder, or inferior epigastric vessels from trocar placement.
- Mesh migration.
- Hernia recurrence.

TEMPLATE OPERATIVE DICTATION

Preoperative diagnosis: *Initial/recurrent* ventral hernia.

Procedure: Laparoscopic ventral hernia repair.

Postoperative diagnosis: Same.

Indications: Patient is a ___-year-old *man/woman* who was evaluated for *an initial/recurrent* ventral hernia. *He/she* complains of *(describe symptoms)*.

Description of procedure: The patient was brought into the operating room and placed on the table in the supine position. General anesthesia was administered. A time-out was completed verifying correct patient, procedure, site, positioning, and implant(s) and/or special equipment prior to beginning this procedure. All bony prominences were padded. Both arms were tucked. A Foley was placed. *An orogastric tube was placed.* The abdomen was prepped from the xiphoid to pubis and table to table with *Chlorhexidine/Betadine/other*. The patient was draped in the usual sterile fashion.

[Choose one:]

*If **Veress needle:** The fascia was elevated and the Veress needle inserted. Proper position was confirmed by aspiration and saline meniscus test. Carbon dioxide was started on low flow. Once it was flowing easily, it was advanced to high flow.*

*If **Hassan cannula:** An incision was made (describe where). Dissection was carried down until the level of the fascia. The fascia was elevated and incised. Entry into the peritoneum was confirmed visually. Two figure-of-eight sutures of 2-0 Vicryl were placed and* *the Hassan cannula inserted under direct vision. The sutures were anchored around the cannula.*

The abdomen was insufflated with carbon dioxide to a pressure of 15 mmHg. The patient tolerated insufflation well. A ___ mm trocar was inserted in the right lower quadrant. The laparoscope was inserted and the abdomen inspected. (Describe normal and abnormal findings). The camera was exchanged to a 30°. Under direct visualization an additional 5-mm trocar was placed in the right lower quadrant below the costal margin. A 12-mm trocar was placed between these two ports. *Additional ports were placed in the left lower quadrant/other.* Care was taken to avoid injury to the bladder or inferior epigastric vessels.

Upon examining the abdominal wall, the hernia appeared to be (describe findings).

[Choose one]

*If **primary repair:** The 30° camera showed a visible defect that was <___cm (describe location). Since the hernia was small, singular, (and other factors such as cirrhosis) primary repair was performed. Using a GraNee needle we placed 0 Ethibond sutures. ___number of sutures were placed approximately 1 cm apart and were on either side of the hernia by approximately 2 cm.*

*If **mesh repair:** A (Proceed/Parietex Composix mesh/other) which measured ___ × ___ cm was used for repair of this ventral hernia. Extracorporeally, the mesh was oriented and the corners were marked with a marking pen. The top and bottom center of the mesh was marked with 0 Ethibond suture to serve as two transfascial anchoring sutures. The mesh was rolled into a tight cigar-like configuration and was introduced through the right upper quadrant 12-mm port. The mesh was placed within the peritoneal cavity without any complications. Then, using the proper orientation and the marks placed initially, the mesh was unraveled using Prestige graspers. The proper orientation of the mesh was maintained throughout the entire procedure, with the nonadherent hydrocellulose-coated side of the mesh facing the bowel. After proper positioning of the mesh, a GraNee needle was used to pull the transfascial sutures out corresponding stab incisions. The suture was adjusted to provide adequate tension on the mesh. This resulted in the placement of the mesh in such a fashion so as to provide gentle trampoline-like formation inside the abdomen covering the hernia defects with an adequate 5 cm overlap along the margins.*

After the transfascial sutures were tied down, the mesh was tacked using a (Tacker/AbsorbaTack/other device). The tacks were placed in a circumferential fashion approximately 0.5 cm from the edge and approximately 1 cm from each other. Crowning was done with a second row of tacks circumferentially, especially in the lower part of the mesh so as to prevent mesh migration and hernia recurrence. After the mesh was tacked in its entirety, we placed multiple additional transfascial sutures 3 cm apart and 2 cm from the edge of the mesh in a circumferential fashion. The abdomen was allowed to collapse to approximately a pressure of 8 mmHg. Next, the sutures were tied.

The abdominal cavity was inspected and the hernia repair appeared satisfactory. The trocars were removed under direct vision. *No bleeding was noted/trocar site bleeding was controlled with electrocautery/suture placement.* The laparoscope was withdrawn and the final trocar removed. The abdomen was allowed to collapse. *All trocar sites greater than 5 mm were closed with _____.*

The skin was closed with 4-0 *Monocryl/Vicryl/other. Benzoin/ Steri-Strips/Glue* was applied. *The port sites and transfascial suture sites were infiltrated with ___ cc of (1% Lidocaine/2% Lidocaine/0.25% Marcaine/other). An abdominal binder was then placed.* The patient tolerated the procedure well and was brought to the PACU in stable condition.

NOTES

Chapter 104

Operations for Infected Abdominal Wound Dehiscence and Necrotizing Soft Tissue Infection of the Abdominal Wall

Kristen C. Sihler, M.D.

INDICATIONS

- Infected fascial dehiscence.
- Infection of abdominal wall not responsive to antibiotics.

ESSENTIAL STEPS

1. *Midline incision/incision that encompasses apparent borders of tissue necrosis.*
2. Widely debride obviously infected tissue with scalpel or electrocautery. Consider sending tissue for quantitative cultures.
3. Secure hemostasis as you debride with judicious and sparing use of electrocautery.
4. Open and debride necrotic tissue, including fascia, taking care not to injure the adherent bowel.
5. Assess the entire abdomen for abscesses. If found, send a sample for gram stain and culture.
6. Irrigate the incision and abdomen copiously.
7. *Close fascia with multiple through-and-through sutures/ if unable to approximate fascia insert biologic mesh or consider doing a damage control closure such as a vacuum dressing and performing a second-look operation in 24–48 h with mesh placement (if needed) at that time.*
8. If fascia is closed or mesh placed, leave the skin and subcutaneous tissue open.

J.J. Hoballah and C.E.H. Scott-Conner (eds.), *Operative Dictations in General and Vascular Surgery*, DOI 10.1007/978-1-4614-0451-4_104,

9. Pack with saline-moistened gauze or place a superficial vacuum dressing if not doing a damage control closure.

NOTE THESE VARIATIONS

- Document extent of debridement including the layers debrided.
- Primary vs. mesh closure.
- Type of mesh placed.

COMPLICATIONS

- Sepsis.
- Ventral hernia.
- Enterocutaneous fistula.

TEMPLATE OPERATIVE DICTATION

Preoperative diagnosis: *Necrotizing soft tissue infection of the abdominal wall/infected abdominal wound dehiscence.*

Procedure: *Debridement of the abdominal wall/wound, drainage of intra-abdominal abscess, washout of the abdomen, insertion of mesh/reapproximation of fascia/temporary closure with planned re-operating.*

Postoperative diagnosis: *Same/intra-abdominal abscess.*

Indications: This ____-year-old *male/female* with a past medical history significant for *diabetes/malignancy/alcohol abuse/malnutrition/obesity/abdominal wound with devitalized tissue/peripheral vascular disease/previous abdominal operation* presented with *spreading erythema/induration/fever/increased white blood cell count/hemodynamic instability/dehiscence/evisceration.* Gram stain showed many *gram-positive/negative/mixed organisms.* Operative debridement, washout, and repair were indicated as an emergency procedure.

Description of procedure: The patient was placed in a supine position and general anesthesia was induced. The abdomen, upper thighs, and chest were prepped and draped in a standard surgical fashion. A time-out was completed verifying correct patient, procedure, site, positioning, and implant(s) and/or special equipment prior to beginning this procedure. A midline incision was carried out through skin and fat, down to the level of the fascia. All grossly infected tissues *including subcutaneous tissue, fat, rectus muscle, etc.,* were sharply excised and hemostasis was achieved with suture ligation of bleeding vessels and judicious use of electrocautery. *Prior fascial sutures were found to have pulled through the* *fascia/broken/suffered knot failure.* Next, the *fascia was incised/prior sutures were removed,* taking care to avoid damaging the underlying bowel. Necrotic fascia was debrided. All four quadrants of the abdomen were explored for intra-abdominal abscesses. *Abscesses were found in (specify locations) and drained.* The abdomen was then irrigated copiously with warmed saline. *The fascia was reapproximated using multiple through-and-through retention sutures of* ____/a Smead-Jones closure with interrupted ____/a ____ (size) sheet of (specify type) mesh was sutured to the fascial edges so as to cover the fascial defect. An abdominal vacuum dressing was placed.* The skin was left open and covered with *saline-moistened gauze/a vacuum dressing.*

The patient was *awakened and taken to the postanesthesia care unit/left intubated and taken to the surgical intensive care unit* in *stable/critical* condition.

NOTES

Section **X**

Breast

Chapter 105

Breast Biopsy

Carol E.H. Scott-Conner, M.D.

INDICATION

- Palpable breast mass with need for removal/definitive diagnosis.

ESSENTIAL STEPS

1. Confirm side of surgery!
2. Local anesthesia.
3. Skin crease incision.
4. Mobilize flaps.
5. Confirm palpable mass.
6. Place traction suture.
7. *If incisional biopsy:*
   - *Remove a generous wedge of tissue using scalpel.*
8. *If excisional biopsy:*
   - *Remove the palpable mass with narrow rim of surrounding normal breast tissue.*
   - *Palpate the cavity for remaining/additional abnormalities, send additional tissue if necessary.*
9. Achieve hemostasis in the cavity.
10. Close subcutaneous tissue with interrupted 3-0 Vicryl.
11. Close the skin with subcuticular suture.

NOTE THESE VARIATIONS

- Site of incision: Circumareolar/skin crease/radial.
- Incisional vs. excisional biopsy.

J.J. Hoballah and C.E.H. Scott-Conner (eds.), *Operative Dictations in General and Vascular Surgery*, DOI 10.1007/978-1-4614-0451-4_105,
© Springer Science+Business Media, LLC 2012

- Frozen section.
- Additional tissue submitted.

COMPLICATIONS
- Hematoma.
- Infection.
- Missed lesion.

TEMPLATE OPERATIVE DICTATION
Preoperative diagnosis: *Right/left* breast mass.
Procedure: *Right/left incisional/excisional* biopsy.
Postoperative diagnosis: Same.
Indications: This ___-year-old *female/male* with a palpable *right/ left* breast mass underwent workup with *ultrasound/mammogram/ fine needle aspiration cytology.* These showed___ and *biopsy was recommended for management/diagnosis/excision was requested by the patient due to fear of cancer.*
Description of procedure: The patient was taken to the operating room and placed supine on the operating table, and after adequate sedation the *right/left* chest and axilla were prepped and draped in the usual sterile fashion. A time-out was completed verifying correct patient, procedure, site, positioning, and implant(s) and/or special equipment prior to beginning this procedure.

A *circumareolar skin incision/skin crease incision/transverse incision* was planned adjacent to the palpable mass. Local anesthesia was infiltrated and a skin incision was made. Additional local anesthesia was infiltrated as needed throughout the case and a total of ___ mL of 1% lidocaine was used. Flaps were raised and the location of the mass confirmed by palpation. A 2-0 silk figure-of-eight stay suture was placed in the mass and used to retract.

[Choose one:]

If incisional biopsy: A generous wedge was cut from the mass and submitted for pathologic examination.

If excisional biopsy: The mass was dissected from surrounding tissues using scalpel. Use of electrocautery was avoided on the specimen. After removing the lump, the cavity was palpated and no additional abnormalities/an additional firm area was palpated. This additional area was similarly excised and submitted separately. The specimen was oriented and submitted to pathology.

Hemostasis was achieved with electrocautery and suture ligatures of 3-0 Vicryl. The subcutaneous tissue immediately under the skin was approximated with interrupted 3-0 Vicryl sutures.

No attempt was made to close the dead space. The skin was closed with a subcuticular suture of running ___. A dressing was applied.

The patient tolerated the procedure well and was taken to the postanesthesia care unit in stable condition.

ACKNOWLEDGMENT

This chapter was contributed by Mazen M. Hashisho, MD, in the first edition.

NOTES

Chapter 106
Breast Ultrasound-Guided Core Biopsy or Cyst Aspiration

Kevin A. Bridge, M.D., M.S.P.H.

INDICATIONS
- Abnormal ultrasound with need for biopsy or aspiration.
- Palpable mass with need for biopsy or aspiration.
  - Ultrasound used to increase precision.

ESSENTIAL STEPS
1. Preoperative time-out and confirmation of surgical site.
2. Prep and drape patient and ultrasound probe.
3. Local anesthesia.
4. Localize mass with ultrasound probe.
5. Advance needle into mass/cyst.
6. Biopsy/aspirate mass.
7. *If Biopsy: Place clip.*
8. Hold pressure over biopsy site.
9. *If Biopsy: Close skin entry site with steri-strips/single inter-rupted suture.*

NOTE THESE VARIATIONS
- Core needle biopsy vs. cyst aspiration.
- Type of biopsy device used.
- Type of clip placed.
- Method of skin closure if biopsy performed.

J.J. Hoballah and C.E.H. Scott-Conner (eds.), *Operative Dictations in General and Vascular Surgery*, DOI 10.1007/978-1-4614-0451-4_106,
© Springer Science+Business Media, LLC 2012

COMPLICATIONS
- Bleeding.
- Hematoma.
- Infection.
- Missed lesion.
- Pneumothorax (rare).

TEMPLATE OPERATIVE DICTATION

Preoperative diagnosis: *Right/left* breast mass.

Procedure: *Right/left* breast ultrasound-guided *core needle biopsy/ cyst aspiration. Placement of clip.*

Postoperative diagnosis: Same.

Indications: This ____-year-old *female/male* with a suspicious breast mass identified by *ultrasound/palpation. Biopsy/aspiration* of mass was indicated for diagnosis of mass. *If palpable mass: Ultrasound was used to increase accuracy. Clip was placed to mark the location of the mass.*

Description of procedure: The patient was placed supine on the exam room table with the arm raised above the head. A time-out was completed verifying correct patient, procedure, site, positioning, and implant(s) and/or special equipment prior to beginning this procedure. The patient and ultrasound probe were then prepped and draped in the usual sterile fashion. Local anesthesia (____ ml of *1% lidocaine with epinephrine/other*) was infiltrated into the overlying skin and region around the mass. The mass was identified on ultrasound. It was located in the *right/left* breast at ____ o'clock ____ cm from the *nipple/areolar border.* It was *isoechoic/hypoechoic/anechoic/other*, had *smooth/microlobulated/ irregular* margins, and measured ____ cm by ____ cm by ____ cm. *It corresponded to the palpable abnormality/the previously noted imaging abnormality.* It exhibited *posterior enhancement/posterior shadowing/other.*

[Choose one:]

If core needle biopsy: A lateral-to-medial/other approach was chosen. A skin entry site was identified and a nick made in the skin with a #11 blade. The ____ automated biopsy needle was advanced to the edge of the mass under ultrasound guidance and the automated core biopsy needle was fired. Multiple samples were taken and submitted for pathology in Formalin. A ____ clip was then advanced into the mass and deployed in the center of the mass under ultrasound guidance.

If cyst aspiration: Using a 22 gauge needle the needle was advanced into the cyst. The contents of the cyst were aspirated.

The needle was withdrawn. Pressure was held over the biopsy site and hemostasis was ensured. *If biopsy: The skin incision was closed with steri-strips/with a single interrupted suture of* _____.

A sterile dressing was applied over the wound. The patient tolerated the procedure well.

NOTES

Chapter 107

Excision of Ducts

Carol E.H. Scott-Conner, M.D.

INDICATIONS
- Nipple discharge, suspicion of intraductal papilloma.
- Mammary fistula.

ESSENTIAL STEPS
1. Confirm side of surgery!
2. Cannulate the draining duct with a lacrimal duct probe.
3. Identify the quadrant to which the probe passes.
4. *Circumareolar incision over that quadrant/radially oriented incision including fistula site.*
5. Elevate flaps.
6. Excise the duct distally to termination on the nipple, proximally as far as possible.
7. Orient the specimen.
8. Achieve hemostasis in the cavity.
9. Close the subcutaneous tissue with interrupted 3-0 Vicryl.
10. Close the skin with subcuticular sutures.

NOTE THESE VARIATIONS
- Total ductal excision on occasion employed.
- When performed for subareolar abscess, use radial incision (including skin over fistula site). Leave tract open if purulence is encountered.

J.J. Hoballah and C.E.H. Scott-Conner (eds.), *Operative Dictations in General and Vascular Surgery*, DOI 10.1007/978-1-4614-0451-4_107,
© Springer Science+Business Media, LLC 2012

COMPLICATIONS
- Hematoma.
- Infection.
- Missed lesion.
- Recurrence.

TEMPLATE OPERATIVE DICTATION
Preoperative diagnosis: *Right/left* nipple discharge.
Procedure: *Right/left* ductal excision.
Postoperative diagnosis: Same.
Indications: This ___-year-old *female/male* with *persistent nipple discharge/mammary fistula* underwent workup with *ultrasound/ mammogram/cytology*. These showed ___ and ductal excision was recommended for *management/diagnosis*.
Description of procedure: The patient was taken to the operating room and placed supine on the operating table and *general anesthesia was induced/sedation was given*. A time-out was completed verifying correct patient, procedure, site, positioning, and implant(s) and/or special equipment prior to beginning this procedure. The *right/left* chest and axilla were prepped and draped in the usual sterile fashion. A lacrimal duct probe was used to cannulate the draining duct. The relevant quadrant was identified *and 1% xylocaine without epinephrine was used to infiltrate the region*. A *circumareolar/radially oriented* incision was made and flaps were elevated. Using the lacrimal duct probe as a guide, the involved duct was excised from its termination on the nipple with a wedge-shaped portion of proximal breast tissue. The specimen was oriented and sent to pathology. *Additional local anesthesia was infiltrated as needed throughout the case and a total of___ mL of 1% lidocaine was used.*

Hemostasis was achieved with electrocautery and suture ligatures of 3-0 Vicryl. The subcutaneous tissue immediately under the skin was approximated with interrupted 3-0 Vicryl sutures. No attempt was made to close the dead space. *The skin was closed with a subcuticular suture of running ___/packed open with ____.* A dressing was applied.

The patient tolerated the procedure well and was taken to the postanesthesia care unit in stable condition.

NOTES

Chapter 108
Needle-Localized Breast Biopsy

Abdi Ahari, M.D.

INDICATIONS

- Abnormal mammogram (nonpalpable lesion) not amenable to image-directed core biopsy.
- Also used (as a lumpectomy) for excision of core biopsy-proven lesions.
  - Ductal carcinoma in situ.
  - Lobular carcinoma in situ.
  - Possible discordant core biopsy.

ESSENTIAL STEPS

1. Confirm side of surgery!
2. Preoperative localizing wire placed under mammographic or ultrasound guidance.
3. Check localizing studies and estimate trajectory of wire and location of mass.
4. *Local/general* anesthesia.
5. *Circumareolar incision/incision over mass/incision midway between mass and needle entry site into the skin.*
6. Develop flaps.
7. Deliver wire into the operative field.
8. Place traction stitch.
9. Carefully remove the mass of tissue around the wire and the tip of the wire.
10. *If methylene blue was injected by mammography: Keep dissection plane away from blue-stained tissues.*

J.J. Hoballah and C.E.H. Scott-Conner (eds.), *Operative Dictations in General and Vascular Surgery*, DOI 10.1007/978-1-4614-0451-4_108,
© Springer Science+Business Media, LLC 2012

11. Avoid using electrocautery on the mass to preserve margins.
12. Orient the specimen.
13. Send to radiology for confirmation.
14. Attain hemostasis.
15. After receiving confirmation, close the wound.

NOTE THESE VARIATIONS
- Location of incision, type of wire.
- Use of methylene blue.

COMPLICATIONS
- Missed lesion.
- Incomplete excision.
- Wire broken/transected during dissection, unable to retrieve.
- Hematoma.

TEMPLATE OPERATIVE DICTATION
Preoperative diagnosis: *Right/left* breast mammographic abnormality.
Procedure: *Right/left* needle-localized breast biopsy.
Postoperative diagnosis: Same.
Indications: This ___-year-old *female/male* with a nonpalpable *right/left breast mass noted on mammography requires needle-localized biopsy for evaluation and treatment/with core biopsy demonstrating* ____ *requires needle-localized lumpectomy for treatment.*
Description of procedure: Preoperative needle localization was performed by radiology. Localization studies were reviewed. The patient was taken to the operating room and placed supine on the operating table, and after adequate sedation the *right/left* chest and axilla were prepped and draped in the usual sterile fashion. A time-out was completed verifying correct patient, procedure, site, positioning, and implant(s) and/or special equipment prior to beginning this procedure.

By comparing the localization studies with the direction and skin entry site of the needle, the probable trajectory and location of the mass was visualized. A *circumareolar skin incision/skin crease incision/transverse incision* was planned in such a way as to minimize the amount of dissection to reach the mass.

Local anesthesia was infiltrated and the skin incision was made. *Additional local anesthesia was infiltrated as needed throughout the case and a total of ___ mL of 1% lidocaine was used.* Flaps were raised and the location of the wire confirmed. *The wire was delivered into the wound.* A 2-0 silk figure-of-eight stay suture was placed around the wire and used for retraction. Dissection was then taken down circumferentially, taking care to include the entire localizing needle and a wide margin of grossly normal tissue. *No methylene blue was encountered.*

The specimen and entire localizing wire were removed. The specimen was oriented and sent to radiology with the localization studies. Confirmation was received that the entire target lesion had been resected. The wound was irrigated. Hemostasis was checked. The wound was closed with interrupted sutures of 3-0 Vicryl and a subcuticular suture of ___. No attempt was made to close the dead space. A dressing was applied.

The patient tolerated the procedure well and was taken to the postanesthesia care unit in stable condition.

NOTES

Chapter 109

Lumpectomy (Partial Mastectomy) and Axillary Node Dissection

Abdi Ahari, M.D.

INDICATIONS
- Carcinoma of the breast amenable to breast-conserving therapy.
- Positive sentinel node biopsy or ultrasound-guided needle biopsy of node.

ESSENTIAL STEPS
1. Confirm side of surgery!
2. General anesthesia.
3. *If re-excision of biopsy site:*
   - *Excise old biopsy scar.*
   - *Develop flaps.*
   - *Resect entire biopsy cavity or selective margins.*
4. *If needle-localized lumpectomy:*
   - *Check localizing studies and estimate trajectory of wire and location of mass.*
   - *Circumareolar incision/incision over mass/incision midway between mass and needle entry site into skin.*
   - *Develop flaps.*
   - *Deliver wire into operative field.*
   - *Place traction stitch.*
   - *Carefully remove mass of tissue around wire and tip of wire.*
   - *If methylene blue injected: Keep dissection plane away from blue-stained tissues.*
   - *Avoid using electrocautery on the mass.*

J.J. Hoballah and C.E.H. Scott-Conner (eds.), *Operative Dictations in General and Vascular Surgery*, DOI 10.1007/978-1-4614-0451-4_109,
© Springer Science+Business Media, LLC 2012

- *Orient the specimen.*
- *Send to radiology for confirmation.*
5. Attain hemostasis.
6. Close the wound.
7. Apply temporary dressing and reprep and drape axilla.
8. Transverse incision below hair-bearing area/oblique incision behind and parallel to the pectoralis major muscle.
9. Develop flaps.
10. Incise the clavipectoral fascia.
11. Dissect under the pectoralis major and minor muscles, removing all fatty tissue but preserving the median pectoral nerve.
12. Identify the axillary vein.
13. Clear of fatty tissue.
14. Ligate the first major branch from the axillary vein to the chest wall.
15. Identify and preserve the thoracodorsal nerve.
16. Identify and preserve the long thoracic nerve.
17. Clear fatty areolar node-bearing tissue from beneath the axillary vein.
18. Orient the specimen and send for pathology.
19. Attain hemostasis.
20. Place closed-suction drain.
21. Close the wound.

NOTE THESE VARIATIONS

- Depending upon previous workup or surgery, lumpectomy may be omitted or performed either as biopsy for palpable lesion or needle-localized excision.
- If nodes are clinically negative, substitute sentinel node biopsy (see Chap. 110 for axillary node dissection).
- Incision for lymphadenectomy *transverse/along pectoralis major muscle.*

COMPLICATIONS

- Failure to attain clean margins on lumpectomy.
- Bleeding.
- Seroma.
- Nerve injury.
- Lymphedema.
- Recurrence, requiring mastectomy.

TEMPLATE OPERATIVE DICTATION

Preoperative diagnosis: Carcinoma of the *right/left* breast.

Procedure: *Lumpectomy and* axillary node dissection, *right/left* side.

Postoperative diagnosis: Same.

Indications: This ___-year-old *female/male developed a breast lump/had an abnormal mammogram* that on workup with *fine needle aspiration cytology/biopsy* was found to be *invasive ductal carcinoma/invasive lobular carcinoma/other* of the breast. Presence of lymph node metastases was confirmed by ____. After discussion of alternatives, the patient elected breast conservation therapy to be followed by radiation therapy to the breast.

If lumpectomy: Accordingly, lumpectomy and axillary node dissection was planned/axillary node dissection was required.

If just axillary node dissection: Because clean margins had been attained at previous lumpectomy (and sentinel node biopsy was positive), axillary node dissection was required to complete the surgical treatment.

Description of procedure: The patient was brought to the operating room and the side of surgery was verified. General anesthesia was induced. The *right/left* breast and axilla were then prepped and draped in the usual sterile fashion.

The lumpectomy was performed first. A circumareolar/skin crease/transverse incision was made overlying the palpable mass/ encompassing the old biopsy incision/overlying the localizing wire.

[Choose one:]

If palpable mass: Flaps were developed and the palpable mass/ biopsy cavity was resected intact, oriented, and sent for pathology. No additional masses were palpated.

If needle-localized lumpectomy: The wire was delivered into the wound. A 2-0 silk figure-of-eight stay suture was placed around the wire and used for retraction. Dissection was then taken down circumferentially, taking care to include the entire localizing needle and a wide margin of grossly normal tissue. (Optional: No methylene blue was encountered.) The specimen and entire localizing wire were removed. The specimen was oriented and sent to radiology with the localization studies. Confirmation was received that the entire target lesion had been resected.

The wound was irrigated. Hemostasis was checked. The wound was closed with interrupted sutures of 3-0 Vicryl and a subcuticular suture of ___. No attempt was made to close the dead space. A temporary dressing was applied.

The patient was then reprepped for the axillary dissection. *A 6-cm horizontal skin incision was made in a skin crease just below the hair-bearing skin of the axilla extending from the lateral edge of the pectoralis major muscle to the anterior edge of the latissimus dorsi muscle/an oblique 6-cm incision was made parallel and just lateral to the edge of the pectoralis major muscle.* Flaps were raised cephalad and caudad to the estimated level of the axillary vein superiorly and the edge of the pectoralis major medially using electrocautery. The clavipectoral fascia was then incised along the edge of the pectoralis major and the pectoralis major and minor were freed from surrounding fat and nodal tissue. Dissection progressed first under the pectoralis major and then under the pectoralis minor muscle.

The pectoral muscles were retracted medially with a Richardson retractor. The medial pectoral neurovascular bundle was identified and preserved. The level II nodal tissue deep to the pectoralis minor was included in the dissection. The axillary vein was then identified and cleared of overlying fat. The first branch off the axillary vein was clamped, divided, and tied with 2-0 silk ties. The thoracodorsal nerve was then identified deep to the ligated vein and preserved. The long thoracic nerve was then identified along the edge of the latissimus dorsi on the chest wall and preserved. The remaining nodal tissue between these nerves was then carefully removed, taking care to protect the nerves. The specimen was then sent to pathology.

The wound was irrigated and hemostasis was achieved. A closed-suction drain was brought into the operative field through a separate stab incision and sutured to the skin with a 3-0 nylon suture. The wound was closed with interrupted 3-0 Vicryl to the subcutaneous layer, followed by a subcuticular layer of ___. The wound was dressed.

The patient tolerated the procedure well and was taken to the postanesthesia care unit in satisfactory condition.

NOTES

Chapter 110

Axillary Sentinel Node Biopsy for Breast Cancer

Michael Bonebrake, M.D.

INDICATIONS

- Breast cancer with clinically negative nodes.
- Desire to avoid lymphadenectomy.

ESSENTIAL STEPS

1. Confirm side of surgery!
2. Inject radioisotope (Tc99 sulfur colloid) *in equal aliquots circumferentially/intradermally around lesion or site of excision/in subareolar region.*
3. Obtain lymphoscintogram.
4. Three to four hours later, take the patient to the operating room.
5. Inject 1–3 mL of isosulfan blue around the tumor and subdermally and gently massage.
6. Use hand-held gamma probe to identify the node and make incision over that spot.
7. Orient incision so it can easily be incorporated into lymphadenectomy incision if necessary.
8. Record counts for 10 s over the node before and after incision, as well as the excised node and the bed from which it was excised.
   - Seek additional nodes if counts on bed are greater than 10% of ex vivo counts on excised node.
9. Before removing the node, check for blue dye.
10. Identify blue lymphatic channels and follow to other nodes.

J.J. Hoballah and C.E.H. Scott-Conner (eds.), *Operative Dictations in General and Vascular Surgery*, DOI 10.1007/978-1-4614-0451-4_110,
© Springer Science+Business Media, LLC 2012

11. Remove any grossly abnormal nodes.
12. Close the incision.

NOTE THESE VARIATIONS

- Amount of isotope, use of isosulfan blue dye.
- More than one node may be identified.
- Isotope may localize to internal mammary nodes as well as or instead of axilla – management then varies with protocol.
- May be combined with lumpectomy; in some circumstances axillary node dissection is done at the same setting.

COMPLICATIONS

- Failure to identify sentinel node.
- Recurrence.

TEMPLATE OPERATIVE DICTATION

Preoperative diagnosis: Carcinoma of breast, *right/left* side.
Procedure: Axillary sentinel node biopsy.
Postoperative diagnosis: Same.
Indications: This ___-year-old *female/male* has invasive carcinoma of the *right/left* breast and desires to avoid lymphadenectomy if possible. Lymph nodes are clinically negative, and sentinel node biopsy was chosen for evaluation and management.
Description of procedure: In the nuclear medicine suite, *the skin surrounding the mass/the breast tissue around the mass/the subareolar region* was injected with Tc-99 sulfur colloid. *Three/four* hours later, the patient and lymphoscintograms were taken to the operating room and general anesthesia was induced.

*(Amount)*____ cc's of isosulfan blue dye were injected into four quadrants around the lesion, with an additional small aliquot injected subdermally over the lesion. This was massaged gently for several minutes. The skin of the *right/left* breast and axilla/arm was prepped and draped in the usual sterile fashion. A time-out was completed verifying correct patient, procedure, site, positioning, and implant(s) and/or special equipment prior to beginning this procedure.

A hand-held gamma probe was used to identify the location of the hottest spot in the axilla. Prior to the incision, the counts were ___. An incision was made and a *blue/not blue/hot/cold* node was identified. The probe was placed in contact with the node and

___ counts were recorded. The node was excised in its entirety. Ex vivo, the node measured ___ counts when placed on the probe. The bed of the node measured ___ counts. *No additional/an additional* hot spot was detected.

If additional hot spot: A second blue node was identified and the following counts registered: ___ prior to excision, ___ ex vivo node, and ___ residual bed. No additional hot spots or blue lymphatics were identified. No clinically abnormal nodes were palpated. The procedure was terminated. Hemostasis was achieved and the wound closed in layers with deep interrupted 3-0 Vicryl and *skin staples/subcuticular suture/other.*

The patient tolerated the procedure well and was taken to the postanesthesia care unit in stable condition.

ACKNOWLEDGMENT

This chapter was contributed by Mazen M. Hashisho, MD, in the first edition.

NOTES

Chapter 111
Modified Radical Mastectomy

Michael C. Fraterelli, M.D.

INDICATION

- Invasive carcinoma of the breast with positive axillary nodes.

ESSENTIAL STEPS

1. Confirm side of surgery!
2. Elliptical incision encompassing the nipple–areolar complex and biopsy scar.
3. Raise flaps in avascular plane between the subcutaneous tissue and breast tissue:
   - Superiorly to the clavicle.
   - Medially to the sternum.
   - Inferiorly to the anterior rectus sheath.
   - Laterally to the anterior border of latissimus dorsi.
4. Remove breast tissue from medial to lateral, including the pectoralis fascia with specimen.
5. *Excise disk of muscle deep to biopsy cavity if tumor is encountered.*
6. At the lateral border of the pectoralis major muscle, allow breast tissue to fall laterally and commence work under the pectoralis major muscle.
7. Incise the clavipectoral fascia.
8. Dissect under the pectoralis major and minor muscles, removing all fatty tissue but preserving the median pectoral nerve.

J.J. Hoballah and C.E.H. Scott-Conner (eds.), *Operative Dictations in General and Vascular Surgery*, DOI 10.1007/978-1-4614-0451-4_111,
© Springer Science+Business Media, LLC 2012

9. Identify the axillary vein.
10. Clear of fatty tissue.
11. Ligate the first major branch from the axillary vein to the chest wall.
12. Identify and preserve the thoracodorsal nerve.
13. Identify and preserve the long thoracic nerve.
14. Clear fatty areolar node-bearing tissue from beneath the axillary vein.
15. Sweep tissue inferiorly to expose muscular boundaries of the axilla, preserving nerves.
16. Remove the specimen by dividing the lateral pedicle of subcutaneous fat.
17. Attain hemostasis.
18. Place closed suction drain(s).
19. Close the wound.

NOTE THESE VARIATIONS

- Skin-sparing mastectomy uses small, specially tailored incisions.
- Sentinel node biopsy rather than axillary node dissection.
- Immediate reconstruction with implants or autogenous tissue.

COMPLICATIONS

- Recurrence.
- Seroma.
- Nerve injury.
- Skin slough.
- Lymphedema.

TEMPLATE OPERATIVE DICTATION

Preoperative diagnosis: Carcinoma of the *right/left* breast.
Procedure: *Right/left* modified radical mastectomy.
Postoperative diagnosis: Same.
Indications: This ___-year-old *female/male developed a breast lump/had an abnormal mammogram* that on workup with *fine needle aspiration cytology/biopsy* was found to be *invasive ductal carcinoma/invasive lobular carcinoma/other* of the breast. She was demonstrated to have axillary node involvement. After discussion of alternatives, the patient elected modified radical mastectomy *with immediate reconstruction.*
Description of procedure: The patient was brought to the operating room and the site of surgery was confirmed. General

anesthesia was induced. A time-out was completed verifying correct patient, procedure, site, positioning, and implant(s) and/or special equipment prior to beginning this procedure. The breast, chest wall, axilla, and upper arm and neck were prepped and draped in the usual sterile fashion.

A skin incision was made that encompassed the nipple–areola complex and the previous biopsy scar and passed in a *generally transverse/oblique direction across the breast/other*. Flaps were raised in the avascular plane between subcutaneous tissue and breast tissue from clavicle superiorly, the sternum medially, the anterior rectus sheath inferiorly, and the anterior border of the latissimus dorsi muscle laterally. Hemostasis was achieved in the flaps. Next, the breast tissue and underlying pectoralis fascia were excised from the pectoralis major muscle, progressing from medially to laterally. At the lateral border of the pectoralis major muscle, the breast tissue was swung laterally and dissection progressed under the muscle.

The clavipectoral fascia was then incised along the edge of the pectoralis major and the pectoralis major and minor were freed from surrounding fat and nodal tissue. Dissection progressed first under the pectoralis major and then under the pectoralis minor muscle. The pectoral muscles were retracted medially with a Richardson retractor. The medial pectoral neurovascular bundle was identified and preserved. The level II nodal tissue deep in the pectoralis minor was included in the dissection. The axillary vein was then identified and cleared of overlying fat. The first branch off the axillary vein was clamped, divided, and tied with 2-0 silk ties. The thoracodorsal nerve was then identified deep to the ligated vein and preserved. The long thoracic nerve was then identified along the edge of the latissimus dorsi on the chest wall and preserved. The remaining nodal tissue between these nerves was then carefully removed, taking care to protect the nerves. The specimen, consisting of breast and attached nodal tissue, was then excised by dividing the remaining lateral pedical and sent to pathology.

The wound was irrigated and hemostasis was achieved.

[Choose one:]

If immediate reconstruction: At this point the plastic surgical team took over to perform the reconstruction. A separate operative note will be dictated for that portion of the surgery.

If no immediate reconstruction: A closed suction drain was/ closed suction drains were brought into the operative field through a separate stab incision and sutured to the skin with a 3-0 nylon suture.

The wound was closed with interrupted 3-0 Vicryl to the subcutaneous layer, followed by a subcuticular layer of ___. The wound was dressed.

The patient tolerated the procedure well and was taken to the postanesthesia care unit in stable condition.

NOTES

Chapter 112
Total (Simple) Mastectomy

Michael C. Fraterelli, M.D.

INDICATIONS
- Ductal carcinoma in situ not amenable to breast conservation.
- Prophylaxis of carcinoma in selected high-risk women.

ESSENTIAL STEPS
1. Confirm side of surgery!
2. *Elliptical incision encompassing nipple–areolar complex and biopsy scar/keyhole incision including nipple–areola and small lateral extension.*
3. Raise flaps in avascular plane between subcutaneous tissue and breast tissue:
   - Superiorly to the clavicle.
   - Medially to the sternum.
   - Inferiorly to the anterior rectus sheath.
   - Laterally just beyond the pectoralis major muscle.
4. Remove breast tissue from medial to lateral, including the pectoralis fascia with specimen.
5. Attain hemostasis.
6. Place closed suction drain(s).
7. Close the wound.

NOTE THESE VARIATIONS
- Sentinel node biopsy is done with mastectomy for DCIS.
- Skin-sparing mastectomy (Chap. 113) uses small, specially tailored incisions.

J.J. Hoballah and C.E.H. Scott-Conner (eds.), *Operative Dictations in General and Vascular Surgery*, DOI 10.1007/978-1-4614-0451-4_112,
© Springer Science+Business Media, LLC 2012

- Immediate reconstruction with implants or autogenous tissue.
- Prophylactic mastectomy commonly a bilateral procedure.

COMPLICATIONS
- Recurrence.
- Seroma.
- Nerve injury.
- Skin slough.

TEMPLATE OPERATIVE DICTATION

Preoperative diagnosis: Ductal carcinoma in situ of the *right/left breast/carcinoma prophylaxis* in high-risk women.

Procedure: *Right/left* total mastectomy.

Postoperative diagnosis: Same.

Indications: ***If DCIS:*** *This ___-year-old female/male developed a breast lump/had an abnormal mammogram that on workup with fine needle aspiration cytology/biopsy was found to be ductal carcinoma in situ.* ***If prophylactic mastectomy:*** *This ___-year-old female was known to be at significantly increased risk of breast cancer due to BRCA1/2 mutation/other.* After discussion of alternatives, the patient elected total (simple) mastectomy *with immediate reconstruction.*

Description of procedure: The patient was brought to the operating room and general anesthesia was induced. A time-out was completed verifying correct patient, procedure, site, positioning, and implant(s) and/or special equipment prior to beginning this procedure. The breast, chest wall, axilla, and upper arm and neck were prepped and draped in the usual sterile fashion.

A skin incision was made that encompassed the nipple–areola complex and the previous biopsy scar and passed in a *generally transverse/oblique direction across the breast/other.* Flaps were raised in the avascular plane between subcutaneous tissue and breast tissue from the clavicle superiorly, the sternum medially, the anterior rectus sheath inferiorly, and past the lateral border of the pectoralis major muscle laterally. Hemostasis was achieved in the flaps. Next, the breast tissue and underlying pectoralis fascia were excised from the pectoralis major muscle, progressing from medially to laterally. At the lateral border of the pectoralis major muscle, the breast tissue was swung laterally and a lateral pedicle identified where breast tissue gave way to fat of axilla. The lateral pedicle was incised and the specimen removed.

Add dictation for sentinel node biopsy, if performed (Chap. 110).

The wound was irrigated and hemostasis was achieved.

[Choose one:]

*If **immediate reconstruction:** At this point the plastic surgical team took over to perform the reconstruction. A separate operative note will be dictated for that portion of the surgery.*

*If **no immediate reconstruction:** A closed suction drain was/ closed suction drains were brought into the operative field through a separate stab incision and sutured to the skin with a 3-0 nylon suture. The wound was closed with interrupted 3-0 Vicryl to the sub-cutaneous layer, followed by a subcuticular layer of ___. The wound was dressed.*

The patient tolerated the procedure well and was taken to the postanesthesia care unit in stable condition.

NOTES

Chapter 113
Skin-Sparing Total Mastectomy

Julie Guidroz, M.D.

INDICATIONS

- DCIS not amenable to breast conservation or patient requesting mastectomy, to be followed with reconstruction.
- Breast cancer treatment in select patients, to be followed with reconstruction.
- Prophylaxis of carcinoma in select high-risk patients, to be followed with reconstruction.

ESSENTIAL STEPS

1. Confirm side of surgery!
2. *SLN biopsy if indicated for staging of the axilla.*
3. *Circumareolar skin incision/incision tailored to geometry of tumor.*
4. Develop skin flaps.
5. Dissect breast from chest wall.
6. Hemostasis.
7. Orient specimen for pathology.
8. Irrigate and pack wounds for hemostasis prior to reconstruction.

NOTE THESE VARIATIONS

- Sentinel lymph node biopsy if patient has breast carcinoma.
- Incision is tailored to allow maximum skin salvage but to excise scar from previous biopsy (if needed).

J.J. Hoballah and C.E.H. Scott-Conner (eds.), *Operative Dictations in General and Vascular Surgery*, DOI 10.1007/978-1-4614-0451-4_113,
© Springer Science+Business Media, LLC 2012

- Prophylactic mastectomy is commonly bilateral.
- Nipple-sparing mastectomy being offered in some centers.

COMPLICATIONS
- Recurrence.
- Seroma.
- Nerve injury.
- Skin slough.
- Wound infection.

TEMPLATE OPERATIVE DICTATION

Preoperative diagnosis: *Invasive carcinoma/DCIS/carcinoma prophylaxis* of the *left/right* breast.

Procedure: *Left/right/bilateral* skin-sparing mastectomy.

Postoperative diagnosis: Same.

Indications: If DCIS/invasive carcinoma: This ___-year-old *female/male* with a *left/right breast mass/abnormality on mammogram that on workup with fine needle aspiration/biopsy was found to be ductal carcinoma in situ/invasive carcinoma.* **If prophylactic:** This ___-year-old *female/male was known to be at significantly high risk of breast cancer due to BRCA1/2 mutation/other.* After discussion of options, the patient requested simple mastectomy with immediate reconstruction.

Description of the procedure: After identifying the patient and verifying the operative site, the patient was brought into the operating room. General anesthesia was induced. A time-out was completed verifying correct patient, procedure, site, positioning, and implant(s) and/or special equipment prior to beginning this procedure. All pressure points were appropriately padded. The *left/right/bilateral* breast(s) was/were then prepped and draped in the usual sterile fashion.

If sentinel lymph node biopsy was performed, include details.

A *circumareolar/____* skin incision was made. Skin flaps were developed in the avascular plane using blunt and sharp dissection with Mayo scissors and electrocautery. The breast was then removed from the chest wall using electrocautery, leaving the pectoral fascia when at all possible. Perforating branches of the internal mammary vessels *were/were not* spared. Hemostasis was obtained with electrocautery. The specimen was oriented and submitted whole to Pathology. The wound was irrigated with sterile saline and packed. The operation was then passed on to Plastic Surgery for immediate reconstruction.

NOTES

Chapter 114
Placement of Balloon Catheter for Brachytherapy

Julie Guidroz, M.D.

INDICATION
- Radiation therapy for invasive breast cancer after lumpectomy.

ESSENTIAL STEPS
1. Confirm side of surgery!
2. Familiarize yourself with the specific device to be used.
3. Localize previous biopsy site with ultrasound, measure cavity size.
4. Select appropriate-sized catheter. Test balloon.
5. *Open cavity through previous incision site/percutaneous entry of cavity with ultrasound guidance.*
6. *Excise wall of seroma cavity to create adequate size for balloon. Assure adequate skin margins.*
7. Irrigate wound, assure hemostasis.
8. If percutaneous entry, confirm entry with seroma fluid. Check for purulence.
9. Remove trocar. Do not allow cavity to completely collapse.
10. Close wound from medial and lateral corners leaving space for catheter.
11. Insert catheter. Inflate catheter with diluted water soluble contrast solution. Verify positioning.

J.J. Hoballah and C.E.H. Scott-Conner (eds.), *Operative Dictations in General and Vascular Surgery*, DOI 10.1007/978-1-4614-0451-4_114,
© Springer Science+Business Media, LLC 2012

NOTE THIS VARIATION
- Entry through old incision/ultrasound-guided percutaneous entry.

COMPLICATIONS
- Recurrence.
- Inadequate skin flap size.
- Balloon rupture.
- Improper positioning.

TEMPLATE OPERATIVE DICTATION
Preoperative diagnosis: Invasive carcinoma of the breast.
Procedure: *Left/right* placement of balloon catheter for brachytherapy.
Postoperative diagnosis: Same.
Indications: This ___-year-old *female/male* with invasive ___ carcinoma underwent lumpectomy with sentinel lymph node biopsy *and axillary lymph node dissection* on ____. After discussion of options, the patient requested brachytherapy for radiation therapy to reduce the risk of recurrence.
Description of the procedure: After identifying the patient and verifying the operative site, the patient was brought into the operating room. General anesthesia was induced. All pressure points were appropriately padded. A time-out was completed verifying correct patient, procedure, site, positioning, and implant(s) and/or special equipment prior to beginning this procedure. The *left/right* breast was then prepped and draped in the usual sterile fashion.

[Choose one:]
If open: The previous lumpectomy scar was reopened with a surgical knife. The incision was carried down to the opening of the seroma. The seroma fluid was inspected for signs of infection. Electrocautery was used for hemostasis. To allow room for the device, select areas of the seroma scar were excised. Care was taken to leave sufficient anterior tissue to preserve an adequate skin bridge.

If percutaneous: The ultrasound probe was sterilely draped and used to identify the seroma cavity. An incision site was chosen superiorly/inferiorly/laterally/medially to the lumpectomy scar. The cavity measured ___.

The appropriate-sized balloon catheter device was then chosen. The balloon was tested by inflation with sterile saline. It filled symmetrically and did not leak. It was deflated and set aside.

[Choose one:]

If open: The wound was irrigated with normal saline and hemostasis was obtained with electrocautery. The device was inserted through a separate, lateral stab wound/through the midportion of the incision. Inverted, interrupted simple sutures with 3-0 vicryl were placed on both the lateral and medial portions of the incision. A running 4-0 monocryl subcuticular stitch was advanced from each edge toward the middle of the incision. The balloon was inflated with the recommended mixture of dilute contrast and sterile saline. A total of ____ ml of dilute contrast was instilled.

If percutaneous: Under ultrasound guidance, the trocar was introduced into the seroma cavity. Seroma fluid was obtained, confirming satisfactory entry. The seroma fluid was inspected for signs of infection. The cavity was not allowed to fully collapse. The trocar was removed. The catheter was then inserted and inflated under ultrasound guidance using the recommended mixture of dilute contrast and sterile saline. A total of ___ ml of dilute contrast was instilled. The placement of the catheter was confirmed with ultrasound.

The wound was then dressed with sterile dressings. The patient was then extubated in the operating room and taken to recovery in stable condition. The patient tolerated the procedure well and without complication.

NOTES

Section **XI**

Lymph Nodes

Chapter 115

Sentinel Node Biopsy for Melanoma

Michael Bonebrake, M.D.

INDICATIONS

- Thin melanoma with *ulceration/involved deep margin/other high-risk features*.
- Intermediate thickness melanoma with clinically negative nodes.
- Thick melanoma with clinically negative nodes.

ESSENTIAL STEPS

1. Inject radioisotope (Tc-99 sulfur colloid) intradermally, circumferentially around the lesion or site of excision.
2. Obtain lymphoscintogram.
3. Three to four hours later, take the patient to the operating room.
4. Inject 1–3 mL of isosulfan blue intradermally and gently massage.
5. Use hand-held gamma probe to identify the node and make an incision over that spot.
6. Orient the incision so it can be easily incorporated into a lymphadenectomy incision if necessary.
7. Record counts for 10 s over the node before and after the incision, as well as the excised node and the bed from which it was excised.
8. Before removing the node, check for blue dye.
9. Identify blue lymphatic channels and follow to other nodes.

J.J. Hoballah and C.E.H. Scott-Conner (eds.), *Operative Dictations in General and Vascular Surgery*, DOI 10.1007/978-1-4614-0451-4_115,
© Springer Science+Business Media, LLC 2012

10. Remove any grossly abnormal nodes.
11. Close the incision.
12. *Perform wide local excision if not previously done.*

NOTE THESE VARIATIONS
- Amount of isotope, use of isosulfan blue dye.
- More than one node may be identified.
- Isotope may localize to more than one nodal basin.
- Wide local excision (Chap. 117) may be done during this procedure.

COMPLICATIONS
- Failure to identify sentinel node.
- Recurrence.

TEMPLATE OPERATIVE DICTATION
Preoperative diagnosis: Melanoma of ___.
Procedure: Sentinel node biopsy *and wide local excision of melanoma.*
Postoperative diagnosis: Same.
Indications: This ___-year-old *male/female* has *Clark's level___/ Breslow level* ___ melanoma of the ___ (specify location) diagnosed on *punch/incisional/excisional biopsy.* Sentinel node biopsy and wide local excision were indicated for evaluation and management.
Description of procedure: In the nuclear medicine suite, the skin surrounding the lesion was injected with Tc-99 sulfur colloid. *Three/four* hours later, the patient and lymphoscintograms were taken to the operating room and general anesthesia was induced. A time-out was completed verifying correct patient, procedure, site, positioning, and implant(s) and/or special equipment prior to beginning this procedure.

The four quadrants of the skin overlying the *melanoma/biopsy* site was injected intradermally with 4 mL of isosulfan blue dye prior to the start of the procedure. This was gently massaged for several minutes. The skin overlying *the right/left axilla/inguinal region* was prepped and draped in the usual sterile fashion.

A hand-held gamma probe was used to identify the location of the hottest spot in the nodal basin. Prior to the incision, the counts were ___. An incision was made and a *blue* node was identified. The probe was placed in contact with the node and ___ counts were recorded. The node was excised in its entirety. Ex vivo, the node measured ___ counts when placed on the probe. The bed of the node measured ___ counts. *No additional/an additional* hot spot was detected. *If additional hot spot*: A second blue node was identified and the following counts registered: ___ prior to excision, ___ ex vivo node, and ___ residual bed. No additional hot spots or blue lymphatics were identified. No clinically abnormal nodes were palpated. The procedure was terminated. Hemostasis was achieved and the wound closed in layers with interrupted 3-0 Vicryl and *skin staples/subcuticular suture/other*.

If wide local excision: *Attention was then turned to the primary site. The patient was repositioned (specify). The region around the primary tumor was prepped and draped in the usual sterile fashion. An elliptical incision was made around the melanoma/biopsy site approximately 2 cm on either side. This incision was deepened to the fascia overlying the muscle. Skin and subcutaneous tissues were removed. Hemostasis was achieved, (if necessary) flaps were raised at the fascial level, and the wound was closed with interrupted 3-0 Vicryl and skin staples/a subcuticular closure/other.*

The patient tolerated the procedure well and was taken to the postanesthesia care unit in stable condition.

ACKNOWLEDGMENT

This chapter was contributed by Mazen M. Hashisho, MD in the first edition.

NOTES

Chapter 116
Superficial Inguinal Lymph Node Dissection

Michael Bonebrake, M.D.

INDICATIONS

- Clinical involvement of inguinal nodes from: melanoma, squamous carcinoma of the anus, carcinoma of the vulva, scrotum, penis, or distal urethra.
- Positive sentinel lymph node biopsy, in the absence of distant metastasis.
- Palliative dissection for control of symptomatic nodal disease.

ESSENTIAL STEPS

1. Oblique/transverse incision.
2. Raise flaps.
3. Identify the femoral vessels.
4. Reflect the lymph nodes off the femoral vessels.
5. Ligate/clip tributaries as they are encountered.
6. Divide and ligate the greater saphenous vein distally.
7. Suture ligate the greater saphenous vein at the fossa ovalis.
8. Identify the inguinal ligament and detach the specimen.
9. Seek Cloquet's node.
10. Check hemostasis.
11. Detach the sartorius muscle and swing medially to cover the defect over the femoral vessels.
12. Secure the sartorius to the external oblique fascia with interrupted 3-0 Vicryl horizontal mattress sutures.
13. Place closed suction drains adjacent to the sartorius.

J.J. Hoballah and C.E.H. Scott-Conner (eds.), *Operative Dictations in General and Vascular Surgery*, DOI 10.1007/978-1-4614-0451-4_116,
© Springer Science+Business Media, LLC 2012

14. Approximate subcutaneous tissues with interrupted 3-0 Vicryl.
15. Close the skin with a subcuticular stitch/staples/other.
16. Apply dressing and compressive Ace bandage to the leg.

NOTE THESE VARIATIONS
- Incision.
- Preservation of the greater saphenous vein.
- Deep dissection may be added if Cloquet's node is positive.

COMPLICATIONS
- Wound breakdown.
- Lymphocele.
- Lymphedema.
- Recurrence.

TEMPLATE OPERATIVE DICTATION

Preoperative diagnosis: Malignant *melanoma/other* metastatic to inguinal nodes.

Procedure: *Right/left* superficial inguinal lymph node dissection.

Postoperative diagnosis: Same.

Indications: This ___-year-old *male/female* was initially diagnosed with malignant *melanoma/other. Fine needle aspiration cytology of palpable node/sentinel lymph node biopsy was positive for metastatic melanoma/other.* Superficial inguinal node dissection was indicated for management.

Description of the procedure: The patient was brought to the operating room and general anesthesia was induced. Preoperative antibiotics were administered. The *right/left* lower extremity was prepped and draped circumferentially in the usual sterile fashion. A time-out was completed verifying correct patient, procedure, site, positioning, and implant(s) and/or special equipment prior to beginning this procedure.

The junction of the sartorius and adductor longus was palpated inferiorly and the middle of the inguinal ligament was palpated superiorly. A thin crescent of skin was then incised, connecting these two points. (Alternatively: *A vertical incision centered over the femoral triangle was made, incorporating a 3–4 cm ellipse of skin over the femoral triangle.*) The subcutaneous tissues were carefully dissected using electrocautery. Flaps were raised from the skin edges deep to Scarpa's fascia to the adductor longus and sartorius muscles. The saphenous vein was identified at the junction of the sartorius and adductor muscles inferiorly, clamped, divided, and ligated. Flaps were raised superiorly to the inguinal ligament, and medial to the pubic tubercle. The *spermatic cord/round ligament* was identified and preserved. The femoral nerve, artery, and vein were identified within the femoral triangle. The lymph nodes were then reflected superiorly off the femoral vessels. Perforating arteries and veins were *ligated using 2-0 and 3-0 silk ties/clipped*. The saphenofemoral junction was then identified within the specimen. The greater saphenous vein was clamped using a pediatric Pott's vascular clamp. The greater saphenous vein was then divided and suture ligated. The dissection was continued superiorly to dissect the lymph nodes off the femoral vessels. The inguinal ligament was then identified and the specimen was completely separated from the vessels and passed off.

The femoral canal was carefully dissected and explored and *Cloquet's node/no node* was identified. The femoral canal was then closed with a figure-of-eight nonabsorbable suture, with care taken not to occlude the femoral vein. *If sartorius flap is performed:* The sartorius muscle was then divided in its superior aspect. It was transposed medially over the vessels and secured to the fascia of the external oblique using 3-0 Vicryl horizontal mattress sutures. The wound was carefully irrigated. There was no evidence of bleeding. Two closed suction drains were placed within the femoral triangle on each side of the sartorius muscle. The subcutaneous tissues were carefully approximated using interrupted 3-0 Vicryl sutures. The skin was closed with *staples/a subcuticular suture/other*. The wound was dressed with sterile gauze and Kerlix wrap. A compressive Ace bandage was applied circumferentially from the toes to the top of the left leg.

The patient tolerated the procedure well and was taken to the postanesthesia care unit in stable condition.

ACKNOWLEDGMENT

This chapter was contributed by Mazen M. Hashisho, MD in the first edition.

NOTES

Chapter 117
Excision of Melanoma

Michael Bonebrake, M.D.

INDICATION
- Incompletely excised melanoma.

ESSENTIAL STEPS
1. Measure desired margin around the lesion.
2. Orient incision in skin line or directed toward the draining lymph nodes.
3. Excise down to fascia.
4. Elevate flaps to facilitate closure.
5. Orient the specimen.
6. Hemostasis.
7. Close.

NOTE THESE VARIATIONS
- Choice of anesthesia.
- Width of margin varies.
- Fascia not always excised.
- May be combined with sentinel node biopsy (Chap. 115).

COMPLICATION
- Recurrence.

J.J. Hoballah and C.E.H. Scott-Conner (eds.), *Operative Dictations in General and Vascular Surgery*, DOI 10.1007/978-1-4614-0451-4_117,
© Springer Science+Business Media, LLC 2012

TEMPLATE OPERATIVE DICTATION

Preoperative diagnosis: *Clark's level/Breslow depth* ___ melanoma of *(location)*, inadequately excised.

Procedure: Wide local excision of melanoma.

Postoperative diagnosis: Same.

Indications: This ___-year-old *male/female* had a pigmented lesion of *(location) biopsied/excised with narrow margins*. Pathology returned *Clark's level/Breslow* depth ___ melanoma. Reexcision was indicated for local control.

Description of procedure: The patient was brought to the *operating room/minor surgery suite and general/regional anesthesia was induced*.

The region around the melanoma was prepped and draped in the usual sterile fashion. A time-out was completed verifying correct patient, procedure, site, positioning, and implant(s) and/or special equipment prior to beginning this procedure.

If sentinel node biopsy: Node biopsy performed before excision.

If local anesthesia: One percent xylocaine without epinephrine (or 50:50 mixture of 1% xylocaine and 0.25–0.5% bupivacaine) was used to infiltrate the region of the proposed incision. The lesion itself was not injected.

An elliptical incision was made around the *melanoma/biopsy site* approximately 1–2*(specify)* cm on all sides. This incision was deepened to the fascia overlying the muscle. Skin and subcutaneous tissues were removed. *The fascia was excised with the specimen.* The specimen was then oriented *with clips/silk suture with a long lateral and short superior stitch.*

Hemostasis was achieved *(if necessary)*, flaps were raised at the fascial level, and the wound was closed with a deep layer of interrupted 3-0 Vicryl and *skin staples/a subcuticular closure/nylon mattress sutures.*

The patient tolerated the procedure well and was taken to the postanesthesia care unit in stable condition. There were no immediate complications.

ACKNOWLEDGMENT

This chapter was contributed by Mazen M. Hashisho, MD in the first edition.

NOTES

Chapter 118

Inguinal and Pelvic Lymphadenectomy (Superficial and Deep Groin Dissection)

Hisakazu Hoshi, M.D.

INDICATIONS

- Metastatic melanoma, carcinoma.
- Positive sentinel node biopsy.

ESSENTIAL STEPS

1. Curvilinear incision crossing the inguinal ligament *(Option: Combined incisions transverse incision above inguinal crease and longitudinal incision in femoral triangle)*.
2. Flaps to expose the femoral triangle and aponeurosis of the external oblique.
3. Identify and preserve the spermatic cord in males.
4. Incise fascia overlying the lateral border of the adductor longus muscle to the crossing of the sartorius.
5. Sweep the nodal tissue medially.
6. Ligate and divide the saphenous vein at the apex of the femoral triangle *(Option: preservation of the greater saphenous vein)*.
7. Incise fascia overlying the sartorius and sweep the nodal tissue off.
8. Clean anterior surfaces of the femoral vessels.
9. Ligate and divide the saphenous vein at the saphenofemoral junction *(Option: preservation of saphenofemoral junction)*.
10. Identify and preserve the branches of the femoral nerve.

J.J. Hoballah and C.E.H. Scott-Conner (eds.), *Operative Dictations in General and Vascular Surgery*, DOI 10.1007/978-1-4614-0451-4_118,
© Springer Science+Business Media, LLC 2012

11. *If pelvic dissection*:
    - *Detach the inguinal ligament from the anterior superior iliac spine and reflect medially/second fascial incision through the inguinal region.*
    - *Dissect the nodal tissue along the external and common femoral vessels and obturator nerve, preserving the nerve, vessels, and ureter.*
12. Hemostasis.
13. Reconstruct inguinal ligament.
14. Transpose the sartorius muscle medially.
15. Place closed suction drains.
16. Close the incision.

NOTE THESE VARIATIONS
- Choice of anesthesia.
- Orientation of incision.
- Inclusion of pelvic dissection; fascial incision.

COMPLICATIONS
- Lymphocele.
- Necrosis of flaps.
- Lymphedema.
- Recurrence.
- Wound infection femoral artery blowout.

TEMPLATE OPERATIVE DICTATION
Preoperative diagnosis: *Metastatic melanoma/carcinoma/positive sentinel node biopsy.*
Procedure: *Inguinal/pelvic lymphadenectomy (Superficial and deep groin dissection) with sartorius muscular flap.*
Postoperative diagnosis: Same.
Indications: This ___-year-old *male/female* with *melanoma/carcinoma of the (detail site)* metastatic to the inguinal nodes required lymphadenectomy for management.
Description of procedure: The patient was brought to the operating room and *general/regional* anesthesia was induced. The right/left groin was prepped and draped in the usual sterile fashion. A time-out was completed verifying correct patient, procedure, site, positioning, and implant(s) and/or special equipment prior to beginning this procedure. *A curvilinear incision was made crossing the inguinal ligament/A longitudinal incision was made in the center portion of femoral triangle and an additional transverse lower abdominal incision was made just above the inguinal crease to avoid*

incision over the inguinal area. Flaps were developed to expose the aponeurosis of the external oblique 5 cm above the inguinal ligament and the femoral triangle. Dissection commenced at the adductor longus muscle just below the inguinal ligament. The fascia of the adductor muscle was incised and fatty and areolar tissue swept medially. *At the apex of the femoral triangle, the greater saphenous vein was doubly ligated with 2-0 silk and divided/The greater saphenous vein was identified, dissected along the entire course up to saphenofemoral junction and preserved.* Dissection then proceeded cephalad up the sartorius muscle by *incising/leaving* investing fascia. The femoral artery and vein were then identified at the apex of the femoral triangle. Dissection on the anterior surface of the femoral vessels was performed toward the inguinal ligament. Areolar and fatty node-bearing tissue was reflected from the vessels proceeding cephalad. The femoral nerve and its branches were identified and protected. *The saphenous vein was identified entering the femoral vein and ligated and divided/The branches of saphenofemoral junction except the greater saphenous vein were ligated and divided.* Soft tissue covering the lower abdominal wall groin area was dissected from the abdominal wall. Remaining attachments were divided and the specimen removed.

If pelvic dissection: *The inguinal ligament was divided from the anterior superior iliac spine and reflected medially then abdominal wall was divided cephalad/an incision was made through the aponeurosis of the external oblique, the internal oblique, and transversus to expose the retroperitoneum. The ureter was seen on the surface of retracted abdominal contents. The dissection started lateral to the iliac vessels and lateral femoral cutaneous nerve was identified and preserved. Soft tissue was dissected off from the common and the external iliac vessels lateral to medial and cephalad to caudad fashion. The internal iliac vessels were exposed and soft tissue between the internal and the external vessels was dissected away from obturator nerve. The specimen was removed en bloc. The inguinal ligament was approximated with interrupted 2-0 PDS/the abdominal wall incision was closed in layers with running 2-0 PDS.*

Hemostasis was checked. The sartorius muscle was detached from its origin from the anterior superior iliac spine and transposed medially. It was brought to lie over the femoral vessels and secured in place with interrupted 3-0 Vicryl. Closed suction drains were placed under the flaps and brought out through separate stab wounds.

The wound was closed with interrupted 3-0 Vicryl and *skin staples/a subcuticular closure/other.*

The patient tolerated the procedure well and was taken to the postanesthesia care unit in stable condition.

NOTES

Section XII
Head and Neck

Chapter 119
Superficial Parotidectomy

Carol E.H. Scott-Conner, M.D.

INDICATIONS

- Tumor of the superficial lobe of the parotid gland.
- *(Rarely, done as part of lymphadenectomy for melanoma.)*

ESSENTIAL STEPS

1. General anesthesia, head turned, cotton wad in ear, corner of mouth, and eyelid draped into field.
2. Y-shaped incision, with extension posterior to the tragus.
3. Develop flaps deep to the platysma and superficial to the parotid (anterior and inferior to the margin of the parotid gland, cephalad to the zygomatic process, and posterior to the sternocleidomastoid muscle).
4. Identify the great auricular nerve and divide the branch that enters the parotid gland.
5. Identify and ligate the external jugular vein just posterior to the parotid gland.
6. Expose the anterior border of the sternocleidomastoid muscle and develop the plane between the muscle and the mastoid.
7. Divide the temporoparotid fascia.
8. Identify the main trunk of the facial nerve *(a small branch of the posterior auricular artery may be encountered and divided)*.
9. Apply traction to the superficial lobe of the parotid gland.

J.J. Hoballah and C.E.H. Scott-Conner (eds.), *Operative Dictations in General and Vascular Surgery*, DOI 10.1007/978-1-4614-0451-4_119,
© Springer Science+Business Media, LLC 2012

10. Dissect in the plane between the parotid gland and facial nerve branches, tracing, and preserving each branch of the facial nerve.
11. Identify and ligate Stensen's duct with absorbable sutures.
12. Remove the superficial lobe.
13. Achieve hemostasis with fine ligatures; avoid use of electocautery close to the nerve.
14. Close with drainage.

NOTE THESE VARIATIONS

- Dissection under the facial nerve and removal of part of the deep lobe.
- Sacrifice of the facial nerve branch with nerve graft reconstruction.
- Use of nerve stimulator

COMPLICATIONS

- Salivary fistula.
- Injury to the facial nerve.
- Gustatory sweating (Frey's syndrome).

TEMPLATE OPERATIVE DICTATION

Preoperative diagnosis: Tumor of the superficial lobe of the *right/left* parotid gland.

Procedure: *Right/left* superficial parotidectomy.

Postoperative diagnosis: Same *with component involving deep lobe*.

Indications: This ___-year-old *male/female* developed a swelling anterior to the *right/left* ear consistent with a parotid tumor on *clinical examination/ultrasound/fine needle aspiration cytology*. Decision was made to proceed with surgical excision.

Description of procedure: The patient was positioned supine with the head turned to the *right/left* side. A time-out was completed verifying correct patient, procedure, site, positioning, and implant(s) and/or special equipment prior to beginning this procedure. A ball of sterile cotton was placed in the external auditory meatus. The field was prepped in the usual fashion and draped so as to include the corner of the mouth and the lateral canthus of the eye. A Y-shaped incision was made in a natural skin crease just anterior to the tragus, progressing inferiorly along a line parallel to the sternocleidomastoid muscle and terminating just below the angle of the mandible with a short extension beneath the tragus to the mastoid process. The incision was deepened through the platysma muscle and hemostasis achieved with electrocautery.

A flap was raised between the anterior surface of the parotid gland and the platysma muscle, taking care not to injure the peripheral branches of the facial nerve, until the medial and inferior borders of the parotid gland were reached. Superiorly the flap was elevated to the zygomatic process and posteriorly the sternocleidomastoid muscle, the mastoid process, and the cartilage of the external auditory canal were exposed.

The great auricular nerve was identified and a small branch entering the substance of the parotid gland was divided sharply. The external jugular vein was identified, doubly ligated with 2-0 silk, and divided.

Dissection then progressed cephalad along the anterior border of the sternocleidomastoid muscle to expose the anterior surface of the mastoid. The temporoparotid fascia was divided and the main trunk of the facial nerve identified.

The main trunk of the facial nerve was traced into the parotid gland and the main branches identified. The superficial lobe of the parotid gland was elevated and dissected free of these branches, removing the tumor completely. Care was taken throughout to avoid injury to the branches of the facial nerve. Stensen's duct was identified and ligated with 2-0 Vicryl and divided. The gland was removed. Hemostasis was achieved with fine ligatures of 4-0 silk.

The facial nerve branches were identified and noted to be intact.

A *closed suction/small Penrose* drain was placed.

The operative field was closed with interrupted 3-0 Vicryl sutures and a running subcuticular suture of 4-0 monocryl.

The patient tolerated the procedure well and was taken to the postanesthesia care unit in stable condition.

NOTES

Chapter 120
Thyroid Lobectomy

Joshua R. French, M.D., and James Howe, M.D.

INDICATIONS

- Enlarging or suspicious thyroid nodule.
- Follicular neoplasm on FNA.
- Toxic nodule.

ESSENTIAL STEPS

1. Develop subplatysmal flaps.
2. Divide the strap muscles in the midline.
3. Ligate and divide the middle thyroid vein.
4. Preserve the external branch of the superior laryngeal nerve.
5. Ligate and divide the superior pole vessels.
6. Mobilize the inferior pole of the thyroid.
7. Identify and preserve the recurrent laryngeal nerve.
8. Divide the inferior thyroid artery and branches distally.
9. Identify and preserve the superior and inferior parathyroid glands.
10. Dissect the thyroid free of the trachea.
11. Divide the thyroid lobe at the isthmus.

NOTE THESE VARIATIONS

- Division of the strap muscles.
- Division of isthmus prior to thyroid dissection.
- Superior pole dissection prior to division of the middle thyroid vein.

J.J. Hoballah and C.E.H. Scott-Conner (eds.), *Operative Dictations in General and Vascular Surgery*, DOI 10.1007/978-1-4614-0451-4_120,
© Springer Science+Business Media, LLC 2012

- Intraoperative recurrent laryngeal nerve monitoring.
- Drain placement.

COMPLICATIONS
- Post-op bleeding, resulting in tracheal compression and airway obstruction.
- Recurrent laryngeal nerve injury.
- Injury to the external branch of the superior laryngeal nerve.
- Hypocalcemia.
- Hypothyroidism.

TEMPLATE OF OPERATIVE DICTATION
Preoperative diagnosis: *Follicular neoplasm/enlarging or suspicious thyroid nodule.*
Procedure: *Right/left* thyroid lobectomy.
Postoperative diagnosis: Same.
Indications: This ___-year-old *male/female* was noted to have a thyroid nodule. On work-up, it was *enlarging/suspicious/a follicular neoplasm on FNA/a toxic nodule.* Thyroid lobectomy is indicated.
Description of procedure: Following induction of general anesthesia, both arms were tucked at the sides and all bony prominences were padded. A roll was placed under the shoulders and the patient was positioned in a modified beach chair position with the neck extended. The neck was prepped and draped in a sterile fashion. A time-out was completed verifying correct patient, procedure, site, positioning, and implant(s) and/or special equipment prior to beginning this procedure.

A ___-cm incision was made in a skin crease positioned approximately two fingerbreadths superior to the sternal notch. The subcutaneous tissues and platysma were divided with electrocautery. Subplatysmal flaps were then raised inferiorly extending to the sternal notch and superiorly extending to the thyroid cartilage. The strap muscles were divided in the midline and retracted laterally.

The *right/left* thyroid lobe was mobilized from its areolar attachments using blunt dissection and electrocautery. The thyroid was gently retracted medially and the middle thyroid vein was identified. It was ligated with 3-0 silk sutures and divided. The thyroid was then gently retracted inferiomedially. The superior pole vessels were ligated with 3-0 silk sutures and divided, with careful attention not to injure the external branch of the superior laryngeal nerve. Attention was turned to the mobilization of the inferior pole using blunt dissection. The vessels in this area were ligated with 3-0 silk sutures and divided.

Next, the thyroid was gently retracted medially and the muscles retracted laterally. The inferior thyroid artery was identified. Using blunt dissection, the recurrent laryngeal nerve was identified and followed superficially along its path to aid in continued safe dissection. The vessels to the thyroid in this vicinity were ligated with 3-0 silk ties and divided with great care to avoid injury to the recurrent laryngeal nerve and to preserve their distal branches. The superior and inferior parathyroid glands were identified and carefully mobilized off of the thyroid gland to preserve their blood supply.

Once the recurrent laryngeal nerve and parathyroid glands were safely dissected free, the thyroid was dissected medially from its attachments to the trachea at the ligament of Berry using electrocautery. Dissection was extended to the isthmus, which was clamped with Kelly clamps, divided, and suture ligated with a 2-0 silk stitch. The specimen was marked with a suture at the superior pole for orientation and handed off to be sent to pathology.

The wound was copiously irrigated and hemostasis was achieved. The strap muscles were reapproximated with interrupted 3-0 Vicryl sutures. The platysma was reapproximated with interrupted 3-0 Vicryl sutures. Approximately 10 cc of 0.25% marcaine was injected subcutaneously. The skin was reapproximated with a running 4-0 Monocryl subcuticular suture. Steri-Strips were placed over the incision and a sterile dressing was applied. The patient tolerated the procedure well and was extubated and taken to the postanesthesia care unit in stable condition.

ACKNOWLEDGMENT

This chapter was contributed by Michael C. Fraterelli, MD in the first edition.

NOTES

Chapter 121
Total Thyroidectomy

Joshua R. French, M.D. and James Howe, M.D.

INDICATIONS

- Thyroid cancer.
- MEN 2A/2B.
- Symptomatic multinodular goiter.
- Grave's disease.

ESSENTIAL STEPS

1. Develop subplatysmal flaps.
2. Divide the strap muscles in the midline.
3. Ligate and divide the middle thyroid vein.
4. Preserve the external branch of the superior laryngeal nerve.
5. Ligate and divide the superior pole vessels.
6. Mobilize the inferior pole of the thyroid.
7. Identify and preserve the recurrent laryngeal nerve.
8. Divide the inferior thyroid artery and branches distally.
9. Identify and preserve the superior and inferior parathyroid glands.
10. Dissect the thyroid from the trachea to the level of the isthmus.
11. Repeat steps 3–9 on the opposite side.
12. Dissect the thyroid free of the trachea.

J.J. Hoballah and C.E.H. Scott-Conner (eds.), *Operative Dictations in General and Vascular Surgery*, DOI 10.1007/978-1-4614-0451-4_121,
© Springer Science+Business Media, LLC 2012

NOTE THESE VARIATIONS
- Division of the strap muscles.
- Division of isthmus prior to thyroid dissection.
- Superior pole dissection prior to division of the middle thyroid vein.
- Intraoperative recurrent laryngeal nerve monitoring.
- Drain placement.
- Reimplantation of a parathyroid gland.
- Central neck dissection.

COMPLICATIONS
- Post-op bleeding, resulting in tracheal compression and airway obstruction.
- Recurrent laryngeal nerve injury.
- Injury to the external branch of the superior laryngeal nerve.
- Hypocalcemia.

TEMPLATE OF OPERATIVE DICTATION
Preoperative diagnosis: *Thyroid cancer/MEN 2/symptomatic multinodular goiter/Grave's disease*.
Procedure: Total thyroidectomy.
Postoperative diagnosis: Same.
Indications: This ___-year-old *male/female* was noted to have *a thyroid cancer on FNA/familial MEN 2/symptomatic multinodular goiter/Grave's disease* on work-up. Total thyroidectomy is indicated.
Description of procedure: Following induction of general anesthesia, both arms were tucked at the sides and all bony prominences were padded. A roll was placed under the shoulders and the patient was positioned in a modified beach chair position with the neck extended. The neck was prepped and draped in a sterile fashion. A time-out was completed verifying correct patient, procedure, site, positioning, and implant(s) and/or special equipment prior to beginning this procedure.

A ___-cm incision was made in a skin crease positioned approximately two fingerbreadths superior to the sternal notch. The subcutaneous tissues and platysma were divided with electrocautery. Subplatysmal flaps were then raised inferiorly extending to the sternal notch and superiorly extending to the thyroid cartilage. The strap muscles were divided in the midline and retracted laterally.

The right thyroid lobe was mobilized from its areolar attachments using blunt dissection and electrocautery. The thyroid was gently retracted medially and the middle thyroid vein was identified. It was ligated with 3-0 silk sutures and divided. The thyroid was then gently retracted inferiomedially. The superior pole vessels were ligated with 3-0 silk sutures and divided, with careful attention not to injure the external branch of the superior laryngeal nerve. Attention was turned to mobilization of the inferior pole using blunt dissection. The vessels in this area were ligated with 3-0 silk sutures and divided.

Next, the thyroid was gently retracted medially and the muscles retracted laterally. The inferior thyroid artery was identified. Using blunt dissection, the right recurrent laryngeal nerve was identified and followed superficially along its path to aid in continued safe dissection. The vessels to the thyroid in this vicinity were ligated with 3-0 silk ties and divided with great care to avoid injury to the recurrent laryngeal nerve and to preserve their distal branches. The right superior and inferior parathyroid glands were identified and carefully mobilized off of the thyroid gland to preserve their blood supply. Once the recurrent laryngeal nerve and parathyroid glands were safely dissected free, the thyroid was dissected medially from its attachments to the trachea at the ligament of Berry using electrocautery. Dissection was extended to the isthmus.

If a pyramidal lobe is identified: *The pyramidal lobe was identified. It was dissected free circumferentially of its attachments to the thyroid cartilage. It was then reflected inferiorly down to the isthmus.*

A similar procedure was then carried out on the left. The left recurrent laryngeal nerve was identified and carefully followed superficially along its course superiorly to ensure it was not injured. The left superior and inferior parathyroid glands were identified and preserved. Dissection was extended to the isthmus, dissecting the thyroid free from the trachea. The specimen was marked with a suture at the right superior pole for orientation and handed off to be sent to pathology.

If a central neck dissection is performed: *A Level VI lymph node dissection was performed by removing the lymphatic tissue in the central neck, extending laterally to the carotid sheath, inferiorly to the sternal notch, and superiorly to the hyoid bone. The specimen was sent to pathology.*

If any parathyroids were reimplanted: *The right/left superior/inferior parathyroid gland was divided into multiple 1-mm sections using a scalpel. Using blunt dissection, two pockets were made in the belly of right/left sternocleidomastoid muscle. Several pieces of parathyroid tissue were place in each pocket. A 4-0 Prolene suture was used to close each pocket and marked with a clip.*

The wound was copiously irrigated and hemostasis was achieved. The strap muscles were reapproximated with interrupted 3-0 Vicryl sutures. The platysma was reapproximated with interrupted 3-0 Vicryl sutures. Approximately 10 cc of 0.25% marcaine was injected subcutaneously. The skin was reapproximated with a running 4-0 Monocryl subcuticular suture. Steri-Strips were placed over the incision and a sterile dressing was applied. The patient tolerated the procedure well and was extubated and taken to the postanesthesia care unit in stable condition.

ACKNOWLEDGMENT

This chapter was contributed by Michael C. Fraterelli, MD in the first edition.

NOTES

Chapter 122
Parathyroidectomy for Adenoma

Joshua R. French, M.D. and James Howe, M.D.

INDICATION
- Parathyroid adenoma.

ESSENTIAL STEPS
1. Develop subplatysmal flaps and divide the strap muscles in the midline.
2. Draw baseline PTH level.
3. Identify and excise the abnormal parathyroid gland.
4. Draw a post-excision PTH level.
5. Verify adequate drop in PTH level.

NOTE THESE VARIATIONS
- PTH drawn from internal jugular vein, peripheral vein, or arterial line.
- Four gland exploration.

COMPLICATIONS
- Hypocalcemia.
- Recurrent laryngeal nerve injury.
- Post-op bleeding, resulting in tracheal compression, and airway obstruction.

J.J. Hoballah and C.E.H. Scott-Conner (eds.), *Operative Dictations in General and Vascular Surgery*, DOI 10.1007/978-1-4614-0451-4_122,
© Springer Science+Business Media, LLC 2012

TEMPLATE OF OPERATIVE DICTATION

Preoperative diagnosis: Parathyroid adenoma.

Procedure: *Right/left superior/inferior* parathyroidectomy with intraoperative PTH.

Postoperative diagnosis: Same.

Indications: This ___-year-old *male/female* was noted to have a parathyroid adenoma on work-up for hypercalcemia. Preoperative studies localized the gland to the *right/left superior/inferior* gland. Parathyroidectomy is indicated.

Description of procedure: Following smooth induction of general anesthesia, both arms were tucked at the sides and all bony prominences were padded. A soft roll was placed under the shoulders and the patient was positioned in a modified beach chair position with the neck extended. The neck and upper chest were prepped and draped in a sterile fashion. A time-out was completed verifying correct patient, procedure, site, positioning, and implant(s) and/or special equipment prior to beginning this procedure. Baseline PTH level was drawn from an IV in the patient's arm.

A ___-cm incision was made in a skin crease positioned approximately two fingerbreadths superior to the sternal notch. The subcutaneous tissues and platysma were divided with electrocautery. Subplatysmal flaps were developed. The strap muscles were divided in the midline and retracted laterally.

The *right/left* thyroid lobe was rotated medially. The loose areolar attachments were dissected bluntly and using electrocautery. An abnormal appearing *right/left superior/inferior* parathyroid gland was noted (*describe location of the gland*). The gland was gently dissected from the surrounding tissues down to its pedicle. The pedicle of the parathyroid gland was clamped and tied with a 3-0 silk suture. The parathyroid gland was excised and sent to pathology. Another PTH level was drawn 10-min post-excision.

Pathology from the gland returned consistent with hypercellular parathyroid and the gland weighed ___-mg. The baseline PTH was (*note value*). The 10-min post-excision PTH was (*note value*). This constituted a (*note percentage*) percent drop from baseline.

If the drop in the PTH was inadequate: The right/left thyroid was retracted medially and exploration was continued inferiorly/superiorly. An abnormal appearing right/left superior/inferior parathyroid gland was noted (describe location of the gland). The gland was gently dissected from the surrounding tissues down to its pedicle. The pedicle of the parathyroid gland was clamped and tied with a 3-0 silk suture. The parathyroid gland was excised and sent to pathology. Another PTH level was drawn 10-min post-excision of

this gland. Pathology from the gland returned consistent with hyper-
cellular parathyroid. Post-excision PTH was (note value), constitut-
ing a (note percentage) percent drop from baseline.

The wound was copiously irrigated and hemostasis was achieved. The strap muscles were reapproximated with interrupted 3-0 Vicryl sutures. The platysma was reapproximated with interrupted 3-0 Vicryl sutures. Approximately 10 cc of 0.25% marcaine was injected subcutaneously. The skin was reapproximated with a running 4-0 Monocryl subcuticular suture. Steri-Strips were placed over the incision and a sterile dressing was applied. The patient tolerated the procedure well and was extubated and taken to the postanesthesia care unit in stable condition.

ACKNOWLEDGMENT

This chapter was contributed by Andrew A. Fedder, MD in the first edition.

NOTES

Chapter 123
Radioisotope-Guided Parathyroidectomy

Joshua R. French, M.D. and James Howe, M.D.

INDICATIONS
- Primary hyperparathyroidism.
- Neck reexploration for primary hyperparathyroidism.
- Persistent hyperparathyroidism.

ESSENTIAL STEPS
1. Nuclear medicine injection of ^{99m}TcMIBI 15–30 min prior to surgery.
2. Use the gamma probe transcutaneously to plan incision.
3. Develop subplatysmal flaps and divide the strap muscles in the midline.
4. Draw baseline PTH level.
5. Use gamma probe to help identify and excise the abnormal parathyroid gland.
6. Obtain ex vivo and background counts.
7. Draw a post-excision PTH level.
8. Verify adequate drop in PTH level.

NOTE THIS VARIATION
- PTH drawn from internal jugular vein, peripheral vein, or arterial line.

J.J. Hoballah and C.E.H. Scott-Conner (eds.), *Operative Dictations in General and Vascular Surgery*, DOI 10.1007/978-1-4614-0451-4_123,
© Springer Science+Business Media, LLC 2012

COMPLICATIONS

- Hypocalcemia.
- Recurrent laryngeal nerve injury.
- Post-op bleeding, resulting in tracheal compression, and airway obstruction.

TEMPLATE OF OPERATIVE DICTATION

Preoperative diagnosis: *Parathyroid adenoma/persistent hyperparathyroidism*.

Procedure: Radioisotope-guided *right/left superior/inferior* parathyroidectomy with intraoperative PTH.

Postoperative diagnosis: Same.

Indications: This ___-year-old *male/female* was noted to have a *parathyroid adenoma/persistent hyperparathyroidism* on work-up for hypercalcemia. Pre-operative studies localized the gland to _____. Radioisotope-guided parathyroidectomy is indicated.

Description of procedure: Prior to surgery, nuclear medicine injection of ^{99m}TcMIBI was performed. Following smooth induction of general anesthesia, both arms were tucked at the sides and all bony prominences were padded. A soft roll was placed under the shoulders and the patient was positioned in a modified beach chair position with the neck extended. The neck and upper chest were prepped and draped in a sterile fashion. A time-out was completed verifying correct patient, procedure, site, positioning, and implant(s) and/or special equipment prior to beginning this procedure. Baseline PTH level was drawn from an IV in the patient's arm.

A ___-cm incision was positioned using the gamma probe to obtain the highest count transcutaneously and made in a skin crease. The subcutaneous tissues and platysma were divided with electrocautery. Subplatysmal flaps were developed. The strap muscles were divided in the midline and retracted.

The *right/left* thyroid lobe was rotated medially. The loose areolar attachments were dissected bluntly and using electrocautery. The gamma probe was used to guide the dissection. An abnormal appearing *right/left superior/inferior* parathyroid gland was noted (*describe location of the gland*). In vivo count was (*note value*). The gland was gently dissected from the surrounding tissues down to its pedicle. The pedicle of the parathyroid gland was clamped and tied with a 3-0 silk suture. The parathyroid gland was excised. The ex vivo count was (*note value*). The gland was sent to pathology. The background count was (*note value*). Another PTH level was drawn 10-min post-excision.

Pathology from the gland returned consistent with hypercellular parathyroid and the gland weighed ___ mg. The baseline PTH was (*note value*). The 10-min post-excision PTH was (*note value*). This constituted a (*note percentage*) percent drop from baseline.

The wound was copiously irrigated and hemostasis was achieved. The strap muscles were reapproximated with interrupted 3-0 Vicryl sutures. The platysma was reapproximated with interrupted 3-0 Vicryl sutures. Approximately 10 cc of 0.25% marcaine was injected subcutaneously. The skin was reapproximated with a running 4-0 Monocryl subcuticular suture. Steri-Strips were placed over the incision and a sterile dressing was applied. The patient tolerated the procedure well and was extubated and taken to the postanesthesia care unit in stable condition.

NOTES

Chapter 124
Parathyroidectomy for Secondary or Tertiary Hyperparathyroidism

Joshua R. French, M.D. and James Howe, M.D.

INDICATION
- Secondary/tertiary hyperparathyroidism.

ESSENTIAL STEPS
1. Develop subplatysmal flaps and divide the strap muscles in the midline.
2. Identify, biopsy, and excise all parathyroid glands, or leave viable remnant of one gland.
3. Verify that pathology of each excised gland is parathyroid tissue.
4. Reimplant small pieces of half a parathyroid gland into the brachioradialis muscle of the non-dominant forearm (for total parathyroidectomy).

NOTE THESE VARIATIONS
- Three-and-a-half gland excision with half gland left on vascular pedicle.
- Cryopreservation of parathyroid tissue.

COMPLICATIONS
- Hypocalcemia.
- Recurrent laryngeal nerve injury.
- Post-op bleeding, resulting in tracheal compression, and airway obstruction.

J.J. Hoballah and C.E.H. Scott-Conner (eds.), *Operative Dictations in General and Vascular Surgery*, DOI 10.1007/978-1-4614-0451-4_124,
© Springer Science+Business Media, LLC 2012

TEMPLATE OF OPERATIVE DICTATION

Preoperative diagnosis: *Secondary/tertiary* hyperparathyroidism.
Procedure: Total parathyroidectomy with autotransplantion into *right/left* forearm (*or three-and-a-half gland parathyroidectomy*).
Postoperative diagnosis: Same.
Indications: This ___-year-old *male/female* developed *secondary/tertiary* hyperparathyroidism unresponsive to medical therapy. *Total/three-and-a-half gland* parathyroidectomy is indicated.
Description of procedure: Following smooth induction of general anesthesia, both arms were tucked at the sides and all bony prominences were padded. A soft roll was placed under the shoulders and the patient was positioned in a modified beach chair position with the neck extended. The neck and upper chest were prepped and draped in a sterile fashion. A time-out was completed verifying correct patient, procedure, site, positioning, and implant(s) and/or special equipment prior to beginning this procedure.

A ___-cm incision was made in a skin crease positioned approximately two fingerbreadths superior to the sternal notch. The subcutaneous tissues and platysma were divided with electrocautery. Subplatysmal flaps were developed. The strap muscles were divided in the midline and retracted laterally.

The right thyroid lobe was rotated medially. The loose areolar attachments were dissected bluntly and using electrocautery. The right *superior/inferior* parathyroid gland was identified (*describe location of the gland*). A biopsy of the gland was sent to pathology. The gland was gently dissected from the surrounding tissues down to its pedicle, which was clamped and tied with a 3-0 silk suture. The parathyroid gland was excised and placed in a labeled cup on ice. The right *superior/inferior* parathyroid gland was identified (*describe location of the gland*). It was biopsied and dissected from the surrounding tissues down to its pedicle, which was clamped and tied with a 3-0 silk suture. The parathyroid gland was excised and placed in a separate labeled cup on ice.

Next the left thyroid lobe was rotated medially and a similar procedure carried out to identify the left parathyroid glands. Each was excised, biopsied, and placed in separate labeled cups on ice. The left superior parathyroid gland was identified (*describe location of the gland*). The left inferior parathyroid gland was identified (*describe location of the gland*). Pathology from each gland returned consistent with parathyroid tissue. The cervical thymus was dissected free on both sides and removed, ligating its inferior veins with 3-0 silk suture.

The *right/left* forearm was extended on an arm board and then prepped and draped in a sterile fashion. An incision was made in the *right/left* lateral forearm. Using blunt dissection, five pockets were carefully made in the belly of the brachioradialis muscle. Approximately half of the *right/left superior/inferior* parathyroid gland was divided into multiple 1–3 mm sections using a scalpel. Several pieces of parathyroid tissue were placed in each pocket. A 4-0 Prolene suture was used to close each pocket and marked with a clip. The deep dermis was reapproximated with interrupted 3-0 Vicryl sutures. The skin was reapproximated with a running 4-0 Monocryl subcuticular suture.

The neck wound was copiously irrigated and hemostasis was achieved. The strap muscles were reapproximated with interrupted 3-0 Vicryl sutures. The platysma was reapproximated with interrupted 3-0 Vicryl sutures. Approximately 10 cc of 0.25% marcaine was injected subcutaneously. The skin was reapproximated with a running 4-0 Monocryl subcuticular suture. Steri-Strips were placed over the incision and a sterile dressing was applied. The patient tolerated the procedure well and was extubated and taken to the postanesthesia care unit in stable condition.

ACKNOWLEDGMENT

This chapter was contributed by Andrew A. Fedder, MD in the first edition.

NOTES

Chapter 125
Cricothyroidotomy

Amy Bobis Stanfill, M.D.

INDICATIONS
- Airway obstruction at or above the level of the larynx.
- Emergency access to the airway when intubation is not possible: Facial trauma or failed intubation and loss of airway.

ESSENTIAL STEPS
1. Have several sizes of tube available (usually a #6 tube for adult male and #5 tube for adult female).
2. Hyperextend the neck *(if no cervical spine fracture)*.
3. Palpate the cricoid and thyroid cartilages.
4. Transverse incision above the cricoid cartilage.
5. *If endotracheal tube in place, withdraw to the level of the cords.*
6. Incision through the cricothyroid membrane.
7. Dilate the tract.
8. Insert tracheostomy tube.
9. Confirm placement.
10. Achieve hemostasis.
11. Secure tube.

NOTE THESE VARIATIONS
- Do not hyperextend the neck if cervical spine injury possible or confirmed.
- Transverse vs. horizontal incision.

J.J. Hoballah and C.E.H. Scott-Conner (eds.), *Operative Dictations in General and Vascular Surgery*, DOI 10.1007/978-1-4614-0451-4_125,
© Springer Science+Business Media, LLC 2012

- Performed over the endotracheal tube or not.
- Size of tube.

COMPLICATIONS
- Bleeding.
- Subglottic stenosis.

TEMPLATE OPERATIVE DICTATION

Preoperative diagnosis: *Airway obstruction/facial trauma/failed intubation and loss of airway/other.*

Procedure: Cricothyroidotomy.

Postoperative diagnosis: Same.

Indications: This ___-year-old *male/female* required *urgent/emergent airway access due to airway obstruction/facial trauma/failed intubation and loss of airway/other.*

Description of procedure: The patient was positioned supine and the neck was *hyperextended/kept in a neutral position to protect the cervical spine.* The neck and anterior chest were prepped and draped in the usual sterile fashion. A time-out was completed verifying correct patient, procedure, site, positioning, and implant(s) and/or special equipment prior to beginning this procedure.

The thyroid and cricoid cartilage were palpated and the skin and subcutaneous tissue in this area were anesthetized with 1% lidocaine *with epinephrine.* The thyroid cartilage was stabilized with the left hand and the cricothyroid space palpated. A 1.5-cm transverse incision was made with a #15 blade over the cricothyroid space. A hemostat was used to bluntly dissect down to the cricothyroid membrane. *The endotracheal tube was withdrawn to the level of the cords.* A #11 scalpel blade was used to puncture the membrane and a tracheal dilator was used to dilate the tract.

A #___ tracheostomy tube was inserted and advanced *as the endotracheal tube was withdrawn completely.* Position was confirmed by *end-tidal CO_2/other.* Hemostasis was achieved in the incision with *electrocautery/ties/packing.* The tracheostomy tube was sutured in place and tracheostomy ties placed and tied around the neck.

The patient tolerated the procedure well and was taken to the postanesthesia care unit in stable condition.

NOTES

Chapter 126
Tracheostomy

Amy Bobis Stanfill, M.D.

INDICATIONS

- Airway obstruction at or above the level of the larynx.
- Chronic respiratory problems.
- Inability to manage secretions.
- Adjunct to major surgery of the mouth, jaw, or larynx.

ESSENTIAL STEPS

1. Best performed as elective procedure over the endotracheal tube.
2. Have several sizes of tubes available:
   - Same size as endotracheal tube.
   - One size smaller in case of difficulty.
3. Hyperextend neck *(if no cervical spine fracture)*.
4. Palpate cricoid and thyroid cartilages.
5. *Vertical midline/transverse* incision.
6. Dissect in midline to the trachea.
7. Partially withdrawn endotracheal tube.
8. Retract the strap muscles laterally and thyroid isthmus superiorly.
9. Palpate the rings.
10. Insert tracheostomy hook between the first and second tracheal rings and retract the trachea superiorly.
11. *Vertical incision through the second and third tracheal rings/transverse incision between the second and third rings/cruciate incision.*

J.J. Hoballah and C.E.H. Scott-Conner (eds.), *Operative Dictations in General and Vascular Surgery*, DOI 10.1007/978-1-4614-0451-4_126,
© Springer Science+Business Media, LLC 2012

12. Dilate the tract.
13. Insert tracheostomy tube as endotracheal tube is withdrawn.
14. Confirm placement.
15. Achieve hemostasis.
16. Secure tube.

NOTE THESE VARIATIONS

- Do not hyperextend the neck if cervical spine injury possible or confirmed.
- Transverse vs. horizontal incision.
- Size of tube.
- Percutaneous dilatational tracheostomy is an increasingly popular alternative (Chap. 127).

COMPLICATIONS

- Bleeding.
- Erosion into the innominate artery with tracheoinnominate artery fistula.

TEMPLATE OPERATIVE DICTATION

Preoperative diagnosis: *Airway obstruction/need for prolonged airway management/other.*
Procedure: Tracheostomy.
Postoperative diagnosis: Same.
Indications: This ___-year-old *male/female* required tracheostomy for *airway obstruction/prolonged airway management/other.*
Description of procedure: The patient was positioned supine and the neck was hyperextended. The neck and anterior chest were prepped and draped in the usual sterile fashion. A time-out was completed verifying correct patient, procedure, site, positioning, and implant(s) and/or special equipment prior to beginning this procedure.

The thyroid and cricoid cartilage were palpated and the skin and subcutaneous tissue in this area were anesthetized with 1% lidocaine *with epinephrine. A vertical midline incision was made from the middle of the thyroid cartilage to just superior to the sternal notch/transverse incision 1.5 cm below the cricoid cartilage was made.* A hemostat was used to bluntly dissect down to the cricothyroid membrane. The strap muscles were retracted laterally and the thyroid isthmus was retracted superiorly *(rarely, divided between hemostats and ligated/oversewn).* The endotracheal tube was withdrawn to the level of the cords. The second tracheal ring was identified. A tracheostomy hook was placed between the first and second tracheal rings and the trachea was retracted superiorly. *A vertical incision was made through the second and third rings/a transverse incision was made between the second and third rings/a cruciate incision was made over the second and third rings* with a #11 scalpel blade. A tracheal dilator was used to dilate the tract.

A #___ tracheostomy tube was inserted and advanced as the endotracheal tube was withdrawn completely. Position was confirmed by *end-tidal CO_2/other*. Hemostasis was achieved in the incision with *electrocautery/ties/packing*. The tracheostomy tube was sutured in place and tracheostomy ties placed and tied around the neck.

The patient tolerated the procedure well and was taken to the postanesthesia care unit in stable condition.

NOTES

Chapter 127
Percutaneous Tracheostomy

Carol E.H. Scott-Conner, M.D.

INDICATIONS
- ■ Airway obstruction at or above the level of the larynx.
- ■ Chronic respiratory problems.
- ■ Inability to manage secretions.

ESSENTIAL STEPS
1. Best performed as an elective procedure over the endotracheal tube.
2. Have several sizes of tube available:
   - • Same size as the endotracheal tube.
   - • One size smaller in case of difficulty.
3. Hyperextend the neck *(if no cervical spine fracture)*.
4. Palpate the cricoid and thyroid cartilages.
5. *Vertical midline/transverse* incision.
6. *Dissect in midline to the trachea.*
7. Partially withdraw the endotracheal tube.
8. Palpate rings.
9. Dilate the tract.
10. Insert the tracheostomy tube as the endotracheal tube is withdrawn.
11. Confirm placement.
12. Achieve hemostasis.
13. Secure the tube.

J.J. Hoballah and C.E.H. Scott-Conner (eds.), *Operative Dictations in General and Vascular Surgery*, DOI 10.1007/978-1-4614-0451-4_127,
© Springer Science+Business Media, LLC 2012

NOTE THESE VARIATIONS

- Do not hyperextend the neck if cervical spine injury possible or confirmed.
- Transverse vs. horizontal incision.
- May be done as totally percutaneous technique or modified with dissection down to the trachea.
- Size of tube.

COMPLICATIONS

- Bleeding.
- Trauma to the back wall of the trachea.
- Improper placement.
- Erosion into the innominate artery with tracheoinnominate artery fistula.

TEMPLATE OPERATIVE DICTATION

Preoperative diagnosis: *Airway obstruction/need for prolonged airway management/other.*

Procedure: Percutaneous tracheostomy.

Postoperative diagnosis: Same.

Indications: This ___-year-old *male/female* required tracheostomy for *airway obstruction/prolonged airway management/other.*

Description of procedure: The patient was positioned supine and the neck was hyperextended. The neck and anterior chest were prepped and draped in the usual sterile fashion. A time-out was completed verifying correct patient, procedure, site, positioning, and implant(s) and/or special equipment prior to beginning this procedure.

The thyroid and cricoid cartilage were palpated and the skin and subcutaneous tissue in this area anesthetized with 1% lidocaine *with epinephrine.*

Next, the bronchoscope was then inserted down through the previously placed endotracheal tube until the carina was well visualized. *Detail the extent of bronchoscopic examination and findings.* The endotracheal tube was slowly withdrawn up to the point where no tracheal rings were visualized.

The trachea was again palpated, stabilized in the midline. A small *transverse/vertical* incision was made *and the soft tissue dissected bluntly down to the trachea at the level of the second and third tracheal rings.* The trachea was then entered using a small finder needle under bronchoscopic visual control.

A larger needle and catheter were then inserted and position confirmed bronchoscopically. The needle was removed and the catheter advanced into the trachea. A guide wire was then inserted and passed distally under bronchoscopic control. The trachea was then dilated using a tapered *#38F Rhino dilator/other*. ___ French tracheostomy tube was then inserted using a #___ French dilator as the inner cannula. The endotracheal tube was then removed and the ventilator connection was switched to the tracheostomy tube. Adequate position was confirmed by bronchoscopy and adequacy of ventilation. The balloon was inflated. No bleeding was noted.

The tracheostomy tube was then fixed in place with two skin sutures and by an umbilical tape around the patient's neck.

The patient tolerated the procedure well and was taken to the postanesthesia care unit in stable condition.

ACKNOWLEDGMENT

This chapter was contributed by Mazen M. Hashisho, MD in the first edition.

NOTES

Section XIII
Miscellaneous Procedures

Chapter 128
Placement of Subclavian Central Venous Catheter

Amy Bobis Stanfill, M.D.

INDICATIONS

- Central venous pressure monitoring.
- Placement of Swan-Ganz catheter.
- Delivery of central venous nutrition or medications.
- Hemodialysis.
- Emergency access when other routes fail.

ESSENTIAL STEPS

1. Position patient supine, in the slight Trendelenburg position, rolled towel between the shoulder blades, and the head turned away from side of placement.
2. Prep the skin with betadine and square off for sterile field: Include the neck on the chosen side in case of change to internal jugular site.
3. Local anesthesia with 1–2% lidocaine: Ensure the skin, subcutaneous tissue, and periosteum are well anesthetized.
4. *Locate the subclavian vein by aspirating blood with small-gauge needle used for local anesthesia.*
5. Locate the subclavian vein with 16-gauge needle (Skin puncture site is in general 1 cm inferior to the distal third of the clavicle).
6. Once the vein is located, place catheter via Seldinger technique.
7. Ensure catheter is working properly: Aspirate from each port and then flush each with heparin.

J.J. Hoballah and C.E.H. Scott-Conner (eds.), *Operative Dictations in General and Vascular Surgery*, DOI 10.1007/978-1-4614-0451-4_128,
© Springer Science+Business Media, LLC 2012

8. Secure catheter in place and apply sterile dressing.
9. Upright chest X-ray to assess line placement and check for pneumothorax.

NOTE THESE VARIATIONS
- Use of ultrasound guidance (see Chap. 129).
- Hickman catheter.
- Subcutaneous port.
- Kits vary; be familiar with the one you are using.
- Passage of Swan-Ganz catheter.

COMPLICATIONS
- Pneumothorax.
- Hemothorax.
- Venous air embolus.
- Cannulation of artery.
- Line infection.
- Bleeding from site.

TEMPLATE OPERATIVE DICTATION
Preoperative diagnosis: *Hemodynamic instability/need for total parenteral nutrition/other*.
Procedure: Placement of central venous catheter via *right/left* subclavian route.
Postoperative diagnosis: Same.
Indications: This ___-year-old *male/female* required central venous access for *hemodynamic monitoring/central venous nutrition/other* due to complications of ___. The subclavian route was chosen.
Description of procedure: The patient was placed supine with a rolled towel between the shoulder blades. The bed was placed in slight Trendelenburg position and the *right/left* chest and neck were prepped and draped with sterile technique. A time-out was completed verifying correct patient, procedure, site, positioning, and implant(s) and/or special equipment prior to beginning this procedure. The central catheter was flushed with heparin to ensure function of each port. Landmarks were identified and a skin entry site was chosen 1–2 cm inferior to the distal third of the clavicle. The skin and subcutaneous tissue were anesthetized with 1% lidocaine. Local anesthesia was carried down to the periosteum of the clavicle.

The vein was then located with a 16-gauge needle with a 10-cc syringe. The needle was inserted at the chosen site with the bevel down and directed toward the sternal notch. With continuous negative pressure in the syringe, the needle was advanced in a stepwise fashion down the clavicle. The vein was located as the needle passed beneath the bone. As soon as the syringe began to fill with venous blood, the needle was rotated 90° so the bevel was pointed at the foot of the bed. The needle position was secured and the syringe removed. The hub was occluded to prevent venous air embolus. The guide wire passed easily and the needle was removed while the wire was held in place. A small incision was then made at the point of wire entry. The dilator was placed over the wire and the tract gently dilated. The catheter was fed over the wire, ensuring the wire exited from the port before advancing the catheter. The catheter was inserted to the desired depth and the wire removed. Each port was aspirated to ensure adequate blood flow and then flushed with heparin. The catheter was secured in place with 2-0 silk sutures and a sterile dressing applied. The patient tolerated the procedure well and was taken to the postanesthesia care unit in stable condition. An upright chest X-ray was obtained to evaluate location of the catheter tip and check for pneumothorax.

NOTES

Chapter 129

Ultrasound-Guided Placement of Subclavian Central Venous Catheter

Timothy D. Light, M.D.

INDICATIONS

- Upper extremity vein sclerosis (this is the only indication for which Medicare will reimburse).
- Central pressure monitoring.
- Delivery of sclerotic medications or agents.

ESSENTIAL STEPS

1. Confirm patient and indication.
2. Review any local protocols or guidelines regarding central venous catheter insertion. Be sure to conform to them or to dictate the justification for varying from them.
3. Gather supplies – always get two kits, confirm ultrasound is functioning, and gather syringes, flushes, and dressing kit.
4. Place ultrasound at shoulder level opposite side of planned insertion site.
5. Place patient supine, in slight Trendelenburg with the head turned to opposite side of planned insertion site.
6. Use ultrasound to confirm vein is in expected location, and is patent, pliable, and has non-pulsatile venous flow. Take photos if the ultrasound machine is so equipped.
7. Prep and drape patient.
8. Have assistant pass onto the field the catheter kit, the ultrasound probe cover and conducting gel, and the ultrasound probe, flushes, syringes, and dressing kits.

J.J. Hoballah and C.E.H. Scott-Conner (eds.), *Operative Dictations in General and Vascular Surgery*, DOI 10.1007/978-1-4614-0451-4_129,
© Springer Science+Business Media, LLC 2012

9. Use the ultrasound probe to identify the vein again. Do not forget your traditional landmarks and positioning. If using the infraclavicular approach, the insertion site will likely be more lateral than expected.

10. Anesthetize the overlying skin and soft tissue with local anesthetic.

11. While holding the ultrasound probe in the non-dominant hand (or using a fully gowned assistant), insert the 16-g needle at a flat angle to the skin about 1–2 cm lateral to the ultrasound probe, in the same plane.

12. The operator should see the tissue of the vein move with the needle insertion. When blood returns, advance the guidewire using typical Seldinger techniques. The guidewire should be seen in the vein. Obtaining a picture at this point is a good practice.

13. Pass off the ultrasound probe and finish the procedure as described in the previous chapter.

14. Remember:
    - Visualizing and cannulating the vein is more challenging than the internal jugular approach.
    - The complication rate increases exponentially with each attempt. Reassess, reposition, and request assistance early.

VARIATIONS

- Kits vary. Be familiar with the one you are using. Include kit name/manufacturer in your dictation.
- Ultrasounds vary. Be familiar with the one you are using. Include ultrasound manufacturer and probe frequency in the dictation.
- Jigs and needle guides are available, but may be cumbersome to use.
- Some operators use a supraclavicular approach which can also be done with ultrasound guidance.
- Some central venous catheters are tunneled, cuffed, or have a port attached. The technique of identifying and accessing the vein is the same.

COMPLICATIONS

- Pneumothorax.
- Hemothorax.
- Arterial puncture, cannulation, or injury.
- Vein laceration.

- Venous air embolus.
- Cardiac perforation with cardiac tamponade.
- Cardiac arrhythmia.

TEMPLATE OPERATIVE DICTATION

Preoperative diagnosis: This _____-year-old *male/female* requires central venous access because peripheral access is neither available nor appropriate for the medications s/he will receive. *(The underlying medical condition or diagnosis might also be added here).*

Procedure: Ultrasound guided left/right subclavian central venous catheter insertion.

Post operative diagnosis: As above.

Indications: The pre-operative diagnosis can be repeated here. Ultrasound guidance was necessary because of anticipated anatomic difficulties due to _____.

Description of procedure: After a review of the indications, consent, and relevant medical record, a team time-out was performed verifying correct patient, procedure, site, positioning, and implant(s) and/or special equipment prior to beginning this procedure. Patient was placed supine, in slight Trendelenburg, with the neck turned to the contralateral side. The *right/left* neck and chest were prepped and widely draped using an approved topical antiseptic and full barrier precautions. A _____ brand ultrasound machine with _____ MHz probe was used to confirm the axillary and subclavian veins were in their usual anatomic location, and were patent, pliable, and had non-pulsatile venous blood flow (see attached photos). A _____ brand central venous catheter kit was used. All parts were flushed and tested prior to use. The skin and subcutaneous tissues were anesthetized with _____ ml of _____% lidocaine.

Using a 16-g needle, the vein was punctured and the guidewire advanced under direct ultrasonic visualization (see attached photos). The guidewire advanced without resistance or difficulty. A skin nick was made at the insertion site, and using Seldinger technique, a dilator was passed over the wire to dilate the subcutaneous tissue. The dilator was exchanged for the catheter and the catheter smoothly advanced. The guidewire was removed without difficulty, and the catheter ports were aspirated, flushed with saline, and capped without complication. The catheter was secured with multiple *sutures/staples* at the desired depth, and a dressing applied. Patient tolerated the procedure well, and a post procedure chest X-ray was ordered.

NOTES

Chapter 130
Placement of Internal Jugular Central Venous Catheter

Amy Bobis Stanfill, M.D.

INDICATIONS
- Central venous pressure monitoring.
- Placement of Swan-Ganz catheter.
- Delivery of central venous nutrition or medications.
- Hemodialysis.
- Emergency access when other routes fail.

ESSENTIAL STEPS
1. Position patient supine, in the slight Trendelenburg position *with a shoulder roll*, and the head turned away from side of placement.
2. Prep skin with betadine and square off for sterile field:
   - Include the chest on the chosen side in case of change to the subclavian site.
3. Local anesthesia with 1–2% lidocaine.
4. *Locate the internal jugular vein by aspirating blood with small-gauge needle used for local anesthesia.*
5. Locate the internal jugular vein with 16-gauge needle: Insert the needle at the apex of the triangle formed by the clavicular and sternal heads of the sternocleidomastoid muscle (with the clavicle as a base) and aim toward the ipsilateral nipple.
6. Once the vein is located, place catheter via Seldinger technique.

J.J. Hoballah and C.E.H. Scott-Conner (eds.), *Operative Dictations in General and Vascular Surgery*, DOI 10.1007/978-1-4614-0451-4_130,
© Springer Science+Business Media, LLC 2012

7. Ensure catheter is working properly.
   - Aspirate from each port and then flush each with heparin.
8. Secure catheter in place and apply sterile dressing.
9. Upright chest X-ray to assess line placement and check for pneumothorax.

NOTE THESE VARIATIONS
- Ultrasound guidance (see Chap. 131).
- Hickman catheter.
- Subcutaneous port.
- Kits vary; be familiar with the one you are using.
- Passage of Swan-Ganz catheter.

COMPLICATIONS
- Pneumothorax.
- Hemothorax.
- Venous air embolus.
- Cannulation of artery.
- Line infection.
- Bleeding from the site.

TEMPLATE OPERATIVE DICTATION
Preoperative diagnosis: *Hemodynamic instability/need for total parenteral nutrition/other.*
Procedure: Placement of central venous catheter via *right/left* internal jugular vein route.
Postoperative diagnosis: Same.
Indications: This ___-year-old *male/female* required central venous access for *hemodynamic monitoring/central venous nutrition/other* due to complications of ___. The internal jugular route was chosen.
Description of procedure: The patient was placed supine with *a shoulder roll and* the head turned to the contralateral side. The bed was placed in slight Trendelenburg position and the *right/left* chest and neck were prepped and draped with sterile technique. A time-out was completed verifying correct patient, procedure, site, positioning, and implant(s) and/or special equipment prior to beginning this procedure. The central catheter was flushed with heparin to ensure function of each port. Landmarks were identified and a skin entry site was chosen at the apex of the triangle formed by the sternal and clavicular heads of the sterno-cleidomastoid muscle (with the clavicle as a base). The skin and subcutaneous tissue were anesthetized with 1% lidocaine.

The vein was then located with a 16-gauge needle with a 10-cc syringe. The carotid pulse was palpated and the needle was inserted with the bevel down at the apex of the triangle, lateral to the carotid artery pulsation. The needle was directed toward the ipsilateral nipple and the vein was entered. The needle position was secured and the syringe removed. The hub was occluded to prevent venous air embolus. The guide wire passed easily and the needle was removed, while the wire was held in place. A small incision was then made at the point of wire entry. The dilator was placed over the wire and the tract gently dilated. The catheter was fed over the wire, ensuring the wire exited from the port before advancing the catheter. The catheter was inserted to the desired depth and the wire removed. Each port was aspirated to ensure adequate blood flow and then flushed with heparin. The catheter was secured in place with 2-0 silk sutures and a sterile dressing applied. The patient tolerated the procedure well and was taken to the postanesthesia care unit in stable condition. An upright chest X-ray was obtained to evaluate location of the catheter tip and check for pneumothorax.

NOTES

Chapter 131

Ultrasound-Guided Placement of Internal Jugular Central Venous Catheter

Timothy D. Light, M.D.

INDICATIONS

- Upper extremity vein sclerosis (this is the only indication for which Medicare will reimburse).
- Central pressure monitoring.
- Hemodialysis (preferred location as it avoids subclavian vein stenosis).
- Delivery of sclerotic medications or agents.

ESSENTIAL STEPS

1. Confirm patient and indication. Review anatomy, history, and relevant lab studies to avoid predictable difficulties – i.e., neck surgery or radiation at planned site, or coagulopathy.
2. Review any local protocols or guidelines regarding central venous catheter insertion. Be sure to conform to them or to dictate the justification for varying from them.
3. Gather supplies – always get two kits, confirm ultrasound is functioning, and gather syringes, flushes, and dressing kit.
4. Place ultrasound between hip and feet on opposite side of planned insertion site.
5. Place patient supine, in slight Trendelenburg with the head turned to opposite side of planned insertion site.
6. Stand at head of bed, slightly to the side of the planned site of insertion.

J.J. Hoballah and C.E.H. Scott-Conner (eds.), *Operative Dictations in General and Vascular Surgery*, DOI 10.1007/978-1-4614-0451-4_131,
© Springer Science+Business Media, LLC 2012

7. Use ultrasound to confirm vein is in expected location, and is patent, pliable, and has non-pulsatile venous flow. Take photos if the ultrasound machine is so equipped.

8. Prep and drape patient.

9. Have assistant pass onto the field the catheter kit, the ultrasound probe cover and conducting gel, and the ultrasound probe, flushes, syringes, and dressing kits.

10. Use the ultrasound probe to identify the vein again. Do not forget your traditional landmarks and positioning.

11. Anesthetize the overlying skin and soft tissue with local.

12. While holding the ultrasound probe in the non-dominant hand (or using a fully gowned assistant), insert the 16-g needle at a 45° angle to the skin about 1–2 cm cephalad to the ultrasound probe, in the same plane. The operator should see the tissue of the vein move with the needle insertion.

13. When blood returns, advance the guidewire using typical Seldinger techniques. The guidewire should be seen in the vein. Obtaining a picture at this point is a good practice.

14. Pass off the ultrasound probe and finish the procedure as described in the previous chapter.

15. Remember that the complication rate increases exponentially with each attempt. Reassess, reposition, and request assistance early.

VARIATIONS

- Kits vary. Be familiar with the one you are using. Include kit name/manufacturer in your dictation.

- Ultrasounds vary. Be familiar with the one you are using. Include ultrasound manufacturer and probe frequency in the dictation.

- Needle guides and jigs are available, but may prove cumbersome.

- Some operators use posterior, anterior, or low approaches which can also be done with ultrasound guidance. These all require slightly different patient, operator, and ultrasound monitor positioning.

- Some central venous catheters are tunneled, cuffed, or have a port attached. The technique of identifying and accessing the vein is the same.

COMPLICATIONS

- Pneumothorax.
- Hemothorax.
- Neck Hematoma.
- Arterial puncture, cannulation, or injury.
- Vein laceration.
- Venous air embolus.
- Cardiac perforation with cardiac tamponade.
- Cardiac arrhythmia.

TEMPLATE OPERATIVE DICTATION

Preoperative diagnosis: This _____-year-old *male/female* requires central venous access because peripheral access is neither available nor appropriate for the medications s/he will receive *(The underlying medical condition or diagnosis might also be added here).*

Procedure: Ultrasound guided *left/right* internal jugular central venous catheter insertion.

Post operative diagnosis: As above.

Indications: The pre-operative diagnosis can be repeated here. *Some commentary about why the IJ site (instead of the subclavian site) was chosen might be useful here.* Ultrasound guidance was used because _____.

Description of procedure: After a review of the indications, consent, and relevant medical record, a team time-out was performed verifying correct patient, procedure, site, positioning, and implant(s) and/or special equipment prior to beginning this procedure. Patient was placed supine, in slight Trendelenburg, with the neck turned to the contralateral side. The *right/left* neck and chest were prepped and widely draped using an approved topical antiseptic and full barrier precautions. A _____ brand ultrasound machine with _____ MHz probe was used to confirm the internal jugular vein was in its usual anatomic location, and was patent, pliable, and had non-pulsatile venous blood flow (see attached photos). A _____ brand central venous catheter kit was used. All parts were flushed and tested prior to use. The skin and subcutaneous tissues were anesthetized with _____ ml of _____% lidocaine.

Using a 16-g needle, the vein was punctured and the guidewire advanced under direct ultrasonic visualization (see attached photos). The guidewire advanced without resistance or difficulty. A skin nick was made at the insertion site, and using Seldinger technique, a dilator was passed over the wire to dilate the subcutaneous tissue. The dilator was exchanged for the catheter and the catheter smoothly advanced. The guidewire was removed without difficulty, and the catheter ports were aspirated, flushed with saline, and capped without complication. The catheter was secured with multiple *sutures/staples* at the desired depth, and a dressing applied. Patient tolerated the procedure well, and a post-procedure chest X-ray was ordered.

NOTES

Chapter 132
Renal Transplantation

Susan Skaff Hagen, M.D., M.S.P.H.

INDICATIONS
- End-Stage Renal Disease due to:
  - Diabetes mellitus.
  - Hypertensive nephropathy.
  - Focal segmental glomerulosclerosis.
  - Reflux nephropathy.
  - Other congenital or acquired diseases.

ESSENTIAL STEPS
1. Verify blood type and UNOS ID.
2. Back table preparation of the kidney.
3. Anesthesia.
4. Insert Foley.
5. Immunosuppression induction therapy and pre-operative antibiotics.
6. Hockey-stick flank incision.
7. Divide abdominal wall muscles and expose the retroperitoneum.
8. Expose the iliac fossa.
9. Dissect the iliac vessels.
10. Occlude the iliac vein.
11. Venotomy and venous end-to-side anastomosis.
12. Occlude the iliac artery.
13. Arteriotomy and arterial end-to side anastomosis.
14. Reperfusion and check hemostasis.

J.J. Hoballah and C.E.H. Scott-Conner (eds.), *Operative Dictations in General and Vascular Surgery*, DOI 10.1007/978-1-4614-0451-4_132,
© Springer Science+Business Media, LLC 2012

15. Ureter to bladder anastomosis.
16. Hemostasis.
17. Close.

NOTE THESE VARIATIONS

- Presence of atherosclerosis or aberrant arteriovenous anatomy.
- Double ureter.
- Cadaveric or living related/unrelated transplant.
- Pediatric to adult transplant: en bloc transplant of two kidneys.
- Spasm requiring verapamil.
- Ureteral stent.
- JP drain.
- Creation of peritoneal window.

COMPLICATIONS

- Hyperacute rejection.
- Hemorrhage.
- Renal artery and/or vein stenosis or thrombosis.
- Ureteral leak.
- Lymphocele.

TEMPLATE OPERATIVE DICTATION

Preoperative diagnosis: End-stage renal disease.
Procedure: Renal transplantation.
Postoperative diagnosis: Same.
Indications: Patient is a ___-year-old *male/female* with end-stage renal disease due to *diabetes mellitus/hypertensive nephropathy/focal segmental glomerulosclerosis/reflux nephropathy/other*. *He/she* presents for a *living related/living unrelated/cadaveric* kidney transplant.
Description of procedure: Prior to the start of the operation, I personally verified that the blood type of the donor was (_) and the recipient is (_) and they are compatible. The UNOS ID was _____.

Patient was brought into the operating room and placed on the table in the supine position. General endotracheal anesthesia was administered. A time-out was completed verifying correct patient, procedure, site, positioning, and implant(s) and/or special equipment prior to beginning this procedure. All bony prominences were padded. The Anesthesia team placed a *right internal jugular central line/an arterial line/and other venous access*. A three-way Foley catheter attached to a GU irrigation set with *methylene blue/antibiotic* impregnated irrigant was inserted. The patient was prepped with *Betadine/Chlorhexadine* from the xiphoid to the mid-thigh. Perioperative antibiotics *Ancef/Other* and immunosuppression *Zenapax/Thymoglobulin/CellCept/Solumedrol* were given.

[Choose one:]

If cadaver: The kidney was prepared on the back table by dissecting free the surrounding connective tissue (*State if double artery or variant anatomy*). The caval and aortic cuff were trimmed and fashioned according to the size of the renal vein and renal artery. Small vessels and lymphatics were ligated with 4-0 silk ties. The ureter and surrounding tissue was left intact to preserve the blood supply. The fatty tissue was removed from the capsule of the kidney. The kidney was sterilely packed in ice and preservation solution.

If living related/unrelated: The kidney was prepared on the back table by dissecting free the surrounding connective tissue from the artery and vein (*State if double artery or variant anatomy*). Small vessels and lymphatics were ligated with 4-0 silk ties. The ureter and surrounding tissue was left intact to preserve the blood supply. The fatty tissue was removed from the capsule of the kidney. The kidney was sterilely packed in ice and preservation solution *and brought into the recipient room.*

If pediatric en bloc: The kidneys were prepared on the back table by dissecting free the surrounding connective tissue from the aorta and inferior vena cava. The proximal end of the aorta and vena cava were closed using 6-0 running Prolene. The branches were ligated and divided. The en bloc kidneys were ready to be anastomosed from the lower cava and aorta. The ureters and surrounding tissue were left intact to preserve the blood supply. The fatty tissue was removed from the capsule of the kidneys. The kidneys were sterilely packed in ice and preservation solution.

A hockey-stick shaped *right/left* flank renal transplant incision was made. The subcutaneous tissues were divided down to the abdominal wall fascia. The fascia was entered lateral to the border of the abdominal rectus.

If male: The spermatic cord was gently retracted medially out of the operative field.

If female: The round ligament was ligated and divided with 2-0 silk ties.

The peritoneum was dissected off the abdominal wall and the insertion of the oblique and transversus abdominus were divided according to the length and direction of the skin incision. The transversalis fascia was divided to access the retroperitoneal tissues, which were retracted medially to expose the iliac vessels. A self-retaining retractor was placed. The iliac fossa was prepared for the transplant. The iliac artery and vein were freed from surrounding tissue. The small perforating vessels were tied with 3-0 silk. Perivascular lymphatic channels were divided with 3-0 silk ties. The external iliac artery and vein were mobilized with sharp dissection to *the bifurcation of the common iliac artery and/or the most distal hypogastric veins,* freeing enough sufficient length of vessels for subsequent anastomosis.

The renal transplant to the right iliac artery and vein was begun by cross-clamping the iliac vein. A longitudinal incision was made in the vein and the vein was flushed with heparinized saline. An end-to-side anastomosis was performed using running 6-0 Prolene. The artery was cross-clamped with a *DeBakey* cross-clamp. An arteriotomy was made. An end-to-side renal artery to iliac artery anastomosis was performed using running 6-0 Prolene. Furosemide and mannitol were administered to the patient to promote diuresis immediately before renal perfusion was established. First the venous cross-clamps were removed and then the arterial cross-clamps. Hemostasis was achieved.

After the anastomoses were made, the abdomen was filled with warm irrigation. The kidney turned a nice pink color. It began to firm up. *Spasm was noted in the vessels and verapamil was injected directly into the iliac artery proximal to the kidney.* Next attention was directed toward the ureter. The bladder was filled with ___ cc of irrigant solution. The ureter was trimmed and spatulated posteriorly. The perivesical fat and muscles were divided with electrocautery at the dome of the bladder. The bladder mucosa was incised. *A double-J ureteral stent was placed in the ureter.* The ureter to bladder end-to-side anastomosis was performed with 6-0 PDS. The anastomosis was checked for any evidence of leak. A second layer of bladder wall detrusor muscles were approximated over the anastomosis with 4-0 PDS.

If double ureter or pediatric en bloc: Two similar ureteral anastomoses were performed.

The abdomen was irrigated with a large amount of saline. Hemostasis was achieved. *A peritoneal window was created. A Jackson Pratt drain was placed.* The abdominal wall was closed in two layers. The dermis was approximated with 3-0 Vicryl. The skin was approximated with *staples/subcuticular suture.*

The transplanted kidney was noted to make urine in the operating room. The patient tolerated the procedure well and was extubated in the operating room. The patient was brought to the

PACU in stable condition. There was approximately ___ hours of cold ischemia time.

ACKNOWLEDGMENT

This chapter was contributed by Gustavo Martinez-Mier, MD in the first edition.

NOTES

Chapter 133

Left Adrenalectomy

Faek R. Jamali, M.D.

INDICATIONS

- Aldosteronoma.
- Cortisol-secreting adenoma (Cushing syndrome or sub-clinical Cushing).
- Pheochromocytoma (sporadic or familial).
- Virilizing or feminizing tumors.
- Nonfunctioning unilateral tumor size >4 cm.
- Adrenal nodule with imaging features atypical for adenoma, myelolipoma, or cyst.
- Adrenocortical carcinoma.
- Solitary unilateral adrenal metastasis.

ESSENTIAL STEPS

1. Prepare the patient adequately (e.g., correct electrolyte abnormalities, control hypertension, preoperative alpha-blockade in pheochromocytoma, stress steroids in Cushing's disease, prophylactic pneumovax administration is recommended in reoperative cases).
2. Enter the abdomen through an extended left subcostal incision. Exposure for this approach may be facilitated by elevating the left flank using a roll under the right side.
3. Explore the abdomen.
4. Mobilize the splenic flexure of the colon.
5. Mobilize the spleen and tail of pancreas (medial visceral rotation).

J.J. Hoballah and C.E.H. Scott-Conner (eds.), *Operative Dictations in General and Vascular Surgery*, DOI 10.1007/978-1-4614-0451-4_133,

6. Dissect retroperitoneal structures including Gerota's fascia, left renal hilum, para-aortic space.
7. Identify, ligate, and divide the left adrenal vein.
8. Dissect all the left supra-renal tissues, including left adrenal gland with en bloc resection of retroperitoneal fat from the superior pole of the left kidney to the diaphragm.

NOTE THESE VARIATIONS
- If the spleen and pancreas cannot be mobilized away from the adrenal because of tumor involvement, then the lesser sac should be opened to allow access to the pancreas and splenic hilum.
- Large malignant tumors on the left may require en bloc resection of the spleen, tail of the pancreas, and even the kidney.
- Adrenal tumors should be removed along with a generous margin of retroperitoneal fat and Gerota fascia.
- In cases of primary adrenal cortical malignancies, periaortic lymph nodes medial to the adrenal should be removed along with the tumor.

COMPLICATIONS
- Tumor rupture with spillage and seeding.
- Bleeding from large raw surface in the retroperitoneum or from accessory lumbar veins.
- Left diaphragmatic injury leading to pneumothorax.
- Splenic injury requiring splenectomy.

TEMPLATE OPERATIVE DICTATION
Preoperative diagnosis: List specific pathology indicating surgery *(see indications above)*, e.g., *pheochromocytoma of the left adrenal gland.*
Procedure: Open left adrenalectomy.
Postoperative diagnosis: List specific intraoperative findings, e.g., *pheochromocytoma of left adrenal gland.*
Indications: This ___-year-old *male/female* patient was found to have a *specific diagnosis of left adrenal gland pathology.* Preoperative biochemical workup showed evidence of *(list specific hormonal activity if present).* Imaging confirmed a ___ cm left adrenal lesion. The patient underwent preoperative preparation *(see point one of essential steps)* and is now presenting for elective left adrenalectomy. The indications, alternatives, risks, and benefits of the surgery were discussed with the patient and informed consent was obtained.

Details of operation: The patient was brought to the operating room and placed on the operating table in the supine position. A roll (or beanbag) was placed under the patient's left flank to allow slight medial rotation of the left side. The abdomen was clipped, prepped with 2% chlorhexidine solution, and draped in the standard fashion. A time-out was completed verifying correct patient, procedure, site, positioning, and implant(s) and/or special equipment prior to beginning this procedure.

The abdomen was approached via a standard extended subcostal incision. The skin was incised two finger breadths below the left costal margin starting from the mid-axillary line and extending to the midline. The incision was deepened through the skin and subcutaneous tissue Scarpa's fascia was opened and the incision taken down to the level of the abdominal wall. Using electrocautery the abdominal wall musculature was divided. The external, internal, and transversalis fascia were divided using electrocautery. The anterior rectus sheath was opened in the left rectus muscle was split using electrocautery with control of the epigastric vessels. The posterior rectus sheath was also divided. Exploration of the abdominal cavity was then carried out to rule out evidence of metastatic disease. The procedure was started by mobilizing the splenic flexure of the colon. This was done starting by mobilization of the white line of told along the descending colon. This mobilization was then carried up to the level of the splenic flexure. The attachment of the omentum to the distal transverse was also divided using electrocautery allowing access into the lesser sac to further facilitate the complete takedown of the splenic flexure. Once the splenic flexure of the colon was completely mobilized, the spleno-renal and retroperitoneal attachments of the spleen were divided with electrocautery. The spleno-phrenic attachments were also divided and the spleen along with the tail of the pancreas rotated medially. Care was taken to avoid any injury to the splenic vein in the course of this dissection. Once the splenic flexure of the colon, the tail of the pancreas and the spleen have been rotated medially, exposure of the adrenal gland in the retroperitoneum was achieved. The suprarenal tissue was then dissected as one block. Gerota's fascia, the upper border of the left kidney and the left renal hilum were identified and dissected. Dissection of the left renal vein and its upper border lead to the identification of the left adrenal vein which was doubly ligated and divided. Using *electrocautery/an appropriate energy device*, the retroperitoneal fat of the left suprarenal region was elevated of the superior pole of the left kidney and gently dissected off the lateral abdominal wall and then posteriorly off the left quadratus lumborum muscle. The arterial supply of the left adrenal gland was controlled and divided as it was encountered along this dissection. It usually consists of three main arterial branches, from the left renal artery, the aorta, and the left phrenic artery. The cephalad attachments of the adrenal and retroperitoneal tissue to the left diaphragm were then divided. The left adrenal gland was then gently retracted laterally to allow for the completion of the medial dissection. The medial dissection was carried as far medially as possible to ensure a negative margin. Care was taken to avoid injury to the capsule of the adrenal gland. The medial dissection was carried out by removing all of the contents of the suprarenal region all the way up to the para-vertebral space. If cancer: *An en bloc dissection of the para-aortic nodes was also carried out as part of the medial extent of the dissection of the suprarenal region. The specimen is then removed en bloc.* Irrigation of the suprarenal region was carried out and confirmation of hemostasis was achieved. The spleen and pancreatic tail were then allowed to return back to their normal anatomical position. Closure of the abdomen and layers was then carried out using number one PDS suture followed by closure of the skin with a skin stapler. The patient tolerated the procedure well. There were no complications and the blood loss was minimal. The instrument and sponge count was correct. The patient was extubated and returned to the recovery room in stable satisfactory condition.

NOTES

Chapter 134
Laparoscopic Left Adrenalectomy

Faek R. Jamali, M.D.

INDICATIONS

- Aldosteronoma.
- Cortisol-secreting adenoma (Cushing syndrome or subclinical Cushing).
- Pheochromocytoma (sporadic or familial).
- Nonfunctioning unilateral tumor >4 cm.
- Adrenal nodule with imaging features atypical for adenoma, myelolipoma, or cyst.
- Solitary unilateral adrenal metastasis.

ESSENTIAL STEPS

1. Prepare the patient (e.g., correct electrolyte abnormalities, control hypertension, preoperative alpha-blockade in pheochromocytoma, stress steroids in Cushing's disease).
2. Position the patient in the full left lateral decubitus position with appropriate padding.
3. Establish pneumoperitoneum and place trocars.
4. Explore the abdomen.
5. Mobilize the splenic flexure of the colon.
6. Mobilize the spleen and tail of pancreas (medial visceral rotation).
7. Dissect retroperitoneal structures including Gerota's fascia, left renal hilum, and para-aortic space.
8. Identify, secure, and divide left adrenal vein.

J.J. Hoballah and C.E.H. Scott-Conner (eds.), *Operative Dictations in General and Vascular Surgery*, DOI 10.1007/978-1-4614-0451-4_134,
© Springer Science+Business Media, LLC 2012

9. Dissect all the left supra-renal tissues, including left adrenal gland and resect the retroperitoneal fat en bloc from the superior pole of the left kidney to the diaphragm.

NOTE THIS VARIATION

- Large malignant tumors on the left may require en bloc resection of the spleen, tail of the pancreas, and even the kidney and should not be approached laparoscopically.

COMPLICATIONS

- Tumor rupture leading to spillage and seeding.
- Bleeding from large raw surfaces in the retroperitoneum or from accessory lumbar veins.
- Left diaphragmatic injury leading to pneumothorax.
- Splenic injury requiring splenectomy.

TEMPLATE OPERATIVE DICTATION

Preoperative diagnosis: List specific pathology indicating surgery *(see indications above)*, e.g., *pheochromocytoma of the left adrenal gland*.

Procedure: Laparoscopic left adrenalectomy.

Postoperative diagnosis: List specific intraoperative findings, e.g., *pheochromocytoma of left adrenal gland*.

Indications: This ___-year-old *male/female* patient was found to have a left adrenal _____. Preoperative biochemical workup showed evidence of *(list specific hormonal activity if present)*. Imaging confirmed a ___ cm left adrenal lesion. The patient underwent preoperative preparation and is now presenting for elective laparoscopic left adrenalectomy. The indications, alternatives, and risks and benefits of the surgery were discussed with the patient and informed consent was obtained.

Details of operation: The patient was brought to the operating room and placed on the operating table in the left lateral decubitus position. The patient was appropriately positioned with padding as well as the use of the beanbag. The abdomen was clipped, prepped with 2% Chlorhexidine solution, and draped in the standard fashion. A time-out was completed verifying correct patient, procedure, site, positioning, and implant(s) and/or special equipment prior to beginning this procedure.

The abdomen was approached *via an open Hasson technique/ placement of Veress needle* and pneumoperitoneum was induced. The first (10 mm) trocar was placed at the mid-level of the subcostal margin on the left side. Two additional 5-mm trocars were placed at the level of the costal margin, 8–10 cm away to the right and left of the camera port. The third 5-mm trocar was placed to at the level of the mid-axillary or posterior axillary line for the assistant's use. Exploration of the abdominal cavity was carried out followed by mobilization of the splenic flexure of the colon by incising the white line of Toldt, facilitated by the left lateral decubitus position. The attention was the turned toward the mobilization of the spleen. The spleno-renal and retroperitoneal attachments of the spleen were divided with electrocautery or an appropriate energy device. This incision of the peritoneum was carried out to the level of the left diaphragm allowing visualization of the fundus of the stomach. Facilitated by the effect of gravity and the weight of the spleen, the spleen and tail of the pancreas were then rotated medially by gentle dissection of the loose areolar space between the pancreas and the retroperitoneum. Care was taken to avoid injury to the splenic vein during the course of this dissection. At this point, the supra-renal tissue and its contents (adrenal gland and retroperitoneal fat) were visible. Gerota's fascia, the upper border of the left kidney and the left renal hilum were then identified and dissected. Dissection of the left renal vein and its upper border led to the identification of the left adrenal vein which was *doubly ligated and divided/clipped and divided/____*. Using *electrocautery/an appropriate energy device*, the retroperitoneal fat of the left suprarenal space was elevated off the superior pole of the left kidney. The dissection was then carried out along the medial aspect of the adrenal gland down to the level of the quadratus lumborum muscle in the retroperitoneum indicating complete removal of all the fat in the suprarenal space. *An accessory adrenal vein running along the medial aspect of the gland and draining into the phrenic vein was encountered and divided.* The dissection of all the supra-renal tissue was then completed in a stepwise fashion. The arterial supply of the left adrenal gland was controlled and divided as it was encountered along this dissection.

Irrigation of the operative bed was then carried with the confirmation of hemostasis. The adrenal gland and all surrounding fat were then placed in a specimen retrieval bag and extracted after enlarging the 10-mm port via a muscle splitting incision. The extraction site was then sutured closed in layers using #1 PDS suture. Re-insufflation of the abdominal cavity was then carried out and hemostasis was confirmed. The trocars were removed under direct vision and the fascia was closed on all trocars sites >10 mm. The skin was closed with 4-0 Monocryl. The patient tolerated the procedure well. There were no complications and the blood loss was minimal. The instrument and sponge count was correct. The patient was extubated and returned to the postanesthesia care unit in stable condition.

NOTES

Chapter 135
Right Adrenalectomy

Faek R. Jamali, M.D.

INDICATIONS

- Aldosteronoma.
- Cortisol-secreting adenoma (Cushing syndrome or subclinical Cushing).
- Pheochromocytoma (sporadic or familial).
- Virilizing or feminizing tumors.
- Nonfunctioning unilateral tumor size >4 cm.
- Adrenal nodule with imaging features atypical for adenoma, myelolipoma, or cyst.
- Adrenocortical carcinoma.
- Solitary unilateral adrenal metastasis.

ESSENTIAL STEPS

1. Prepare the patient adequately (e.g., correct electrolyte abnormalities, control hypertension, preoperative alpha-blockade in pheochromocytoma, stress steroids in Cushing's disease).
2. Enter the abdomen through an extended right subcostal incision. Exposure for this approach may be facilitated by elevating the right flank using a roll under the right side.
3. Explore the abdomen.
4. Mobilize the triangular ligament of the liver and medial rotation of the right liver lobe to expose IVC.
5. Dissect the right border of the IVC.
6. Identify, dissect, and clip the right adrenal vein.

J.J. Hoballah and C.E.H. Scott-Conner (eds.), *Operative Dictations in General and Vascular Surgery*, DOI 10.1007/978-1-4614-0451-4_135,
© Springer Science+Business Media, LLC 2012

7. Dissect all the right supra-renal tissue, including right adrenal gland and en bloc resection of retroperitoneal fat and any attached organ (liver, kidney, diaphragm) as needed to ensure complete tumor resection.

NOTE THESE VARIATIONS

- Large malignant tumors on the right may require en bloc resection of a liver segment (Segment VIII) and even the kidney.
- Adrenal tumors should be removed along with a generous margin of retroperitoneal fat and Gerota fascia.
- In cases of primary adrenal cortical malignancies, periaortic lymph nodes medial to the right renal hilum should be removed along with the tumor.

COMPLICATIONS

- Tumor rupture leading to spillage and seeding.
- Bleeding from large raw surface in the retroperitoneum or from accessory lumbar veins.
- Right diaphragmatic injury leading to pneumothorax.

TEMPLATE OPERATIVE DICTATION

Preoperative diagnosis: List specific pathology indicating surgery *(see indications above)*, e.g., *pheochromocytoma of the right adrenal gland*.

Procedure: Open right adrenalectomy.

Postoperative diagnosis: List specific intraoperative findings, e.g., *pheochromocytoma of right adrenal gland*.

Indications: This ___-year-old *male/female* patient was found to have a *specific diagnosis of right adrenal gland pathology*. Preoperative biochemical workup showed evidence of *(list specific hormonal activity if present)*. Imaging confirmed a ___ cm right adrenal lesion. The patient underwent preoperative preparation *(see point one of essential steps)* and is now presenting for elective right adrenalectomy. The indications, alternatives, risks, and benefits of the surgery were discussed with the patient and informed consent was obtained.

Details of operation: The patient was brought to the operating room and placed in the supine position. A roll (or beanbag) was placed under the patient's right flank to allow slight medial rotation of the right side. The abdomen was clipped, prepped with 2% chlorhexidine solution, and draped in the standard fashion. A time-out was completed verifying correct patient, procedure, site, positioning, and implant(s) and/or special equipment prior to beginning this procedure.

The abdomen was approached via a standard extended subcostal incision. The skin was incised two finger breadths below the right costal margin starting from the mid-axillary line and extending to the midline. The incision was deepened through the skin and subcutaneous tissue Scarpa's fascia was opened and the incision taken down to the level of the abdominal wall. The anterior rectus sheath was opened in the right rectus muscle was split using electrocautery with control of the epigastric vessels. The posterior rectus sheath was also divided. Using electrocautery, the lateral abdominal wall musculature was divided. The external, internal, and transversalis fascia were divided using electrocautery. Exploration of the abdominal cavity was then carried out to rule out evidence of metastatic disease. The procedure was started by mobilizing the triangular ligament of the liver and rotating the right hepatic lobe medially to allow exposure of the IVC and of the adrenal gland in the retroperitoneum. Dissection of the right border of the IVC was then carried out by incising the peritoneal reflection overlying the suprarenal lodge along the right border of the IVC all the way up to the diaphragm. Care was taken not to injure the right hepatic vein. Gentle dissection along the right border of the IVC led to the identification of the right adrenal vein which was then ligated and divided. The dissection along the right border of the IVC was then carried further posteriorly until reaching the Quadratus Lumborum muscle and then inferiorly until reaching the right renal hilum. The right suprarenal lodge was then dissected and removed as one block. Using *electrocautery/ an appropriate energy device*, the retroperitoneal fat of the right suprarenal lodge was elevated off the superior pole of the right kidney and gently dissected off the lateral abdominal wall, posteriorly off the right Quadratus Lumborum muscle and superiorly off the diaphragm.. The arterial supply of the right adrenal gland was controlled and divided as it was encountered along this dissection. *(It usually consists of three main arterial branches, from the right renal artery, the aorta, and the right phrenic artery)*. Care was taken not to injure any accessory right renal arteries that may easily be confounded for adrenal arterial branches originating from the renal artery. Care was also taken to avoid injury to the capsule of the adrenal gland. If cancer: *An en bloc dissection of the para-aortic nodes was also carried out as part of the medial extent of the dissection of the suprarenal tissue. The specimen is then removed en bloc (when indicated for ACC).* Irrigation of the suprarenal region was carried out and confirmation of hemostasis was achieved.

The right lobe of the liver was then allowed to return back to its normal anatomical position. Closure of the abdomen and layers was then carried out using number one PDS suture followed by closure of the skin with a skin stapler. The patient tolerated the procedure well. There were no complications and the blood loss was minimal. The instrument and sponge count was correct. The patient was extubated and returned to the recovery room in stable satisfactory condition.

NOTES

Chapter 136
Laparoscopic Right Adrenalectomy

Faek R. Jamali, M.D.

INDICATIONS

- Aldosteronoma.
- Cortisol-secreting adenoma (Cushing syndrome or subclinical Cushing).
- Pheochromocytoma (sporadic or familial).
- Nonfunctioning unilateral nodule >4 cm.
- Nodule with imaging features atypical for adenoma, myelolipoma, or cyst.
- Solitary unilateral adrenal metastasis.

ESSENTIAL STEPS

1. Prepare the patient (e.g., correct electrolyte abnormalities, control hypertension, preoperative alpha-blockade in pheochromocytoma, stress steroids in Cushing's disease).
2. Position the patient in the full right lateral decubitus position with appropriate padding.
3. Establish pneumoperitoneum and place trocars.
4. Explore the abdomen.
5. Mobilize the triangular ligament of the liver and elevate the right lobe of the liver.
6. Dissect the right border of the inferior vena cava.
7. Identify, Dissect, secure, and divide the right adrenal vein.
8. Dissect all the right supra-renal tissues, including right adrenal gland and perform en bloc resection of retroperitoneal fat from the superior pole of the right kidney to the diaphragm.

J.J. Hoballah and C.E.H. Scott-Conner (eds.), *Operative Dictations in General and Vascular Surgery*, DOI 10.1007/978-1-4614-0451-4_136,

NOTE THIS VARIATION

- Large malignant tumors on the right may require en bloc resection of the segment VIII of the liver and even the kidney and should not be approached laparoscopically.

COMPLICATIONS

- Massive bleeding can occur if the adrenal vein is torn or avulsed.
- Tumor rupture leading to spillage and seeding.
- Bleeding from large raw surfaces in the retroperitoneum or from accessory lumbar veins.
- Right diaphragmatic injury leading to pneumothorax.

TEMPLATE OPERATIVE DICTATION

Preoperative diagnosis: List specific pathology indicating surgery *(see indications above)*, e.g., *pheochromocytoma of the right adrenal gland*.

Procedure: Laparoscopic right adrenalectomy.

Postoperative diagnosis: List specific intraoperative findings, e.g., *pheochromocytoma of right adrenal gland*.

Indications: This ___-year-old *male/female* patient was found to have a right adrenal ___. Preoperative biochemical workup showed evidence of ____ *(list specific hormonal activity if present)*. Imaging confirmed a ___cm right adrenal lesion. The patient underwent preoperative preparation *(see point one of essential steps)* and is now presenting for elective laparoscopic right adrenalectomy. The indications, alternatives, and risks and benefits of the surgery were discussed with the patient and informed consent was obtained.

Details of operation: The patient was brought to the operating room and placed on the operating table in the right lateral decubitus position. The patient was appropriately positioned with padding as well as the use of a beanbag. The abdomen was clipped, prepped with 2% Chlorhexidine solution, and draped in the standard fashion. A time-out was completed verifying correct patient, procedure, site, positioning, and implant(s) and/or special equipment prior to beginning this procedure.

The abdomen was approached via an *open Hasson/Veress needle* technique and pneumoperitoneum was created. The first (10 mm) trocar was placed at the mid-level of the subcostal margin on the right side. Two additional 5-mm trocars at the level of the costal margin, 8–10 cm away to the right and right of the camera port. The third 5-mm trocar was placed to at the level of the mid-axillary or posterior axillary line for the assistant's use.

Exploration of the abdominal cavity was carried out followed by mobilization of the triangular ligament of the liver and elevation/ rotation of the right hepatic lobe medially using a 5-mm curved tip retractor and hook electrocautery to allow exposure of the IVC and the adrenal gland in the retroperitoneum. Dissection of the right border of the IVC was then carried out by incising the peritoneal reflection overlying the suprarenal tissues along the right border of the IVC all the way up to the diaphragm using *hook electrocautery/energy device*. Care was taken not to injure the right hepatic vein. Gentle dissection along the right border of the IVC led to the identification of the right adrenal vein which was then *ligated and divided/secured with an endoscopic stapler with a vascular load/M/L clipper or Hemolocks*. The dissection along the right border of the IVC was then carried further posteriorly until reaching the quadratus lumborum muscle and then inferiorly until reaching the right renal hilum with clear identification of the right renal vein. The right suprarenal tissues were then dissected and removed en bloc. Using *electrocautery/energy device*, the retroperitoneal fat of the right suprarenal space was elevated off its superior attachments to the diaphragm, the superior pole of the right kidney and gently dissected off the lateral abdominal wall. The posterior dissection was carried out to the level of the right quadratus lumborum muscle ensuring complete removal of the all the adrenal gland and suprarenal tissue as one block. The arterial supply of the right adrenal gland was controlled and divided using an appropriate energy source, as it was encountered along this dissection. Care was taken not to injure any accessory right renal arteries. Care was also taken to avoid injury to the capsule of the adrenal gland. The adrenal gland and all surrounding fat were then placed in a specimen retrieval bag and extracted after enlarging the 10-mm port via a muscle splitting incision. The extraction site was then sutured closed in layers using #1 PDS suture. Re-insufflation of the abdominal cavity was then carried out and hemostasis was confirmed. The trocars were removed under direct vision and the fascia was closed on all trocars sites >10 mm. The skin was closed with 4-0 Monocryl. The patient tolerated the procedure well. There were no complications and the blood loss was minimal. The instrument and sponge count was correct. The patient was extubated and returned to the postanesthesia care unit in stable condition.

NOTES

Chapter 137
Insertion of Peritoneal Dialysis Catheter

Philip M. Spanheimer, M.D. and Thomas E. Collins, M.D.

INDICATION
- Long-term access for peritoneal dialysis.

ESSENTIAL STEPS
1. Access the peritoneal cavity.
2. Insert the catheter into the peritoneal cavity.
3. Place the proximal cuff in the pre-peritoneal space.
4. Create a tunnel from the catheter entrance to exit site.
5. Place the distal cuff in the subcutaneous tissue.
6. Close the abdomen.
7. Flush the catheter and allow contents to run out.

NOTE THESE VARIATIONS
- Laparoscopic versus open.
- Type and size of catheter.
- Positioning of exit site.

COMPLICATIONS
- Bacterial or fungal peritonitis bowel perforation.
- Catheter site infection.
- Catheter migration.
- Catheter obstruction.

J.J. Hoballah and C.E.H. Scott-Conner (eds.), *Operative Dictations in General and Vascular Surgery*, DOI 10.1007/978-1-4614-0451-4_137,
© Springer Science+Business Media, LLC 2012

TEMPLATE OPERATIVE DICTATION
Preoperative diagnosis: *End-stage renal disease.*
Procedure: Insertion of peritoneal dialysis catheter.
Postoperative diagnosis: Same.
Indications: This ___-year-old *male/female* required dialysis for end-stage renal disease secondary to _____. Peritoneal access was chosen for dialysis.
Description of procedure: The patient was placed in the supine position and general endotracheal anesthesia was induced. Preoperative antibiotics were given. The abdomen was prepped and draped in the usual sterile fashion. A time-out was completed verifying correct patient, procedure, site, positioning, and implant(s) and/or special equipment prior to beginning this procedure.

If Open: A 4 cm vertical incision was made in the midline approximately 2–3 cm below the umbilicus. The incision was deepened through the subcutaneous tissues using electrocautery. Hemostasis was assured. The anterior rectus sheath was opened and the muscle fibers bluntly dissected. The posterior rectus sheath was sharply incised and the abdominal cavity entered. *Adhesions were lysed sharply under direct vision with Metzenbaum scissors.* Adequate area for peritoneal dialysis was visualized within the abdominal cavity. The patient was placed in the Trendelenburg position and the catheter was placed over a stylet and advanced into the peritoneal cavity. The intraperitoneal segment was advanced into the peritoneal cavity and the cuff into the pre-peritoneal space. The peritoneum and rectus sheaths were closed with __-0 *absorbable suture* ensuring that the catheter was not caught in the suture line. A tunnel was created to the exit site *lateral/caudal* to the entrance site. The distal cuff was placed subcutaneously ___ cm from the exit site. The wound was copiously irrigated. Scarpa's fascia was closed with *3/4-0 Vicryl*. The skin was closed with *4/5-0 Monocryl/Vicryl/Staples*.

If Laparoscopic: A 2–3 cm infraumbilical incision was made in the midline using a scalpel. The umbilicus was grasped with *forceps/coker* and elevated. The anterior and posterior rectus sheaths were opened sharply in the midline and the abdominal cavity entered. A 5-mm trocar was inserted and insufflated with CO_2. The patient was placed in Trendelenburg position and a 5-mm 0° scope was inserted and diagnostic laparoscopy performed. A 5-mm port was inserted under direct vision into the pre-peritoneal space at the planned catheter exit site *lateral/caudal* to the insertion site. *Adhesions were lysed using Ligasure/Harmonic Scalpel/Other.* A double-cuffed peritoneal dialysis catheter was inserted through the infraumbilical port. *Placement of the catheter was not satisfactory and an additional 5-mm port was placed. The catheter was grasped and positioned into the pelvis.* The periumbilical port was removed and the catheter was tunneled to the exit site with the proximal cuff positioned in the tunnel. All trocars were removed and hemostasis was assured. The fascia was closed with *3/4-0 Vicryl* and the skin with *4/5-0 Monocryl/Vicryl.*

The catheter was flushed with saline and the incision was inspected for leakage. The saline was allowed to drain and showed no evidence of hemoperitoneum or fecal contamination.

The patient tolerated the procedure well and was taken to the postanesthesia care unit in stable condition.

NOTES

Chapter 138

Pediatric Inguinal Hernia Repair (Herniotomy*)

Graeme Pitcher, M.B.B.Ch.

INDICATION
- Patency of the processus vaginalis with hydrocele or hernia.

ESSENTIAL STEPS
1. Supine position.
2. Prep the operative site from the upper thighs to above the umbilicus.
3. Make a curvilinear incision in the skin crease centered over the mid-inguinal point.
   - Correct placement of the incision is important for reasons of cosmesis as well as affording good access to the structures in the inguinal canal. This incision satisfies both requirements.
4. Elevate Scarpa's fascia with toothed forceps and divide it with electrocautery.
5. When the window of fibro-areolar tissue above the external oblique aponeurosis is seen, develop this plane further by blunt dissection.
   - Visualize the inguinal ligament as well as the external ring at this stage.

---

*Note that in children the operation is more properly referred to as a herniotomy as no reparative operation (as in herniorrhaphy) is performed on the inguinal canal. The operation in the vast majority of cases entails the high ligation of the sac, which results in a solid repair for the vast majority of children.

J.J. Hoballah and C.E.H. Scott-Conner (eds.), *Operative Dictations in General and Vascular Surgery*, DOI 10.1007/978-1-4614-0451-4_138,
© Springer Science+Business Media, LLC 2012

- This allows you to exclude the rare femoral hernia.
- It also ensures that you open the external oblique in the proper position to allow good access to the structures in the inguinal canal.

6. Identify the sac.
   - Look inferior to the ilioinguinal nerve beneath the curving fibers of the internal oblique.
   - Slight downwards pressure on the two retractors providing exposure can make the sac more prominent at this stage.

7. Elevate the sac by separating the cremaster fibers and grasping it with a forcep.
   - Further exposure is best achieved at this stage by holding it up and peeling the cremaster fibers away from it bluntly with a DeBakey forcep.

8. At this stage, there are two options to proceed:
   - In patients with large, thin-walled sacs, especially in small babies, one may deliberately open the sac and perform further dissection from within. This is the author's preference.
   - In patients with more manageable sacs, the sac can be dissected from the cord structures without the need to open it.
   - Note that in females it is important to open the sac in all cases to ensure that the operator is not ligating a fallopian tube (which may loop into the sac) in error.

9. **If the sac is opened:** Open the sac between two hemostats. Dissect posteriorly toward the cord structures while serially applying small hemostats to the proximal sac margin. Ultimately one will have a narrow bridge of sac between the last two hemostats that can be safely negotiated with the vessels and vas in the background and the dissection accomplished safely under direct vision.

10. **If the sac is left closed sac**: Seek a plane between the posterior wall of the sac and the vessels and vas deferens. This can be achieved either by dissection with the tip of a hemostat or scissors or by rolling the sac over ones nondominant hand index finger and entering the plane with a scissors in that way. If the sac is inadvertently opened, one can revert to the open sac approach if the operation becomes difficult.

11. Once the sac is dissected free and controlled, clamp it with a single hemostat. Further dissection both superiorly

and inferiorly around the internal ring with sustained traction on the sac will allow identification of the proper site of suture ligation flush with the fascia transversalis and lateral to the inferior epigastric vessels.

12. In girls, the round ligament can be ligated with the same suture as the sac and affords a sound closure. The distal portion of the round ligament is usually ligated for hemostasis.

13. Transfix the sac with a 4.0 Vicryl suture and suture ligate it. High-risk hernias can be double ligated.

14. Pull the scrotal contents down into the scrotum at this stage to prevent iatrogenic ascending testis and to allow easier closure of the external oblique.

15. In a boy with a communicating hydrocele, drain the distal entrapped fluid by presenting it up to the incision with pressure from below and creating a wide fenestration in the tunica vaginalis.
    • If this step is omitted, this postoperative hydrocele will cause parental anxiety and will require later drainage or aspiration.

16. Close the external oblique aponeurosis with a running suture of 4.0 Vicryl starting at the external ring and running laterally to the end.
    • Place the bites at varying depths to avoid weakening the aponeurosis with a parallel line of sutures – the "tear off postage stamp effect."
    • Avoid entrapping the ilioinguinal nerve in the suture line.

17. Close Scarpa's fascia with one to three buried interrupted sutures of 4.0 Vicryl.

18. Close the skin with a running subcuticular suture.

NOTE THESE VARIATIONS

■ In babies with extremely large internal rings expanded by giant hernias, it may be necessary to bolster the fascia transversalis with some fine prolene sutures (in the form of a medial interfoveolar ligament or Marcy repair) to minimize recurrence.
   ○ This is controversial.

■ Occasionally, a sliding hernia involving the cecum or sigmoid will form the wall of the sac.
   ○ Under these circumstances, it can be dissected off the sac, returned to the abdominal cavity and the sac closed

with a running suture of 5.0 prolene or equivalent to achieve sound closure.

- In certain situations, it may be advisable to rule out contralateral hernia by laparoscopy.
  - To do this, a modified purse-string suture is placed around the open sac. A 2/3 mm port is placed in the sac into the peritoneal cavity and the sac tied temporarily around it. A pneumoperitoneum of 8–10 mmHg is achieved and a 2.7-mm 70° lens is introduced. This is passed horizontally across the abdomen and usually affords a good view of the opposite internal ring.
- When faced with strangulated bowel in an indirect inguinal hernia, the initial steps are the same.
  - The sac is opened and the bowel inspected and returned to the abdominal cavity if intact.
  - In some cases, the internal ring will have to be opened slightly with a lateral incision to release the strangulated bowel.
  - If the operator is comfortable, bowel resection, anastomosis, and hernia repair can all be carried out through the groin access. Alternatively, a small laparotomy can be helpful.

COMPLICATIONS

- Recurrence.
- Testicular atrophy.
- Injury to vas deferens.
- Superficial wound infection.

TEMPLATE OPERATIVE DICTATION

Preoperative diagnosis: Inguinal hernia or hydrocele.
Procedure: Inguinal herniotomy.
Postoperative diagnosis: Same.
Indications: This ___day-, week-, month-, or year-old *male/female* presented with a groin bulge or inguinal hernia or hydrocele.
Description of procedure: The patient was brought into the operating room, and placed supine on the operating table. General anesthesia was induced. All pressure points were padded. The groin and lower abdomen was prepped and draped in a sterile fashion. A time-out was completed verifying correct patient, procedure, site, positioning, and implant(s) and/or special equipment prior to beginning this procedure.

An incision was then made in a skin crease over the mid-inguinal point. The external oblique aponeurosis was opened longitudinally parallel to the inguinal ligament. The sac was identified and carefully dissected free from the other structures of the spermatic cord. The sac contained ____ which was reduced into the peritoneal cavity. A high ligation was performed with a transfixing suture of 4.0 Vicryl. The external oblique aponeurosis was closed with a running suture of 4.0 Vicryl from medial to lateral. The scarpas fascia was approximated by two (three) buried 4.0 vicryl interrupted sutures. The skin was closed with a running subcuticular suture of 5.0 monocryl. The patient tolerated the procedure well and was awakened from anesthesia and taken to the postanesthesia care unit in a satisfactory condition.

NOTES

Chapter 139

Laparoscopic Pyloromyotomy

Graeme Pitcher, M.B.B.Ch.

INDICATION

- Infantile hypertrophic pyloric stenosis.

ESSENTIAL STEPS

1. Supine position. The patient is orientated transversely across operating table.
2. The anesthesiologist places a size 8- or 10-F nasogastric tube.
3. Palpate the pylorus while the patient is anesthetized.
4. Prep the abdomen in the usual sterile manner from the pubis to the nipple line.
5. Obtain pneumoperitoneum by a modified Hasson technique by dilating the umbilical cicatrix and passing a blunt instrument into the peritoneal cavity, ensuring that no injury is made to the liver.
6. Place a size 2/3-mm or 5-mm port in the umbilical position and obtain a pneumoperitoneum of 7–10 mmHg.
7. Pass a short 30° laparoscope into the abdomen and confirm the presence of a hypertrophic pylorus is confirmed.
8. Rotate the lens to view the anterior abdominal wall and make a stab incision using a number 11 blade approximately in the right mid-clavicular line, 2–3 cm below the costal margin.

J.J. Hoballah and C.E.H. Scott-Conner (eds.), *Operative Dictations in General and Vascular Surgery*, DOI 10.1007/978-1-4614-0451-4_139,

9. Introduce an atraumatic grasper through this incision without the use of a port.

10. Make a similar incision at the same level on the patients left side just medial to the mid-clavicular line.
    - Make this incision sufficiently lateral enough so as not to allow the formation of muscular defects, which can occur if the incision is made too close to the midline.

11. Introduce the arthrotomy knife or electrocautery device that will be used to divide the pyloric muscle through this incision without the use of a port.

12. Grasp the duodenum distal to the hypertrophic area with the left hand, with a grip that is firm yet gentle and not too tight, and bring it forward into view.

13. Determine the limits of the hypertrophic muscle by palpating with the blunt tip of the arthrotomy knife in the right hand with the blade protected.

14. Make a longitudinal incision from just short of the distal limit of the muscle to the level of the gastric wall using the blade protruding to approximately 2 mm.

15. Withdraw the blade and insert the blunt tip of the arthrotomy knife into the incision in the muscle and rotate it to begin spreading the fibers.

16. Insert the specialized spreader into the pyloric muscle incision and open it.
    - This usually allows the first visualization of the mucosa.
    - Errant fibers will sometimes require the repeated passage of the knife to divide them followed by repeated spreading.

17. Take great care not to divide the distal fibers too close to the distal extent of division, as it is there that the duodenal mucosa is most superficial and where inadvertent mucosal injuries are most likely to occur.

18. Examine the mucosa to determine that it is intact.

19. Remove the blade and exchange it for a second atraumatic grasper.

20. Grasp the upper and lower leaves of muscle in the two graspers.

21. The pyloromyotomy is complete when the two halves can be moved independently from one another.

22. Carefully remove the instruments in the stab incisions and check these incisions for hemostasis.

23. Desufflate the abdomen and remove the port from the umbilicus.

24. Close the defect in the sheath of the umbilicus with a horizontal, vertical, or figure of eight type suture of 4.0 Vicryl.
25. Close the skin with tissue glue at the umbilicus as well as at the site of the two stab incisions.
    • No deep closure is performed at these two sites.

NOTE THESE VARIATIONS
■ A 5-mm lens may be used if no smaller lens is available.
■ The operator may elect to grasp the stomach with the right hand and to perform the pyloromyotomy with the left hand. This allows grasping on the more robust stomach wall as apposed to the more vulnerable duodenal wall.
■ A standard protected electrocautery tip may substitute for the arthrotomy blade. The incision is then made on a low blend setting with a power of 10. The extent of the incision is usually scored first on the surface using the coagulation mode. The blade doubles as a blunt spreader very effectively. Care must be taken to coordinate activation of the current so as not to cause inadvertent injury during spreading.
■ An air insufflation test can be performed to test the mucosal integrity by the passage of 40–60 cc of air into the nasogastric tube by the anesthesiologist. The mucosal surface is inspected for bubbling.

COMPLICATIONS
■ Mucosal perforation.
■ Incomplete pyloromyotomy.
■ Injury to the liver or duodenum.
■ Port site hernias or dehiscence (rare).

TEMPLATE OPERATIVE DICTATION
Preoperative diagnosis: Hypertrophic pyloric stenosis.
Procedure: Laparoscopic pyloromyotomy.
Postoperative diagnosis: Same.
Indications: This ___-week-old *male/female* presented with forceful vomiting and was found to have clinical, radiological, and ultrasound features to support the diagnosis.
Description of procedure: The patient was brought into the operating room, and placed supine on the operating table. General anesthesia was induced. A nasogastric tubes was placed. All pressure points were padded. The abdomen was prepped and draped

in a sterile fashion. A time-out was completed verifying correct patient, procedure, site, positioning, and implant(s) and/or special equipment prior to beginning this procedure.

An incision was then made within the umbilicus. A trocar was introduced into the abdomen under direct vision. The abdomen was insufflated with carbon dioxide to a pressure of 8 mmHg. The patient tolerated insufflation well. The laparoscope was then inserted and the abdomen was inspected. There was no injury noted from initial trocar placement. The stomach was identified and the pylorus could also easily be seen and appeared hypertrophic. A stab incision was then made on the right side of the abdomen within the rectus sheath under direct vision. An atraumatic grasper was placed into the abdomen and the duodenum was grasped. A second stab incision was then made on the left side of the abdomen and an arthrotomy knife was introduced. The pyloric muscle was incised extending from just proximal to the duodenum and onto the stomach for approximately 2 cm. The blade was retracted and the sheath was used to start the myotomy. The pyloric spreader was then used to complete the pyloromyotomy. The mucosa was seen bulging but intact. Both halves were independently movable indicating an adequate pyloromyotomy. There was no gross bleeding. Instruments were then removed and the abdomen desufflated. The umbilical fascia was then using 4-0 Vicryl sutures. The skin was closed using 5-0 Vicryl. The patient tolerated the procedure well and was awakened from anesthesia and taken to the postanesthesia care unit in a satisfactory condition.

NOTES

Chapter 140
Pediatric Laparoscopic Nissen Fundoplication

Joel Shilyansky, M.D.

INDICATIONS

- Patients with GERD complicated by:
  - Failure to thrive.
  - Aspiration.
  - Laryngospasm associated with reflux and leading to severe cyanotic or apneic events.
- Failure of medical therapy of GERD:
  - Persistent esophagitis.
  - Pain.
  - Regurgitation and vomiting resulting in significant impact on the quality of life.
- Barrett's esophagus (intestinal metaplasia).
- Hiatal or paraesophageal hernia.

ESSENTIAL STEPS

1. Supine position or low lithotomy position to allow the surgeon to stand at the foot of the bed, moderate reverse Trendelenberg (~20° head up).
2. Port placement:
   - (a) Port size is variable and depends on surgeon's preference and the size of the child. Five 5-mm port can accommodate most circumstances. Some surgeons prefer 3-mm trocars in a small baby.
   - (b) 30° Laparoscope.
3. Elevate the left lateral segment of the liver using a retractor placed through the right lateral port.

J.J. Hoballah and C.E.H. Scott-Conner (eds.), *Operative Dictations in General and Vascular Surgery*, DOI 10.1007/978-1-4614-0451-4_140,

4. Divide the short gastric vessels *(this maneuver is not always needed and performed based on surgeon preference)*.
   (a) Enter the lesser sac along the greater curve of the stomach through an avascular window to the left of the body or fundus.
   (b) Take great care not to injure the spleen especially as the vessel get shorter superiorly.
5. Retract the stomach inferiorly.
6. Incise the gastrohepatic and the phrenoesophageal ligament.
7. Dissect the right crus.
   (a) Make sure enough crus is exposed.
8. Dissect the esophagus posteriorly and create a large enough window to accommodate the fundus.
   (a) Take great care not to injure the:
      (i) Esophagus
      (ii) Vagus nerve
      (iii) Aorta
   (b) Avoid extensive dissection in the mediastinum:
      (i) By identifying the junction of the right and left crura one can avoid getting lost.
      (ii) Some dissection of the mediastinal esophagus may be needed to gain greater intraabdominal length of the esophagus.
   (c) Avoid dissecting into the left pleural space, as it may result in tension pneumothorax. If pneumothorax occurs place a chest tube on the left. Tube may be removed at the end of procedure after pneumoperitoneum is evacuated.
9. Close the crus with a bougie in the esophagus.
   (a) Place the crural stitch.
   (b) Ask anesthesia to insert the bougie.
      (i) Protect the airway since accidental extubation during passage of bougie can occur.
   (c) Make sure that the thick part of the bougie is past the gastroesophageal junction.
   (d) Withdraw the bougie into the thoracic esophagus to facilitate the next step.
10. Bring a fold of the fundus behind the esophagus.
   (a) Bring a fold of the fundus anteriorly to the esophagus.
11. Place three fundoplication sutures spanning 1–1.5 cm from the superior to the inferior.

- (a) Place the first, superior suture, then advance the bougie and tie it over the bougie.
- (b) If the tie is not perfect, you can replace it later.
- (c) Place the remaining sutures.
    - (i) Incorporate the anterior esophagus in the fundoplication sutures to prevent is from sliding down. Take a bite of anterior fold of fundus, then the anterior wall of the esophagus, and then the posterior fold of fundus.
    - (ii) If the first suture is too loose, replace it.
- (d) The fundoplication should surround the intraabdominal esophagus.
- (e) Remove the bougie.
- (f) Tack the fundoplication to the crus to prevent the wrap from herniating into the chest.
12. Withdraw instruments.
13. Close umbilical fascial defect.

COMPLICATIONS

- Patient selection is critical for the success of the procedure. The procedure is very effective at preventing retrograde flow of gastric contents, gastroesophageal reflux disease. Patients with gastric outlet obstruction, severely delayed gastric emptying, retching, aspiration of saliva, and obesity have less than satisfactory outcomes and may suffer exacerbation of their symptoms and early failure of fundoplication.
- Injury to esophagus.
- Injury to spleen.
- Injury to vagus nerves.
- Injury to aorta.
- Pneumothorax.
- Failed fundoplication.
- Dysphagia.

TEMPLATE OPERATIVE DICTATION

Preoperative diagnosis: *Refractory gastroesophageal reflux/hiatus hernia/paraesophageal hernia*.

Procedure: Laparoscopic Nissen fundoplication.

Postoperative diagnosis: Same.

Indications: This _____-*month/year*-old *male/female* had *refractory gastroesophageal reflux with* _____*/hiatus hernia/paraesophageal* *hernia.* Medical management failed and laparoscopic Nissen fundoplication was indicated for definitive treatment.

Description of procedure: The patient was positioned supine in the operating room table. General endotracheal anesthesia was administered. A time-out was completed verifying correct patient, procedure, site, positioning, and implant(s) and/or special equipment prior to beginning this procedure. An orogastric tube was inserted. The child was then placed at the end of the table *(optional: in low lithotomy position).* The abdomen was prepped and draped. The patient was then placed in reverse Trandelenburg at 20° angle.

An umbilical incision was created. The fascia was incised and traction sutures were placed in the fascia. *(Optional: An occult umbilical hernia defect was chosen for entry site into fascia). A 5-mm port was introduced into the peritoneal cavity under direct vision/a Veress needle was inserted* and the abdomen was insufflated. *If Veress needle: A 5-mm port was then placed.*

The abdomen was examined. Four additional 5-mm ports were placed, the two operating ports in subcostal position at the mid-clavicular line on both the left and on the right, and two retracting ports along the right and left anterior axillary line. *To mobilize the fundus, short gastric vessels were divided using the ligasure/harmonic scalpel.* The gastrohepatic ligament was divided. The presence of a replaced left hepatic artery was evaluated *(and if present: it was avoided).* The stomach was retracted inferiorly. The esohago-phrenic ligament was divided. The right diaphragmatic crus was identified and dissected. The cardia and esophagus were freed at the hiatus using a combination of blunt and sharp dissection. The posterior dissection was carried out from right to left taking great care not to injure the esophagus. The anterior and posterior Vagus nerves were visualized and spared. The left diaphragmatic crus were identified. The posterior aspect of the esophagus was freed for sufficient length to allow the fundus to pass without tension. Dissection of the mediastinal esophagus was performed to allow for sufficient intra-abdominal esophageal length.

A _____ French bougie was atraumatically passed into the esophagus. Crural repair was performed posteriorly using 2-0 Ethibond sutures. The sutures were tied with a bougie placed within the esophagus. Next a 360° fundoplication was performed. The bougie was partially withdrawn into the thoracic esophagus. A fold of the fundus was passed behind the esophagus. The remainder of the fundus was folded anteriorly to the esophagus. The twofold of the fundus were brought together to create a 1–1.5 cm long fundoplication. The superior fundoplication suture was placed. 2-0 Ethibond is commonly used. The bougie was passed back into the stomach prior to tying the first fundoplication suture. Two additional fundoplication sutures were then placed and tied with the bougie in the esophagus. The two superior sutures incorporated the esophagus at the hiatus. The most inferior suture was at or just above the level of the gastroesophageal junction. The bougie was removed. The fundoplication was tacked to the diaphragmatic crus using two 2-0 Ethibond sutures to prevent the wrap from migrating into the chest.

The laparoscopic instruments were then withdrawn. The umbilical fascial defect was closed with _____. The skin incisions were closed with absorbable ____ sutures and a dressing was applied. The patient tolerated the procedure well and was taken to the postanesthesia care unit in satisfactory condition.

NOTES

Section XIV
Cerebrovascular Occlusive Disease

Chapter 141
Carotid Endarterectomy

Jamal J. Hoballah, M.D., M.B.A.

INDICATIONS
- Asymptomatic stenosis >60%.
- Symptomatic stenosis >50%. In the absence of high medical risk patients or high surgical risk patient (recurrent stenosis, tracheostomy, neck radiation) where carotid stenting will be considered.

ESSENTIAL STEPS
1. Incise the skin and platysma.
2. Retract the sternocleidomastoid laterally.
3. Identify the internal jugular and facial veins.
4. Transect and suture ligate the facial vein.
5. Expose and dissect the common, internal, and external carotid arteries.
6. Identify and preserve the vagus and hypoglossal nerve.
7. Anticoagulate with heparin.
8. Cross-clamp the internal, common, and external carotid arteries.
9. Insert shunt if needed.
10. Perform the endarterectomy.
11. Assess the endarterectomized surface and the endpoints.
12. Close the arteriotomy.
13. Backbleed the internal and external carotid arteries and forwardbleed the common carotid artery.
14. Resume flow into the external then internal carotid arteries.

J.J. Hoballah and C.E.H. Scott-Conner (eds.), *Operative Dictations in General and Vascular Surgery*, DOI 10.1007/978-1-4614-0451-4_141,
© Springer Science+Business Media, LLC 2012

15. Assess reconstruction.
16. Secure hemostasis.
17. Close the wound.

NOTE THESE VARIATIONS

- Carotid endarterectomy is most commonly performed by opening the carotid artery longitudinally and removing the plaque. The artery is then closed primarily or with a patch as described in this chapter. The patch used can be prosthetic (polyester and PTFE) or autogenous (greater saphenous and jugular vein). Alternatively, the internal carotid artery is transected obliquely at its origin and the endarterectomy is performed using an eversion technique as described in Chapter 142.

- During carotid endarterectomy, the need for shunting can be determined by performing the procedure with the patient awake under regional/local anesthesia, by using EEG monitoring or measuring internal carotid stump pressure. Alternatively, routine shunting may be carried out.

COMPLICATIONS

- Stroke.
- Hematoma.
- Thrombosis.
- Cranial nerve injury.
- Infection.
- Recurrent Stenosis.

TEMPLATE OPERATIVE DICTATION

Preoperative diagnosis: *Right/left* carotid stenosis.

Procedure: *Right/left carotid endarterectomy; primary closure; patch angioplasty; vein/Dacron/*PTFE.

Postoperative diagnosis: Same.

Indications: This ___-year-old *male/female* was *asymptomatic/had prior transient monocular blindness/transient ischemic attacks/stroke. Duplex scan/angiography/MRA/CTA* revealed stenosis of the *right/left* internal carotid artery. The risks and benefits of carotid endarterectomy were explained to the patient who elected to proceed with the surgical intervention.

Description of procedure: The patient was placed in the supine barber chair position. The procedure was performed under *general endotracheal/regional/local anesthesia.*

The *right/left neck and right/left upper thigh* were prepped and draped in a standard fashion.

Electroencephalogram (EEG) monitoring was commenced.

A longitudinal skin incision was made overlying the anterior border of the sternocleidomastoid muscle. The incision was deepened through the platysma with electrocautery. The sternocleidomastoid muscle was retracted laterally.

The internal jugular vein was identified. Dissection along the medial border of the jugular vein revealed the facial vein. The facial vein was transected and suture ligated using a 3-0 silk suture.

The common carotid, the internal carotid, the superior thyroid, and the external carotid arteries were exposed and dissected.

The vagus and hypoglossal nerves were identified and preserved. Traction over the angle of the mandible was avoided to protect the mandibular branch of the facial nerve. The ansa cervicalis was transected to improve the exposure of the internal carotid artery.

Five thousand units of heparin were administered intravenously 75 UI/kg and an activated clotting time (ACT) was checked.

Five minutes after heparin administration, the internal carotid artery was clamped with a Yasargil clamp. The common carotid artery was clamped with a DeBakey vascular clamp. The external carotid and superior thyroid arteries were controlled with silastic vessel loops.

No EEG changes were noted/EEG slowing was noted immediately after cross-clamping the internal carotid artery. An arteriotomy was performed on the anterolateral surface of the common carotid artery with a #11 blade scalpel and extended into the internal carotid artery using a Pott's scissors.

A Javid/Sundt/Pruitt-Inahara/inlying/outlying shunt was inserted in the common and internal carotid arteries. The EEG returned to normal after shunt placement.

The endarterectomy plane was developed with a Freer elevator. The plaque was transected proximally in the common carotid artery. In the distal internal carotid artery, the plaque was feathered off, leaving a smooth endpoint. Eversion endarterectomy of the external carotid artery was performed and the carotid plaque was removed.

The endarterectomized surface was gently irrigated with heparinized saline solution. All remaining free debris was removed with a fine forceps.

The distal endarterectomy endpoint was inspected. *Tacking sutures were not deemed necessary/few interrupted 6-0 prolene sutures were used to tack down the distal endpoint to secure the distal intima.*

[Choose one:]

*If **primary closure:*** The arteriotomy was closed primarily using a continuous 6-0 prolene suture.

*If **patch closure:*** The arteriotomy was closed using a patch angioplasty. *A Dacron/PTFE/vein* patch was used.

A 6-cm segment of greater saphenous vein was harvested from the right upper thigh. The vein segment was slit longitudinally. The patch was trimmed and the patch angioplasty was performed using a continuous 6-0 prolene suture. The suture was started at the apex of the arteriotomy in the internal carotid artery and ran on each side. The patch was trimmed to the appropriate size and another suture was started at the other end of the patch and ran on each side to meet the first suture.

Prior to tying the last sutures, the shunt was removed.

The internal carotid, external carotid, and superior thyroid arteries were backbled. The common carotid was forwardbled. The carotid lumen was again irrigated with heparinized saline.

Flow was first reestablished into the external carotid artery and then into the internal carotid artery.

No EEG changes were noted during the removal of the shunt/ EEG changes were noted during the removal of the shunt; however, the EEG quickly returned to normal. The suture line was checked for hemostasis. Needle hole bleeding was controlled with the topical application of Surgical.

Doppler/duplex evaluation revealed excellent flow signals through the common carotid, internal carotid, and external carotid arteries.

After ensuring hemostasis, the wounds were closed using 3-0 Vicryl for the platysma and soft tissues. The skin was closed with staples. Sterile dressings were applied.

The patient was awakened, noted to have no gross neurological deficits, and taken to the postanesthesia care unit in stable condition.

Chapter 142
Carotid Endarterectomy Using the Eversion Technique

Dale Maharaj, M.D. and R. Clement Darling III, M.D.

INDICATIONS
- Asymptomatic stenosis >60%.
- Symptomatic carotid stenosis >50% (as for standard carotid endarterectomy).

CONTRAINDICATIONS
- Previous carotid endarterectomy with patch closure (relative).
- Prior irradiation, radical neck dissection, extensive high lesions.
- Carotid bypass.

COMPLICATIONS
- Stroke, hematoma, thrombosis, cranial nerve injury, infection.
- Recurrent laryngeal nerve/hoarseness, ipsilateral tongue deviation, marginal mandibular branch – ipsilateral lip drop.

ADVANTAGES OF EVERSION
- Less chance of closure-related stenosis. No need for patch.
- Plaque extraction is simpler and clamp time minimized.
- Better visualization and management of endpoint.
- Quick, simple reanastomosis.

J.J. Hoballah and C.E.H. Scott-Conner (eds.), *Operative Dictations in General and Vascular Surgery*, DOI 10.1007/978-1-4614-0451-4_142,
© Springer Science+Business Media, LLC 2012

- Lower incidence of recurrent carotid stenosis.
- Lower incidence of cranial nerve injury.

ESSENTIAL STEPS

1. Skin incision at the anterior border of the sternocleiodomastoid.
2. Divide platysma and retract the sternocleiodomastoid laterally.
3. Identify and then retract internal jugular laterally.
4. Transect and suture-ligate the facial vein (branch of internal jugular vein crossing over carotid bifurcation).
5. Expose the common, internal and external carotid arteries.
6. Identify and preserve the vagus and hypoglossal nerves.
7. Anticoagulate (30 U/kg) heparin.
8. Cross-clamp the internal, external, and common carotid arteries.
9. Transect the internal carotid artery at the bulb obliquely and dissect circumferentially.
10. Insert Javid type shunt (only for neurological deterioration) before or after the endarterectomy.
11. Extend arteriotomy on the internal and common carotid cephalad and caudally, respectively, as needed.
12. Evert the internal carotid artery while holding the plaque in place with a forceps.
13. Remove the common and external carotid plaque as with a standard endarterectomy (transect the plaque and deal with the common carotid and external carotid plaques individually).
14. Assess the endarterectomised surface and the endpoints, remove atherosclerotic debris.
15. Reconstruct the internal and common carotid using a continuous 6/0 polypropylene suture starting at the cephalad corner.
16. Backbleed the internal and external carotid arteries and forward bleed the common carotid artery just before complete closure and flush with heparinized saline.
17. Resume flow into the external, common, then internal carotid arteries.
18. Assess reconstruction – Doppler, Duplex scan.
19. Ensure hemostasis.
20. Close the platysma and skin.

OPERATIVE NOTE

Preoperative diagnosis	Rt/Lt; Carotid stenosis
Procedure	Rt/Lt; Eversion Carotid Endarterectomy with/without shunt
	Cervical block/general anesthesia
Postoperative diagnosis	Same
Indications	___year old man/woman
	Asymptomatic/TIAs/Stroke
	Duplex/Angiography/MRA: ___% stenosis of the Rt/Lt internal carotid artery.

Description of the procedure: The patient was placed in the supine position with the neck extended and lateral.

The procedure was performed under Cervical block/general anesthesia.

The Rt/Lt neck was prepped and draped in a standard surgical fashion.

A longitudinal incision was made overlying the anterior border of the sternocleidomastoid muscle and continued through the platysma.

The sternocleidomastoid muscle was retracted laterally.

The internal jugular vein was identified and dissection proceeded along the medial border of this vessel.

The facial vein was transected and suture ligated.

The common carotid, the internal carotid, external carotid, and the superior thyroid arteries were exposed and dissected.

The vagus and hypoglossal nerves were identified and preserved.

30 U/kg of heparin was administered intravenously.

The internal carotid and external carotid arteries were clamped with Yasargil clips and the common carotid artery was clamped with a Cooley vascular clamp.

The internal carotid artery was transected from the carotid bulb initially using a # 11 blade and a Metzenbaum scissors, in an oblique fashion.

An arteriotomy was carried cephalad and caudally on the internal and carotid artery, respectively, for 5–10 mm.

*Shunting as needed for neurologic deterioration.

The internal carotid artery was everted using ring forceps while the plaque was held stable with a DeBakey's forceps.

The plaque was "feathered" from the endpoint, ensuring that there was no residual plaque or debris.

Attention was now shifted to the common/external carotid artery.

The endarterectomy plane was developed with a Staphylor-rhaphy elevator within the carotid bulb.

The plaque was transected proximally in the common carotid artery.

In the distal internal carotid artery the plaque was feathered leaving a very smooth endpoint. Eversion endarterectomy of the external carotid artery was performed leaving disease-free vessel just proximal to the superior thyroid artery.

The endarterectomized surface was gently irrigated with heparinized saline solution.

All remaining free debris was removed with a fine forceps and the endpoint re-inspected.

Tacking sutures of 7-0 or 8-0 polypropylene were used to secure the distal endpoint (rarely needed).

The internal carotid artery and the carotid bulb were reconstructed using a continuous 6-0 polypropylene suture, commencing at the heel (cephalad apex)of the internal carotid artery.

Prior to placement of the last three sutures, the carotid vessels were "flushed" and irrigated with heparinized saline.

Flow was re-established to the external carotid artery and then into the internal carotid artery.

The suture line was inspected for hemostasis and Gelfoam Thrombin/Additional sutures were placed. Doppler/Duplex assessment revealed triphasic flow signals through the internal carotid, external carotid, and common carotid arteries.

The platysma was closed using 3-0 Vicryl.

The skin was closed with staples.

Throughout the procedure, and at the completion of the procedure the patient remained neurologically stable.

He was transferred to the postanesthesia care unit in a satisfactory state.

Chapter 143
Redo Carotid Endarterectomy

David C. Corry, M.D. and Mark Adelman, M.D.

INDICATIONS

- Asymptomatic stenosis >80% (higher than ACAS for primary endarterectomy to balance risk of cranial nerve injury).
- Symptomatic carotid stenosis >70% (per standard NASCET criteria).
- In the presence of contraindication of carotid stenting.

ESSENTIAL STEPS

1. Mark the old incision prior to prepping; prep the thigh if planning to use vein reconstruction.
2. Incise the skin and platysma.
3. Retract the sternocleidomastoid laterally.
4. Identify the internal jugular vein and retract laterally.
5. Expose and control the common carotid artery.
6. Identify and preserve the vagus nerve.
7. Identify and preserve the hypoglossal nerve.
8. Expose and control the internal carotid artery as required for test-clamping only.
9. Test-clamp the internal carotid; evaluate for selective shunt placement.
10. Mobilize the carotid artery as necessary proximally and distally.
11. Control the external carotid artery.
12. Fully anticoagulate with heparin.

J.J. Hoballah and C.E.H. Scott-Conner (eds.), *Operative Dictations in General and Vascular Surgery*, DOI 10.1007/978-1-4614-0451-4_143,

13. Test patient's tolerance of internal carotid artery cross-clamping.
14. Selective shunt placement:
    - Shunt not required
      - Cross-clamp the internal, external, and common carotid arteries sequentially.
      - Create an arteriotomy and extend with Pott's scissors.
      - Complete endarterectomy and decide on repair type.
    - Shunt required
      - Select shunt type.
      - Further expose proximal and distal carotid as required to place shunt.
      - Cross-clamp the internal, external, and common carotid arteries sequentially.
      - Create an arteriotomy and extend with Pott's scissors. Insert shunt and secure.
      - Verify flow in shunt and check for ischemic changes [electroencephalogram (EEG)/cognitive–motor exam].
      - Complete endarterectomy and decide on repair type.
15. Repair type:
    - Patch angioplasty
      - Select type of patch (vein/Dacron/PTFE); harvest saphenous from the thigh if vein to be used.
      - Fashion patch to fit arteriotomy.
      - Complete anastomosis with running suture, removing shunt if used.
    - Interposition graft
      - Select type of conduit (vein/Dacron/PTFE); harvest saphenous from the thigh if vein to be used.
      - Complete distal anastomosis with running suture.
      - Measure length and complete proximal anastomosis.
      - If shunt required, make appropriate provisions (see below in "if interposition graft" section). Suture ligate the external carotid artery.
16. Backbleed from the external, common, and internal carotid arteries.
17. If interposition graft used, back- and forwardbleed via proximal anastomosis.

18. Flush copiously in the lumen before tying final anastomosis.
19. Release flow into the external carotid first then common and internal carotid arteries sequentially.
20. Assess reconstruction for proper conformation and flow.
21. Secure hemostasis.
22. Close the wound and apply dressing.
23. Assess neurological status before removing patient from operating room.

NOTE THESE VARIATIONS

- During redo carotid endarterectomy, a patch angioplasty closure is usually possible if the original carotid endarterectomy was closed primarily. If a patch closure was performed in the original procedure, another patch angioplasty closure may not be possible and an interposition vein graft will be needed.

COMPLICATIONS

- Stroke.
- Hematoma.
- Thrombosis.
- Cranial nerve injury.
- Myocardial infarction.

TEMPLATE OPERATIVE DICTATION

Preoperative diagnosis: *Right/left* recurrent carotid stenosis.
Procedure: *Right/left* redo carotid endarterectomy *patch angioplasty/interposition graft (vein/Dacron/PTFE)*.
Postoperative diagnosis: Same.
Indications: This ___-year-old *male/female* had a carotid endarterectomy with *primary/patch* closure in __ for an *asymptomatic/symptomatic* carotid stenosis. She has been *asymptomatic/has recently developed transient monocular blindness/transient ischemic attacks/stroke. Duplex scan/angiography/MRA* revealed ___% stenosis of the *right/left* internal carotid artery.

The risks and benefits of carotid endarterectomy were explained to the patient who elected to proceed with the surgical intervention. Carotid stent was not an option.
Description of procedure: The patient was placed in the supine, "beach-chair" position.

The procedure was performed under *general endotracheal/ regional/local anesthesia*.

The *right/left* neck and *right/left* upper thigh were prepped and draped in a standard surgical fashion.

EEG monitoring was initiated (if used).

A longitudinal incision was made in the previous skin incision and extended proximally in the neck (thus making the initial dissection of anatomic landmarks in virgin tissue planes). The incision was deepened through the platysma with electrocautery.

The anterior border of the sternocleidomastoid muscle was located and retracted laterally.

The medial border of the internal jugular vein was identified and retracted laterally.

The common carotid artery was located in a virgin tissue plane in the proximal neck and controlled with a silastic vessel loop.

The vagus nerve was identified and protected while dissecting in the carotid sheath.

Before further dissection of the carotid artery was performed distally, the posterior digastric muscle tendon was located near the angle of the mandible to aid in localizing the hypoglossal nerve. Traction over the angle of the mandible was avoided to protect the marginal mandibular branch of the facial nerve. The hypoglossal nerve was identified as it crossed over the internal carotid and protected.

The internal carotid artery was exposed with minimal dissection (only as required to allow test clamping) and controlled with a vessel loop.

The remainder of the interposing carotid artery was freed from surrounding scar and lymphatic tissue.

The external carotid artery was exposed at its origin and controlled with a vessel loop.

The patient was given ____ units of heparin intravenously and an activated clotting time (ACT) was checked to be greater than 200 s. The ACT was maintained above 200 s throughout the operation with intermittent heparin boluses as required.

The internal carotid artery was clamped and the patient was assessed for signs of cerebral ischemia *[decreased motor and cognitive response (if awake)/EEG changes/mean internal carotid backpressure <50 mmHg (if under general anesthesia)]*. The patient was/ was not shunt dependent.

The common and internal carotid arteries were further mobilized as needed to insert a shunt (if required).

The external and common carotid arteries were clamped sequentially after the internal carotid to prevent distal embolization.

An arteriotomy was created on the anterolateral surface of the common carotid with a #11 blade and extended into the internal carotid artery using a Pott's scissors.

A *Javid/Sundt/Pruitt-Inahara inlying or outlying* shunt was inserted in the common and internal carotid arteries (if required). The patient was closely monitored for signs of cerebral ischemia and any changes were noted to dissipate with established blood flow through the shunt.

An endarterectomy plane was developed with a Freer elevator. The plaque was transected proximally in the common carotid artery. In the distal internal carotid artery, the plaque was feathered to leave a smooth endpoint. Eversion endarterectomy of the external carotid artery was performed and the carotid plaque was removed.

The endarterectomy surface was gently irrigated with heparinized saline solution. All remaining free debris was removed with a fine forceps.

The endarterectomy was inspected and assessed to require *patch angioplasty/interposition* graft.

[Choose one:]

If patch angioplasty: The arteriotomy was closed using a patch angioplasty of *Dacron/PTFE/vein*.

A vein patch was fashioned from a 6-cm segment of greater saphenous vein harvested from the upper thigh.

The patch angioplasty was performed using continuous 6-0 monofilament suture starting in the apex of the internal carotid, using care not to narrow the lumen.

The lumen was flushed periodically with heparinized saline to prevent buildup of stasis clot during the remainder of the repair and anastomosis.

The internal carotid and external carotid arteries were back-bled and the common carotid was forwardbled.

Clamps were released to first reestablish flow from the common carotid into the external carotid artery, with flow thereafter allowed into the internal carotid artery.

The patient was examined for signs of cerebral ischemia, and none were present.

[If the patient was shunt dependent: The shunt was removed after near-completion of the anastomosis and internal carotid flow resumed thereafter in a timely fashion (as described above)].

If interposition graft: An interposition graft of appropriately sized *Dacron/PTFE/vein (harvested from the upper thigh)* was sutured to healthy carotid artery end-to-end using 6-0 monofilament suture, beginning with the distal anastomosis.

Care was used not to narrow the lumen of the internal carotid artery.

Proximally, the common carotid anastomosis was completed in a similar fashion.

Prior to tying the last anastomosis, the graft was irrigated with copious amounts of heparinized saline and bleeding was allowed into the graft (with the internal carotid artery clamp in place) to vent any remaining debris or air.

Internal carotid artery flow was then reestablished and the patient was noted to be free of any signs of cerebral ischemia.

The external carotid artery was suture ligated.

[If the patient was shunt dependent: A separate shunt was inserted through the interposition conduit prior to its anastomosis to the carotid artery. A shunt exchange was then performed, and the interposition conduit was sewn into place (end-to-end, as described above). The shunt was removed after the majority of each anastomosis was completed, and internal carotid flow resumed thereafter in a timely fashion].

The suture lines were checked for hemostasis. Needle hole bleeding was controlled with the application of a topical thrombogenic agent *Surgicel/Gelfoam/thrombin.*

After hemostasis was assured, the wounds were closed using 3-0 Vicryl for the platysma and soft tissues. The skin was closed with staples. Sterile dressings were applied.

The patient tolerated the procedure well and was taken to the postanesthesia care unit in stable condition and neurologically intact.

Chapter 144
Carotid Artery Balloon Angioplasty and Stenting

Munier M.S. Nazzal, M.D.

INDICATIONS

- Symptomatic carotid artery stenosis greater than 50% in high-risk patients for carotid endarterectomy, recurrent internal carotid artery stenosis, patients with prior neck radiation, presence of a tracheostomy, high-carotid bifurcation (C2 level).
- Asymptomatic patients with carotid stenosis greater than 70%, as part of a study or registry.

CONTRAINDICATIONS

- Absence of adequately experienced operator.
- Lack of adequate imaging.
- Thrombus within the internal carotid artery.
- Tortuous common carotid and/or internal carotid arteries that might interfere with the procedure.
- Shaggy aortic arch.
- Lack of femoral access due to iliofemoral occlusive disease.

ESSENTIAL STEPS

1. Loading with Clopidogrel prior to procedure (patient should be on Clopidogrel 75 mg once per day for at least 48 h before the procedure, or 300 mg at the day of the procedure).
2. Percutaneous access to the femoral artery.

J.J. Hoballah and C.E.H. Scott-Conner (eds.), *Operative Dictations in General and Vascular Surgery*, DOI 10.1007/978-1-4614-0451-4_144,
© Springer Science+Business Media, LLC 2012

3. Diagnostic angiogram of the carotid and cerebral circulations noting any intracerebral occlusive disease.
4. Calculation of the degree of stenosis. Calculation of the lesion length and segment to be stented.
5. Careful manipulation of the wires and catheters within the carotid artery and ascending aorta.
6. Insertion of the 0.035 wire within the external carotid artery for a better purchase to facilitate next step.
7. Placement of shuttle sheath tip (or guiding catheter) within the common carotid artery proximal to the carotid bifurcation.
8. Crossing the stenosis with filter wire and placement of the filter within the internal carotid artery distal to the lesion.
9. Predilatation of severely stenosed internal carotid artery with a small balloon (3 mm×2 cm balloon).
10. Stent deployment in the internal carotid artery covering the lesion into adjacent normal segments proximally and distally.
11. Balloon dilatation of the stented segment. Avoid over sizing of the balloon. Accept residual stenosis up to 30%.
12. Filter export out of the internal carotid artery.
13. Avoid crossing the carotid lesion with 0.035 wires and catheters.
14. Completion angiogram to evaluate for complications and residual stenosis.
15. Careful and continuous neurological monitoring throughout the procedure and in the postoperative period.
16. Adequate anticoagulation with ACT kept over 250 s during the procedure.
17. Be ready for immediate administration of atropine, vasopressors and fluids when necessary.

NOTE THESE VARIATIONS

- Various protection devices are available. Filters require crossing the lesion with a 0.014 wire carrying the filter. Examples: Angioguard, Accunet, Spider, and Emboshield systems. Proximal cerebral protection devices do not require crossing the lesion. Examples: Gore Flow reversal, Mo.Ma ultraproximal systems. Use the system you are most familiar with.
- Avoid doing an arch aortogram if previously evaluated (MRA, CTA, or angiogram).
- Avoid predilatation of the lesion if the stenosis is not severe.

COMPLICATIONS

- Stroke.
- Carotid dissection/thrombosis/distal embolization.
- Bradycardia/hypotension/MI.
- Hematoma.

TEMPLATE OPERATIVE DICTATION

Preoperative diagnosis: *Right/left* carotid stenosis.

Procedure: *Right/left carotid angiogram; Right/Left Carotid stenting with protection device.*

Postoperative diagnosis: Same.

Indications: This ___-year-old *male/female had prior transient monocular blindness/transient ischemic attacks/stroke. Duplex scan/angiography/MRA/CTA* revealed stenosis of the *right/left* internal carotid artery. S/he was considered to be a high-risk patient for carotid endarterectomy due to *her/his recurrent stenosis/high-level lesion/prior neck radiation/tracheostomy/significant cardiac morbidity.* The patient was offered carotid stenting. The risks and benefits of carotid stenting were explained to the patient who elected to proceed with the intervention. All complications were discussed with the patient including stroke, cardiac complications, and hematoma at the site of access.

Description of procedure: The patient was brought to the angiography suite and placed in the supine position. The right/left groins were prepped and draped in the usual fashion.

The right/left groin was infiltrated (1% lidocaine/0.5% marcaine). *Under ultrasound guidance and* using Seldinger technique, a size 5/6 French sheath was introduced percutaneously in the right/left common femoral artery.

Heparin sulfate (dose: 75–100 U/kg) was administered intravenously to the patient. The heparin dose was adjusted throughout the procedure to maintain an activated clotting time greater than 250 s.

A J wire was advanced under fluoroscopic guidance into the ascending aorta. A 5-French pigtail catheter was advanced over the wire and placed in the ascending aorta. An aortic arch angiogram was performed under 45° of left anterior oblique position. The catheter was exchanged for a 5-French *Headhunter/Vertebral/ Bernstein/SIM/or other catheters*. The catheter was selectively placed in the right common carotid artery and then in the left common carotid artery. A total of (*volume/type of contrast media*) was injected in the *right/left* carotid and cerebral circulation. Images were obtained in different angles to assess both the extracranial and intracranial circulations. The degree of the stenosis was calculated in the *right/left* internal carotid artery and a decision was made to proceed with carotid artery stenting. The diameters of the internal and common carotid arteries were calculated. The lengths of the segment with stenosis and the segment to be stented were measured.

The Headhunter/Vertebral/Bernstein/SIM2 catheter was placed in the common carotid artery on the site to be stented. A stiff Glidewire (Terumo) was navigated into the common carotid artery and then into the external carotid artery. The catheter and sheath were exchanged for a 6-French shuttle sheath. A (*headhunter, JB2*) slip catheter was used within the shuttle sheath to facilitate shuttle advancement within the carotid artery. The tip of the shuttle sheath was placed in the common carotid artery proximal to the carotid bifurcation.

The location of the carotid bifurcation and area of stenosis were *marked/noted* on the screen using an erasable marker and a bony landmark. A marking ruler was used to help localize the area of stenosis and the segment to be stented.

A (size) *Angioguar/Spider/Accunet* was advanced through the sheath and placed in the internal carotid artery distal to the area of stenosis. The filter was deployed under fluoroscopy. Its location was noted on the screen. Contrast was injected to confirm placement within the *right/left* internal carotid artery.

Predilatation of the stenotic segment was done using a 3×2 Maverick Balloon (or any similar type). During dilatation, blood pressure and pulse rate were noted. Then a (*type and size x length*) stent was advanced and placed in the internal/common carotid artery segment. Location was confirmed by fluoroscopy before deployment. The stent was carefully deployed within the segment of stenosis as previously marked.

The stent delivery device was removed. A 4.5/5 mm (type and length) balloon was advanced over the wire to post-dilate the stented segment carefully watching for blood pressure and pulse variations. *1 mg atropine was administered to the patient because of bradycardia (if occurred). Intravenous fluid (NS/Ringer's solution) was infused in the patient for hypotension (if occurred). Dopamine (5 mics/kg/min) started and titrated because of persistent hypotension (if given).* Hemodynamic parameters and neurological status were continuously monitored during the procedure.

An angiogram was done following the post-stent dilatation to evaluate both the carotid and cerebral circulations.

An export sheath was introduced over the wire. The filter was captured under fluoroscopy and carefully withdrawn through the stented segment and removed out of the sheath. The filter was inspected for any captured material (mention if any).

A final completion angiogram was done. The residual stenosis was found to be (*percentage*).

ACT was checked and found to be second.

The shuttle sheath was removed and exchanged for a (French size) short sheath.

The femoral arteries were evaluated for possible closure by injecting (volume and type of contrast). The access site was successfully sealed (closed) using (type of closure device) or sheath was removed and manual compression was applied to the groin for (time in minutes) until the bleeding was controlled.

Patent was taken to the recovery room. Neurological and hemodynamic parameters were continuously monitored in the recovery room. The patient was transferred to the intensive care unit for an overnight observation.

NOTES

- ➢ Avoid unnecessary manipulation of the wires and catheters within the aorta and carotid arteries.
- ➢ Use proper catheters for different arch types.
- ➢ Use a slip catheter within the shuttle sheath instead of the dilator for difficult angles.
- ➢ Use long wires (260 cm) for exchange of catheters and shuttle sheath.
- ➢ Use monorail and rapid exchange catheters and balloons.
- ➢ In difficult angles, place the wire in the external carotid artery for easier control and easier advancement of the sheath or guide catheters into the common carotid artery.
- ➢ Keep the tip of the shuttle sheath within the field of imaging during the procedure.
- ➢ Use supporting wires (body wires) in difficult angles of the internal carotid artery to facilitate passage of the filter.
- ➢ Change the position of the neck with extension, flexion, and rotation to help advance wire, balloon, and stent if stuck during the procedure.
- ➢ Never force the stent into the area with stenosis. Predilate the area when necessary.
- ➢ Never inject blood-contaminated contrast in the cerebral circulation. Repeated flushing of the syringe is advisable.

Chapter 145
Carotid Subclavian Bypass

Julie Freischlag, M.D. and John Lane, M.D.

INDICATIONS

- Symptomatic proximal subclavian stenosis, "subclavian steal syndrome."
- Vertebrobasilar symptoms: Visual disturbances, vertigo, ataxia, dysphagia, dysarthria, transient hemiparesis, and hemisensory disturbances.
- Upper-extremity ischemic symptoms: Fatigue on exertion, rest pain, microembolic disease.
- "Coronary steal syndrome" [associated with left internal mammary artery (LIMA) coronary grafts].
- Debranching procedure prior to TEVAR.

OPTIONAL STEPS

1. Institute electroencephalogram (EEG) monitoring and general anesthesia.
2. Incise the skin/platysma (supraclavicular).
3. Divide the lateral head of the sternocleidomastoid (SCM).
4. Reflect the scalene fat pad superiorly.
5. Dissect and retract the phrenic nerve from the anterior surface of the anterior scalene muscle.
6. Double ligate and divide the thoracic duct.
7. Divide the anterior scalene.
8. Dissect the subclavian artery.
9. Control the subclavian arterial branches (thyrocervical/costocervical trunks, internal mammary, and vertebral).

J.J. Hoballah and C.E.H. Scott-Conner (eds.), *Operative Dictations in General and Vascular Surgery*, DOI 10.1007/978-1-4614-0451-4_145,
© Springer Science+Business Media, LLC 2012

10. Dissect the common carotid artery.
11. Heparinize.
12. Cross-clamp the subclavian artery.
13. Perform distal anastomosis between the subclavian artery and graft (PTFE/Dacron/vein).
14. Clamp graft and reestablish flow to the subclavian artery.
15. Cross-clamp the common carotid artery.
16. Insert shunt if necessary.
17. Tunnel bypass beneath the phrenic nerve and internal jugular vein.
18. Perform proximal anastomosis between the common carotid artery and graft.
19. Back- and forwardbled the carotid artery and graft.
20. Resume flow to the graft and then the common carotid artery.
21. Assess reconstruction.
22. Secure hemostasis and place drain.
23. Reapproximate scalene fat pad and SCM.
24. Close wound.

NOTE THIS VARIATION

- Endovascular treatment (angioplasty/stenting) is becoming a popular method for subclavian revascularization. Subclavian revascularization can be achieved by transposing the subclavian artery into the common carotid artery or by creating a bypass from the common carotid artery to the subclavian artery. The procedure can be performed through a single supraclavicular incision or by adding an additional cervical incision along the anterior border of the sternocleidomastoid muscle for the carotid exposure. The conduit can be an autogenous vein (greater saphenous vein), a polyester graft (Dacron), or a ringed polytetrafluoroethylene graft (PTFE).

COMPLICATIONS

- Death.
- Stroke.
- Bleeding.
- Hematoma.
- Lymphatic leak.
- Nerve injury (phrenic, recurrent, laryngeal, vagus, and brachial plexus).

TEMPLATE OPERATIVE DICTATION

Preoperative diagnosis: *Right/left* symptomatic proximal subclavian stenosis.

Procedure: *Right/left* carotid subclavian bypass using *PTGE/ Dacron/vein*.

Postoperative diagnosis: Same.

Indications: This __-year-old *male/female* presented with *verte-brobasilar/upper-extremity ischemic* symptoms. Evaluation with *duplex/angiography/MRA/CTA* revealed ___ stenosis of the *right/left* subclavian artery.

Description of procedure: EEG electrodes were placed preoperatively and baseline brainwave activity was recorded.

General anesthesia was induced.

The patient was positioned supine on the operating table with the neck extended and rotated away from the side of interest.

Skin preparation was performed in the normal sterile fashion.

Intravenous antibiotics were administered.

A supraclavicular incision was performed extending 10 cm medial to the sternocleidomastoid and 2 cm superior to the clavicle.

The subcutaneous tissue and platysma were divided with electrocautery.

The lateral head of the sternocleidomastoid was divided with electrocautery.

The scalene fat pad was separated from its attachments to the clavicle inferiorly and retracted superiorly.

The phrenic nerve was dissected and retracted medially from the anterior surface of the anterior scalene muscle.

The thoracic duct was double-ligated and divided.

The anterior scalene muscle was divided with electrocautery and retracted to gain exposure to the subclavian artery.

Dissection of the subclavian artery was performed medially until 1–2 cm of subclavian artery was accessible proximal to the vertebral artery.

The subclavian, vertebral, internal mammary, and thyrocervical arteries were controlled with vessel loops.

The carotid sheath was opened with care not to injure the vagus nerve.

The internal jugular vein was retracted superomedially, gaining exposure to the common carotid artery.

The carotid artery was dissected for a distance of 3–4 cm and was encircled with moistened umbilical tapes.

Intravenous heparin was administered (5,000 U) and the subclavian artery was clamped using vascular clamps.

A *6/8-mm PTFE* vs. *Dacron* vs. *vein* graft was selected and spatulated appropriately.

An end-to-side anastomosis was performed between the graft and the subclavian artery with 6-0 polypropylene suture.

The graft was clamped near the anastomosis and flow was reestablished to the upper extremity.

The graft was tunneled beneath the phrenic nerve and internal jugular vein.

The common carotid was clamped with vascular clamps.

Carotid shunting was selectively performed on the basis of changes in EEG activity.

The graft was trimmed and spatulated appropriately.

An end-to-side anastomosis was performed between the common carotid artery and graft using 6.0 polypropylene suture.

The common carotid artery and graft were back- and forward-bled.

Flow was reestablished to the subclavian artery, then the vertebral and carotid arteries.

Hemostasis was achieved.

Drain placement and wound closure were performed. The patient tolerated the procedure well and was taken to the postanesthesia care unit in stable condition.

Chapter 146
Carotid Subclavian Transposition

Julie Freischlag, M.D. and John Lane, M.D.

INDICATIONS

- Symptomatic proximal subclavian stenosis, "subclavian steal syndrome."
- Vertebrobasilar symptoms: Visual disturbances, vertigo, ataxia, dysphagia, dysarthria, transient hemiparesis, and hemisensory disturbances.
- Upper-extremity ischemic symptoms: Fatigue on exertion, rest pain, microembolic disease.
- "Coronary steal syndrome" [associated with left internal mammary artery (LIMA) coronary grafts].
- Debranching prior to TEVAR.

OPTIONAL STEPS

1. Institute electroencephalogram (EEG) monitoring and general anesthesia.
2. Incise the skin/platysma (supraclavicular).
3. Divide the lateral head of the sternocleidomastoid (SCM).
4. Reflect the scalene fat pad superiorly.
5. Dissect and retract the phrenic nerve from the anterior surface of the anterior scalene.
6. Double ligate and divide the thoracic duct.
7. Divide the anterior scalene.
8. Dissect the subclavian artery 1–2 cm proximal to the vertebral artery.

J.J. Hoballah and C.E.H. Scott-Conner (eds.), *Operative Dictations in General and Vascular Surgery*, DOI 10.1007/978-1-4614-0451-4_146,
© Springer Science+Business Media, LLC 2012

9. Control the subclavian arterial branches (thyrocervical/costocervical trunks, internal mammary, and vertebral).
10. Dissect the common carotid artery.
11. Heparinize.
12. Divide the subclavian artery proximal to the vertebral artery between vascular clamps.
13. Oversew the proximal subclavian arterial stump.
14. Cross-clamp the common carotid artery.
15. Insert shunt if necessary.
16. Transpose the subclavian artery beneath the phrenic nerve and internal jugular vein.
17. Perform anastomosis between the common carotid and subclavian arteries.
18. Resume flow to the subclavian, then the vertebral, and then the carotid.
19. Assess reconstruction.
20. Secure hemostasis and place drain.
21. Reapproximate the scalene fat pad and SCM.
22. Close the wound.

NOTE THESE VARIATIONS

- Endovascular treatment (angioplasty/stenting) is becoming a popular method for subclavian revascularization.
- When angioplasty/stenting is not desired, subclavian revascularization can also be achieved by transposing the subclavian artery into the common carotid artery or by creating a bypass from the common carotid artery to the subclavian artery. The advantage of subclavian carotid transposition includes a single arterial anastomosis and the lack of graft utilization. It tends to require more proximal dissection and mobilization of the subclavian artery to allow a tension-free anastomosis.

COMPLICATIONS

- Death.
- Stroke.
- Bleeding.
- Hematoma.
- Lymphatic leak.
- Nerve injury (phrenic, recurrent laryngeal, vagus, and brachial plexus).

TEMPLATE OPERATIVE DICTATION

Preoperative diagnosis: *Right/left* symptomatic proximal subclavian stenosis.

Procedure: *Right/left* carotid subclavian transposition.

Postoperative diagnosis: Same.

Indications: This __-year-old *male/female* was found to have symptomatic subclavian stenosis with *vertebrobasilar/upper-extremity ischemic symptoms* upon *duplex/angio/MRA/CTA* with ___ stenosis of the *right/left* subclavian artery.

Description of procedure: EEG electrodes were placed preoperatively and baseline brainwave activity was recorded. General anesthesia was induced.

The patient was positioned supine on the operating table with the neck extended and rotated away from the side of interest.

Skin preparation was performed in the normal sterile fashion.

Intravenous antibiotics were administered.

A supraclavicular incision was performed extending 10 cm medial to the SCM and 2 cm superior to the clavicle.

The subcutaneous tissue and platysma were divided with electrocautery.

The lateral head of the SCM was divided with electrocautery.

The scalene fat pad was separated from its attachments to the clavicle inferiorly and retracted superiorly.

The phrenic nerve was dissected and retracted medially from the anterior surface of the anterior scalene muscle.

The thoracic duct was double-ligated and divided.

The anterior scalene muscle was divided with electrocautery and retracted to gain exposure to the subclavian artery.

Dissection of the subclavian artery was performed medially until 1–2 cm of subclavian artery was accessible proximal to the vertebral artery.

The subclavian, vertebral, internal mammary, and thyrocervical arteries were controlled with vessel loops.

The carotid sheath was opened with care not to injure the vagus nerve.

The internal jugular vein was retracted superomedially, gaining exposure to the common carotid artery.

The carotid artery was dissected for a distance of 3–4 cm and was encircled with moistened umbilical tapes.

Intravenous heparin was administered (5,000 U).

The branches of the subclavian artery were controlled and the subclavian artery was doubly clamped proximal to the vertebral artery.

The subclavian artery was divided between the clamps using a surgical scalpel.

The proximal stump of the subclavian artery was oversewn using two rows of 4-0 polypropylene sutures in a horizontal mattress fashion.

The proximal clamp was carefully removed and hemostasis was assessed.

The subclavian artery was tunneled below the phrenic nerve and internal jugular vein to the common carotid artery.

The common carotid artery was controlled using two angled vascular clamps.

Carotid shunting was performed due to slowing noted on EEG monitoring.

A longitudinal arteriotomy was created using a #11 scalpel and the arteriotomy was extended using Pott's scissors.

An end-to-side anastomosis was performed between the subclavian and common carotid artery using 6-0 polypropylene suture.

The subclavian and carotid arteries were back- and forward-bled.

Flow was reestablished to the subclavian artery, then the vertebral and carotid arteries.

Assessment of flow was determined in the carotid, subclavian, and vertebral arteries using a hand-held Doppler probe.

Hemostasis was achieved.

A silastic, closed suction drain was placed in the supraclavicular fossa.

The scalene fat pad was returned to its anatomic location and secured to the clavicle using interrupted 3.0 absorbable sutures.

The lateral head of the SCM was reapproximated using absorbable sutures.

The platysma was closed using running 3-0 absorbable suture and the skin was closed using a 5-0 subcuticular suture.

Sterile dressings were applied.

The patient awoke from anesthesia without neurological deficits.

The patient tolerated the procedure well and was taken to the postanesthesia care unit in stable condition.

Chapter 147
Vertebral Artery Reconstruction

David C. Corry, M.D. and Mark Adelman, M.D.

INDICATIONS

- Vertebrobasilar insufficiency with bilateral vertebral stenosis/occlusion.
- Symptomatic subclavian steal syndrome.

ESSENTIAL STEPS

1. Incise the skin and platysma.
2. Incise the scalene fat pad and retract superiorly.
3. Identify the phrenic nerve.
4. Divide the scalenus anticus muscle (in some cases, this may be preserved).
5. Identify and divide the vertebral veins.
6. Identify the stellate ganglion (preserve).
7. Control the subclavian artery proximal and distal to the vertebral artery.
8. Control the internal mammary artery.
9. Decide on the type of repair.
10. Anticoagulate with heparin.
11. Clamp the vertebral artery.
12. Clamp the proximal and distal subclavian artery.
13. Repair type:
    - For angioplasty:
        - Make arteriotomy in the subclavian artery extending up onto the vertebral artery.
        - Perform plication of the vertebral artery.

J.J. Hoballah and C.E.H. Scott-Conner (eds.), *Operative Dictations in General and Vascular Surgery*, DOI 10.1007/978-1-4614-0451-4_147,
© Springer Science+Business Media, LLC 2012

- Harvest 3 cm of greater saphenous vein from the thigh.
- Prepare a vein patch angioplasty.
- Sew patch angioplasty over the vertebral arterial plication and arteriotomy.
- Backbleed the vertebral artery.
- Backbleed the subclavian artery.
- Forwardbleed the subclavian artery.
- Complete the anastomosis.
- Unclamp the distal subclavian artery.
- Unclamp the proximal subclavian artery.
- Unclamp the vertebral artery.
- Place small closed suction drain.
- Wound closure.
- For vertebral transposition:
  - Retract the sternocleidomastoid (this may need to be divided).
  - Control the common carotid artery proximally and distally.
  - Systemically anticoagulate.
  - Clamp the vertebral artery.
  - Clamp the distal subclavian artery.
  - Clamp the proximal subclavian artery.
  - Divide the vertebral artery just distal to origin.
  - Oversew the proximal vertebral artery stump.
  - Mobilize the vertebral artery and prepare for transposition.
  - Plan the arteriotomy.
  - Clamp the common carotid artery distally.
  - Clamp the common carotid artery proximally.
  - Make small common carotid artery arteriotomy.
  - End-to-side vertebral to common carotid anastomosis using 7-0 prolene.
  - Backbleed the vertebral artery.
  - Backbleed the common carotid artery.
  - Forwardbleed the common carotid artery.
  - Tie suture line with vertebral artery backbleeding.
  - Unclamp the proximal common carotid artery.
  - Unclamp the distal common carotid artery.
14. Check for hemostasis.
15. Place closed suction drainage catheter.
16. Wound closure.

NOTE THESE VARIATIONS

- Vertebral revascularization can be achieved by performing a vein patch angioplasty of the origin of the vertebral artery or by vertebral carotid transposition. If the atherosclerotic pathology is limited to the origin of the vertebral artery and in the presence of vertebral artery redundancy, plication and vein patch angioplasty can be the preferred procedure. If the atherosclerotic disease is also affecting the origin of the subclavian artery, a vertebral carotid transposition is performed especially if the carotid artery is disease free.

COMPLICATIONS

- Stroke.
- Hematoma.
- Thrombosis.
- Phrenic nerve injury.
- Thoracic duct injury (left side).
- Recurrent laryngeal nerve injury (right side).
- Myocardial infarction.

TEMPLATE OPERATIVE DICTATION

Preoperative diagnosis: Vertebrobasilar insufficiency, subclavian steal syndrome, *right/left* vertebral artery stenosis.

Procedure: *Right/left vertebral plication and vein patch angioplasty/right/left vertebral carotid transposition.*

Postoperative diagnosis: Same.

Indications: This ___-year-old *male/female* presented with *vertebrobasilar/subclavian steal* symptoms. Evaluation with *duplex/angiography/magnetic resonance angiography* revealed ___ stenosis of the *right/left* vertebral artery.

Description of procedure: The patient was placed in the supine position.

The procedure was performed under general endotracheal anesthesia.

The *right/left* neck and *right/left* upper thigh were prepped and draped in the usual sterile fashion.

A transverse curvilinear skin incision was made from the lateral edge of the medial head of the sternocleidomastoid muscle for a distance of 5–6 cm. The platysma muscle was divided with electrocautery.

The scalene fat pad was identified. The scalene fat pad was divided inferiorly and retracted superiorly.

The phrenic nerve was identified and gently mobilized medially.

The scalenus anticus muscle was divided and the *right/left* vertebral artery was identified. Prior to identifying this vessel, the vertebral veins were divided between ligatures. (On the left side, the thoracic duct was identified and *preserved/ligated*. On the right side, the recurrent laryngeal nerve was identified and preserved.) Care was taken to identify the stellate ganglion and preserve it.

The vertebral artery was assessed to require plication and patch angioplasty or transposition repair.

[Choose one:]

If vertebral artery plication and patch angioplasty: The vertebral artery was mobilized and found to be redundant.

The proximal and distal subclavian arteries were identified and controlled.

The internal mammary was identified and controlled.

The patient was systemically heparinized and the vertebral artery and distal subclavian artery were clamped sequentially, followed by the proximal subclavian artery.

A keyhole-shaped arteriotomy was placed in the subclavian artery and extended up onto the vertebral artery.

Using 6-0 monofilament suture in a running fashion, the vertebral artery was plicated to reduce its redundancy. After completion of the plication, saphenous vein was harvested from the thigh and a saphenous vein patch was fashioned. The saphenous vein patch angioplasty was performed using 6-0 monofilament suture in a running fashion.

After forward- and backbleeding, the anastomosis was completed and flow was initiated first down the subclavian artery and then up the vertebral artery.

If vertebral artery to common carotid artery transposition: The sternocleidomastoid was retracted medially.

The common carotid artery was identified and controlled proximally and distally.

The vertebral artery was clamped, followed sequentially by the distal subclavian and proximal subclavian arteries.

The vertebral artery was divided just distal to its origin and the vertebral artery stump was oversewn with 6-0 monofilament suture.

The remaining end of the vertebral artery was extensively mobilized up to its bony insertion.

The distal common carotid artery was cross-clamped, followed by the proximal common carotid artery.

After careful planning, an arteriotomy along the posterolateral border of the carotid artery was performed. The arteriotomy was extended up the vertebral artery along its anteromedial border. This was extended for a distance of approximately 5–6 mm.

Using 6-0/7-0 monofilament suture, an end-to-side running anastomosis was performed between the vertebral artery and common carotid artery.

Prior to tying the anastomosis, the vertebral artery was backbled and the common carotid artery was backbled. The proximal common carotid artery was then forwardbled and the suture line was tied with the vertebral artery backbleeding.

The proximal common carotid artery was unclamped, followed by the distal common carotid artery.

Hemostasis was achieved.

A 7-mm closed suction drain was placed deep in the wound.

The scalene fat pad was placed gently over the phrenic nerve.

The platysma muscle was closed with 3-0 absorbable sutures in a running fashion.

The skin was closed with 4-0 subcuticular absorbable sutures *(for vein patch angioplasty, the thigh incisions were closed in layers)*.

The patient tolerated the procedure well and was taken to the postanesthesia care unit in stable condition and neurologically intact.

NOTES

Chapter 148
Subclavian Artery Angioplasty Stenting

Rabih Houbballah, M.D. and Jamal J. Hoballah, M.D., M.B.A.

INDICATIONS
- Subclavian artery steal syndrome manifested by dizziness and arm pain on exercise.
- Angina pectoris in the presence of an LIMA graft.

ESSENTIAL STEPS
1. Ipsilateral Brachial artery access using a micropuncture sheath.
2. Replacement of the micropuncture sheath with a size 5-French Sheath.
3. Placement of a diagnostic catheter in the axillary artery.
4. Heparinization: 50–75 UI/kg.
5. Performance of angiogram to delineate the location of the stenosis and relationship to the origins of subclavian, vertebral, and internal mammary arteries.
6. Replacement of the 5-French Sheath with a 6-F guiding catheter or long (55 cm) sheath.
7. Performance of another angiogram under magnification.
8. Crossing the lesion under road-map and identification of the location of the stenosis and the size of the stent to be used.
9. Angioplasty/stenting using size 8×3 self-expending stent.
10. Post-stent in dilatation of the stenotic segment.
11. Angiogram documenting patency and absence of dissection.
12. Reversal of the heparin and removal of the sheath.

J.J. Hoballah and C.E.H. Scott-Conner (eds.), *Operative Dictations in General and Vascular Surgery*, DOI 10.1007/978-1-4614-0451-4_148,
© Springer Science+Business Media, LLC 2012

NOTE THESE VARIATIONS

- The procedure can also be performed through a femoral approach. A long sheath/guiding catheter (90 cm) will be place in the proximity of the stenosis.

COMPLICATIONS

- Injury to the subclavian artery (Dissection, pseudoaneurysm, and perforation).
- Occlusion of the internal mammary or vertebral artery.
- Access artery thrombosis (brachial).
- Bleeding/false aneurysm of the brachial artery.

TEMPLATE DICTATION

Preoperative diagnosis: Right/left subclavian artery stenosis with subclavian artery steal syndrome.

Procedure: Aortogram; left/right subclavian angiogram; subclavian artery angioplasty; and subclavian artery stent placement.

Postoperative diagnosis: Right/left subclavian artery stenosis.

Indications: This is a ___-year-old *male/female* patient presented with *arm numbness and pain/angina following coronary artery bypass grafting*. Evaluation revealed the presence of a *right/left* significant subclavian artery stenosis.

Details of the operation: The patient was brought to the operating room and placed on the angiography table in the supine position. The right anticubital/femoral area were prepped and draped in a standard session. The area over the brachial/femoral artery was anesthetized with 1% Xylocaine. Percutaneous cannulation of the right brachial artery was achieved using an 18-gauge vascular access needle. A 0.035" Standard Hydrophilic Guidewire soft angled, 180 cm was advanced through the needle and under fluoroscopy up the brachial and axillary arteries, into the subclavian artery. The needle was removed and a 5-French short Pinnacle sheath was first placed over the glide wire. The patient was given 5,000 U of heparin intravenously (75–100 U/kg). A *multipurpose MP 4F, Angled Glide Catheter* was introduced over the wire into the proximal axillary artery and an angiogram was performed. The angiogram revealed the presence of a *very tight stenosis/occlusion* ___cm distal to the origin of the subclavian artery. On evaluation of this stenosis, decision was made to treat this interventionally. The MP catheter was advanced to the area of pathology and after gentle manipulation the Glide wire successfully crossed the lesion. The MP catheter was advanced over the Glide wire. The glide wire was exchanged for a 0.035" Stiff angled wire, 260 cm wire.

The sheath was then removed and replaced by a 6-French or 7-French 45-cm long valved anti-kinking sheath, which was parked just few centimeters from the location of the subclavian artery stenosis. Pre-dilation with a size 3×4 cm non-compliant balloon was performed. A self-expanding/balloon mounted stent measuring 8×4 cm was then introduced and used to cross the lesion under road-map imaging. The stent was then deployed in the desired location.

Variation: For balloon-mounted stent, the balloon was inflated using an Endoflator device, thus expanding the stent. There was noted to be a tight calcific lesion with a waist created in the balloon. Based on the waist size in the balloon, the stenosis was felt to be about 80% of luminal diameter. The balloon and stent expanded to profile, up to 10 atmospheres on the Endoflator device.

Post-stenting dilatation was performed using a size 8 mm × 4 cm balloon. Completion arteriogram demonstrates a stent in good position. It was fully deployed. There was good flow across the stented lesion. Both vertebral and internal mammary arteries were patent. There was/wasn't a mild poststenotic dilatation in the subclavian artery. There was no evidence of dissection. There was no evidence of extravasation. The Heparin was then reversed (Optional) and the catheter, wire, and sheath were removed when the ACT was below 150 s. Gentle pressure was applied on the brachial artery, while monitoring of distal flow into the radial artery until hemostasis was achieved.

If a femoral artery approach was preferred, closure of the arteriotomy could be performed using a percutaneaous closure device such as a 6F Angioseal (St Jude medical) or a Starclose (Abbott Vascular).

Chapter 149
Aorto-Innominate Artery Bypass

Christian Bianchi, M.D. and Jeffrey L. Ballard, M.D.

INDICATIONS

- Symptomatic innominate artery stenosis >50%.
- Asymptomatic stenosis >70% or deep ulcerated plaque lesion associated with >50% stenosis.
- Debranching procedure prior to TEVAR.

ESSENTIAL STEPS

1. Limited skin incision from the sternal notch to the third intercostal space.
2. Divide the sternum to the third intercostal space, creating an upside-down T-shaped incision.
3. Push aside or transect the thymus in midline plane.
4. Open the pericardium and place pericardial stay sutures.
5. Expose and dissect the ascending aorta.
6. Divide venous tributaries to fully mobilize the left brachiocephalic vein.
7. Expose and thoroughly dissect the innominate artery and the proximal aspects of right subclavian and common carotid arteries.
8. Construct end-to-side proximal aortic anastomosis (reinforce suture line with Teflon felt).
9. Construct end-to-end distal innominate artery anastomosis.
10. Backbleed subclavian and common carotid arteries and forward flush bypass graft.

J.J. Hoballah and C.E.H. Scott-Conner (eds.), *Operative Dictations in General and Vascular Surgery*, DOI 10.1007/978-1-4614-0451-4_149,
© Springer Science+Business Media, LLC 2012

11. Resume prograde blood flow in this order: The subclavian first, followed by the common carotid artery.
12. Place #19F Blake drain deep in the pericardial space and bring out the second intercostal space lateral to the internal mammary artery.
13. Wire close sternal incision after adequate wound hemostasis.
14. Close the fascia, subcutaneous tissue, and skin in separate layers.

NOTE THESE VARIATIONS
- The sternotomy may be extended beyond the third intercostal space to include the entire sternum.
- Additional graft may be added to bypass the left common carotid artery in the presence of significant disease.
- Endovascular treatment (angioplasty/stenting) is gaining popularity as another revascularization option.

COMPLICATIONS
- Stroke.
- Transient ischemia attacks (TIAs).
- Upper-extremity embolism.
- Recurrent laryngeal nerve injury.
- Pneumothorax.
- Aortic arch dissection.
- Internal mammary artery injury.
- Mediastinitis.
- Mediastinal bleeding.

TEMPLATE OPERATIVE DICTATION
Preoperative diagnosis: Symptomatic innominate artery stenosis.
Procedure: Ascending aorta-to-innominate artery bypass with 10/12-mm Dacron tube graft.
Postoperative diagnosis: Same.
Indications: This ___-year-old *male/female was asymptomatic/presented with TIA, stroke, or upper-extremity embolism.* Preoperative arch aortogram demonstrated severe stenosis of the proximal innominate artery. Endovascular treatment was not an option.
Description of procedure: The procedure was performed under general anesthesia with the patient in supine position.

The neck and anterior chest were prepped and draped in a standard fashion.

A midline incision was made from the sternal notch to the third intercostal space and deepened to the sternum with electrocautery. An oscillating blade mounted on a redo sternotomy saw was used to make a sternal incision from the notch to the third intercostal space. The sternal incision was "Td" at the third intercostal space to facilitate exposure of the upper mediastinum. Hemostasis was obtained at the periosteal edges, follow by placement of a pediatric sternal retractor. The thymus was divided in the midline with cautery and the pericardium was opened longitudinally to expose the ascending aorta. Silk stay sutures were placed in the pericardial edges and secured to the skin.

The left brachiocephalic vein was dissected circumferentially and isolated with a silastic vessel loop. The ascending aorta was gently dissected free from surrounding tissue with care not to injure pulmonary or neurolymphatic structures. The innominate artery was identified and circumferentially dissected to its bifurcation into the subclavian and common carotid arteries. The origin of each of these arteries was exposed and then controlled with a silastic vessel loop. Systemic anticoagulation was then achieved using an intravenous bolus of heparin (100 U/kg). Approximately 3 min later, a partially occluding clamp was placed on the anterolateral aspect of the ascending aorta. An aortotomy was created with a #11 blade and lengthened appropriately with angled Pott's scissors. A 10/12-mm Dacron tube graft was anastomosed in an end-to-side fashion to the ascending aorta using 4-0 prolene sutures in a running fashion. The suture line was reinforced with a strip of Teflon felt. An atraumatic clamp was then placed on the graft near the proximal anastomosis, and the side-biting clamp on the ascending aorta was released.

Next, vascular occluding clamps were applied to the proximal innominate, right subclavian, and common carotid arteries. The innominate artery was transected distally and the proximal innominate artery was oversewn in two separate layers using 4-0 prolene sutures. The Dacron graft was *passed over/tunneled under* the left brachiocephalic vein to facilitate an end-to-end anastomosis at the level of the distal innominate artery. The anastomosis was created using 4-0 prolene sutures in a continuous running fashion. Just prior to completion of the anastomosis, the subclavian and common arteries were backbled and the bypass graft was flushed to clear all potential air and debris from the lumens. Prograde blood flow was first established to the subclavian artery, followed by the right common carotid. Immediate intraoperative duplex ultrasound was used to confirm a widely patent innominate artery reconstruction with no compromise in the graft lumen diameter.

Heparin was reversed with protamine sulfate and hemostasis was obtained throughout the upper mediastinum using cautery and thrombin-soaked Gelfoam. A #19F drain was placed within the pericardium and brought out through a separate stab incision made in the second intercostal space. The drain was secured at the skin exit site using a 3-0 nylon suture. The wound was then closed after verification of hemostasis, using sternal wires followed by reapproximation of the pectoral fascia using 3-0 Vicryl in a continuous running fashion. The subcutaneous tissue was closed using 3-0 Vicryl, followed by subcuticular skin closure with a 3-0 monocryl suture. Sterile dressing was applied and the drain was placed to bulb suction.

The patient tolerated the procedure well was awakened in the operating room and noted to have no gross neurological deficits and was taken to the postanesthesia care unit in stable condition.

NOTES

Chapter 150

Innominate/Common Carotid Artery Angioplasty Stenting Using Hybrid Open Technique

Jamal J. Hoballah, M.D., M.B.A.

INDICATIONS

- Symptomatic innominate/right/left common carotid artery stenosis (transient ischemic attacks, stroke, finger/hand ischemia) in the presence of arch/iliac anatomy that precludes percutaneous femoral approach.

ESSENTIAL STEPS

1. Five centimeters neck incision along the sternocleidomastoid muscle border under local anesthesia.
2. Exposure of the common carotid artery.
3. Placement of a size 6-French Sheath with marked tip using Seldinger technique.
4. Heparinization: 50–75 UI/kg.
5. Performance of angiogram to delineate the location of the stenosis and relationship to the aortic arch and origins of the right subclavian (in the case of innominate stenosis).
6. Crossing the lesion using a multipurpose catheter and glide wire in the common carotid artery.
7. Performance of another angiogram under magnification.
8. Identification of the location of the stenosis and the size of the stent to be used.
9. Applying a vascular clamp on the common carotid artery distal to the insertion of the 6-French sheath to protect from embolization.

J.J. Hoballah and C.E.H. Scott-Conner (eds.), *Operative Dictations in General and Vascular Surgery*, DOI 10.1007/978-1-4614-0451-4_150,
© Springer Science+Business Media, LLC 2012

10. Angioplasty/stenting using balloon expandable stent/self-expending under road-map.
11. Post-stent dilatation of the stenotic segment.
12. Angiogram documenting patency and absence of dissection.
13. Removal of the balloon and flushing any debris through the size 6-French sheath.
14. Reversal of the heparin and removal of the sheath.

NOTE THESE VARIATIONS

- For innominate pathology, the procedure can also be performed through a brachial approach; however this does not provide any cerebral protection.
- A ballon expandable stent can provide very precise deployment location and may also be used.
- The common carotid exposure can be performed under cervical block or local anesthesia.

COMPLICATIONS

- Common carotid/innominate (dissection, pseudoaneurysm, perforation, and rupture).
- Distal embolization (Brain or hand).

TEMPLATE DICTATION

Pre-operative diagnosis: Symptomatic innominate; *right/left* common carotid artery.

Procedure: Aortogram; innominate; *right/left* common carotid artery angioplasty and stent placement.

Post-operative diagnosis:

Indications: This is a ...-year-old *male/female* patient presenting with *right/left TIA, stroke, transient monocular blindness arm numbness, and pain/angina following coronary artery bypass grafting*. Evaluation revealed the presence of a significant *right/left* common carotid artery/innominate stenosis. The anatomy of the aortic arch/iliac arteries was felt inappropriate for percutaneous approach through the femoral or brachial approach. The decision was to perform a carotid/innominate stenting through an open neck approach.

Details of the operation: The patient was brought to the operating room and placed on the angiography table in the supine position. With the patient in the supine position, and after administration of *cervical block* anesthesia, the neck was prepped and draped in the usual sterile fashion. A 5-cm skin incision was then performed along the medial edge of the sternocleidomastoid. The platysma was incised and the sternocleidomastoid was mobilized laterally exposing the internal jugular vein. The internal jugular vein was then mobilized laterally exposing the common carotid artery. This was freely dissected for a 5-cm segment. The patient was then given 5,000 U of intravenous Heparin, and using the Seldinger technique, the common carotid artery was punctured and a size 6-French sheath was introduced. A retrograde angiogram of the *carotid/innominate* artery was performed through the sheath and revealed the area of the stenosis. Using an MP catheter and a glide wire, the stenosis was negotiated, allowing the wire to traverse the stenosis into the aortic arch. This was followed by the advancement of the catheter over the wire into the aortic arch. The glide wire was then exchanged to a stiff wire. A repeat angiogram was then performed under magnification. The size of the vessel and the size of the stent to be used were then selected. The common carotid artery was then cross-clamped and the stent was introduced over the wire into the desired location. A *self-expanding stent/balloon expandable stent* was inserted into the desired location and the stent was deployed. Post-deployment angioplasty was performed (for self-expanding stent). An angiogram revealed excellent placement without any extravasation. The catheter and wire were then removed. Aspiration through the sheath was performed to flush out any debris from the angioplasty site. The sheath was then removed allowing the artery to flush out any debris. A vascular clamp was then reapplied proximal to the sheath insertion site and the hole in the common carotid artery was over sewn with a 5-0 Prolene suture. The clamps were then removed and flow was resumed into the internal and external carotid arteries.

Hemostasis was secured and the wound was then irrigated. The wound was closed with 3-0 Vicryl for the platysma and 4-0 Monocryl for the skin.

The patient tolerated the procedure well and was transferred to the recovery room in good condition.

Section XV

Mesenteric and Renal Artery Occlusive Disease

Chapter 151

Antegrade Aortoceliac/Mesenteric Bypass for Chronic Mesenteric Ischemia

Roderick T.A. Chalmers, M.D.

INDICATIONS

- Patient with classic symptoms (abdominal pain, weight loss, postprandial pain, diarrhea, and fear of food) with two of three visceral vessel occlusions.
- Angiograms reveal extent of and length of occlusion(s).

ESSENTIAL STEPS

1. Midline abdominal incision.
2. General laparotomy to exclude other relevant pathologies.
3. Incise the left triangular ligament and retract the left lobe of the liver to the right.
4. Enter the lesser omentum and retract the stomach inferiorly and to the left.
5. Identify the esophagus (nasogastric tube helpful) and gently mobilize to the left.
6. Divide the median arcuate ligament and crural fibers in the midline to gain access to the anterior surface of the supra-celiac aorta.
7. Expose several centimeters of the supraceliac aorta.
8. Trace the anterior aorta inferiorly until the origin of the celiac axis is encountered.
9. Dissect out the celiac axis and its three main branches.
10. Expose and dissect the superior mesenteric artery (SMA).
11. Administer systemic heparin 50–75 U/kg.

J.J. Hoballah and C.E.H. Scott-Conner (eds.), *Operative Dictations in General and Vascular Surgery*, DOI 10.1007/978-1-4614-0451-4_151,
© Springer Science+Business Media, LLC 2012

12. Apply side-biting Sitinsky clamp to the supra-celiac aorta.
13. Create the proximal anastomosis with an 8-mm knitted Dacron/PTFE graft.
14. Create the distal anastomosis to the celiac artery or hepatic artery.
15. Create a side limb.
16. Create the distal anastomosis to the SMA.
17. Check for celiac and SMA flow and for bowel viability.
18. Confirm viability of the gut and distal extremities.
19. Ensure hemostasis.
20. Close the abdominal wall with mass closure.
21. Recheck distal pulses and urine output.

NOTE THESE VARIATIONS

- Endovascular treatment (angioplasty/stenting) is an acceptable option when possible though associated with a higher recurrence rate.
- A bifurcated graft with a limb to the celiac and another to the SMA is often used. Alternatively, an aortoceliac bypass is constructed and the bypass to the SMA is constructed as a side arm of the aortoceliac graft.
- Aortic control is typically achieved with a side-biting clamp. On occasion, aortic disease may dictate using proximal and distal clamps.
- The site for the celiac anastomosis can be either the distal celiac or one of its proximal branch arteries, usually the common hepatic artery.
- The site for anastomosis on the SMA is dictated by the distal extent of disease. For the origin and most proximal segment of the SMA, exposure is achieved by gently retracting the upper border of the pancreas inferiorly. For the mid- and distal segments of the SMA in the root of the small bowel mesentery, exposure is achieved by first reflecting the transverse colon superiorly (much easier). Bypass to the SMA at this level needs to be tunneled with care, usually behind the pancreas and in front of the left renal vein. The graft may be also tunneled anterior to the pancreas, especially if a vein graft is used.

COMPLICATIONS

- Bleeding.
- Graft thrombosis with recurrent ischemia.
- Renal failure.

- Lower limb embolism.
- Spinal cord ischemia.
- Myocardial infarction.

TEMPLATE OPERATIVE DICTATION

Preoperative diagnosis: Chronic mesenteric ischemia secondary to celiac and mesenteric occlusive disease.

Procedure: Antegrade aortoceliac and/or aortomesenteric bypass with 8-mm Dacron.

Postoperative diagnosis: Same.

Indication: This is a ___-year-old *male/female* with a history of *weight loss, postprandial abdominal pain and diarrhea, and a fear of food*. Angiography showed occlusion of the proximal celiac artery, tight stenosis of the origin of the SMA, and occlusion of the inferior mesenteric artery. The patient consented to surgical *celiac/mesenteric revascularization* having been fully informed of the risks and benefits of the procedure.

Description of procedure: The patient was placed supine on the operating table with arms *tucked in/at 80°*. Large-bore intravenous and central venous lines were placed by anesthesia and general anesthesia achieved with endotracheal intubation. A Foley urethral catheter was placed under sterile conditions. The entire anterior chest, abdomen, and both legs to knee level were prepared and draped. Routine antibiotic prophylaxis was administered prior to the skin incision.

A skin incision was fashioned from the xiphisternum to symphysis pubis. The subcutaneous tissues were divided in the midline with electrocautery. The peritoneum was entered sharply and the abdominal wall incision completed.

There were no *adhesions/moderate adhesions* that were lysed.

General laparotomy revealed *no/the following abnormalities (detail)*.

The left triangular ligament of the liver was incised and the left hepatic lobe retracted to the right. The lesser omentum was incised and the stomach gently retracted inferiorly. Using a combination of blunt and sharp dissection, the esophagus was identified and protected. The esophagus was mobilized to the left and the median arcuate ligament and fibers of the right crus incised, allowing exposure of the supraceliac aorta. Several small bleeding vessels were controlled with *electrocautery/ligatures*. The anterior and lateral surfaces of the aorta were cleared of surrounding tissues for several centimeters proximally. Next, the dissection was continued distally and the origin of the celiac artery dissected clear of surrounding tissues. The left gastric, splenic, and common hepatic arteries were individually dissected and slung with vessel slings. The distal celiac artery was soft and suitable for the location of the distal anastomosis.

The proximal superior mesenteric artery was exposed and slung via an incision in the peritoneum at the root of the small bowel mesentery. A tunnel was created behind the pancreas with care being taken to protect the left renal vein and its tributaries. The SMA was a pulseless vessel of good caliber.

The patient received 5,000 U of heparin intravenously.

A Sitinsky clamp was applied to the supraceliac aorta and the aorta opened with a #15 blade. An 8-mm *knitted Dacron PTFE* graft was anastomosed end-to-side with 3-0 polypropylene sutures. One extra suture was required to ensure hemostasis. The graft was clamped and the Sitinsky removed. Aortic clamp time was ___ min. The vessel slings around the celiac branch arteries were tensed and the celiac artery was opened longitudinally. Backbleeding from distally was brisk. The graft was cut to length and anastomosed end-to-side with 5-0 polypropylene sutures. The graft was flushed and vessels backbled before completing the suture line and releasing clamps. There was an excellent pulse in the common hepatic and splenic arteries.

A second length of 8-mm *knitted Dacron/PTFE/vein* graft was then placed in the retro-pancreatic tunnel. The aortoceliac graft was reclamped and opened longitudinally. The second graft was anastomosed end-to-side to this with 5-0 polypropylene. This second graft was clamped proximally and the clamp removed from the first graft. Using slings to control the SMA, an arteriotomy was made on this vessel. Heparinized saline was injected distally with ease. The graft was cut to length and sutured end-to-side to the SMA again with 5-0 polypropylene. There was good flow with clamps removed. Hemostasis was carefully assessed and found to be satisfactory. The small and large bowels were carefully inspected and found to be well vascularized and exhibiting active peristalsis. There was a palpable pulse in the ileocolic vessels and also in the marginal artery. Using a hand-held Doppler, there was a biphasic signal throughout the small and large bowel vessels.

A final check of hemostasis was made. The divided crural fibers were reconstituted with interrupted 2-0 Vicryl sutures. The abdominal content was returned to the peritoneal cavity. Abdominal closure was with mass 0 polypropylene sutures. The skin was closed with staples.

The patient tolerated the procedure well and was taken to the postanesthesia care unit in stable condition.

Chapter 152
Celiac and SMA Stenting

Raphael C. Sun, M.D.

INDICATIONS
- Acute mesenteric ischemia.
- Chronic mesenteric ischemia.

ESSENTIAL STEPS
1. Femoral or brachial access.
2. Anticoagulate with IV heparin sulfate (3,000–7,000 U).
3. Control access with 6-French sheath.
4. Aortogram for SMA/CA anatomy evaluation.
5. Cannulation of the SMA/CA.
6. Exchange of guide wire.
7. Pre-dilate the stenotic lesion.
8. Advance introducer sheath or guiding sheath up to or across the lesion.
9. Position stent across lesion.
10. Retract sheath and recheck position with angiogram.
11. Deploy stent across lesion.
12. Post-stent placement angiogram.
13. Check ACT.
14. Remove all sheaths, wires, and catheters.
15. Apply pressure.
16. Secure hemostasis.

NOTE THESE VARIATIONS
- Femoral approach most commonly used.
- Brachial approach is especially useful for the SMA.

J.J. Hoballah and C.E.H. Scott-Conner (eds.), *Operative Dictations in General and Vascular Surgery*, DOI 10.1007/978-1-4614-0451-4_152,
© Springer Science+Business Media, LLC 2012

- Size of wires, sheaths, catheters, and stents will vary depending on access and degree of stenosis and patient's anatomy.

COMPLICATIONS
- Nephrotoxicity.
- Artery dissection.
- Thrombosis.
- Artery perforation and hemorrhage.
- Embolization.
- Pseudoaneurysm.

TEMPLATE OPERATIVE DICTATION

Preoperative diagnosis: Mesenteric ischemia.

Procedure: Mesenteric angiogram, SMA/celiac balloon angioplasty, and SMA/celiac stent placement.

Postoperative diagnosis: Mesenteric ischemia.

Indications: This ___-year-old male/female was found to have a history of nausea, vomiting, and pain after eating with significant weight loss. Angioplasty and stenting was indicated.

Description of procedure: The patient was brought to the operative suite and placed on the operating table in the supine position. A proper time-out was taken. The right/left groin/arm was shaved, prepped, and draped in the usual sterile fashion. Monitored anesthesia was provided. Prophylactic antibiotics were given by the anesthesiologist. The area over the common femoral artery/brachial artery was anesthetized with 1% lidocaine solution. Heparin 3,000–7,000 IU was given intraoperatively.

A micropuncture needle was used to access the femoral/brachial artery and exchanged for a micropuncture sheath. This was exchanged for a 5–7 French sheath using the Seldinger technique. An angled Glide wire/Bentson wire and angled catheter were used to advance into the descending aorta down into the abdominal aorta. The angled Glidewire was then exchanged for an Omni Flush catheter. Using the catheter, an aortogram was obtained that demonstrated ____(findings)____. The SMA/CA was cannulated. This was done with an MPA catheter and an angled Glidewire to cross the occlusion. The MPA catheter was removed and occlusion was crossed with a Glide catheter. A 0.014 Mailman wire/TAD wire was exchanged and placed into the SMA/CA and the lesion was dilated with a 2.5-mm VascuTrak cutting balloon and dilated with an ____mm × ____mm angioplasty balloon under fluoroscopy. A self-expandable/balloon-expandable stent with a 0.014 wire was used and deployed without difficulty at the origin of the stenosis.

Completion angiogram revealed a widely patent SMA/CA that demonstrated brisk flow across the previous stenotic segment and showed filling of the branches of the SMA/CA. Both AP and Lateral views were obtained. There was no residual stenosis, dissection, or thrombosis noted. All balloons, wires, sheaths, and catheters were after the ACT was less than 150–180. Direct manual pressure was held for 10 min over the access site to achieve hemostasis. There were no complications. The patient tolerated the procedure well and was brought back to the postanesthesia care unit in stable condition.

Chapter 153

Superior Mesenteric Artery Embolectomy with Primary/ Patch Closure for Acute Embolic Mesenteric Ischemia

Roderick T.A. Chalmers, M.D.

INDICATION

- Acute abdominal pain, atrial fibrillation/other arrhythmia, with no other obvious cause.

ESSENTIAL STEPS

1. Midline abdominal incision.
2. Thorough exploration of the peritoneal cavity.
3. Careful inspection of the small and large bowel to determine extent of ischemia; investigation of the pulse in the superior mesenteric artery (SHA) from its origin to the distal vasculature.
4. Expose the proximal SMA by incising the peritoneum at the root of the small bowel mesentery.
5. Control the vessel and its branches with slings.
6. Perform a *transverse/longitudinal* arteriotomy.
7. Remove embolic material with forceps.
8. Pass a #4 (red) Fogarty embolectomy catheter proximally to establish good inflow.
9. Pass a smaller (#3, green) Fogarty embolectomy catheter distally and retrieve all *embolus/thrombus*.
10. Allow for one pass of the catheter with no clot retrieved.
11. Inject heparinized saline distally.
12. Close arteriotomy *primarily/patch*.
13. With flow restored to the SMA, allow for 10 or 15 min with the intestine returned to the abdominal cavity.

J.J. Hoballah and C.E.H. Scott-Conner (eds.), *Operative Dictations in General and Vascular Surgery*, DOI 10.1007/978-1-4614-0451-4_153,
© Springer Science+Business Media, LLC 2012

14. Assess pulsation in the distal small bowel mesentery and color and contractility of the bowel.
15. If all the bowel looks viable return it to the abdomen.
16. Close the abdomen in usual fashion.
17. Monitor the patient carefully in intensive care unit (serial blood gas analysis, lactate levels, etc.).
18. Perform relook laparotomy 12–24 h later no matter what the clinical scenario is.

NOTE THIS VARIATION

- If the SMA is of reasonable caliber and an embolic etiology is suspected, perform a transverse arteriotomy; otherwise, perform a longitudinal arteriotomy.
- The transverse arteriotomy is typically closed with interrupted 6-0 or 5-0 polypropylene sutures. The longitudinal arteriotomy is closed with a patch (a segment of saphenous vein should be harvested simultaneously from one of the groins to minimize the duration of bowel ischemia).

COMPLICATIONS

- High-associated mortality.
- Bowel infarction.
- Multiorgan failure.

TEMPLATE OPERATIVE DICTATION

Preoperative diagnosis: Embolic occlusion of the SMA with acute bowel ischemia.

Procedure: Fogarty catheter embolectomy of the SMA with saphenous vein patch closure.

Postoperative diagnosis: Same.

Indications: This is a ___-year-old *male/female* who presented with acute onset of abdominal pain. *Clinically, the patient was in fast atrial fibrillation. Biochemistry revealed a low-grade metabolic acidosis.* A clinical diagnosis of acute embolic mesenteric occlusion was made. A CTA confirmed the diagnosis. *The patient* was taken to the operating room with a view to performing an SMA *embolectomy/revascularization* procedure. *The patient* was apprised of the risks of the condition and of the surgical procedure.

Description of procedure: The patient was placed supine on the operating table. The arms were *tucked in/placed at 80°* at the sides. Anesthesia placed peripheral and central venous lines, a Swan-Ganz catheter, and arterial lines and the patient was intubated. A Foley urinary catheter was inserted under sterile conditions. The anterior abdominal wall and right thigh were draped and prepped in the usual manner. The patient received intravenous cefuroxime and metronidazole prior to skin incision.

A midline abdominal skin incision was made. The subcutaneous tissues were divided with electrocautery. The linea alba was opened with electrocautery. The peritoneum was opened along the length of the wound.

Abdominal exploration revealed the small intestine from the proximal jejunum to terminal ileum and the right colon to the mid-transverse level to be ischemic looking, flaccid with no evidence of peristalsis. There was no palpable pulsation within the vessels in the small bowel mesenteric arcades and *a monophasic/ no Doppler* signal. The remainder of the colon and the other abdominal viscera appeared normal. The SMA was exposed and slung by opening the peritoneum at the root of the small bowel mesentery. The SMA was pulseless at this level but was a soft, disease-free artery with a diameter of 5 mm. A transverse arteriotomy was fashioned with a #15 blade. Fresh embolus was retrieved with forceps, giving rise to a little inflow. A #4 Fogarty catheter was passed proximally and further thrombus/embolus was obtained and the inflow was excellent. The proximal SMA was double slung to control bleeding. A #3 Fogarty catheter was passed distally and further thrombus was retrieved and there was some backbleeding. Heparinized saline was injected with ease. The SMA was closed with interrupted 6-0 polypropylene sutures.

(*If longitudinal SMA: A portion of greater saphenous vein was harvested from the right groin. At the same time, a #4 Fogarty catheter was passed proximally and further thrombus/embolus was obtained and the inflow was excellent. The proximal SMA was double slung to control bleeding. A #3 Fogarty catheter was passed distally and further thrombus was retrieved and there was some backbleeding. Heparinized saline was injected with ease. The harvested vein was opened and cut to size and shape. It was sutured to the SMA with 6-0 polypropylene.*)

Flow was restored to the SMA and, after ensuring that the anastomosis was hemostatic, the intestines were returned to the abdominal cavity, taking all stretch off the small bowel mesentery. After a 15-min interval, there was an easily palpable pulse in the SMA and ileocolic vessels. Also there appeared to be a palpable pulse in the marginal artery. The Doppler signal was biphasic in the distal SMA and marginal artery. The previously ischemic small bowel had become pink and there were areas of active peristalsis. The entire colon also appeared satisfactorily vascularized.

After a final check for hemostasis, the intestines were returned to the peritoneal cavity. The abdominal wall was closed with a mass closure of 0 polypropylene sutures. The skin was closed with staples.

The patient tolerated the procedure well and was taken to the intensive care unit in stable condition. Serial arterial blood gas analysis and serum lactate levels will be measured. A relook laparotomy will be performed in 24 h.

Chapter 154

Superior Mesenteric Artery Thrombectomy with Retrograde Aortomesenteric Bypass for Acute Thrombotic Mesenteric Ischemia

Roderick T.A. Chalmers, M.D.

INDICATION

- Acute abdominal pain, evidence of bowel ischemia (acidosis, elevated lactate, clinical evidence of occlusive arterial disease), with other causes of pain excluded.

ESSENTIAL STEPS

1. Midline abdominal incision.
2. Abdominal exploration reveals ischemia of the small bowel beyond the proximal jejunum.
3. Pulseless superior mesenteric artery (SMA) with evidence of occlusive disease (palpable calcification, calcification of aorta, and iliac arteries).
4. Expose the SMA in the root of the small bowel mesentery as before.
5. Confirm its patency distally and proximal occlusion.
6. Expose the infrarenal aorta by incising the posterior peritoneum to the left of the duodenojejunal (DJ) flexure, distal to the inferior mesenteric vein.
7. Find a soft portion of the aorta that can be clamped safely and used as the site for a graft anastomosis.
8. Be prepared to harvest a length of saphenous vein for use as a graft (preferable to prosthetic graft where ischemic bowel is present).

J.J. Hoballah and C.E.H. Scott-Conner (eds.), *Operative Dictations in General and Vascular Surgery*, DOI 10.1007/978-1-4614-0451-4_154,
© Springer Science+Business Media, LLC 2012

9. Administer systemic heparin intravenously (75–100 U/kg) and wait a few minutes.
10. Control the SMA with slings.
11. Perform longitudinal arteriotomy distal to the middle colic artery takeoff.
12. Attempt to pass # Fogarty embolectomy catheter proximally (confirms proximal occlusion/tight stensosis with supervening thrombosis).
13. Pass #3 Fogarty embolectomy catheter distally, removing all clot.
14. Side-bite clamp on the infrarenal aorta.
15. Longitudinal aortotomy to the right of the midline of 2-cm length.
16. Reverse harvested long saphenous vein and suture end-to-side to the aorta with 4-0 polypropylene sutures.
17. Lay graft in "cleft" between the aorta and vena cava.
18. Cut vein graft to length and anastomose so that heel of graft lies distally and toe proximally on the SMA. This avoids the kinking associated with other techniques.
19. Anastomose the vein graft to the SMA with 6-0 polypropylene sutures.
20. Check that anastomoses are hemostatic.
21. Return the intestines to the peritoneal cavity for 15 min.
22. Reinspect the entire small and large intestine for viability.
23. Palpate for pulses in the SMA, distal ileocolic arteries, and marginal artery.
24. Resect the obviously infarcted bowel.
25. Do not anastomose the bowel, bring out end stoma(s).
26. Close the abdomen as usual.
27. Plan for a relook laparotomy in 12–24 h.
28. Monitor patient in intensive care unit with blood gases, electrolytes, and serum lactate levels.

NOTE THIS VARIATION

- If the aorta is extremely calcified, the iliac arteries can serve as an inflow source.

COMPLICATIONS

- Bowel infarction.
- Myocardial infarction.
- Multiorgan failure.
- Lower limb ischemia.
- Pneumonia.

TEMPLATE OPERATIVE DICTATION

Preoperative diagnosis: Acute mesenteric ischemia.

Procedure: Thrombectomy of the SMA with retrograde aortomesenteric reversed saphenous vein bypass.

Postoperative diagnosis: Same.

Indications: This is a ___-year-old *male/female* who presented with a short history of acute abdominal pain. There was a history of recent weight loss and epigastric pain after eating. Peptic ulcer and other upper gastrointestinal pathologies had been ruled out previously. *The patient* was thought to have acute mesenteric ischemia and consented to laparotomy with a view to mesenteric revascularization if possible. *The patient* was aware of the risks of the procedure, including the possible need for *colostomy/ileostomy*.

Description of procedure: The patient was placed supine on the operating table. The arms were *tucked in/placed at 80°* at the sides. Anesthesia placed peripheral and central venous lines, a Swan-Gantz catheter, and arterial lines and the patient was intubated. A Foley urinary catheter was inserted under sterile conditions. The anterior abdominal wall and right thigh were draped and prepped in the usual manner. The patient received intravenous cefuroxime and metronidazole prior to skin incision.

A midline abdominal skin incision was made. The subcutaneous tissues were divided with electrocautery. The linea alba was opened with electrocautery. The peritoneum was opened along the length of the wound.

Abdominal exploration revealed the small intestine from the proximal jejunum to terminal ileum and the right colon to the mid-transverse level to be pale and flaccid with no evidence of peristalsis. There was no palpable pulsation within the vessels in the small bowel mesenteric arcades. The SMA was exposed in the root of the small bowel mesentery. It was pulseless and more proximally was obviously calcified and occluded. It was deduced that the acute bowel ischemia was due to acute thrombosis of a heavily diseased proximal SMA. As there was bowel salvageable, it was decided to attempt SMA thrombectomy and aortomesenteric bypass.

The SMA was dissected just distal to the middle colic artery takeoff and slings were passed around the vessel and its branches for control.

The infrarenal aorta was exposed by incising the posterior peritoneum overlying it. The aorta had obvious areas of calcification but there was a length of soft aorta found at the level of the inferior mesenteric artery.

While these arteries were being dissected, a 30-cm length of greater saphenous vein was harvested from the right thigh.

The patient was given 5,000 U of intravenous heparin.

A 1.5-cm longitudinal arteriotomy was fashioned on the proximal SMA with a #15 blade. There was fresh thrombus within the vessel lumen and this was removed with forceps. There was no inflow and the vessel was clearly occluded proximally. A #3 Fogarty embolectomy catheter was passed distally and a small amount of fresh thrombus was retrieved. *A #2 Fogarty embolectomy catheter was also passed in the larger SMA branches and a small amount of fresh thrombus was also retrieved.* There was some backbleeding. Heparinized saline was injected distally.

The soft portion of the infrarenal aorta was isolated using two clamps and a 2-cm aortotomy performed. It was clear that the inferior mesenteric artery was chronically occluded over several centimeters from its origin. The harvested saphenous vein was placed in reversed orientation and anastomosed end-to-side to the aorta with a continuous 4-0 polypropylene suture. This anastomosis was hemostatic when the clamps were removed from the aorta. With a ligaclip placed on the distal end of the graft, it was placed in the gutter between the aorta and the vena cava so that it lay without kinks, in retrograde orientation. Attention was turned to the SMA. The vein graft was cut to length so that the toe of the planned anastomosis to the SMA was at the proximal end of the SMA arteriotomy and the heel at the distal end. The graft was anastomosed to the SMA with continuous 6-0 polypropylene. When flow was restored to the graft, there was a palpable pulse in the distal SMA and, within 1 or 2 min, the color of the small bowel began to improve. The intestines were replaced carefully in the peritoneal cavity and packs soaked in warm saline placed over them. After a 15-min interval, the intestines were reinspected. The entire small and large bowels appeared viable. There were palpable pulsations in the distal SMA and ileocolic and ascending colic arteries and evidence of peristalsis.

After a final check for hemostasis, the intestines were returned to the peritoneal cavity. The abdominal wall was closed with 0 polypropylene and staples to skin.

The patient tolerated the procedure well and was taken to the intensive care unit in stable condition. Serial arterial blood gas analysis and serum lactate levels will be measured. A relook laparotomy will be performed in 24 h.

Chapter 155
Bilateral Aortorenal Bypass

Jamal J. Hoballah, M.D., M.B.A.

INDICATIONS

- Renal artery occlusive disease: Asymptomatic, renovascular hypertension, and renal insufficiency.
- Recurrent renal artery stenosis following angioplasty/stenting.

ESSENTIAL STEPS

1. Midline xiphoid to pubis incision; *transverse/bilateral* subcostal incision.
2. Abdominal exploration for unexpected findings.
3. Retract the transverse colon anteriorly and to the right.
4. Retract the splenic flexure posteriorly and laterally.
5. Divide the peritoneal periaortic attachment of the duodenum.
6. Wrap the small bowel in a wet towel and retract to the right.
7. Incise the retroperitoneum overlying the aorta and continue proximally.
8. Identify the left renal vein.
9. Dissect and mobilize the left renal vein and divide its branches.
10. Expose and dissect the left renal artery.
11. Expose and dissect the right renal artery.
12. Anticoagulate with heparin 75–100 U/kg and wait 5 min.
13. Cross-clamp the aorta and perform the proximal anastomosis of the left aortorenal bypass.

J.J. Hoballah and C.E.H. Scott-Conner (eds.), *Operative Dictations in General and Vascular Surgery*, DOI 10.1007/978-1-4614-0451-4_155,
© Springer Science+Business Media, LLC 2012

14. Perform the proximal anastomosis of the right aortorenal bypass.
15. Give 12.5 g mannitol intravenously.
16. Construct the distal anastomosis to the left renal artery.
17. Evaluate the reconstruction with *Doppler/duplex*.
18. Construct the distal anastomosis to the right renal artery.
19. Evaluate the reconstruction with *Doppler/duplex*.
20. Reevaluate hemostasis.
21. Close the abdomen.
22. Recheck distal pulses.

NOTE THESE VARIATIONS
- Renal artery angioplasty/stenting has gained popularity as the first line of intervention.
- The right renal artery may be accessed by exposing the pararenal aorta and the origin of the right renal artery and tracing it distally posterior to the vena cava. Alternatively, the right renal artery is approached by performing a Kocher maneuver and exposing it lateral to the vena cava.
- Vein or prosthetic grafts may be used to construct the bypass.
- The renal artery anastomosis can be constructed using end-to-end or end-to-side configuration.

COMPLICATIONS
- Bleeding.
- Myocardial infarction.
- Pneumonia.
- Renal failure.
- No postoperative improvement in renal function or blood pressure control.
- Leg ischemia.

TEMPLATE OPERATIVE DICTATION
Preoperative diagnosis: Bilateral renovascular occlusive disease.
Procedure: Bilateral aortorenal bypasses.
Postoperative diagnosis: Same.
Indications: This ___-year-old *male/female* was found to have poorly controlled hypertension despite maximal medical therapy. *The patient* has *no/mild/moderate/severe* renal dysfunction with blood urea nitrogen ___ and creatinine ___.

Angiogram/CTA/MRA revealed ___% right renal artery stenosis and___% left renal artery stenosis. The risks and benefits of surgical intervention were discussed with the patient and *he/she* elected to undergo surgical intervention.

Description of procedure: The patient was placed supine on the operating table. The arms were *tucked in/placed at 80°*. Normal bony prominences were padded. Anesthesia placed appropriate lines and induced and intubated the patient without complications. A Foley catheter was then placed under sterile technique. The patient's anterior abdomen and both lower extremities were circumferentially prepped and draped in the usual sterile fashion. Preoperative antibiotics were administered prior to skin incision.

The skin incision was then made from the subxiphoid to the suprapubic region. The subcutaneous tissue was divided with electrocautery. The linea alba was exposed and incised. The peritoneum was elevated and entered sharply. The abdominal wall incision was then extended to the full length of the skin incision.

There were *no/moderate number* of adhesions requiring lysis.

Abdominal exploration revealed no/the following incidental findings (detail).

The transverse colon was then elevated superiorly out of the wound, wrapped in a moist towel. A moist rolled laparatomy pad was placed in the bed of the splenic flexure of the colon, which was retracted laterally and posteriorly. The remainder of the small bowel was then deflected to the right, exposing the aorta. Sharp dissection of the ligament of Treitz and the distal fourth portion of the duodenum allowed further exposure of the aorta and retraction of the small bowel to the right. The small bowel was then wrapped in a moistened towel and held in place using the Omni retractor.

The retroperitoneum overlying the aorta was incised and continued proximally to the level of the left renal vein and distally toward the aortic bifurcation. The inferior mesenteric vein was encountered, ligated, and divided. The lymphatics overlying the infrarenal aortic neck were ligated and divided.

The abdominal aorta was then sharply dissected.

The infrarenal aorta appeared to be adequate for clamping and constructing the proximal anastomoses.

Further mobilization of the left renal vein was performed. The left *gonadal, lumbar, and adrenal veins* were ligated and divided. The left renal vein was circumferentially mobilized and retracted proximally, exposing the renal arteries.

The left renal artery was dissected distally toward its segmental branches.

The right renal artery was dissected distally posterior to the inferior vena cava for a 3-cm segment. This necessitated division of few venous branches draining into the medial aspect of the vena cava.

(*Alternatively:* *The peritoneum lateral to the second part of the duodenum was incised and the duodenum and head of pancreas were reflected medially and anteriorly performing a Kocher maneuver. The right renal vein draining into the inferior vena cava was exposed posterior to the duodenum. The right renal vein was mobilized cephalad, exposing the right renal artery. The right renal artery was then exposed and encircled with a vessel loop. The right renal artery was dissected proximally and distally until it divided into its segmental branches.*)

The greater saphenous vein was exposed and two 15-cm segments were harvested.

The patient was given 5,000 U or 75 UI/kg of heparin intravenously along with 12.5 g of mannitol. The aorta was clamped proximally and distally and a soft part of the aorta was identified. A 1-cm incision was performed on the left anterolateral aspect of the aorta. The vein was used in a *reversed/nonreversed* manner. One end was spatulated. An anastomosis was then performed between the spatulated end of the vein and the aortotomy using a 5-0 prolene running suture. At the completion of the anastomosis, the aorta was backbled and forwardbled and irrigated with heparinized saline. The suture line was then completed.

A 1-cm incision was performed on the right anterolateral aspect of the aorta and a similar procedure was performed on that side.

The left renal artery was then *ligated/suture ligated* as proximal as possible toward its origin from the aorta. The distal part of the artery was controlled with a Yasargil clip. The renal artery was then transected and its distal end spatulated. The end of the vein was spatulated to match the arteriotomy. An end-to-end anastomosis was then performed using a 5-0 prolene running suture. At the completion of the anastomosis, the renal artery was allowed to backbleed and the graft was forward flushed. The anastomosis was irrigated with heparinized saline. The sutures were tied and the anastomotic suture line was checked for hemostasis, which was adequate. There were excellent Doppler signals in the kidney.

The same was then performed on the other side.

The renal artery cross-clamp time was ___ min.

The proximal and distal anastomoses were reinspected for hemostasis.

The renal artery was evaluated using intraoperative *duplex/Doppler ultrasound*. The reconstruction appeared to be patent without any defects and there were excellent Doppler signals in the kidney.

The abdominal wall was then closed using #1 prolene *interrupted/continuous* sutures. The skin was closed with staples. The feet were inspected and there was evidence of strong Doppler signals. The patient tolerated the procedure well and was transferred to the postanesthesia care unit in stable condition, making good urine output.

Chapter 156
Hepatorenal Artery Bypass

Jamal J. Hoballah, M.D., M.B.A.

INDICATIONS

- Renal artery occlusive disease: Asymptomatic, renovascular hypertension, renal insufficiency, recurrent following angioplasty/stenting.
- Aortic disease precluding the use of the aorta as ain inflow. As part of aortic debranching procedure.

ESSENTIAL STEPS

1. Rule out via a lateral aortogram the presence of any stenosis at the origin of the celiac artery.
2. *Right subcostal incision/midline xyphoid to pubis incision.*
3. Abdominal exploration for unexpected findings.
4. Stomach retracted to the left, and the lesser omentum entered.
5. The common hepatic, proper hepatic, and gastroduodenal arteries dissected and encircled with silastic vessel loops.
6. Kocher maneuver performed.
7. The right renal vein exposed.
8. The right renal artery exposed and encircled with a vessel loop.
9. Greater saphenous vein segment harvested.
10. Anticoagulation with intravenous heparin.

J.J. Hoballah and C.E.H. Scott-Conner (eds.), *Operative Dictations in General and Vascular Surgery*, DOI 10.1007/978-1-4614-0451-4_156,
© Springer Science+Business Media, LLC 2012

11. Proximal end-to-side anastomosis constructed to the common hepatic artery.
12. 12.5 g of mannitol given intravenously.
13. Distal anastomosis performed (end-to-end or end-to-side) to the renal artery.
14. Hemostasis established.
15. Revascularization checked with *Doppler/duplex.*
16. Incisions closed.

NOTE THESE VARIATIONS
- The vein can be used in a reversed or nonreversed fashion.
- The renal artery anastomosis can be done in an end-to-end or end-to-side manner.

COMPLICATIONS
- Bleeding.
- Myocardial infarction.
- Pneumonia.
- Renal failure.
- No postoperative improvement in renal function or blood pressure control.

TEMPLATE OPERATIVE DICTATION
Preoperative diagnosis: Renovascular occlusive disease.
Procedure: Right hepatorenal bypass.
Postoperative diagnosis: Same.
Indications: This ___-year-old *male/female* was found to have poorly controlled hypertension despite maximal medical therapy. The patient has *no/mild/moderate/severe* renal dysfunction with blood urea nitrogen ___ and creatinine ___.
Angiogram revealed ___% right renal artery stenosis and a severely calcified and diseased infrarenal aorta. The risks and benefits of surgical intervention were discussed with the patient and *he/she* elected to undergo surgical intervention. The patient has prior angioplasty/stenting with recurrent stenosis.
Description of procedure: The patient was placed supine. The procedure was performed under general anesthesia. The abdomen and upper thighs were prepped and draped in the standard fashion.

A right subcostal incision was then performed. The incision was deepened through the subcutaneous tissue and fat. The anterior rectus sheath was identified and divided. The rectus muscle was divided with electrocautery. The posterior rectus sheath and the peritoneum were then lifted and the abdominal cavity entered. The muscle incision was then extended for the full length of the skin incision.

Exploration revealed no evidence of any unexpected findings. The stomach was retracted to the left and the lesser omentum entered. Palpation along the upper border of the pancreas revealed the location of the hepatic artery. The common hepatic artery was dissected and encircled with a silastic vessel loop. The common hepatic artery was traced distally toward its bifurcation into the proper hepatic and the gastroduodenal arteries, which were also dissected and encircled with silastic vessel loops.

Attention was then directed to expose the right renal artery. The peritoneum lateral to the second part of the duodenum was incised and the duodenum and head of pancreas were reflected medially and anteriorly performing a Kocher maneuver. The right renal vein draining into the inferior vena cava was exposed posterior to the duodenum. The right renal vein was mobilized cephalad, exposing the right renal artery. The right renal artery was then exposed and encircled with a vessel loop. The right renal artery was dissected proximally and distally until it divided into its segmental branches.

Attention was then directed to harvesting of the greater saphenous vein in the thigh. An upper thigh incision was performed over the greater saphenous vein, which had been evaluated and marked preoperatively by duplex ultrasonography. The vein was mobilized toward the saphenofemoral junction, and its branches were ligated and divided. A segment measuring 15 cm was harvested. The patient was given 5,000 U of heparin intravenously.

Atraumatic vascular clamps were applied on the common hepatic, proper hepatic, and gastroduodenal arteries. A 1.0-cm incision was then performed in the common hepatic artery. The vein was used in a reversed manner. The end of the vein was spatulated to match the hepatic arteriotomy. The proximal anastomosis was then constructed using a running 5-0 prolene suture. At the completion of the anastomosis, forward- and back-bleeding from the hepatic arteries were performed, and the anastomosis was irrigated with heparinized saline. The sutures were tied and the anastomosis was checked for hemostasis, which was adequate.

The patient was then given 12.5 g of mannitol intravenously.

[Choose one:]

If end-to-end anastomosis: The right renal artery was then ligated as proximally as possible to its origin. The distal end was controlled with a Yasargil clip. The renal artery was transected and the distal end was spatulated. The bypass was measured to the appropriate length and transected. The distal end of the bypass was spatulated to match the size of the renal artery. An end-to-end anastomosis was then constructed using a running 5-0 prolene.

__If end-to-side anastomosis:__ The right renal artery was then controlled distally and proximally as close as possible to its origin using Yasargil clips/vascular clamps/vascular Bulldog clamps/silastic loops. A 1-cm arteriotomy was then performed in the renal artery. The bypass was measured to the appropriate length and transected. The distal end of the bypass was spatulated to match the size of the renal arteriotomy. An end-to-side anastomosis was then constructed using a running 5-0 prolene suture.

At the completion of the anastomosis, back-bleeding from the renal artery was obtained and the graft was forward flushed. The anastomosis was irrigated with heparinized saline, and the sutures were tied. The suture line was checked for hemostasis and was adequate. The renal artery cross-clamp time was ___ min.

The proximal and distal anastomoses were reinspected for hemostasis.

The renal artery was evaluated using intraoperative *duplex/Doppler ultrasound*. The reconstruction appeared to be patent without any defects and there were excellent Doppler signals in the kidney.

The wound was then closed in layers using #1 Vicryl sutures. The skin was closed with staples. The patient tolerated the procedure well and was transferred to the postanesthesia care unit in good condition, making good urine output.

Chapter 157

Transaortic Celiac and Superior Mesenteric Artery Endarterectomy

Christian Bianchi, M.D. and Jeffrey L. Ballard, M.D.

INDICATION

- Chronic mesenteric ischemia due to atherosclerotic occlusive disease of the celiac and superior mesenteric arteries (usually ostial lesions).

ESSENTIAL STEPS

1. Retroperitoneal aortic exposure via left flank incision.
2. Identify and expose the left renal artery to use as a landmark for further dissection.
3. Divide the median arcuate ligament and left crus of the diaphragm to expose the supraceliac aorta.
4. Ligate the iliolumbar venous tributary immediately inferior to the left renal artery.
5. Divide the neurovascular tissue around and superior to the left renal artery to facilitate exposure of origins of the superior mesenteric and celiac arteries.
6. Dissect out each mesenteric artery in a similar fashion.
7. Administer intravenous bolus of mannitol (12.5 g) and heparin (100 U/kg) prior to application of supraceliac cross-clamp.
8. Create a curvilinear aortotomy in the paravisceral aorta.
9. Create an appropriate endarterectomy plane just superior to the celiac artery and use curved scissors to transect the paravisceral aortic plaque around the origins of the mesenteric arteries.

J.J. Hoballah and C.E.H. Scott-Conner (eds.), *Operative Dictations in General and Vascular Surgery*, DOI 10.1007/978-1-4614-0451-4_157,
© Springer Science+Business Media, LLC 2012

10. Complete meticulous plaque extraction at the level of the celiac and superior mesenteric arteries using eversion endarterectomy technique.
11. Sharply transect distal paravisceral plaque without creating a flap.
12. Back-bleed the mesenteric arteries into the aorta and flush the proximal and distal abdominal aorta.
13. Close aortotomy using 4-0 prolene bolstered with Teflon felt strips.
14. Perform immediate intraoperative duplex ultrasound examination of the celiac and superior mesenteric arteries.
15. Achieve meticulous hemostasis.
16. Close the surgical wound in layers.

NOTE THESE VARIATIONS

- Endovascular treatment (angioplasty/stenting) is an option especially in high-risk patient even though it is associated with higher recurrence rate.
- Revascularization of the mesenteric vessels can be achieved using aortoceliac–mesenteric bypasses or transaortic celiac and superior mesenteric artery endarterectomy.
- Transaortic endarterectomy can be performed using a retroperitoneal approach as described in this chapter or through a transperitoneal approach with medial visceral notation.
- If the plaque in the superior mesenteric artery (SMA) extends distally and does not lend itself to a smooth endpoint, an additional longitudinal arteriotomy is carried in the SMA to complete the endarterectomy. The arteriotomy is then closed using a vein patch angioplasty.

COMPLICATIONS

- Acute mesenteric artery occlusion, dissection, or thrombosis.
- Hepatobiliary or small bowel ischemia.
- Distal aortic, renal, or lower-extremity embolization.
- Acute tubular necrosis or renal failure.

TEMPLATE OPERATIVE DICTATION

Preoperative diagnosis: Chronic mesenteric ischemia.
Procedure: Transaortic celiac and superior mesenteric artery endarterectomy.

Postoperative diagnosis: Same.

Indications: This ___-year-old *male/female* has a ___-month history of postprandial abdominal pain associated with significant and unintended weight loss. Duplex ultrasound suggested severe atherosclerotic disease at the origins of the celiac and superior mesenteric arteries and arteriography confirmed this finding.

Description of procedure: The procedure was performed under general anesthesia with the patient placed in a modified right lateral decubitus position. The chest, abdomen, and groin were prepped and draped in a standard fashion. An incision was made across the left flank extending from just lateral to the umbilicus toward the tip of the twelfth rib posteriorly. The incision was deepened through abdominal fascia and musculature to the peritoneum. The twelfth rib was partially resected to improve this extraperitoneal exposure of the left retroperitoneal space. The peritoneal contents and left kidney including Gerota's fascia were rotated medially off the psoas muscle and diaphragm to expose the abdominal aorta. The left renal artery was identified and neurovascular tissue surrounding this vessel was divided between silk ligatures. Division of median arcuate ligament and the left diaphragmatic crus facilitated exposure and dissection of the distal descending thoracic and supraceliac aorta. Inferior to the left renal artery, iliolumbar venous tributaries to the left renal vein were divided to allow superomedial retraction of the renal vein off the infrarenal aorta. This maneuver facilitated exposure of the aorta below the level of the renal arteries.

Attention was then turned to the paravisceral aorta, where the celiac and superior mesenteric arteries were individually dissected free of surrounding tissue for approximately 1 cm beyond grossly palpable atherosclerotic disease. The left and right renal arteries were also dissected free of surrounding tissue at their origins. All these vessels were encircled with a silastic loop for vascular control. Mannitol (12.5 g) and heparin (100 U/kg) were administered intravenously and after 3 min the vessel loops were gently snugged around the uninvolved aspects of each mesenteric vessel and the origins of the renal arteries. Supraceliac and infrarenal vascular occluding clamps were then placed to facilitate a bloodless operative field.

A curvilinear aortotomy was then created that began just below the level of the left renal artery and coursed posterolaterally around the origins of the mesenteric arteries to end just superior to the origin of the celiac artery. An endarterectomy plane was developed just superior to the celiac artery and curved scissors were used to transect the paravisceral aortic plaque around to origins of the mesenteric arteries. Meticulous plaque extraction then took place at the level of the celiac and superior mesenteric arteries using a Freer elevator and eversion endarterectomy technique. Neat endpoints were visualized prior to release of the everted vessel. Distally, the paravisceral plaque was sharply transected superior to the left renal artery without creating a flap. The aortotomy was then closed using a running 4-0 prolene suture. This suture line was reinforced using longitudinal strips of Teflon felt. The mesenteric and renal arteries, infrarenal aorta, and supraceliac aorta were all back-bled/flushed just prior to completion of the suture line. Supraceliac clamp time was ____ min.

Immediate intraoperative duplex ultrasound interrogation of the celiac and superior mesenteric arteries was then performed. This demonstrated widely patent mesenteric vessels with normal flow velocities. After meticulous hemostasis, wound closure was accomplished in layers using #1 Vicryl suture for the posterior rectus sheath, transversalis fascia, transversus abdominus, and internal oblique muscle layers. The anterior rectus sheath and external oblique aponeurosis were closed with #1 PDS suture. Subcuticular skin closure was accomplished with 3-0 monocryl.

The patient tolerated the procedure well and was taken to the postanesthesia care unit in stable condition.

Chapter 158
Transaortic Renal Artery Endarterectomy

Christian Bianchi, M.D. and Jeffrey L. Ballard, M.D.

INDICATIONS

- Primary: Renovascular hypertension due to unilateral or bilateral ostial renal artery stenosis >60%.
- Secondary: Preservation of kidney parenchyma in cases of severe unilateral or bilateral renal artery stenosis in conjunction with infrarenal aortic aneurysm or aortoiliac occlusive disease.

ESSENTIAL STEPS

1. Retroperitoneal aortic exposure via left flank incision.
2. Identify and expose the left renal artery.
3. Divide the median arcuate ligament and left crus of the diaphragm.
4. Ligate the iliolumbar venous tributary.
5. Expose the proximal aspect of the right renal artery.
6. Grossly palpate the pararenal aorta to determine level of clamp (supraceliac/suprarenal).
7. Administer intravenous bolus of mannitol (12.5 g) and heparin (100 U/kg) prior to application of aortic cross-clamp.
8. Create curvilinear aortotomy that courses posterolaterally around the left renal artery ending at or below the level of the superior mesenteric artery (SMA).
9. Create appropriate endarterectomy plane beginning in the pararenal aorta and complete plaque extraction using eversion endarterectomy technique for both renal arteries.

J.J. Hoballah and C.E.H. Scott-Conner (eds.), *Operative Dictations in General and Vascular Surgery*, DOI 10.1007/978-1-4614-0451-4_158,
© Springer Science+Business Media, LLC 2012

10. Back-bleed the renal arteries into the aorta and flush the proximal and distal abdominal aorta.
11. Close aortotomy using 4-0 prolene bolstered with Teflon felt strips.
12. Perform immediate intraoperative duplex ultrasound examination of the renal arteries.
13. Achieve meticulous hemostasis.
14. Close the surgical wound in layers.

NOTE THESE VARIATIONS

- Endovascular treatment (angioplasty/stenting) is often performed as first line of interventional therapy.
- Renal vascularization can be achieved using bypasses to the renal arteries or transaortic renal endarterectomy.
- Transaortic renal endarterectomy can be performed using a retroperitoneal approach as described in this chapter or through a transperitoneal approach.
- In the transabdominal approach, the aorta is ideally clamped above the SMA. The renal endarterectomy can be performed through a longitudinal aortotomy in the pararenal aorta or through a transverse aortotomy that extends from the proximal anterior wall of the right renal artery to the proximal anterior wall of the left renal artery. The longitudinal aortotomy is closed primarily while the transverse is closed with a patch.
- When renal endarterectomy is performed in conjunction with the placement of an aortic graft, the aorta is transected 1 cm below the origin of the renal arteries and the endarterectomy is performed through the transected aorta.

COMPLICATIONS

- Acute renal artery occlusion, dissection, or thrombosis.
- Acute tubular necrosis, transient or permanent renal failure.
- Distal aortic, mesenteric, or lower-extremity embolization.

TEMPLATE OPERATIVE DICTATION

Preoperative diagnosis: Renovascular hypertension with severe bilateral renal artery stenosis.
Procedure: Bilateral transaortic renal artery endarterectomy.
Postoperative diagnosis: Same.

Indications: This ___-year-old *male/female* has uncontrolled hypertension and new-onset of renal insufficiency. Preoperative imaging demonstrates severe bilateral renal artery stenosis without associated aortoiliac occlusive disease.

Description of procedure: The procedure was performed under general anesthesia with the patient placed in a modified right lateral decubitus position. The chest, abdomen, and groin were prepped and draped in a standard fashion. An incision was made across the left flank extending from just lateral to the umbilicus toward the tip of the twelfth rib posteriorly. The incision was deepened through the abdominal fascia and musculature to the peritoneum. The twelfth rib was partially resected to improve this extraperitoneal exposure of the left retroperitoneal space. The peritoneal contents and left kidney including Gerota's fascia were rotated medially off the psoas muscle and diaphragm to expose the abdominal aorta. The left renal artery was identified and neurovascular tissue surrounding this vessel was divided between silk ligatures. The median arcuate ligament and a portion of the left diaphragmatic crus were divided to facilitate exposure of the suprarenal and supraceliac aorta. Inferior to the left renal artery, iliolumbar venous tributaries to the left renal vein were divided to allow superomedial retraction of the renal vein off the infrarenal aorta. This maneuver facilitated identification and exposure of the proximal right renal artery and facilitated exposure of the abdominal aorta from the diaphragmatic crura through the aortic bifurcation.

Gross palpation of the extent of atherosclerotic disease at the juxtarenal aorta demonstrated significant plaque through the level of the proximal SMA. Therefore, the supraceliac aorta was dissected free of surrounding tissue. In addition, the left and right renal arteries were exposed for at least 1 cm beyond the gross extent of palpable disease. Silastic vessel loops were then passed around each renal artery in a Pott's loop fashion for vascular control. Mannitol (12.5 g) and heparin (100 U/kg) were administered intravenously and after 3 min the vessel loops were gently snugged around the distal aspect of each renal artery. The infrarenal aorta was then cross-clamped, followed by supraceliac clamp application.

Longitudinal aortotomy was initiated below the level of the left renal artery and gently curved posterolaterally around the left renal artery origin to end directly opposite the SMA. Entry into the appropriate endarterectomy plane was made just inferior to the SMA and curved scissors were used to transect the pararenal aortic plaque circumferentially. With meticulous control of the mobilized plaque and gentle manipulation of the renal artery away from the plaque using a Freer elevator, vessel loops about each renal artery were loosened temporarily so that a clean endarterectomy breakpoint could be individually accomplished without creating a flap within the renal artery. The aortotomy was then closed using a running 4-0 prolene suture. This suture line was reinforced using longitudinal strips of Teflon felt. The renal arteries, infrarenal aorta, and suprarenal aorta were flushed just prior to completion of the suture line. Supraceliac clamp time was ____ min.

Immediate intraoperative duplex ultrasound interrogation of each renal artery was then performed. This demonstrated widely patent renal arteries with normal flow velocities.

After meticulous hemostasis, wound closure was accomplished in layers using #1 Vicryl sutures for the posterior rectus sheath, transversalis fascia, transversus abdominus, and internal oblique muscle layers. The anterior rectus sheath and external oblique aponeurosis were closed with #1 PDS suture. Subcuticular skin closure was accomplished with 3-0 monocryl.

The patient tolerated the procedure well and was taken to the postanesthesia care unit in stable condition.

Chapter 159

Renal Artery Angioplasty and Stenting

F. Ezequiel Parodi, M.D. and Murray L. Shames, M.D.

INDICATIONS

- Cure or improve renovascular hypertension that has failed to respond to a combination of medications.
- To improve or stabilize renal function.
- Focal renal artery stenosis.

ESSENTIAL STEPS

1. Femoral access.
2. Aortogram for renal artery anatomy evaluation and artery sizing.
3. Cannulation of the renal artery (SOS, Simmons catheter).
4. Exchange of guide wire to floppy-tip wire (0.035 or 0.018 in. depending on stent to be used).
5. Predilate the stenotic lesion.
6. Advance introducer sheath or guiding sheath *up to or across* the lesion over a guide wire.
7. Position stent across the lesion.
8. Retract sheath and check position with angiogram.
9. Deploy stent.
10. Completion angiogram.

NOTE THIS VARIATION

- After predilating the renal artery stenosis, the guiding sheath may be introduced across the stenosis or kept in the aorta just below the renal artery. In the latter situation, the balloon-mounted stent will be advanced across the

J.J. Hoballah and C.E.H. Scott-Conner (eds.), *Operative Dictations in General and Vascular Surgery*, DOI 10.1007/978-1-4614-0451-4_159,
© Springer Science+Business Media, LLC 2012

renal artery stenosis without the protection of the guiding sheath.

COMPLICATIONS

- Vascular injury (dissection, thrombosis, perforation, embolization).
- Renal parenchymal injury (embolization, perforation).
- Contrast nephropathy.

TEMPLATE OPERATIVE DICTATION

Preoperative diagnosis: *Right/left* renal artery stenosis with *hypertension/renal insufficiency*.

Procedure: Aortogram, renal angiogram, renal angioplasty, and renal stent placement.

Postoperative diagnosis: *Right/left* renal artery stenosis with *hypertension/renal insufficiency*.

Indications: This ___-year-old *male/female* patient was found to have symptomatic *right/left* renal artery stenosis.

Details of operation: The patient was brought to the operating room and placed on the operating table in the supine position. The *right/left* groin was shaved, prepped with povidone–iodine solution, and draped in the standard fashion. The area over the common femoral artery was anesthetized with *1% lidocaine/0.25% bupivacaine* solution. A Seldinger needle was used to access the common femoral artery. A Bentson wire was advanced into the needle and tracked with fluoroscopy into the descending thoracic aorta. The needle was removed and a 6–8 French arterial sheath advanced into the external iliac artery. A pigtail catheter was positioned at the level of the renal arteries and an arteriogram was performed to evaluate the vessels and their diameters. The pigtail was then exchanged for a *Simmons/SOS/Cobra* catheter. A guide wire *(Glide/Bentson/V18[0.018])* was used to cannulate the affected renal artery. A selective renal angiogram confirmed the focal high-grade stenosis with a normal renal artery distally. The wire was advanced across the lesion and the patient was anticoagulated with heparin (1,000–3,000 U). The wire was exchanged for a *TAD wire/Rosen wire* (or the 0.018 in., wire left in position), making sure to keep the tip in view and in a renal branch vessel. The lesion was predilated with a ___-mm angioplasty balloon. A ___-mm guiding catheter was then advanced to or across the stenotic lesion. A ___-mm stent was introduced through the guiding sheath. The guiding *catheter/sheath* was then retracted. The position of the lesion was then confirmed with an angiogram and the ____ stent placed across the stenosis and deployed by balloon inflation. The postdeployment angiogram demonstrated brisk flow across the previously stenotic segment, without any intrastent stenosis or arterial dissection. The sheaths and wires were sequentially removed. Pressure was applied for hemostasis for 15 min.

The patient tolerated the procedure well and was transferred to the postanesthesia care unit in stable condition.

RADIOLOGY SUPERVISION AND INTERPRETATION

1. *Aortogram:* High-grade focal, *nonostial/ostial* stenosis of the *right/left* renal artery.
2. *Postdeployment angiogram:* A stent has been placed across renal artery stenosis, brisk flow, and no residual stenosis.

NOTES

Anatomic Requirements

Focal renal artery stenosis

Necessary Equipment

X-ray compatible operating table

Angled C-arm

Seldinger needle

Selection of 0.035" and 0.018" guidewires (Bentson, Amplatz, Glide)

Selection of catheters (Simmons, SOS, Cobra)

Guiding sheaths (6F-8F)

Sheaths (6F-8F)

Angioplasty balloons (4–8 mm)

Selection of short balloon-expandable stems (4–8 mm)

Section XVI

Aortoiliac Occlusive Disease

Chapter 160
Thoracofemoral Bypass

Kelly S.A. Blair, M.D. and Hisham Bassiouny, M.D.

INDICATIONS

- Presence of an abdominal stoma.
- Radiation therapy.
- Aortic occlusion.
- Symptomatic (disabling claudication, rest pain, ulceration, gangrene, or limb salvage) lower-extremity occlusive disease.
- Revascularize lower extremities where standard aortofemoral bypass grafts cannot be used due to severe patient comorbidities (chronic obstructive pulmonary disease, etc.) or hostile abdomen.
- Revascularize lower extremities before or after removal of infected aortic grafts.
- Revascularize lower extremities after exclusion of infrarenal aortic aneurysm.

ESSENTIAL STEPS

1. Place a double-lumen endotracheal tube.
2. Position the patient on a beanbag with shoulders at a 45° angle and the pelvis as flat as possible.
3. Perform an incision at the level of the sixth intercostal space.
4. Deepen the incision, switch to single-lung ventilation, and enter the pleural cavity.
5. Transect the pulmonary ligament and free the lung.

J.J. Hoballah and C.E.H. Scott-Conner (eds.), *Operative Dictations in General and Vascular Surgery*, DOI 10.1007/978-1-4614-0451-4_160,
© Springer Science+Business Media, LLC 2012

6. The descending aorta below the level of the pulmonary vein was selected for an inflow. Dissect a segment of the descending aorta below the pulmonary vein and encircle it with umbilical tape.
7. Perform bilateral vertical groin incisions overlying each common femoral artery.
8. Dissect the common femoral, superficial femoral, and profunda femoris arteries on both sides.
9. Create a small left retroperitoneal incision and then a retroperitoneal tunnel from the chest to the left groin through the diaphragm with a tunneler.
10. Create a subcutaneous tunnel between each groin incision with a tunneler from the left retroperitoneal to the right groin.
11. Anticoagulate with 75–100 U/kg of intravenous heparin.
12. Clamp the thoracic aorta using a side-biting clamp.
13. Create an incision in the aorta and construct the proximal anastomosis using an appropriately sized bifurcated PTFE or Dacron graft.
14. Place a Fogarty graft clamp on the distal graft and slowly remove the aortic clamps.
15. Pass the graft through the retroperitoneal tunnel, avoiding any twists.
16. Construct the left femoral anastomosis.
17. Construct the right femoral anastomosis.
18. Re-evaluate hemostasis in all anastomoses.
19. Assess the distal vessels by both palpation and Doppler exam.
20. Place a left chest tube and close left thoracotomy.
21. Close groin incisions.

NOTE THESE VARIATIONS

■ *A unilateral aorto-left femoral bypass with a femorofemoral cross-over bypass can be used as described in the template dictation. Alternatively, a bifurcated graft may be used as described in the essential steps. The latter will require an additional small left retroperitoneal exposure to ensure adequate retropubic tunneling, to the right groin. It will also require one less anastomosis.*

■ When constructing the proximal anastomosis, a side-biting clamp is often used to control the descending thoracic aorta yet maintain distal flow into the visceral vessels. On occasion, proximal and distal control with separate clamps may be necessary.

COMPLICATIONS

- Graft infection.
- Ureter injury.
- Bleeding.
- Distal embolization.
- Renal failure.
- Mesenteric infarction.
- Myocardial infarction.

TEMPLATE OPERATIVE DICTATION

Preoperative diagnosis: Bilateral lower-limb ischemia.
Procedure: Thoracofemoral bypass.
Postoperative diagnosis: Same.
Indications: The patient is a ___-year-old *male/female* with bilateral symptomatic lower-extremity occlusive disease (disabling claudication, rest pain, ulceration, gangrene, or limb salvage). *The patient has had multiple failed previous aortic revascularization/ hostile abdomen abdominal stoma/radiation therapy/aortic occlusion/infected aortic grafts.*
Description of procedure: The patient was placed in the supine position on a beanbag. The patient was connected to general anesthesia-monitoring equipment and induced with general endotracheal anesthesia. An arterial line and pulmonary artery catheter were placed. A Foley catheter was placed. A double-lumen endotracheal tube was placed.

After intubation, the patient was positioned on a beanbag with shoulders at a 45° angle toward the patient's right side. The left arm was supported on a sling anteriorly and superiorly. The pelvis was as flat as possible.

An incision was performed with a scalpel in the left chest at the level of the sixth intercostal space. The incision was taken down through the subcutaneous tissue as well as the intercostal muscles with electrocautery. Single-lung ventilation was introduced with deflation of the left lung. The pleural cavity was incised, with care taken to avoid injury to the underlying lung. A rib retractor was utilized for exposure. The lung was freed at the inferior aspect by transecting the pulmonary ligament with electrocautery.

The left lung was retracted cephalad.

The descending aorta below the level of the pulmonary vein was selected for an inflow site. The aorta was dissected from surrounding tissue and encircled with umbilical tape for proximal and distal control.

A linear vertical groin skin incision was performed overlying each common femoral artery with a scalpel. This incision was taken down through the subcutaneous tissue and the femoral sheath with electrocautery. The common femoral, superficial femoral, and profunda femoris arteries were identified and dissected from surrounding tissue. Proximal distal control was obtained with vessel loops.

A retroperitoneal tunnel was created through the diaphragm and retroperitoneum extending into the groin incision with a tunneler. In addition, a subcutaneous tunnel was performed between each groin incision with the tunneler. Appropriately sized PTFE was selected and passed through the retroperitoneal tunnel. A second PTFE graft was placed through the subcutaneous tunnel between the groin incisions. Care was taken to ensure that no twisting of the grafts occurred. The patient was heparinized with 100 U/kg of intravenous heparin.

An aortic clamp was placed on the encircled thoracic aorta proximally. A second aortic clamp was placed on the thoracic aorta distally. A linear aortotomy was performed with a scalpel between the clamps. The arteriotomy was enlarged with Pott's scissors or curved Metzenbaum scissors.

The proximal PTFE graft was beveled and an end-to-side anastomosis was performed with a *running/continuous* 3-0 monofilament nonabsorbable suture, beginning at the inferior heel of the graft. The running suture was carried up each side of the arteriotomy and completed in the middle of the arterotomy on the operator's side. Prior to completion of the anastomosis, the aorta was back-bled proximally and distally. The aorta was then flushed with heparinized saline. The anastomosis was completed.

A Fogarty graft clamp was placed on the distal graft after it was flushed with heparinized saline. Aortic clamps were slowly removed in the usual sequence to prevent hypotension and distal embolization. All excess graft was pulled through the retroperitoneal tunnel.

Attention was now focused on the distal anastomosis. Vascular clamps were placed on the ipsilateral common femoral, superficial femoral, and profunda femoral vessels. A longitudinal arteriotomy was performed in the common femoral with a scalpel. The arteriotomy was extended with Pott's scissors. The graft was cut to appropriate length and beveled in the usual manner. The graft was anastomosed to the arteriotomy in a *running/continuous* fashion with a 5-0 monofilament nonabsorbable suture.

After completion of the femoral anastomosis, a window of graft was removed from the hood of the anastomosis. The end of the femorofemoral bypass graft was beveled and anastomosed to the PTFE hood in an end-to-side manner with a *continuous/running* 5-0 monofilament nonabsorbable suture. This anastomosis was performed as distally as possible to maximize the volume flow through the long proximal limb of the bypass graft. Prior to completion of the anastomosis, all vessels were back-bled and flushed with heparinized saline. The anesthesiologist was informed of impending revascularization of each limb so that bicarbonate and extra intravenous fluids could be administered for acid washout and to prevent hypotension. Clamps were removed from the graft and the vessels in the usual sequence to prevent distal embolization. Hemostasis was assured. A Fogarty graft clamp was placed on the femorofemoral bypass PTFE graft.

Attention was now focused on the contralateral groin anastomosis. Vascular clamps were placed on the common femoral, superficial femoral, and profunda femoral vessels. A longitudinal arteriotomy was performed in the common femoral with a scalpel. The arteriotomy was extended with Pott's scissors. The graft was cut to appropriate length and beveled in the usual manner. The graft was anastomosed to the arteriotomy in a *running/continuous* fashion with a 5-0 monofilament nonabsorbable suture. Prior to completion of the anastomosis, all vessels and grafts were back-bled and flushed with heparinized saline. The anastomosis was completed. The Fogarty graft clamp was removed from the PTFE graft and vascular clamps were removed in the usual sequence.

Hemostasis of all anastomoses was assured. Distal vessels were examined by both palpation and Doppler exam and then documented. Capillary refill of each foot was examined and assured. Evaluation of distal embolization was noted.

Incisions were copiously irrigated. All instruments, lap pads, and retractors were removed. A #32 French chest tube was placed in the left chest through a stab incision in the usual manner and secured with 1-0 nylon. The chest tube was connected to a pleurovac and the lung reinflated. The chest incision was closed in layers with interrupted 1-0 maxon to reapproximate the ribs after a rib approximator was placed. The muscle and fascia were closed in layers with *continuous/running* 2-0 Vicryl. The skin was reapproximated with a continuous 4-0 Vicryl subcuticular closure. Each groin wound was closed in two layers with *running/continuous* 2-0 Vicryl. The skin was reapproximated with a continuous 4-0 Vicryl subcuticular closure. Steristrips and sterile dressing were placed.

The patient awoke in the operating room, was extubated, and was taken to the *postanesthesia care unit/intensive care unit* in hemodynamically stable condition. A chest X-ray was obtained.

NOTES

Chapter 161
Aortobifemoral Bypass

Rabih A. Houbballah, M.D. and Jamal J. Hoballah, M.D., M.B.A.

INDICATIONS
- Disabling claudication.
- Ischemic rest pain.
- Nonhealing ulcers.
- Foot gangrene.

ESSENTIAL STEPS
1. Bilateral groin incisions.
2. Expose the right common femoral, superficial femoral, and profunda femoris arteries and prepare them for clamping.
3. Expose the left common femoral, superficial femoral, and profunda femoris arteries and prepare them for clamping.
4. Midline subxyphoid to suprapubic incision.
5. Abdominal exploration for unexpected findings.
6. Retract the transverse colon anteriorly and to the right.
7. Retract the splenic flexure posteriorly and laterally.
8. Divide the peritoneal periaortic attachment of the duodenum.
9. Wrap the small bowel in a wet towel and retract to the right.
10. Incise the retroperitoneum overlying the aorta and continue proximally.
11. Identify the left renal vein.

J.J. Hoballah and C.E.H. Scott-Conner (eds.), *Operative Dictations in General and Vascular Surgery*, DOI 10.1007/978-1-4614-0451-4_161,
© Springer Science+Business Media, LLC 2012

12. Dissect the aorta at the level of the left renal vein and prepare it for clamping.
13. Incise the retroperitoneum overlying the aorta and continue distally to the level of the aortic bifurcation.
14. Create a tunnel from each common femoral artery to the aortic bifurcation, staying posterior to the ureters.
15. Anticoagulate with heparin 75–100 U/kg and wait for 5 min.
16. Apply the proximal clamp on the aorta below the renal arteries.
17. Apply the distal clamp on the aorta at the level of the inferior mesenteric artery.
18. Create a longitudinal arteriotomy measuring 2.5–3 cm.
    - *Alternative: Transect the aorta 2–3 cm below the infrarenal clamp.*
    - *Oversew the distal aortic end using a 3-0 prolene running suture.*
19. Construct the proximal anastomosis and check for hemostasis.
20. Pass the right limb into the right tunnel.
21. Cross-clamp the common femoral, superficial femoral, and profunda femoris arteries.
22. Create a longitudinal arteriotomy in the common femoral artery.
    - *Alternative: Extend the arteriotomy into the profunda femoris with possible endarterectomy.*
23. Construct the right distal anastomosis and check for hemostasis.
24. Back-bleed the femoral bifurcation and forward-flush the graft.
25. Perfuse into the lower extremity.
26. Repeat the same on the left.
27. Check sigmoid viability.
28. Re-evaluate hemostasis.
29. Close the periaortic tissues.
    - *Alternative: Create omental flap for graft coverage.*
30. Close the abdomen.
31. Recheck distal pulses.

NOTE THESE VARIATIONS

- The femoral arteries may be exposed first, followed by the aorta, or vice versa.
- The proximal control is typically carried at the infrarenal level. If the aortic disease precludes infrarenal clamping,

the aorta can be controlled at the suprarenal or supraceliac level.

- The proximal anastomosis can be performed in an end-to-end or end-to-side fashion depending on the best means to preserve pelvic perfusion and the quality of the aorta at the infrarenal level.
- In severely calcified vessels, limited endarterectomy may be necessary to conduct the proximal or distal anastomoses.
- The periaortic tissue may not be adequate to cover the graft, necessitating coverage with an omental flap.

COMPLICATIONS

- Bleeding.
- Myocardial infarction.
- Pneumonia.
- Renal failure.
- Wound infection.
- Wound dehiscence.
- Limb ischemia.
- Trash foot.
- Bowel ischemia.
- Buttock ischemia.
- Spinal cord ischemia.
- Ureteral injury.
- Graft occlusion.
- Anastomotic false aneurism.
- Impotence.
- Aortoenteric fistula.
- Graft infection.

TEMPLATE OPERATIVE DICTATION

Preoperative diagnosis: Aortoiliac occlusive disease.
Procedure: (1) Aortobifemoral bypass with *20×10/18×9/16×8 PTFE/Dacron* graft; (2) endarterectomy of the right common femoral and profunda femoris arteries.
Postoperative diagnosis: Same.
Indications: This is a ___-year-old *male/female* with *disabling claudication/ischemic rest pain/nonhealing ulcers/foot gangrene.* Evaluation revealed aortoiliac occlusive disease. The risks and benefits of the surgical options were discussed with the patient and *he/she* elected to proceed with surgical intervention.
Description of procedure: The patient was placed supine on the operating table. The arms were *tucked in/placed at 80°.* Normal bony prominences were padded. Anesthesia placed appropriate

lines and induced and intubated the patient without complications. A Foley catheter was then placed under sterile technique. A nasogastric tube was inserted in the stomach and placed under aspiration. The patient's anterior abdomen and both lower extremities were circumferentially prepped and draped in the usual sterile fashion. Preoperative antibiotics were administered prior to skin incision.

1. Bilateral exposure of the femoral arteries

A vertical skin incision was started in the right groin midway between the pubic tubercle and the anterior superior iliac spine and extended for approximately 10–12 cm. The incision was deepened through the subcutaneous tissues with electrocautery. The encountered lymphatics were ligated and divided. The common femoral artery was then exposed and sharply dissected circumferentially. The dissection was extended proximally to the inguinal ligament and distally to include the superficial femoral and profunda femoris arteries. The common femoral, superficial femoral, and profunda femoris arteries were encircled with silastic vessel loops. Minor branches of the common femoral artery were identified and spared. The same was performed on the left side. The groin wounds were then packed bilaterally with antibiotic-soaked sponge.

2. Infrarenal aortic exposure

Attention was then focused on the abdominal part of the operation. A skin incision was made from the subxiphoid to the suprapubic region. The subcutaneous tissue was then divided with electrocautery. The linea alba was exposed and incised. The peritoneum was elevated and entered sharply. The abdominal wall incision was then extended to the full length of the skin incision.

There was *no/moderate amount* of adhesions requiring lysis.

Abdominal exploration revealed *no/the following incidental findings (detail)*.

The transverse colon was then elevated superiorly out of the wound, wrapped in a moist towel. A moist rolled lap pad was placed in the bed of the splenic flexure of the colon, which was retracted laterally and posteriorly. The remainder of the small bowel was then reflected to the right, exposing the infrarenal aorta. Sharp dissection of the ligament of Treitz and the distal fourth portion of the duodenum allowed further exposure of the aorta and retraction of the small bowel to the right. The small bowel was then wrapped in a moistened towel and held in place using the Omni retractor.

The retroperitoneum overlying the aorta was incised. The incision continued proximally to the level of the left renal vein. The inferior mesenteric vein was encountered, ligated, and divided. The lymphatics overlying the aortic neck were ligated and divided.

The infrarenal aorta was then sharply dissected for a 6-cm segment and appeared adequate for clamping.

[Choose one:]

If infrarenal aorta inadequate: The infrarenal aorta appeared to be inadequate for clamping and constructing the proximal anastomosis (in cases of complete infrarenal aortic occlusion or if the aorta was extremely calcified, not allowing an area of safe clamping). Thus, further mobilization of the left renal vein was performed. The left gonadal, lumbar, and adrenal veins were ligated and divided. The left renal vein was circumferentially mobilized and retracted proximally, exposing the renal arteries. The left and right renal arteries were identified at their origin from the aorta and encircled with silastic vessel loops. The suprarenal aorta was sharply dissected and appeared adequate for clamping.

If para/suprarenal aorta inadequate: The para/suprarenal aorta was felt to be inadequate for clamping; the supraceliac aorta was exposed and dissected. This was performed by incising the lesser omentum, mobilizing the esophagogastric junction to the left and dividing the right crus of the diaphragm.

The dissection was then carried distally toward the aortic bifurcation. A tunnel from each common femoral artery to the aortic bifurcation was then created bluntly with the index fingers staying posterior to the ureters.

3. Heparinization

The patient was given heparin 75–100 U/kg and mannitol 12.5 g intravenously. After 5 min from the heparin administration, the proximal vascular clamp was applied on the *aorta below the renal arteries/suprarenal aorta* after controlling the renal arteries with *Yasargil clamp/Bulldog clamp/supraceliac aorta*. The distal vascular clamp was applied on the aorta at the level of the inferior mesenteric artery.

4. Proximal anastomosis

A longitudinal arteriotomy in the anterior wall of the aorta was created measuring 2.5–3 cm.

Alternative: The aorta was transected 2–3 cm below the level of the renal arteries. The distal aortic end was oversewn with 3-0 prolene sutures; a localized endarterectomy of the proximal stump was performed.

The aortic lumen was irrigated with heparinized saline solution and all debris was removed.

A *20 × 10/18 × 9/16 × 8 Dacron/PTFE* graft was then soaked in antibiotic solution. The body of the graft was trimmed and tailored for the proximal anastomosis. The anastomosis was constructed in a running fashion using 3-0 prolene sutures. At the completion of the suture line, the sutures were tied and the anastomosis checked for hemostasis. Hemostasis was *adequate/except for a suture line bleeding controlled with an interrupted mattress suture/needle hole bleeding controlled with the topical application of Gelfoam soaked with thrombin.*

5. Distal anastomosis

Attention was focused on the femoral anastomoses. The right limb of the graft was then passed in the preformed tunnel posterior to the ureter, maintaining alignment and avoiding any kinks. The common femoral, superficial femoral, and profunda femoris arteries were cross-clamped.

A longitudinal arteriotomy in the anterior wall of the common femoral artery was created.

(Alternative: Extend arteriotomy into the profunda femoris with possible endarterectomy.)

The right limb of the graft was then sized and cut. The anastomosis was then performed with 5-0 prolene running sutures. Prior to completing the anastomosis the distal clamps were released, allowing for back-bleeding of the superficial and profunda femoris arteries. The aortic clamp was released for forward-flushing of the graft. The anastomosis was copiously irrigated with heparinized saline solution. The clamps were then released, allowing flow into the profunda femoris artery first, followed by the superficial femoral artery. There were strong Doppler signals in the right superficial femoral and profunda femoris arteries.

Attention was then focused on the left femoral anastomosis. The left limb of the graft was passed in the preformed tunnel anterior to the left common iliac artery and posterior to the ureter. The left common femoral, superficial femoral, and profunda femoris arteries were cross-clamped. A longitudinal arteriotomy in the anterior wall of the left common femoral artery was created and extended into the profunda femoris artery. *The atherosclerotic plaque was extensive and an endarterectomy was deemed necessary. Using a Freer elevator, the plaque in the common femoral artery was elevated and circumferentially dissected. The plaque was transected proximally and elevated. The plaque was feathered at the distal end in the profunda femoris artery.*

The left graft limb was then sized and cut. The left femoral anastomosis was then constructed into the profunda femoris artery with 5-0 prolene running sutures. Prior to completing the anastomosis, the graft limb was forward-flushed, the femoral bifurcation back-bled, and the anastomosis copiously irrigated with heparin saline solution. The anastomosis was then completed and blood flow resumed into the left profunda femoris artery. The left profunda femoris artery had a strong pulse distal to the anastomosis with a strong Doppler signal.

Reinspection of all the suture lines was performed and revealed adequate hemostasis.

The field was then irrigated with antibiotic solution.

The periaortic soft tissues were then sutured over the aortic graft using 3-0 Vicryl sutures.

The periaortic tissue was inadequate to cover the aortic graft and an omental flap was deemed necessary. A tongue of omentum based on the left omental artery was created. The flap was allowed to gently fold over the transverse colon mesentery and was placed over the aortic prosthesis. The flap was then secured in place with a running 3-0 silk suture.

The bowel was then placed back in the anatomic position.

Abdominal wall closure was then performed with *running/ interrupted* 0 prolene sutures.

The groin wounds were then re-evaluated, ensuring adequate hemostasis. The soft tissues in the groin were then closed over the graft limbs in two layers of 3-0 Vicryl. A redon drain was left in each groin wounds .The skin edges were opposed with skin staples.

The peri-incisional prep and drape were cleaned and dried, followed by 4×4 gauze, silk tape.

The feet were inspected and appeared well perfused. There were good Doppler signals in the pedal vessels bilaterally.

The patient tolerated the procedure well and was taken to the postanesthesia care unit in stable condition.

NOTES

Chapter 162
Retroperitoneal Aortofemoral Bypass

Kelly S.A. Blair, M.D. and Hisham Bassiouny, M.D.

INDICATIONS

- Symptomatic (disabling claudication, rest pain, ulceration, gangrene, or limb salvage) aortic/aortoiliac occlusive disease.
- "Shaggy" aorta with recurrent distal embolization.

ESSENTIAL STEPS

1. The patient is positioned with the shoulders at a 45° angle toward the patient's right side and the pelvis as flat as possible.
2. Perform a left flank incision extending from two finger breadths below the umbilicus to the tip of the twelfth rib.
3. Divide the external and internal oblique and transverse abdominus muscles.
4. Separate and mobilize the peritoneum to the costal cartilage and to the anterior iliac spine.
5. Retract the peritoneum to the right.
6. Identify the iliopsoas muscle and ureter.
7. Develop a plane between the colon anteriorly and the ureter posteriorly.
8. Mobilize the colon to the right, keeping the left kidney and ureter posteriorly.
9. Identify the left renal vein and the level of the infrarenal aorta.

J.J. Hoballah and C.E.H. Scott-Conner (eds.), *Operative Dictations in General and Vascular Surgery*, DOI 10.1007/978-1-4614-0451-4_162,
© Springer Science+Business Media, LLC 2012

10. Dissect the infrarenal aorta to the level of the aortic bifurcation.
11. Encircle the proximal aorta with an umbilical tape.
12. Perform linear vertical groin incision overlying each common femoral artery.
13. Dissect the common femoral, superficial femoral, and profunda femoris arteries.
14. Create a retroperitoneal tunnel from the aortic bifurcation, over the iliac artery, and beneath each ureter, extending into the groin incision.
15. Pass an umbilical tape through each retroperitoneal tunnel.
16. Administer 100 U/kg of intravenous heparin.
17. Create the proximal anastomosis (end-to-side vs. end-to-end).
18. Pass each graft limb through the retroperitoneal tunnel.
19. Clamp the femoral arteries on one side and create the femoral anastomosis.
20. Repeat the same on the opposite side.
21. Reassess all anastomoses for hemostasis.
22. Close abdominal and groin incisions with surgical staples. Each groin wound was closed in two layers with *running/ continuous* 2-0 Vicryl. The skin was reapproximated.

NOTE THESE VARIATIONS

- The plane of the retroperitoneal dissection may be anterior to the kidney as described above or posterior to the kidney. In the latter situation, the kidney is mobilized and retracted anteriorly. The lumbar vein will serve to identify the level of the left renal vein.
- The proximal (aortic) anastomosis may be performed using an end-to-end or end-to-side configuration.

COMPLICATIONS

- Graft infection.
- Ureter injury.
- Graft-enteric fistula.
- Bleeding.
- Distal embolization.
- Renal failure.
- Mesenteric failure.
- Myocardial infarction.

TEMPLATE OPERATIVE DICTATION

Preoperative diagnosis: Aortoiliac occlusive disease.

Procedure: Retroperitoneal aortofemoral bypass.

Postoperative diagnosis: Same.

Indications: This is a ___-year-old *male/female* with *disabling claudication/ischemic rest pain/nonhealing ulcers/foot gangrene.* Evaluation revealed aortoiliac occlusive disease. The risks and benefits of the surgical options were discussed with the patient and *he/she* elected to proceed with surgical intervention.

Description of procedure: The patient was placed in the supine position on a beanbag. The patient was connected to general anesthesia monitoring equipment and induced with general endotracheal anesthesia. An arterial line and pulmonary artery catheter were placed. A Foley catheter was placed.

The patient was then repositioned with the shoulders at a 45° angle toward *his/her* right side. The left arm was supported on a sling anteriorly and superiorly. The pelvis was as flat as possible.

A skin incision was performed in the left flank extending from two finger breadths below the umbilicus to the tip of the twelfth rib. The external and internal oblique muscles were divided with electrocautery. The left rectus muscle was divided with electrocautery. The transversus abdominus muscle fibers were split. The peritoneum, which lies directly below the transversus abdominus muscle, was separated from the muscle laterally and from the posterior rectus sheath medially with a moist gauze. The peritoneum was mobilized superiorly to the costal cartilage and inferiorly to the anterior iliac spine.

The peritoneum was retracted to the right until the iliopsoas muscle and ureter were visualized. The plane between the colon anteriorly and the ureter posteriorly were developed. The colon was mobilized to the right. The left kidney and ureter remained posteriorly. The left renal vein was visualized as it crosses the aorta, thus identifying the level of the infrarenal aorta. An Omni retractor was utilized for exposure.

The infrarenal aorta was dissected from surrounding tissue, with Metzenbaum scissors, down to the level of the aortic bifurcation. The proximal aorta was encircled with umbilical tape for proximal control.

A linear vertical groin was performed overlying each common femoral artery with a scalpel. This incision was taken down through the subcutaneous tissue and the femoral sheath with electrocautery. The common femoral, superficial femoral, and profunda femoris arteries were identified and dissected from surrounding tissue. Proximal distal control was obtained with vessel loops.

A retroperitoneal tunnel was created by blunt finger dissection from the aortic bifurcation, over the iliac artery, extending into the groin incision. Care was taken to create the tunnel beneath each ureter. An umbilical tape was passed through each retroperitoneal tunnel.

The patient was heparinized with 100 U/kg of intravenous heparin. After the appropriately sized bifurcated graft was obtained, it was pulled through the retroperitoneal tunnels to the groin incisions. Care was taken to ensure that no twisting of the grafts occurred.

An aortic clamp was placed on the encircled infrarenal aorta proximally. A second aortic clamp *or bilateral proximal common iliac artery clamps were placed distally*. A small Bulldog clamp was placed on the inferior mesenteric artery (IMA), which was removed after the anastomosis was completed.

A linear aortotomy was performed with a scalpel above the level of the IMA and below the level of the renal arteries. The arteriotomy was enlarged with Pott's scissors or curved Metzenbaum scissors. Any loose debris or thrombus was removed from the aorta.

Posterior bleeding lumbar arteries were clipped retroperitoneally with stainless steel surgical clip (or excluded by oversewing from within the aorta with a simple interrupted suture).

A *20 × 10/18 × 9/16 × 8/14 × 7 polyester/PTFE* graft was used. The proximal bifurcated graft was beveled and an end-to-side anastomosis was performed with a *running/continuous* 3-0 monofilament nonabsorbable suture, beginning at the inferior heel of the graft. The running suture was carried up each side of the arteriotomy and completed in the middle of the arteriotomy on the operator's side. Prior to completion of the anastomosis, the aorta was forward- and back-bled. The aorta was then flushed with heparinized saline. The anastomosis was completed and checked for hemostasis.

Fogarty graft clamps were placed on each limb of the bifurcated graft. Aortic clamps were slowly removed in the usual sequence to prevent hypotension and distal embolization. The IMA clamp was removed. Blood was flushed through one limb of the graft; then, each limb was flushed with heparinized saline and reclamped. All excess graft was pulled through the retroperitoneal tunnels.

In each groin, vascular clamps were placed on the common femoral, superficial femoral, and profunda femoris arteries. A linear arteriotomy was performed with a scalpel and enlarged with Pott's scissors. Each limb of the graft was cut to the appropriate length and then beveled in the usual manner. Each limb of the graft was anastomosed to the femoral artery with a 5-0 monofilament nonabsorbable in a *continuous/running* manner as previously described. Prior to completion of the anastomosis, all vessels were back-bled and flushed with heparinized saline. The anastomosis was completed. The anesthesiologist was informed of impending revascularization of each limb *so that bicarbonate and extra intravenous fluids could be administered for acid washout and to prevent hypotension.* Clamps were removed from the graft limbs and the vessels in the usual sequence to prevent distal embolization.

Hemostasis of all anastomoses was assured. Distal vessels were examined by both palpation and Doppler exam and then documented. Capillary refill of each foot was examined and assured. Evaluation of distal embolization was noted if present.

Incisions were copiously irrigated. All instruments, lap pads, and retractors were removed. The abdominal incision was closed in layers with *running/continuous* 1-0 maxon. The skin was reapproximated with surgical staples. Each groin wound was closed in two layers with *running/continuous* 2-0 Vicryl. The skin was reapproximated with surgical staples. Sterile dressings were placed.

There were no complications.

The patient awoke in the operating room, was extubated, and was taken to the *postanesthesia care unit/intensive care unit* in hemodynamically stable condition with excellent *pedal signals/pulses.*

NOTES

Chapter 163
Axillobifemoral Bypass

Kelly S.A. Blair, M.D. and Hisham Bassiouny, M.D.

INDICATIONS
- Disabling claudication.
- Ischemic rest pain.
- Nonhealing ulcers.
- Foot gangrene.
- Aortic graft infection.

ESSENTIAL STEPS
1. Infraclavicular incision.
2. Incise the pectoralis muscle fascia and spread the muscle along its fibers.
3. *May divide partially or completely the pectoralis minor close to its insertion.*
4. Identify the axillary vessels.
5. Mobilize the axillary vein and identify the axillary artery.
6. Circumferentially dissect the first portion of the axillary artery.
7. Bilateral groin incisions.
8. Expose the right common femoral, superficial femoral, and profunda femoris arteries and prepare them for clamping.
9. Expose the left common femoral, superficial femoral, and profunda femoris arteries and prepare them for clamping.
10. Create a tunnel from the right common femoral artery to the axillary artery along the midaxillary line starting

J.J. Hoballah and C.E.H. Scott-Conner (eds.), *Operative Dictations in General and Vascular Surgery*, DOI 10.1007/978-1-4614-0451-4_163,
© Springer Science+Business Media, LLC 2012

subcutaneously in the groin and continuing on the chest wall posterior to the pectoralis major.

11. Create a subcutaneous tunnel between both groins.
12. Anticoagulate with heparin 75–100 U/kg and wait 5 min.
13. Proximal and distal control of the axillary artery.
14. Create a 1-cm arteriotomy in the axillary artery.
15. Construct the proximal anastomosis and check for hemostasis.
16. Pass the graft in the axillary tunnel.
17. Cross-clamp the common femoral, superficial femoral, and profunda femoris arteries.
18. Create a longitudinal arteriotomy in the common femoral artery.
    - *Alternative: Extend the arteriotomy into the profunda femoris with possible endarterectomy.*
19. Construct the right distal anastomosis and check for hemostasis.
20. Create a 1- to 1.2-cm incision in the hood of the *femoral anastomosis/(or a more proximal area in the axillofemoral graft).*
21. Construct an end-to-side anastomosis with the femorofemoral bypass.
22. Back-bleed femoral bifurcation and forward-flush the graft.
23. Perfuse into the lower extremity.
24. Pass the femorofemoral graft in its tunnel.
25. Repeat the same on the left.
26. Re-evaluate hemostasis.
27. Close the incision.

NOTE THESE VARIATIONS

- The femoral arteries may be exposed first, followed by the axillary artery, or vice versa, or simultaneously using a double-team approach. In the presence of groin infection the femoral artery can be exposed through an incision lateral to the sartorius muscle.
- Numerous variations are possible for the femoral anastomoses of the axillofemoral and femorofemoral graft. The proximal anastomosis of the femorofemoral bypass can be performed in the hood of the femoral anastomosis of the axillofemoral bypass or in a more proximal segment of the axillofemoral bypass. Another alternative is to connect the femorofemoral graft directly to the femoral artery and then connect the axillofemoral artery to the hood of the femoral anastomosis of the femorofemoral graft.

COMPLICATIONS

- Bleeding.
- Wound infection.
- Wound dehiscence.
- Limb ischemia.
- Graft thrombosis.

TEMPLATE OPERATIVE DICTATION

Preoperative diagnosis: Bilateral aortoiliac occlusive disease.

Procedure: Axillobifemoral bypass: Right axillobifemoral artery bypass with distal anastomoses to the profunda femoris bilaterally, using 8-mm ringed PTFE graft.

Postoperative diagnosis: Same.

Indications: This is a ___-year-old *male/female* with *disabling claudication/ischemic rest pain/nonhealing ulcers/foot gangrene*. Evaluation revealed aortoiliac occlusive disease. The patient had significant medical comorbidities. The risks and benefits of the surgical options were discussed with the patient and *he/she* elected to proceed with surgical intervention.

Description of procedure: The patient was placed in the supine position. The procedure was performed under general anesthesia. The patient's right shoulder, chest, groin, and lower extremities were prepped and draped in the usual sterile fashion. A 10- to 12-cm transverse incision a finger breadth inferior and parallel to the right clavicle was performed and deepened through the subcutaneous tissues. The pectoralis major fascia was identified and incised. The incision was deepened through the pectoralis major bluntly by separating the muscle along its fibers. The underlying pectoral fat was incised, exposing the axillary vessels. A short segment of the axillary vein was mobilized and its tributaries were ligated and divided to expose the axillary artery. The first portion of the axillary artery just medial to the pectoralis minor was identified and encircled with a silastic vessel loop. A 3- to 4-cm segment of the axillary artery was circumferentially dissected. *The pectoralis minor muscle was partially/completely divided close to its insertion to facilitate the exposure.*

A vertical skin incision was then performed overlying the right common femoral artery. The incision was deepened through the subcutaneous tissue. Encountered venous and lymphatic tributaries were ligated and divided. The common femoral, superficial femoral, and profunda femoris arteries were dissected. The same was performed on the opposite side. A tunnel from the right groin to the infraclavicular incision along the anterior axillary line was made. This tunnel was subcutaneous except for its upper part, where it coursed posterior to the pectoralis major and anterior to the chest wall. A subcutaneous tunnel was then performed between the two groin incisions. Intravenous heparin at 75 U/kg was then administered. An 8-mm ringed PTFE graft was then passed through the axillary tunnel. Vascular clamps were applied on the axillary artery and a 1-cm arteriotomy was created. The end of the PTFE graft was spatulated to match the arteriotomy. An end-to-side anastomosis was then constructed with a 5-0 prolene suture. At the completion of the anastomosis, forward-flushing and back-bleeding of the axillary artery were performed. The anastomosis was checked for hemostasis, which was adequate.

Attention was then directed to the right groin. The common femoral, superficial femoral, and profunda femoral arteries were controlled. A 1- to 1.5-cm arteriotomy was started in the common femoral and extended into the *profunda femoris/superficial femoral artery*. The distal end of the graft was measured to appropriate length and transected obliquely to match the arteriotomy. An end-to-side anastomosis was then performed between the PTFE graft and the arteriotomy using 5-0 prolene sutures. A 1-cm arteriotomy was then performed in the hood of the femoral anastomosis. Another 8-mm ringed PTFE graft was then used to construct the femorofemoral bypass. The end of the graft was spatulated and then sutured with *5-0/6-0* prolene to the incision in the axillofemoral graft. At the completion of the anastomosis, the graft was forward-flushed and the femoral vessels were allowed to back-bleed. The anastomosis was irrigated with heparinized saline and the sutures were tied. The suture lines were then inspected for hemostasis, which was adequate except for needle hole bleeding controlled by Gelfoam soaked with thrombin. The femorofemoral graft was then passed in its tunnel. The left common femoral, superficial femoral, and profunda femoral arteries were controlled. A 1- to 1.5-cm arteriotomy was started in the common femoral and extended into the *profunda femoris/superficial femoral artery*. The distal end of the graft was measured to appropriate length and transected obliquely to match the arteriotomy. An end-to-side anastomosis was then performed between the PTFE graft and the arteriotomy using 5-0 prolene sutures. At the completion of the anastomosis, the graft was forward-flushed and the femoral vessels were allowed to back-bleed. The anastomosis was irrigated with heparinized saline and the sutures were tied. The suture lines were then inspected for hemostasis, which was adequate.

The patient had good continuous Doppler signals in both profunda femoris arteries as well as the pedal vessels. All the wounds were irrigated with antibiotic solution. Hemostasis was secured. In the right subclavicular incision, the subcutaneous layers were reapproximated with a running 3-0 Vicryl suture and the skin was closed with staples. The investing femoral fascia and the subcutaneous layers were closed with running 3-0 Vicryl sutures and the skin was closed with staples. Dressings were applied.

The patient tolerated the procedure well and was awakened in the operating room and taken to the postanesthesia care unit in stable condition.

Chapter 164
Iliofemoral Bypass

Munier M.S. Nazzal, M.D.

INDICATIONS
- Disabling claudication.
- Ischemic rest pain.
- Nonhealing ulcers.
- Foot gangrene with unilateral iliac occlusive disease, in the presence of normal or near-normal aorta and proximal common iliac artery.

ESSENTIAL STEPS
1. Incise the skin and subcutaneous tissue to expose the common femoral, superficial femoral, and profunda femoris arteries.
2. Incise the skin and external oblique muscle over the lower quadrant of the abdomen.
3. Divide the internal oblique and transverse muscles.
4. Develop retroperitoneal space and expose the iliac vessels to the bifurcation.
5. Develop a tunnel between the common iliac artery and common femoral artery.
6. Anticoagulate with heparin.
7. Pass synthetic graft, 8 mm.
8. Perform proximal anastomosis.
9. Perform distal anastomosis.
10. Assess the retroperitoneum and groin for bleeding.
11. Close both wounds.

J.J. Hoballah and C.E.H. Scott-Conner (eds.), *Operative Dictations in General and Vascular Surgery*, DOI 10.1007/978-1-4614-0451-4_164,

NOTE THESE VARIATIONS

- May start with the iliac exposure, followed by the femoral exposure, or vice versa.
- The proximal (iliac anastomosis) may be performed using an end-to-side or end-to-end configuration depending on the status of the artery and the need to maintain hypogastric flow.

COMPLICATIONS

- Retroperitoneal hematoma.
- Distal embolization.
- Thrombosis.
- Wound infection.

TEMPLATE OPERATIVE DICTATION

Preoperative diagnosis: *Right/left* leg claudication with iliac artery occlusion.

Procedure: *Right/left* iliofemoral bypass with PTFE/Dacron 8-mm graft.

Postoperative diagnosis: Same.

Indications: This is a ___-year-old *male/female* presenting with claudication. Evaluation *(angiography/MRA/___)* revealed occlusion of the *right/left* iliac arteries with reconstitution of the *common femoral/profunda/superficial femoral artery*.

Description of procedure: The patient was placed in a supine position. The procedure was performed under *general/epidural/spinal* anesthesia. The abdomen, both groins, and lower extremities were prepped and draped.

A vertical skin incision was made over the *right/left* groin. The subcutaneous tissues were incised and encountered lymphatics were ligated and divided. The common femoral, superficial femoral, and profunda femoral arteries were dissected and isolated with silastic vessel loops.

A curvilinear incision was made in the *right/left* lower quadrant of the abdomen. The external oblique aponeurosis was incised in the direction of its fibers. The tendinous part of the internal oblique muscle and transversus abdominis muscle were incised.

The retroperitoneum was exposed and retracted with the assistance of a self-retaining retractor.

The proximal common iliac artery was dissected and encircled with silastic tapes. A 1-in. segment of the artery was cleared of the surrounding tissue.

A tunnel was constructed deep to the inguinal ligament between the retroperitoneal space and the groin incision.

An 8-mm *PTFE/Dacron* graft was tunneled between the incisions.

Intravenous heparin 70–100 U/kg was administered to the patient and after 3–5 min a vascular clamp was applied to each end of the dissected segment of the common iliac artery.

A 1.0–1.5 cm arteriotomy was created in the common iliac artery. An anastomosis was constructed between the end of the graft and the side of the common iliac artery using *4-0/5-0* prolene.

A clamp was applied to the graft, followed by removal of the common iliac artery clamps.

Clamps were applied to the common femoral, profunda femoris, and superficial femoral arteries.

A longitudinal arteriotomy was made in the common femoral artery and*/extended into the/profunda femoris/superficial femoral artery.*

An anastomosis was constructed between the end of the graft and the side of the common femoral artery using 5-0 prolene.

Before completing the anastomosis, the lumen was flushed with heparinized saline and forward-bleeding and back-bleeding were allowed from all arteries.

The anastomosis was completed and blood was allowed to flow in the graft and the distal vessels.

Blood flow in the superficial femoral and profunda femoris arteries was checked by both palpation and Doppler probe.

Hemostasis was secured in both wounds.

The retroperitoneal wound was closed in layers, the first layer using Vicryl-0 to close the transverse and internal oblique muscles in *interrupted/continuous* fashion. The second layer used Vicryl-0 to close the *external oblique muscle/aponeurosis* in *interrupted/continuous* fashion.

The skin was closed with staples. The groin was closed in three layers: The first layer with 3-0 Vicryl for the fascia, the second layer with 3-0 Vicryl for the subcutaneous tissue, and the skin with staples. Dressings were applied.

Pulse and Doppler flow were checked in the arteries distally.

The patient tolerated the procedure well and was awakened and taken to the postanesthesia care unit in stable condition.

NOTES

Chapter 165
Femorofemoral Bypass

Munier M.S. Nazzal, M.D.

INDICATIONS

- Ischemia of the lower extremity.
- Disabling claudication.
- Ischemic rest pain.
- Nonhealing ulcers.
- Foot gangrene with unilateral stenotic/obstructive lesion of the iliac artery not amenable to endovascular procedures.
- Occlusion of a limb of an aortobifemoral bypass that could not be opened by thrombectomy or thrombolysis.

ESSENTIAL STEPS

1. Incision of the skin over both groins.
2. Dissection of the common femoral, superficial femoral, and profunda femoris arteries bilaterally.
3. Creation of a tunnel between both groin incisions.
4. Passing a PTFE graft (preferably reinforced with rings) in the tunnel.
5. Anticoagulate with heparin.
6. Clamping of the common, profunda, and superficial femoral arteries.
7. Arteriotomy in the donor common femoral artery made obliquely toward the profunda femoris artery.
8. Performance of the anastomosis in the donor femoral artery.

J.J. Hoballah and C.E.H. Scott-Conner (eds.), *Operative Dictations in General and Vascular Surgery*, DOI 10.1007/978-1-4614-0451-4_165,
© Springer Science+Business Media, LLC 2012

9. Back-bleeding of the profunda and superficial femoral arteries bilaterally.
10. Repeat the same on the opposite limb.
11. Femoral endarterectomy and profundoplasty may be necessary.
12. Resume flow to the lower extremity.
13. Secure hemostasis.
14. Close the wound.

NOTE THESE VARIATIONS

- The femorofemoral bypass is usually constructed using a C configuration. In the presence of severe calcifications in the donor femoral artery, a lazy S configuration may be used. In this configuration, the proximal anastomosis is performed as proximal as possible after starting at the junction with the external iliac artery. Alternatively, a localized endarterectomy of the femoral artery may be necessary.

- In the presence of occlusive disease in the donor iliac vessel, an intraoperative angioplasty/stenting of the stenotic pathology can be combined with the femorofemoral bypass.

COMPLICATIONS

- Infections.
- Bleeding.
- Hematoma.
- Steal syndrome of the donor leg.

TEMPLATE OPERATIVE DICTATION

Preoperative diagnosis: Ischemia of the *right/left* lower extremity.
Procedure: Femorofemoral bypass with reinforced PTFE graft.
Postoperative diagnosis: Same.
Indications: This is a ___-year-old *male/female* who presents with ischemia of the *right/left* lower extremity. The patient was found to have occlusion of the *right/left* common iliac artery. The contralateral iliac artery and common femoral artery were normal without any evidence of stenosis.
Description of procedure: The patient was placed in a supine position. The procedure was performed under *general endotracheal/spinal/epidural/local* anesthesia. Both lower extremities were prepped and draped in a standard surgical fashion.

A vertical incision was made over the *right/left* femoral artery. Fascia and lymphatic tissue were bisected. The *common femoral/ superficial femoral/profunda femoris* arteries were dissected and isolated with silastic vessel loops.

A tunnel was created subcutaneously between both groin incisions. The *PTFE/ring-enforced PTFE/Dacron* graft was passed in the tunnel.

The patient was given 5,000 U of heparin intravenously. Five minutes after heparin administration, the common femoral, profunda femoris, and superficial femoral arteries were clamped on the donor side using vascular clamps.

An arteriotomy was performed in the common femoral artery obliquely toward the profunda femoris artery using a #11 blade scalpel and extended using Pott's scissors. The end of the graft was fashioned to fit the arteriotomy. An anastomosis was constructed between the end of the graft and the side of the femoral artery using 5-0 prolene in a continuous fashion. Before completing the anastomosis, the lumen was irrigated. An atraumatic vascular clamp was applied to the graft and the profunda femoris and superficial femoral arteries were allowed to back-bleed. The common femoral artery was allowed to forward-bleed. The anastomosis was completed and blood was allowed to flow into the donor leg.

The recipient femoral artery was prepped in the same fashion as the donor side. An arteriotomy was made in the common femoral artery *and extended toward the profunda femoris artery.* Anastomosis was constructed between the end of the graft and the side of the common femoral artery in a similar fashion. Blood was allowed to back-bleed from the profunda femoris and superficial femoral arteries and the graft was allowed to forward-bleed. The lumen was irrigated and the anastomosis was completed.

Blood flow in the superficial femoral and profunda femoris arteries was checked by both palpation and Doppler probe.

Hemostasis was secured in both groins.

Both groins were closed in three layers: The first layer with 3-0 Vicryl for closing the fascia, the second layer with 3-0 Vicryl for closing the subcutaneous tissue, and the skin with staples.

Pulse was checked in both donor and recipient legs postoperatively.

Dressing was applied to both groins.

The patient tolerated the procedure well, was awakened, the lower extremities were noted for the presence of pulsations by *Doppler/palpation*, and the patient was taken to the postanesthesia care unit in stable condition.

NOTES

Chapter 166
Iliac Artery Angioplasty and Stenting

F. Ezequiel Parodi, M.D. and Murray L. Shames, M.D.

INDICATION

- Short (<5 cm) stenosis or occlusion of the iliac artery with symptoms (claudication, rest pain, nonhealing ulcer, and gangrene).

ESSENTIAL STEPS

1. Percutaneous or open access of the common femoral artery on the affected side.
2. Control access with 5-French sheath.
3. Anticoagulate with IV heparin sulfate (5,000 U).
4. Place guide wires through the lesion into the abdominal aorta under fluoroscopic guidance.
5. Perform diagnostic aortogram with femoral runoff.
6. Measure gradient across the lesion (optional).
7. Measure length and degree of the stenotic lesion using DSA.
8. Dilate with appropriately sized balloon.
9. Deploy stent across the lesion.
10. Remeasure gradient and completion angiogram to evaluate for residual stenosis and potential complications.

NOTE THESE VARIATIONS

- The sheath size will vary depending on the stent and balloon used.
- Predilation of the lesion may be performed.

J.J. Hoballah and C.E.H. Scott-Conner (eds.), *Operative Dictations in General and Vascular Surgery*, DOI 10.1007/978-1-4614-0451-4_166,
© Springer Science+Business Media, LLC 2012

COMPLICATIONS
- Artery dissection.
- Artery rupture with hemorrhage.
- Embolization.
- Thrombosis.

TEMPLATE OPERATIVE DICTATION

Preoperative diagnosis: Claudication (or other symptoms) secondary to iliac artery stenosis.

Procedure: Iliac angioplasty and stent placement.

Postoperative diagnosis: Same.

Indications: The patient is a ___-year-old *male/female* with lifestyle-limiting claudication (or other symptoms of peripheral arterial occlusive disease (PUD)) with diminished *right/left* femoral pulse. Preoperative duplex evaluation is consistent with *right/left* iliac stenosis. The patient has been informed of the risks and benefits of angiography and balloon angioplasty and stenting of the iliac vessels, and has agreed to the procedure.

Description of procedure: The patient was brought to the operating room and positioned on the operating table in the supine position. *Prophylactic antibiotics were administered by the anesthesiologist if required.* The *right/left* groin was shaved, prepped with povidone–iodine solution, and draped in the usual fashion. *Local/regional* anesthetic (*1% lidocaine/0.25% bupivacaine*) was infiltrated in the region of the common femoral artery. A small cut was made in the skin overlying the common femoral artery. The Seldinger needle was inserted into the common femoral artery and a guide wire advanced into the iliac artery under fluoroscopic guidance. A short 5–7-French sheath was then placed over the wire. An angiogram was performed through the sheath and the stenosis identified. The stenosis was then crossed with a *Glide/Bentson* guide wire and guiding catheters. An aortogram with runoff was performed. Using the images from the angiogram, the length and diameter of the stenotic iliac artery was measured. Intravenous heparin sulfate (5,000 U) was administered by the anesthesiologist. A ___-mm angioplasty balloon was then passed over the wire and centered across the lesion. The lesion was dilated while observing the vessel with fluoroscopy. An angiogram was performed through the femoral sheath; there was no evidence of dissection or vessel rupture. A ___-mm *self-expandable/balloon-expandable* stent was then placed over the wire and advanced across the lesion. The stent was deployed without difficulty. Angiography was performed with contrast and no residual stenosis, dissection, or thrombus was noted. All balloons, catheters, sheaths, and wires were then removed. Manual compression of the common femoral artery was performed for 10–15 min for hemostasis. A strong ipsilateral femoral pulse was noted at the completion of the procedure.

The patient tolerated the procedure well and was taken to the postanesthesia care unit in stable condition.

RADIOLOGY SUPERVISION AND INTERPRETATION

1. *Aortogram with runoff:* Patent distal aorta with high-grade stenosis of the common/external iliac artery on the right/left.
2. *Angiogram postangioplasty and stent:* Stent placed in right/left common/external iliac artery, brisk flow, no residual stenosis.

NOTES

Section **XVII**

Infrainguinal Occlusive Disease

Chapter 167

Femoropopliteal Bypass with PTFE Graft

Jamal J. Hoballah, M.D., M.B.A.

INDICATIONS
- Tissue loss.
- Gangrene.
- Rest pain.
- Disabling claudication.

ESSENTIAL STEPS
1. Expose the popliteal artery.
2. Expose the inflow femoral vessels.
3. Create graft tunnel.
4. Construct the proximal anastomosis.
5. Check for hemostasis.
6. Pass graft through tunnel.
7. Construct the distal anastomosis.
8. Completion angiogram.
9. Wound closure.
10. Pulses re-evaluation.

NOTE THESE VARIATIONS
- Endovascular treatment (angioplasty/stenting/recanalization) is often attempted as a first revascularization option.
- The graft can be tunneled in various ways, most commonly in a subsartorial tunnel to the above-knee popliteal level and then anatomic between the heads of the gastrocnemius muscle for the below-knee popliteal level.

J.J. Hoballah and C.E.H. Scott-Conner (eds.), *Operative Dictations in General and Vascular Surgery*, DOI 10.1007/978-1-4614-0451-4_167,
© Springer Science+Business Media, LLC 2012

COMPLICATIONS

- Bleeding.
- Gangrene.
- Thrombosis of graft.
- Infection.
- Myocardial infarction.

TEMPLATE OPERATIVE DICTATION

Preoperative diagnosis: Infrainguinal arterial occlusive disease with *right/left* leg *disabling claudication, right/left foot rest pain, right/left foot/toe ulcerations/gangrene.*

Procedure: *Right/left* common femoral artery to above-knee popliteal artery PTFE bypass; completion intraoperative arteriogram.

Postoperative diagnosis: Same.

Indications: The patient is a ___-year-old *male/female* with *right/left* leg disabling claudication, *right/left* foot rest pain, *right/left foot/toe ulcerations/gangrene.*

Preoperative evaluation revealed infrainguinal occlusive disease with reconstitution of the *suprageniculate/infrageniculate* popliteal artery with good tibial runoff. Endovascular revascularization was not deemed appropriate.

The risks and benefits of revascularization were explained to the patient and *he/she* elected to undergo surgical intervention.

Description of procedure: The patient was placed supine on the operating table. The arms were *tucked in/placed at 80°.* Normal bony prominences were padded. The anesthesia team placed appropriate lines and *regional/general* anesthesia was induced. A Foley catheter was placed under sterile technique. The patient's lower abdomen and both lower extremities were circumferentially prepped and draped in the usual sterile fashion. Preoperative antibiotics were administered prior to skin incision.

[Choose one:]

If above-knee popliteal artery: A 10- to 12-cm longitudinal skin incision was performed on the medial aspect of the thigh along the anticipated anterior border of the sartorius muscle. The skin incision was deepened through the subcutaneous tissue, exposing the adductor tendon anteriorly and the sartorius muscle posteriorly. The fascia between these two muscles was incised and the popliteal fossa entered. A self-retaining retractor was placed deeper in the wound and the popliteal artery was palpated and exposed. A 2-cm segment of the popliteal artery was sharply dissected. Attention was then directed to the groin.

If below-knee popliteal artery: A 10- to 12-cm longitudinal skin incision was performed 1–2 cm posteromedial and parallel to the tibia. The incision was deepened through the subcutaneous tissue, exposing the fascia. Attention was made to avoid injuring the great saphenous vein. The fascia was incised and the popliteal space was entered. A self-retaining retractor was applied, retracting the gastrocnemius muscle posteriorly and laterally. The tendons of the semimembranosus and semitendinosus muscles were divided to further facilitate the exposure. The popliteal vessels were identified. A 2-cm segment of the popliteal artery was sharply dissected. Attention was then directed to the groin.

A vertical curvilinear skin incision overlying the right common femoral artery pulse was made. The incision was deepened through the subcutaneous tissues with electrocautery. The encountered lymphatics were ligated and divided. The common femoral artery was then exposed and sharply dissected circumferentially. The dissection was extended proximally to the inguinal ligament and distally to include the superficial femoral and profunda femoris arteries. The common femoral, superficial femoral, and profunda femoris arteries were encircled with silastic vessel loops. Minor branches of the common femoral artery were identified and spared.

If above-knee popliteal bypass: A *subfascial/subsartorial* tunnel was then created using a *Zepplin/Kelly weck/Gortex tunneler.*

If below-knee popliteal bypass: A 5-cm longitudinal skin incision was performed on the medial aspect of the thigh along the anticipated anterior border of the sartorius muscle. The skin incision was deepened through the subcutaneous tissue, exposing the adductor tendon anteriorly and the sartorius muscle posteriorly. The fascia between these two muscles was incised and the above-knee popliteal fossa entered. The tunnel was created bluntly between the heads of the gastrocnemius muscle connecting the infrageniculate popliteal space with the suprageniculate popliteal space. A *subsartorial/subfascial tunnel* was then created between the suprageniculate popliteal space and the inguinal incision using a *Zepplin/Kelly weck/Gortex tunneler.*

The patient was given 5,000 U of heparin intravenously and after 5 min elapsed, the common femoral artery, profunda, and superficial femoral artery were clamped. A longitudinal arteriotomy in the common femoral artery was performed and extended with Pott's scissors for 1 cm. A PTFE graft 6/8 mm with rings was used and its end was fashioned to match the femoral arteriotomy. The proximal anastomosis was constructed between the PTFE graft and the femoral arteriotomy with a running *5-0/6-0 prolene/*

Gortex suture. Prior to completing the suture line, back-bleeding of the popliteal artery, forward-flushing of the graft, and irrigation of the anastomosis with heparinized solution were performed. The anastomosis was then completed and checked for hemostasis, which was *adequate/revealed needle hole bleeding. This was controlled with the application of Gelfoam soaked with thrombin.* The PTFE graft was then passed distended through the tunnel, avoiding any twists.

Atraumatic *vascular clamps/Bulldog clamps/Yasargil clips* were placed proximally and distally on the dissected popliteal artery. A 1-cm arteriotomy was then created in the anterior wall of the popliteal artery.

The PTFE graft was transected at the appropriate length. The transected end was incised along its posterior aspect, spatulating the vein. The distal anastomosis to the popliteal artery was constructed with a running *5-0/6-0* prolene suture. Prior to completing the suture line, back-bleeding, forward-flushing, and irrigation of the anastomosis with heparinized solution was performed. The anastomosis was then completed and checked for hemostasis, which was adequate. A 20-gauge angiocatheter was then introduced into the PTFE graft near the proximal anastomosis and an intraoperative arteriogram was performed. This revealed a widely patent anastomosis and no evidence of filling defects or kinks. The angiocatheter was removed and its puncture site repaired with a 6-0 prolene suture. The suture lines and the wounds were then rechecked for hemostasis. There was good *Doppler signal/palpable pulses* in the foot and a good augmentation of the signal with compressing and releasing the PTFE graft. The wounds were all irrigated with antibiotic solution. The subcutaneous tissue in the groin wound was closed in two layers of 3-0 Vicryl sutures. The fascia overlying the sartorius muscle was approximated with 3-0 Vicryl sutures. The skin was closed with staples.

The patient tolerated the procedure well and was transferred to the postanesthesia care unit in stable condition.

Chapter 168
Femoroinfrapopliteal PTFE Bypass with Adjunctive AVF or Vein Cuff

Sujata Subramanian, M.D., Keith D. Calligaro, M.D., and Matthew J. Dougherty, M.D.

INDICATION

- Limb-threatening ischemia (rest pain, ischemic ulcer, gangrene), in the presence of native autogenous vein.

ESSENTIAL STEPS

1. Incise the skin and enter the appropriate muscle plane for proximal and distal arterial anastomosis.
2. Identify the para-arterial veins and divide venous tributaries anterior to the artery.
3. Expose the appropriate arterial site for proximal arterial anastomosis.
4. Expose the appropriate arterial site for distal arterial anastomosis (less length required if tourniquet used; more if proximal and distal clamps or vessel loops).
5. Expose the adjacent tibial vein for construction of arteriovenous anastomosis or identify other venous segment (greater saphenous vein, etc.) for vein patch.
6. If necessary, make additional skin incisions and enter the appropriate tissue plane for tunneling graft.
7. Anticoagulate with heparin.
8. Clamp the inflow artery and perform proximal anastomosis with prosthetic graft.
9. Tunnel the graft to the distal anastomotic site.
10. Apply clamps (preferably small Bulldog clamps or vessel loops) to the outflow artery.

J.J. Hoballah and C.E.H. Scott-Conner (eds.), *Operative Dictations in General and Vascular Surgery*, DOI 10.1007/978-1-4614-0451-4_168,
© Springer Science+Business Media, LLC 2012

11. Incise the artery approximately 10 mm long.
12. *If arteriovenous fistula:*
    - *Ligate the distal vein and place vessel loop or small Bulldog clamp on the proximal vein, divide the vein distally and incise the ventral surface of the vein the same length as arteriotomy.*
        - *Suture the end of the vein to arteriotomy.*
        - Incise the hood of the vein and extend proximally approximately 10 mm long.
        - Suture the end of the graft onto the longitudinal venotomy.
    - *If vein patch/cuff:*
        - Excise appropriate length of adequate-diameter vein and fashion cuff/patch.
        - Suture vein cuff/patch onto arteriotomy.
        - Suture the end of the graft onto cuff/patch.
13. Remove clamps/vessel loops.
14. Completion arteriography.
15. Secure hemostasis.
16. Close wound.

NOTE THIS VARIATION

- Prosthetic grafts can be anastomosed to infrapopliteal vessels directly or with the addition of adjunctive procedures devised in an attempt to improve patency rates. These adjunctive procedures include the incorporation of a vein patch or cuff in the distal anastomosis or the creation of an arteriovenous fistula. A side-to-side arteriovenous fistula can be created at the site of the distal anastomosis and the prosthetic graft is sutured directly to the AV fistula. Alternatively, an end-to-side AV fistula can be created and the graft is sutured to the hood of the vein as described in this chapter. This technique will provide a combination of a vein patch and an AV fistula.

COMPLICATIONS

- Graft thrombosis.
- Amputation.
- Bleeding.
- Local nerve injury.
- Cardiac and pulmonary complications.

TEMPLATE OPERATIVE DICTATION

Preoperative diagnosis: *Right/left* foot ischemia.

Procedure: *Right/left common/superficial/deep femoral-to-anterior tibial/posterior tibial/peroneal artery* with PTFE graft and adjunctive *arteriovenous fistula/vein cuff/patch.*

Postoperative diagnosis: Same.

Indications: This ___-year-old *male/female* was found to have *rest pain/ischemic ulcer/gangrene.* Noninvasive arterial studies showed ___. *Arteriography/duplex/MRA* showed ___.

Description of procedure: The patient underwent *epidural/general* anesthesia and placement of a radial artery catheter. Intravenous antibiotics were administered within 30 min of the incision. The patient was placed in the supine position. The *right/left* leg was prepped and draped in the usual sterile fashion.

The skin was incised over the *common/superficial* femoral artery and the plane medial to the sartorius muscle was entered. The skin was incised over the *anterior tibial/posterior tibial/ peroneal artery* and the muscles were freed away. The para-arterial veins were identified and any venous tributaries anterior to the artery were divided.

The appropriate arterial site for proximal arterial anastomosis was exposed. The appropriate arterial site for distal arterial anastomosis was exposed. *An adjacent tibial vein was dissected free for construction of arteriovenous anastomosis/another venous segment (greater saphenous vein, etc.) was freed away for vein patch.*

Additional skin incisions were made (if necessary) and appropriate tissue planes were entered for tunneling graft. A *subcutaneous/subfascial/anatomic* tunnel was then created.

The patient was given heparin 100 U/kg intravenously and ACTs were followed and maintained >200 s.

Angled DeBakey clamps were applied proximally and distally to the inflow artery. An arteriotomy was made 15 mm long. The PTFE graft was sutured to the artery with a running 6-0 *prolene/ Gortex* suture. The graft was clamped proximally. The distal and then the proximal arterial clamps were removed.

There was good hemostasis after Surgicel was applied.

The graft was tunneled to the distal anastomotic site *through a Gortex tunneler subcutaneously/with a Kelly clamp anatomically. Small Bulldog clamps were applied proximally and distally to the outflow artery/(if extremely calcified artery) Esmarch bandage applied from the toes to the distal thigh; a tourniquet was inflated to 300 mmHg at the distal thigh and the bandage removed.* The distal artery was incised 10 mm longitudinally.

[Choose one:]

If arteriovenous fistula: The adjacent vein was ligated distally and a small Bulldog clamp was applied proximally. The vein was divided distally and the ventral surface of the vein was incised 10 mm longitudinally. The end of the vein was anastomosed to the artery with a running 6-0 prolene suture. The hood of the vein was incised longitudinally and extended proximally 10 mm. The end of the graft was sutured to the longitudinal venotomy with a running 6-0 prolene suture.

If vein patch/cuff: An appropriate length of adequate-diameter vein was excised and a *cuff/patch* was fashioned. The vein *cuff/patch* was sutured onto arteriotomy with a running 6-0 prolene suture. The end of the graft was sutured onto the vein *cuff/patch.*

The Bulldog clamps were removed from the proximal vein and artery, the clamp on the graft was removed, and *the distal Bulldog clamp on the artery was removed/the tourniquet was deflated.*

A completion arteriogram was performed by injecting 20 cc of dye through a butterfly needle inserted into the graft and performing fluoroscopy of the distal graft and outflow artery (and AVF). The needle was removed and the site oversewn with a 6-0 prolene suture.

There was good hemostasis after Surgicel was applied to the distal anastomosis.

The wounds were irrigated with antibiotic solution. The wounds were closed with a running 2-0 Vicryl suture in the fascia and the skin was closed with staples.

The wounds were dressed.

The patient tolerated the procedure well and was taken to the postanesthesia care unit in stable condition.

Chapter 169

Femoroposterior Tibial Bypass with Reversed Greater Saphenous Vein

Rabih Houbballah, M.D. and Jamal J. Hoballah, M.D., M.B.A.

INDICATIONS
- Tissue loss.
- Gangrene.
- Rest pain.
- Disabling claudication.

ESSENTIAL STEPS
1. Expose the target tibial vessel.
2. Expose the inflow femoral vessels.
3. Harvest the greater saphenous vein.
4. Create graft tunnel.
5. Heparinize the patient with one bolus of 50 units/kg.
6. Reverse the vein.
7. Construct the proximal anastomosis.
8. Check for hemostasis.
9. Mark the vein with methylene blue to avoid twist
10. Pass graft through the tunnel.
11. Check for twist and kink
12. Construct the distal anastomosis.
13. Completion angiogram.
14. Wound closure.
15. Pulses re-evaluation.

J.J. Hoballah and C.E.H. Scott-Conner (eds.), *Operative Dictations in General and Vascular Surgery*, DOI 10.1007/978-1-4614-0451-4_169,
© Springer Science+Business Media, LLC 2012

NOTE THESE VARIATIONS
- Grafts to the posterior tibial artery may be tunneled in various ways, including subcutaneous, subfascial, or anatomic tunnels.
- Control of the target vessels can be achieved in various ways, such as tourniquet, internal occluders, silastic vessel loops, vascular clamps, or Yasargil clips.

COMPLICATIONS
- Bleeding.
- Gangrene.
- Thrombosis of graft.
- Infection.
- Myocardial infarction.

TEMPLATE OPERATIVE DICTATION
Preoperative diagnosis: Infrainguinal arterial occlusive disease with, *right/left foot rest pain, right/left foot/toe ulcerations/gangrene.*
Procedure: *Right/left* common femoral artery to posterior tibial artery vein bypass with reversed right greater saphenous vein; completion intraoperative arteriogram.
Postoperative diagnosis: Same.
Indications: The patient is a ___-year-old *male/female* with *right/left foot rest pain, right/left foot/toe ulcerations/gangrene.*

Preoperative evaluation revealed infrainguinal occlusive disease with reconstitution of the posterior tibial artery in the *proximal/mid/distal* leg. Duplex mapping of the right leg revealed a good saphenous vein which was marked.

The risks and benefits of revascularization were explained to the patient and *he/she* elected to undergo surgical intervention.
Description of procedure: The patient was placed supine on the operating table. The arms were *tucked in/placed at 80°*. Normal bony prominences were padded. The anesthesia team placed appropriate lines and *regional/general* anesthesia was induced. A Foley catheter was placed under sterile technique. The patient's lower abdomen and both lower extremities were circumferentially prepped and draped in the usual sterile fashion. Preoperative antibiotics were administered prior to skin incision.

1. Exposure of the posterior tibial artery
A 10- to 12-cm vertical skin incision was performed on the medial aspect of the leg, 2 cm posteromedial and parallel to the tibia. The incision was located directly over the saphenous vein.

The skin incision was deepened through the subcutaneous tissue, the saphenous vein was carefully reflected posteriorly. The deep muscular fascia was incised, exposing the medial head of gastrocnemius muscle which is reclined posteriorly. The soleus muscle is then exposed and incised along its attachment down to its posterior deep fascia. This fascia was incised, exposing the posterior tibial and flexor muscles. Gentle dissection between these two muscles was performed and a self-retaining retractor was placed deeper in the wound, exposing the posterior tibial artery and veins. The artery is palpated to assess the feasibility of the distal anastomosis. A 2-cm segment of the posterior tibial artery was sharply dissected. Crossing venae comitantes were ligated and divided.

2. Exposure of the common femoral artery

A vertical curvilinear skin incision overlying the right common femoral artery was made extending down the upper medial thigh along the preoperatively mapped greater saphenous vein. The incision was deepened through the subcutaneous tissues with electrocautery. The encountered lymphatics were ligated and divided. The common femoral artery was then exposed and sharply dissected circumferentially. The dissection was extended proximally to the inguinal ligament and distally to include the superficial femoral and profunda femoris arteries. The common femoral, superficial femoral, and profunda femoris arteries were encircled with silastic vessel loops. Minor branches of the common femoral artery were identified and spared. The greater saphenous vein was then identified. The vein was exposed from the saphenofemoral junction to the *mid/lower* leg through one *continuous incision/multiple incisions separated by skin bridges*. Dextran–heparin–papaverin solution was infused into the saphenous vein through a blunt needle that was placed in a side branch in the most distal aspect of the vein. The saphenous vein was harvested and its tributaries ligated with *3-0/4-0* silk ties.

3. Creation of the tunnel

A tunnel was then created using a *Zepplin/Kelly weck/Gortex tunneler.*

The tunnel was subcutaneous parallel to the course of the saphenous vein to the level of the exposed posterior tibial artery.

The tunnel was subfascial along the medial aspect of the thigh and knee.

The tunnel was subfascial/subsartorial along the medial aspect of the thigh and then anatomic at the knee level passing between both heads of the gastrocnemius muscle. Below the knee the tunnel was posterior to the soleus muscle.

4. Anticoagulation

The patient was given 50 UI/Kg of heparin intravenously. The saphenous vein was transected at the saphenofemoral junction and its stump suture ligated with 2-0 silk sutures. The distal end was double ligated and transected.

5. Proximal anastomosis

The common femoral artery, profunda, and superficial femoral artery were clamped. A longitudinal arteriotomy in the common femoral artery was performed and extended with Pott's scissors for 1 cm. The vein was then reversed and its distal end was incised along its posterior wall/*incorporating a side branch, creating a T junction shape.* The proximal anastomosis was constructed between the spatulated vein and the femoral arteriotomy with a running 5-0/6-0 prolene suture. Prior to completing the suture line, back-bleeding, forward-flushing, and irrigation of the anastomosis with heparinized solution was performed. The anastomosis was then completed and checked for hemostasis, which was adequate. The flow through the vein was checked and was pulsatile. The end of the vein was ligated with a 2-0 silk tie. The vein was rechecked for hemostasis. The vein was marked with methylene blue and then passed distended through the tunnel, avoiding any twists.

6. Distal anastomosis

A tourniquet was placed above the knee and an Esmarch rubber bandage was applied to the foot and wrapped proximally to exsanguinate the leg. The tourniquet was then inflated to 350 mmHg.

[Choose one:]

*If **internal occluder:** A 1-cm arteriotomy was then created in the anterior wall of the posterior tibial artery. A 2.0/2.25/2.50-mm internal occluder (flowrestor) was introduced into the lumen to achieve proximal and distal control.*

*If **loops or clamps:** Proximal and distal control of the posterior tibial artery was then performed using vessel loops/vascular clamps/Bulldog clamp. A 1-cm arteriotomy was then created in the anterior wall of the posterior tibial artery.*

The vein was transected at the appropriate length and was incised along its posterior aspect, spatulating the vein. The distal anastomosis to the posterior tibial artery was constructed with a running 7-0 prolene suture. Prior to completing the suture line, back-bleeding, forward-flushing, and irrigation of the anastomosis with heparinized solution was performed. The anastomosis was then completed and checked for hemostasis, which was adequate.

7. Completion angiogram

A 20-gauge angiocatheter was then introduced into a side branch in the vein near the proximal anastomosis and an intraoperative arteriogram was performed. The angiogram revealed a widely patent anastomosis and no evidence of filling defects or kinks. The angiocatheter was removed and its puncture site repaired with a 6-0 prolene suture.

8. Closure

The suture lines and wounds were then rechecked for hemostasis. There was good Doppler signal in the foot at the posterior tibial artery level and a good augmentation of the signal with compressing and releasing the vein graft. The wounds were all irrigated with antibiotic solution and a redon's drain was left in each wound. The subcutaneous tissue in the groin wound was closed in two layers of 3-0 Vicryl sutures. The fascia overlying the distal part of the soleus muscle was approximated with 3-0 Vicryl sutures. The skin was closed with staples.

The patient tolerated the procedure well and was taken to the postanesthesia care unit in stable condition.

Chapter 170

Femoroanterior Tibial Bypass with Nonreversed Greater Saphenous Vein

Sung Woon Chung, M.D. and Jamal J. Hoballah, M.D., M.B.A.

INDICATIONS
- Tissue loss.
- Gangrene.
- Rest pain.
- Disabling claudication.

ESSENTIAL STEPS
1. Expose the target tibial vessel.
2. Expose the inflow femoral vessels.
3. Harvest the greater saphenous vein.
4. Create graft tunnel.
5. Construct the proximal anastomosis.
6. Incise the valves.
7. Check for hemostasis.
8. Pass graft through the tunnel.
9. Construct the distal anastomosis.
10. Completion angiogram.
11. Wound closure.
12. Pulse re-evaluation.

NOTE THESE VARIATIONS
- Tibial bypass are very rarely performed for intermittent claudication.
- Endovascular recanalization may be attempted first prior to creating a bypass.

J.J. Hoballah and C.E.H. Scott-Conner (eds.), *Operative Dictations in General and Vascular Surgery*, DOI 10.1007/978-1-4614-0451-4_170,
© Springer Science+Business Media, LLC 2012

- Grafts to the anterior tibial artery may be tunneled in various ways, including subcutaneous, subfascial, or anatomic tunnels. These grafts typically originate in the medial aspect of the groin. They cross to the lateral aspect of the extremity in the thigh or below the knee. Below the knee, they may cross anterior to the tibia subcutaneously or posterior to the tibia through the interosseous membrane.
- Control of the target vessels can be achieved in various ways, such as tourniquet, internal occluders, silastic vessel loops, vascular clamps, or Yasargil clips.
- Various valvulotomes may be used to incise the valves.

COMPLICATIONS
- Bleeding.
- Gangrene.
- Thrombosis of graft.
- Infection.
- Myocardial infarction.

TEMPLATE OPERATIVE DICTATION

Preoperative diagnosis: Infrainguinal arterial occlusive disease with *right/left leg disabling claudication, right/left foot rest pain, right/left foot/toe ulcerations/gangrene.*

Procedure: *Right/left* common femoral artery to anterior tibial artery vein bypass with nonreversed right greater saphenous vein; completion intraoperative arteriogram.

Postoperative diagnosis: Same.

Indications: The patient is a ___-year-old *male/female* with *right/left foot rest pain, right/left foot/toe ulcerations/gangrene.* Endovascular recanalization was not possible/deemed appropriate.

Preoperative evaluation revealed infrainguinal occlusive disease with reconstitution of the anterior tibial artery in the *proximal/mid/distal* leg.

The risks and benefits of revascularization were explained to the patient and *he/she* elected to undergo surgical intervention.

Description of procedure: The patient was placed supine on the operating table. The arms were *tucked in/placed at 80°.* Normal bony prominences were padded. The anesthesia team placed appropriate lines and *regional/general* anesthesia was induced. A Foley catheter was placed under sterile technique. The patient's lower abdomen and both lower extremities were circumferentially prepped and draped in the usual sterile fashion. Preoperative antibiotics were administered prior to skin incision.

A 10- to 12-cm vertical skin incision was performed 2 cm lateral and parallel to the tibia. The skin incision was deepened through the subcutaneous tissue until the fascia was identified. The fascia was incised, exposing the tibialis anterior and extensor hallucis muscles. Gentle blunt dissection between these two muscles was performed and a self-retaining retractor was placed deeper in the wound, exposing the anterior tibial artery and veins. A 2-cm segment of the anterior tibial artery was sharply dissected. Crossing venae comitantes were ligated and divided.

Attention was then directed to the groin. A *vertical/curvilinear* skin incision overlying the right common femoral artery was made extending down the upper medial thigh along the preoperatively mapped greater saphenous vein. The incision was deepened through the subcutaneous tissues with electrocautery. The encountered lymphatics were ligated and divided. The common femoral artery was then exposed and sharply dissected circumferentially. The dissection was extended proximally to the inguinal ligament and distally to include the superficial femoral and profunda femoris arteries. The common femoral, superficial femoral, and profunda femoris arteries were encircled with silastic vessel loops. Minor branches of the common femoral artery were identified and spared. The greater saphenous vein was then identified. The vein was exposed from the saphenofemoral junction to the *mid/lower* leg through *one continuous incision/multiple incisions separated by skin bridges.* Dextran–heparin–papaverin solution was infused into the saphenous vein through a blunt needle that was placed in a side branch in the most distal aspect of the vein. The saphenous vein was harvested and its tributaries ligated with 3-0/4-0 silk ties.

A tunnel was then created using a *Zepplin/Kelly weck/Gortex tunneler.*

The tunnel was subcutaneous, crossing from medial to lateral in the thigh and continuing laterally in the leg.

The tunnel was subcutaneous along the medial aspect of the thigh and knee and crossed from medial to lateral below the knee anterior to the tibia.

The tunnel was subcutaneous/subfascial along the medial aspect of the thigh and knee. Below the knee, the tunnel crossed from medial to lateral through the interosseous membrane.

The patient was given 5,000 U of heparin intravenously. A side-biting clamp was applied on the common femoral vein and the saphenous vein was transected, incorporating the saphenofemoral junction and a 1-mm rim of the femoral vein. The femoral venotomy was then closed with a running 5-0 prolene suture.

The saphenofemoral valve was then excised under direct vision using Pott's scissors. The common femoral artery, profunda, and superficial femoral artery were clamped. A longitudinal arteriotomy in the common femoral artery was performed and extended with Pott's scissors for 1 cm. The proximal anastomosis was constructed between the hood of the saphenofemoral junction and the femoral arteriotomy with a running 6-0 prolene suture. Prior to completing the suture line, back-bleeding, forward-flushing, and irrigation of the anastomosis with heparinized solution was performed. The anastomosis was then completed and checked for hemostasis, which was adequate. The remaining valves were then lysed using a retrograde valvulotome introduced through side branches and the distal end of the saphenous vein. The flow through the vein was checked and was pulsatile. The end of the vein was ligated with a 2-0 silk tie. The vein was rechecked for hemostasis. The vein was then passed through the tunnel, avoiding any twists.

A tourniquet was placed above the knee and an Esmarch rubber bandage was applied to the foot and wrapped proximally to exsanguinate the leg. On completion of this the tourniquet was inflated to 250–350 mmHg. A 1-cm arteriotomy was then created in the anterior wall of the anterior tibial artery.

[Choose one:]

If internal occluder: A 1-cm arteriotomy was then created in the anterior wall of the anterior tibial artery and a 2.0/2.25/2.50-mm internal occluder was introduced into the lumen.

If loops or clamps: Proximal and distal control of the anterior tibial artery was then performed using vessel loops/vascular clamps/ Bulldog clamps.

The vein was transected at the appropriate length. The transected end was incised along its posterior aspect, spatulating the vein. The distal anastomosis to the anterior tibial artery was constructed with a running 7-0 prolene suture. Prior to completing the suture line, back-bleeding, forward-flushing, and irrigation of the anastomosis with heparinized solution was performed. The anastomosis was then completed and checked for hemostasis, which was adequate.

A 20-gauge angiocatheter was then introduced into a side branch in the vein near the proximal anastomosis and an intraoperative arteriogram was performed. The angiogram revealed a patent anastomosis with no evidence of any retained valves, filling defects, or kinks. The angiocatheter was removed and its puncture site repaired with a 6-0 prolene suture. The suture lines and the wounds were then rechecked for hemostasis. There was good Doppler signal in the foot at the dorsalis pedis with a good augmentation of the signal with compressing and releasing the vein graft. The wounds were all irrigated with antibiotic solution. The subcutaneous tissue in the groin wound was closed in two layers of 3-0 Vicryl sutures. The fascia overlying the anterior tibial muscle and extensor hallucis muscles was partially closed with 3-0 Vicryl sutures. The skin was closed with staples.

The patient tolerated the procedure well and was transferred to the postanesthesia care unit in stable condition.

Chapter 171
In Situ Femoroperoneal Bypass

Jamal J. Hoballah, M.D., M.B.A.

INDICATIONS
- Tissue loss.
- Gangrene.
- Rest pain.
- Disabling claudication.

ESSENTIAL STEPS
1. Expose the target peroneal vessel.
2. Expose the greater saphenous vein (GSV).
3. Expose the inflow femoral vessels.
4. Transect the GSV at the saphenofemoral junction.
5. Excise the saphenofemoral valve under direct vision.
6. Construct the proximal anastomosis.
7. Incise the valves.
8. Identify and ligate arteriovenous (AV) fistulae.
9. Construct the distal anastomosis.
10. Completion angiogram.
11. Recheck for hemostasis.
12. Wound closure.
13. Pulses re-evaluation.

NOTE THESE VARIATIONS
- Femeroperoneal bypass are very rarely done for intermittent claudication.
- Numerous variations exist in performing in situ bypasses. Instead of exposing the entire saphenous vein, only the

805

J.J. Hoballah and C.E.H. Scott-Conner (eds.), *Operative Dictations in General and Vascular Surgery*, DOI 10.1007/978-1-4614-0451-4_171,
© Springer Science+Business Media, LLC 2012

proximal and distal ends of the vein may be exposed. Various long valvulotomes (some with detachable heads) can be used and are usually introduced from the most distal end of the vein. The venous side branches are identified by preoperative vein mapping or intraoperative angiography/angioscopy. Direct cutdowns are performed over these branches to ligate them. Alternatively, the branches are occluded by endovascular embolization.

- The peroneal artery can be exposed through a medial approach or through a lateral approach that involves excising a segment of the fibula.
- Control of the target vessels can be achieved in various ways, such as tourniquet, internal occluders, silastic vessel loops, vascular clamps, or Yasargil clips.

COMPLICATIONS

- Wound complications (infection/skin necrosis).
- Bleeding.
- Gangrene.
- Graft thrombosis.
- Myocardial infarction.

TEMPLATE OPERATIVE DICTATION

Preoperative diagnosis: Infrainguinal arterial occlusive disease with *right/left foot rest pain, right/left foot/toe ulcerations/gangrene.*

Procedure: In situ *right/left* common femoral artery to peroneal artery vein bypass; completion intraoperative arteriogram.

Postoperative diagnosis: Same.

Indications: The patient is a ___-year-old *male/female* with *right/left foot rest pain, right/left foot/toe ulcerations/gangrene.* Endovascular revascularization was not successful/deemed appropriate.

Preoperative evaluation revealed infrainguinal occlusive disease with reconstitution of the peroneal artery in the proximal/*mid/distal* leg.

The risks and benefits of revascularization were explained to the patient and *he/she* elected to undergo surgical intervention.

Description of procedure: The patient was placed supine on the operating table. The arms were *tucked in/placed at 80°.* Normal bony prominences were padded. The anesthesia team placed appropriate lines and *regional/general* anesthesia was induced. A Foley catheter was placed under sterile technique. The patient's lower abdomen and both lower extremities were circumferentially prepped and draped in the usual sterile fashion. Preoperative antibiotics were administered prior to skin incision.

[Choose one:]

If medial exposure of peroneal artery: *A 10- to 12-cm vertical skin incision was performed overlying the preoperatively mapped GSV at the level chosen for the construction of the distal anastomosis. The saphenous vein was identified and protected. The incision was deepened through the subcutaneous tissue, exposing the underlying fascia. The fascia was incised, exposing the soleus muscle. The soleus muscle was incised along its attachment down to its posterior deep fascia. This fascia was incised, exposing the posterior tibial and the flexor muscles. Gentle blunt dissection between these two muscles was performed and a self-retaining retractor was placed deeper in the wound, exposing the posterior tibial artery and veins. The posterior tibial vascular bundle was then retracted anteriorly and the dissection continued toward the fibula along the intermuscular septum, exposing the peroneal vessels.*

If lateral exposure of peroneal artery: *A 10- to 12-cm vertical skin incision was performed on the lateral aspect of the leg overlying the fibula. The incision was deepened until the fibula was exposed. A 6- to 8-cm segment of the fibula was isolated. A right-angle clamp was passed carefully behind the fibula, freeing its posterior border. The freed segment of fibula was then excised using a Gigli/electric saw. The underlying tissue was then incised, exposing the underlying peroneal vessels.*

The peroneal vein was then identified and mobilized, exposing the peroneal artery. A 2-cm segment of the peroneal artery was sharply dissected. Crossing venae comitantes were ligated and divided. Attention was then directed to the groin. A vertical curvilinear skin incision was started overlying the right common femoral artery. The incision was extended down the upper medial thigh along the preoperatively mapped GSV. The GSV was then identified and traced toward the saphenofemoral junction. The saphenofemoral junction and an adjacent 5-cm segment of the saphenous vein were circumferentially dissected. Venous branches originating from this segment were isolated and divided. The anterior aspect of the saphenous vein was then exposed from the saphenofemoral junction to the *mid/lower* leg through one continuous incision. Attention was then directed toward the common femoral artery. The subcutaneous tissues overlying the femoral pulse were incised with electrocautery. The common femoral artery was then exposed and sharply dissected circumferentially. The encountered lymphatics were ligated and divided. The dissection was extended proximally to the inguinal ligament and distally to include the superficial femoral and profunda femoris arteries.

The common femoral, superficial femoral, and profunda femoris arteries were encircled with silastic vessel loops. Minor branches of the common femoral artery were identified and spared.

The patient was given 5,000 U of heparin intravenously. A side-biting clamp was applied on the common femoral vein and the saphenous vein was transected, incorporating the saphenofemoral junction and a 1-mm rim of the femoral vein. The femoral venotomy was then closed with a running 5-0 prolene suture.

The saphenofemoral valve was then excised under direct vision using Pott's scissors. The common femoral artery, profunda, and superficial femoral artery were clamped. A longitudinal arteriotomy in the common femoral artery was performed and extended with Pott's scissors for 1 cm. The proximal anastomosis was constructed between the hood of the saphenofemoral junction and the femoral arteriotomy with a running 5-0 prolene suture. Prior to completing the suture line, back-bleeding, forward-flushing, and irrigation of the anastomosis with heparinized solution was performed. The anastomosis was then completed and checked for hemostasis, which was adequate. With the vein arterialized, the skin overlying the vein was incised and the vein sequentially exposed. The remaining valves were then disrupted using a retrograde valvulotome introduced through side branches and the distal end of the saphenous vein. Vein branches identified during dissection and by Doppler exam were ligated. The flow through the vein end was checked and was pulsatile. The distal end of the vein was controlled with a *Yasargil/Bulldog* clamp.

If tourniquet: A tourniquet was placed above the knee and an Esmarch rubber bandage was applied to the foot and wrapped proximally to exsanguinate the leg. Following leg exsanguination, the tourniquet was inflated to 250–350 mmHg.

If clamps or loops: Proximal and distal control of the peroneal artery was then performed using *Yasargil clamps, vascular clamps, Bulldog clamps, or silastic vessel loops.*

A 1-cm arteriotomy was then created in the anterior wall of the peroneal artery. The vein was transected at the appropriate length. The transected end was incised along its posterior aspect, spatulating the vein. The distal anastomosis to the peroneal artery was constructed with a running 7-0 prolene suture. Prior to completing the suture line, back-bleeding, forward-flushing, and irrigation of the anastomosis with heparinized solution was performed. The anastomosis was then completed and checked for hemostasis, which was adequate. A 20-gauge angiocatheter was then introduced into a side branch in the vein near the proximal anastomosis and an intraoperative arteriogram was performed.

The angiogram revealed a patent anastomosis with no evidence of any retained valves, filling defects, or kinks. The angiocatheter was removed and its puncture site repaired with a 6-0 prolene suture. The suture lines and the wounds were then rechecked for hemostasis. There was good Doppler signal in the foot at the level of the dorsalis pedis and posterior tibial arteries and a good augmentation of the signal with compressing and releasing the vein graft. The wounds were all irrigated with antibiotic solution. The subcutaneous tissue in the groin wound was closed in two layers of 3-0 Vicryl sutures. The fascia overlying the soleus muscle was partially closed with 3-0 Vicryl sutures. The skin was closed with staples.

The patient tolerated the procedure well and was transferred to the postanesthesia care unit in stable condition.

Chapter 172

Femoroplantar Composite Vein Bypass

Jamal J. Hoballah, M.D., M.B.A.

INDICATIONS
- Tissue loss.
- Gangrene.
- Rest pain.

ESSENTIAL STEPS
1. Expose the target plantar vessel.
2. Expose the inflow femoral vessels.
3. Harvest the vein segments.
4. Construct an end-to-end anastomosis between the two vein segments.
5. Create graft tunnel.
6. Reverse composite vein graft.
7. Construct the proximal anastomosis.
8. Check for hemostasis.
9. Pass graft through the tunnel.
10. Construct the distal anastomosis.
11. Completion angiogram.
12. Wound closure.
13. Pulses re-evaluation.

NOTE THESE VARIATIONS
- The vein segments can be connected with both being in a reversed direction. Alternatively, one segment can be reversed and the other nonreversed to provide a better

J.J. Hoballah and C.E.H. Scott-Conner (eds.), *Operative Dictations in General and Vascular Surgery*, DOI 10.1007/978-1-4614-0451-4_172,
© Springer Science+Business Media, LLC 2012

match between the size of both ends. The valves of the non-reversed segment will be disrupted with a valvulotome.

- Grafts to the plantar artery may be tunneled in various ways, including subcutaneous, subfascial, or anatomic tunnels.
- Control of the target vessels can be achieved in various ways, such as tourniquet, internal occluders, silastic vessel loops, vascular clamps, or Yasargil clips.

COMPLICATIONS
- Bleeding.
- Gangrene.
- Thrombosis of graft.
- Infection.
- Myocardial infarction.

TEMPLATE OPERATIVE DICTATION

Preoperative diagnosis: Infrainguinal arterial occlusive disease with *right/left foot rest pain, right/left foot/toe ulcerations/gangrene.*

Procedure: *Right/left* common femoral artery to posterior tibial artery vein bypass with reversed right greater saphenous vein; completion intraoperative arteriogram.

Postoperative diagnosis: Same.

Indications: The patient is a ___-year-old *male/female* with *right/left leg disabling claudication, right/left foot rest pain, right/left foot/toe ulcerations/gangrene.* Endovascular revascularization was not successful/deemed appropriate.

Preoperative evaluation revealed infrainguinal occlusive disease with reconstitution of the lateral plantar artery at the ankle.

The risks and benefits of revascularization were explained to the patient and *he/she* elected to undergo surgical intervention.

Description of procedure: The patient was placed supine on the operating table. The arms were *tucked in/placed at 80°*. Normal bony prominences were padded. The anesthesia team placed appropriate lines and *regional/general* anesthesia was induced. A Foley catheter was placed under sterile technique. The patient's lower abdomen and both lower extremities were circumferentially prepped and draped in the usual sterile fashion. Preoperative antibiotics were administered prior to skin incision.

A 6- to 8-cm vertical skin incision was performed on the medial aspect of the ankle 2 cm posteromedial to the medial malleolus. The skin incision was deepened through the subcutaneous tissue until the fascia was identified. The fascia was incised, exposing the posterior tibial artery and veins. The artery was traced distally toward its bifurcation into the medial and lateral plantar vessels. A 2-cm segment of the lateral plantar artery was sharply dissected. Crossing venae comitantes were ligated and divided. Attention was then directed to the groin. A vertical curvilinear skin incision overlying the right common femoral artery was made extending down the upper medial thigh along the preoperatively mapped greater saphenous vein. The incision was deepened through the subcutaneous tissues with electrocautery. The encountered lymphatics were ligated and divided. The common femoral artery was then exposed and sharply dissected circumferentially. The dissection was extended proximally to the inguinal ligament and distally to include the superficial femoral and profunda femoris arteries. The common femoral, superficial femoral, and profunda femoris arteries were encircled with silastic vessel loops. Minor branches of the common femoral artery were identified and spared.

An incision over the preoperatively mapped vein segments was performed. Two vein segments of appropriate length were harvested. The vein ends were spatulated and then sutured together *with both veins in the same direction/with one vein reversed and the other in a nonreversed direction.*

A tunnel was then created using a *Zepplin/Kelly weck/Gortex tunneler.*

The tunnel was subcutaneous parallel to the course of the saphenous vein to the level of the exposed posterior tibial artery.

The tunnel was subcutaneous/subfascial along the medial aspect of the thigh and knee.

The tunnel was subfascial/subsartorial along the medial aspect of the thigh and then anatomic at the knee level passing between both heads of the gastrocnemius muscle. Below the knee the tunnel was posterior to the soleus muscle.

The patient was given 5,000 U of heparin intravenously.

The common femoral artery, profunda, and superficial femoral artery were clamped. A longitudinal arteriotomy in the common femoral artery was performed and extended with Pott's scissors for 1 cm. The vein graft was then reversed and its distal end was incised along its *posterior wall/incorporating a side branch creating a T junction shape.* The proximal anastomosis was constructed between the spatulated vein and the femoral arteriotomy with a running *5-0/6-0* prolene suture. Prior to completing the suture line, back-bleeding, forward-flushing, and irrigation of the anastomosis with heparinized solution was performed. The anastomosis was then completed and checked for hemostasis, which was adequate.

The flow through the vein graft was checked and was pulsatile/*except for the nonreversed segment. A valvulotome was introduced through the distal end of the composite graft and used to disrupt the valves.* The end of the vein graft was ligated with a 2-0 silk tie. The vein was rechecked for hemostasis. The vein graft was then passed distended through the tunnel, avoiding any twists.

A tourniquet was placed above the knee and an Esmarch rubber bandage was applied to the foot and wrapped proximally to exsanguinate the leg. The tourniquet was then inflated to 350 mmHg.

[Choose one:]

If internal occluder: A 1-cm arteriotomy was then created in the anterior wall of the plantar artery. A 2.0/2.25/2.50-mm internal occluder (flowrestor) was introduced into the lumen to achieve proximal and distal control.

If loops or clamps: Proximal and distal control of the plantar artery was then performed using vessel loops/vascular clamps/ Bulldog clamp. A 1-cm arteriotomy was then created in the anterior wall of the plantar artery.

The vein graft was transected at the appropriate length. The transected end was incised along its posterior aspect, spatulating the transected vein. The distal anastomosis to the posterior tibial artery was constructed with a running 7-0 prolene suture. Prior to completing the suture line, back-bleeding, forward-flushing, and irrigation of the anastomosis with heparinized solution was performed. The anastomosis was then completed and checked for hemostasis, which was adequate. A 20-gauge angiocatheter was then introduced into a side branch in the vein near the proximal anastomosis and an intraoperative arteriogram was performed. The angiogram revealed a widely patent anastomosis and no evidence of filling defects or kinks. The angiocatheter was removed and its puncture site repaired with a 6-0 prolene suture. The suture lines and wounds were then rechecked for hemostasis. There was a good Doppler signal in the foot at the plantar artery level and a good augmentation of the signal with compressing and releasing the vein graft. The wounds were all irrigated with antibiotic solution. The subcutaneous tissue in the groin wound was closed in two layers of 3-0 Vicryl sutures. The fascia overlying the distal part of the soleus muscle was approximated with 3-0 Vicryl sutures. The skin was closed with staples.

The patient tolerated the procedure well and was transferred to the postanesthesia care unit in stable condition.

Chapter 173
Superficial Femoral Artery/Popliteal Artery/Tibial Angioplasty Stenting

Jamal J. Hoballah, M.D., M.B.A.

INDICATIONS
- Disabling claudication.
- Rest pain.
- Tissue loss.
- Gangrene.

ESSENTIAL STEPS
1. Percutaneous contralateral access of the common femoral artery.
2. Control access with 5-French sheath.
3. Anticoagulate with IV heparin sulfate (3,000 U).
4. Place guide wire into the abdominal aorta under fluoroscopic guidance.
5. Perform diagnostic aortogram with contralateral distal leg runoff.
6. Decide about continuing the procedure from the contralateral approach by crossing the bifurcation and placing a cross-over sheath or guiding catheter into the common femoral artery of the affected limb. Antegrade percutaneous or open access on the ipsilateral side.
7. Insertion of a long sheath or guiding catheter to the proximity of the lesion.
8. Measure length and degree of the stenotic/occluded lesion using DSA.
9. Additional anticoagulation at 75 UI/kg to keep ACT greater than 250seconds.

J.J. Hoballah and C.E.H. Scott-Conner (eds.), *Operative Dictations in General and Vascular Surgery*, DOI 10.1007/978-1-4614-0451-4_173,
© Springer Science+Business Media, LLC 2012

10. Crossing the stenosis with a glide wire/crossing the occlusion using subintimal technique/occlusion crossing catheters.
11. Predilation with a 3 mm × 4 cm balloon for the superficial femoral or popliteal arteries or a 1.5mm balloon for the tibial arteries; this will also serve as an additional method to measure the length of the stenosis and the diameter of the vessel to select the appropriate size balloon/stent.
12. Angioplasty and stenting.
13. Dilate with appropriately sized balloon.
14. Deploy stent across the lesion.
15. Post-stent dilatation.
16. Completion angiogram.

NOTE THESE VARIATIONS

- Preoperative MRA or CTA may guide the choice of the access and provide better planning.
- For lesions of the proximal superficial femoral artery (SFA), a contralateral approach with crossing of the aortic bifurcation is usually preferred.
- For crossing occlusion in the mid or distal SFA or tibial artery an antegrade puncture may provide better control and ability to cross chronic occlusions.
- Chronic occlusion may be crossed by navigating the wire through the occlusion, using sub-intimal angioplasty technique, or special catheters with lumen re-entry capability.
- In chronic occlusions, predilation may be useful prior to introducing the stent.
- In chronic occlusions, primary stenting may be desirable.
- With subintimal technique, stenting may be limited to the distal re-entry segment or may be used for the entire segment.
- In tibial disease, angioplasty is usually carried without the need for stenting.
- In tibial disease or popliteal disease adjacent to significant branches, atherectomy may be used instead of balloon angioplasty once the lesion is crossed in the hope of preserving the branches.
- Tibial occlusion that could not be crossed using standard wire techniques may be crossed using laser recanalization.

COMPLICATIONS

- Inability to cross the occlusion.
- Distal embolization.

- Dissection thrombosis.
- Vessel rupture.
- Renal failure.

TEMPLATE OPERATIVE DICTATION

Preoperative diagnosis: Infrainguinal arterial occlusive disease with *right left foot disabling claudication, right/left foot rest pain, right/left foot/toe ulcerations/gangrene.*

Procedure: *Right/left* SFA/popliteal/anterior tibial/peroneal/posterior tibial angioplasty/stenting.

Postoperative diagnosis: Same.

Indications: The patient is a ___-year-old *male/female* with *right / left foot disabling claudication, right/left foot rest pain, right/left foot/ toe ulcerations/gangrene.*

Preoperative evaluation revealed infrainguinal occlusive disease:

Superfical femoral artery/popliteal/anterior tibial/peroneal/posterior tibial stenosis/occlusion.

The risks and benefits of revascularization were explained to the patient and *he/she* elected to undergo surgical intervention.

Description of procedure: The patient was placed on the angiography table. Both groins were prepped and draped in the usual sterile fashion. The contralateral femoral artery was punctured using Seldinger technique with a micropuncture set which was exchanged to a size 5 French sheath. A 0.035" Standard Hydrophilic Guidewire soft angled, 180 cm was introduced into the aorta and an Omni Flush catheter was introduced over the wire to the aorta to the level of L1 vertebra. An aortogram with iliac runoff was performed. There was no evidence on any significant aorto-iliac occlusive disease. The Omni flush catheter was then used to cross over the aortic bifurcation to the contralateral side of interest. The tip of the catheter was then advanced to the level of the distal external iliac artery. A distal leg angiogram and runoff was then obtained through the Omni flush catheter. This revealed *superficial femoral artery/popliteal/anterior tibial/peroneal/ posterior tibial stenosis/occlusion.*

The decision was to proceed with the procedure from the contralateral side. A stiff wire was introduced into the Omni flush catheter and the Omni flushed was removed. The 5-French sheath was then replaced by a size 6-French Balkin sheath/6-French guiding catheter which was parked in the common femoral artery. The patient was administered 75 UI/Kg of Heparin intravenously. A road map/angiogram under magnification was performed of the area of *stenosis/occlusion*. Using of a size 4-French angled Glide catheter and a *straight/angled* glide wire, the glide catheter was advanced to the level of the *stenosis/occlusion* in the SFA. *The wire was negotiated across the stenosis/occlusion and the lesion was crossed; A subintimal angioplasty technique/re-entry catheter was used to cross the lesion.* The Glide catheter was advanced across and then distal to the lesion into the popliteal artery. An angiogram through the catheter was then performed documenting intraluminal placement. A 0.035 wire, 260 cm long was then introduced into the catheter and the catheter removed. The stenotic/occluded segment of the SFA were identified and predilated with size 4 mm×4 cm balloon. A *size* ____ self expending stent was then advanced and deployed at the desired location. The delivery system was removed and then an appropriately sized balloon ____ was used to postdilate the stent. An angiogram was performed and showed no evidence of any residual stenosis with no distal embolization.

Ipsilateral approach: ideal for tibial disease

Using a Seldinger technique and a micropuncture set, the ipsilateral common femoral artery was punctured. The micropuncture sheath was replaced by a size 5 French short sheath. An angiogram was performed revealing *stenotic/occlusive* disease in the *posterior tibial/anterior tibial/peroneal* artery. A size 6 French Guiding Catheter was then used to replace the 5-French sheath and advanced to the popliteal artery. Heparin 75 UI/Kg was then administered intravenously. The size 4 French Angled Glide Catheter was advanced into *the posterior tibial/anterior tibial/peroneal artery*. A 0.014″ × 190 cm Hydrophilic guidewire was negotiated across the stenosis. An angiogram under magnification was performed to further delineate the segment to be treated. An appropriate size balloon ____ was then inserted and inflated for 30 seconds. An angiogram revealed *no/minimal residual* stenosis with no extravasation. The catheter and wire were then removed and the sheath was removed when the ACT drifted below 150.

NOTES

Chapter 174
Midbypass Revision

Jamal J. Hoballah, M.D., M.B.A.

INDICATIONS
- Failing bypass.
- Vein bypass stenosis identified during duplex surveillance.

ESSENTIAL STEPS
1. Mark the area of stenosis preoperatively under duplex guidance.
2. Perform a longitudinal skin incision over the bypass.
3. Identify the bypass and dissect the area of stenosis.
4. Confirm the site of stenosis by Doppler ultrasound.
5. Harvest an appropriate segment of vein.
6. Anticoagulate.
7. Proximal and distal control.
8. Create a longitudinal incision in the graft.
9. *Alternative 1: Perform a vein patch angioplasty.*
   - *Alternative 2: Excise the disease vein segment and replace it with the harvested vein.*
10. Angiogram to confirm the adequacy of the reconstruction.
11. Wound closure.

NOTE THESE VARIATIONS
- Endovascular treatment (balloon angioplasty) is often attempted as a first revascularization option except if the stenotic segment is very long.

J.J. Hoballah and C.E.H. Scott-Conner (eds.), *Operative Dictations in General and Vascular Surgery*, DOI 10.1007/978-1-4614-0451-4_174,
© Springer Science+Business Media, LLC 2012

- A vein patch angioplasty is typically used with focal stenoses. If the stenosis is diffuse the vein segment is excised and replaced.

COMPLICATIONS
- Recurrent stenosis.
- Graft thrombosis.
- Bleeding.
- Infection.

TEMPLATE OPERATIVE DICTATION

Preoperative diagnosis: Failing vein bypass with midgraft stenosis.

Procedure: Vein bypass revision with *vein patch angioplasty/interposition vein graft.*

Postoperative diagnosis: Same.

Indications: This is a ___-year-old *male/female* with a failing *femoro/popliteal/tibial* vein bypass identified on routine duplex surveillance. The stenotic area is at the midgraft level and extends for 1 cm. The risks of thrombosis and benefits and risks of surgical intervention were discussed with the patient, who elected to undergo surgical intervention. Percutaneous intervention was not successful/deemed appropriate.

Description of procedure: The patient was placed in a supine position. The procedure was performed under *local/regional/general* anesthesia. The *right/left* lower extremity was prepped and draped in a sterile manner. A longitudinal skin incision was performed over the anticipated marked area of stenosis. The incision was deepened in the subcutaneous tissue until the graft was identified. The graft was dissected and exposed for 1.5 cm proximal and distal to the area of stenosis. *Doppler ultrasonography/angiogram* was used to confirm the site of stenosis. A skin incision was then performed over the preoperatively marked *cephalic/basilic/short saphenous/long saphenous* vein. A ___-cm segment of vein was harvested. The patient was given 75 U/kg of heparin intravenously. Proximal and distal control of the bypass was then performed and a longitudinal incision in the graft through the area of stenosis was then performed.

[Choose one:]

If vein patch angioplasty: The harvested vein segment was then incised longitudinally, creating a patch. The patch was then sutured using a continuous running suture of 6-0/7-0 prolene.

If interposition vein graft: A long segment of vein appeared to be stenotic with severe neointimal hyperplasia. The decision was made to replace that segment of vein. The disease segment was excised and remaining ends were spatulated. The harvested vein was reversed and then spatulated to match the bypass. An end-to-end anastomosis between the proximal part of the graft and the vein segment was then performed using a continuous running 6-0/7-0 prolene suture. Upon the completion of the anastomosis the suture line was checked for hemostasis and was adequate. The distal end of the vein segment was then spatulated to match the distal end of the bypass. The distal anastomosis was then performed using a running suture of 6-0/7-0 prolene.

The suture line was checked for hemostasis, which was adequate.

A 20-gauge *angiocath/butterfly* was then inserted in the graft proximal to the reconstruction and an angiogram was obtained. The angiogram revealed patent reconstruction without any additional areas of stenosis.

Hemostasis was secured. The wound was irrigated with saline solution.

The wound was then closed using 3-0 Vicryl for the subcutaneous tissue and staples for the skin.

The patient tolerated the procedure well and was transferred to the postanesthesia care unit in stable condition.

NOTES

Chapter 175

Distal Bypass Revision

Jamal J. Hoballah, M.D., M.B.A.

INDICATIONS

- Failing bypass.
- Distal vein bypass stenosis identified during duplex surveillance.

ESSENTIAL STEPS

1. Mark the area of stenosis preoperatively under duplex guidance.
2. Perform a longitudinal skin incision over the bypass.
3. Identify the bypass and dissect a segment proximal to the area of stenosis.
4. Expose the target artery distal to the stenotic area.
5. Confirm the site of stenosis by Doppler ultrasound.
6. Harvest an appropriate segment of vein.
7. Anticoagulate.
8. Proximal and distal control.
9. *Alternative 1: Vein patch angioplasty.*
   - *Alternative 2: Interposition/jump graft. Create the proximal anastomosis end-to-end/end-to-side configuration; construct the distal anastomosis end-to-side configuration.*
10. Angiogram to confirm the adequacy of the reconstruction.
11. Wound closure.

NOTE THESE VARIATIONS

- Percutaneous balloon angioplasty is often attempted first.

J.J. Hoballah and C.E.H. Scott-Conner (eds.), *Operative Dictations in General and Vascular Surgery*, DOI 10.1007/978-1-4614-0451-4_175,
© Springer Science+Business Media, LLC 2012

- Distal anastomotic stenoses can be treated by vein patch angioplasty, which requires tedious dissection of the anastomosis, or interposition of a vein segment. If a long segment of the distal bypass is stenotic, replacement of that segment is carried. The proximal anastomosis may be performed in an end-to-end or end-to-side fashion. The latter is typically used when the retrograde flow into the target vessel is preserved and the stenotic area is in the most distal part of the distal anastomosis toward the target vessel.

COMPLICATIONS

- Recurrent stenosis.
- Graft thrombosis.
- Bleeding.
- Infection.

TEMPLATE OPERATIVE DICTATION

Preoperative diagnosis: Failing vein bypass with distal graft stenosis.

Procedure: Vein bypass revision with *vein patch angioplasty/interposition/jump vein graft.*

Postoperative diagnosis: Same.

Indications: This is a ___-year-old *male/female* with a failing *femoro/popliteal/tibial* vein bypass identified on routine duplex surveillance. The stenotic area is at the level of the distal anastomosis and extends for ___ cm. Endovascular revascularization was not successful/deemed appropriate. The risks of thrombosis and benefits and risks of surgical intervention were discussed with the patient, who elected to undergo surgical intervention.

Description of procedure: The patient was placed in a supine position. The procedure was performed under *local/regional/general* anesthesia. The *right/left* lower extremity was prepped and draped in a sterile manner. A longitudinal skin incision was performed over the anticipated marked area of stenosis. The incision was deepened in the subcutaneous tissue until the graft was identified. The graft was dissected and exposed for 1.5 cm proximal to the area of stenosis.

The dissection was then continued distally, exposing the anastomosis and the target vessel distal to it. Doppler ultrasonography/angiogram was used to confirm the site of stenosis. A skin incision was then performed over the preoperatively marked *cephalic/basilic/short saphenous/long saphenous* vein. A ___-cm segment of vein was harvested. The patient was given 75 U/kg of heparin intravenously. Proximal and distal control of the bypass was then performed.

[Choose one:]

If vein patch angioplasty: A longitudinal incision in the graft through the area of stenosis was then performed. The harvested vein segment was then incised longitudinally, creating a patch. The patch was then sutured using a continuous running suture of 6-0/7-0 prolene.

If interposition/jump graft: A long segment of the distal bypass was stenotic with severe neointimal hyperplasia. The decision was made to replace that segment of vein. The disease segment was excised by transecting the bypass proximal to the stenotic segment and just proximal to the distal anastomosis. The distal end of the bypass was oversewn with a running 6-0 prolene suture. The proximal end was spatulated. The harvested vein was then spatulated to match the bypass. An end-to-end anastomosis between the proximal part of the graft and the vein segment was then performed using a continuous running 6-0/7-0 prolene suture. Upon the completion of the anastomosis the suture line was checked for hemostasis and was adequate. Proximal and distal control of the target vessel was then obtained and a ___-cm arteriotomy was performed. The distal end of the vein segment was then spatulated to match the arteriotomy. The distal anastomosis was then performed using a running suture of 6-0/7-0 prolene.

The suture line was checked for hemostasis, which was adequate.

A 20-gauge *angiocath/butterfly* was then inserted in the graft proximal to the reconstruction and an angiogram was obtained. The angiogram revealed patent reconstruction without any additional areas of stenosis.

Hemostasis was secured. The wound was irrigated with saline solution. The wound was then closed using 3-0 Vicryl for the subcutaneous tissue and staples for the skin.

The patient tolerated the procedure well and was transferred to the postanesthesia care unit in stable condition.

NOTES

Chapter 176
Bypass Stenosis Angioplasty

Fady F. Haddad, M.D. and Ahmad Zaghal, M.D.

INDICATION

■ Salvage of patent but hemodynamically failing bypass because of in-graft stenosis, inflow or outflow stenosis (usually detected on Duplex surveillance).

ESSENTIAL STEPS

1. If target lesion or plan is unclear from the preoperative duplex, we favor prepping and draping the patient from the start umbilicus to toes bilaterally in preparation for potential cut-down or open repair.
2. Get access from the contralateral leg if possible (refer to alternative below).
3. Advance angiographic catheter into aorta and perform aorto iliac and bilateral femoral imaging.
4. Manipulate catheter and wire to get cross-over access to the contralateral iliac.
5. Perform selective angiography of the target extremity and bypass.
   • Decision to proceed with percutaneous angioplasty vs. open repair.
   • Select lesions to be treated (we recommend during these procedures the use of marked "Glow and Tell Tape," Le Maitre or other, taped directly on the index limb).
6. Anticoagulate patient with systemic heparin. Target ACT ~250–300.

J.J. Hoballah and C.E.H. Scott-Conner (eds.), *Operative Dictations in General and Vascular Surgery*, DOI 10.1007/978-1-4614-0451-4_176,

7. Exchange catheter for a long cross-over sheath parked usually in the distal external iliac artery EIA (unless bypass originate from the popliteal, than longer sheath may be needed). 6 French is usually satisfactory.

8. Access the bypass using 0.014 wire, which should be advanced beyond all lesions to be treated.

9. Image again through the sheath; keep the reference image; select and advance appropriate balloon and proceed with angioplasty.

NOTE THESE VARIATIONS

- Alternatively: If access from contralateral side is deemed impossible for some reason(bypass from the groin, severe tortuosity, iliac occlusion…), than either proceed with brachial approach if the stenosis is proximal in the thigh and reachable, or consider an open cut-down on the bypass which can be used for imaging proximal and distally and access for the angioplasty as well.

- Antegrade access may also be possible if the graft originates from or distal to the superficial femoral artery.

For any of the reasons above, or other anatomic consideration (very long stenosis, multiple stenosis, etc.), decision could be made to proceed with open repair of the bypass; this is done typically using a vein patch angioplasty or an interposition vein graft if the stenosis is long.

TEMPLATE DICTATION

Preoperative diagnosis: Right/Left lower extremity bypass graft stenosis.

Postoperative diagnosis: Same.

Operation:

Contralateral femoral artery puncture.

Selective lower extremity angiography.

Proximal/distal/mid bypass graft balloon angioplasty using (balloon size and diameter) and or proximal/distal anastomotic stenosis PTA.

Indication: Patient, co-morbidities, a case of right critical limb ischemia, S/P right/Left autogenous bypass (from-to-), done around __ months ago, follow-up duplex scan showed the presence of a tight Stenosis at __ (location), and an another Stenosis at (level), (or alternatively a hemodynamically failing bypass), planned for angiography and angioplasty for assisted primary patency.

Procedure: Under local anesthesia using 1% lidocaine, (with or without sedation), both lower extremities and groins were prepped and scrubbed in the usual fashion from the umbilicus down to the ankles.

Retrograde access to the contralateral femoral artery was achieved using a micropuncture system, which was then exchanged to a 5-French sheath. Pigtail catheter (or preferably a VCF or Omni flush 65 cm) was introduced over a starter wire (or hydrophilic wire) into the distal infrarenal aorta. Angiographic runs of the aorto iliac and proximal femoral arteries were taken bilaterally. A Glide wire (Terumo) was manipulated and advanced into the contralateral iliac down to the femoral artery and the catheter was advanced over it *(alternatively, the flush catheter may need to be changed to a Glide catheter if it does not progress as needed).* Selective images of the contralateral extremity and the bypass are taken, and the pathology identified. At this point an exchange wire was advanced into the catheter (typically a Rosen wire or equivalent, or an Amplatz wire if significant tortuosity) and the sheath exchanged to a long 6-French sheath that is parked into the distal external iliac artery (typically a Balkan sheath from Cook or alternative). Patient is given systemic IV Heparin to keep ACT ~300. Road map or reference images of the bypass origin are taken in the appropriate orientation to open the anastomosis. Glide wire and a 4-French angled glide catheter are used to negotiate and get selective access to the bypass. Catheter is gently advanced in the bypass origin, and the wire is typically exchanged at this point to a 0.014" wire (example Nitrix-angled tip from EV3 or a Floppy II or a BMW). The wire is advanced without difficulty into the bypass as needed, for a good distance beyond all stenotic lesions and across the distal anastomosis when needed, especially if this one is to be treated as well. At this point, after all target lesions are identified, an appropriately sized low profile balloon is used (typically anywhere between 2.5 and 4 mm depending on bypass size, starting with a conservatively lower estimate), and a 2- to 3-min inflation is done. Control angiography through the sheath is performed, and depending on the result a larger balloon maybe used. In lesions which do not respond to regular balloon, a cutting balloon, undersized, is used initially, followed by a regular balloon dilatation. After satisfactory control, attention is given to the next stenosis. Following a final control of the totality of the bypass including the run off vessel, wire access is lost from the bypass; the long sheath is exchanged to a short 11 cm 6-French sheath. An ACT is checked, and more often than not it is still prolonged at this point, and the sheath is left in place to be removed later in the recovery area. Alternatively, a closure system could be used and the sheath removed directly following the procedure.

At the end of the procedure pulse in the DP/PT and Doppler's are checked.

Section XVIII

Thromboembolectomy

Chapter 177
Aortic Saddle Embolus

Theodore H. Teruya, M.D., and Ahmed M. Abou-Zamzam, M.D.

INDICATION
- Acute bilateral lower-extremity ischemia due to embolus.

ESSENTIAL STEPS
1. Prep the patient (be prepared to do an axillary femoro-femoral bypass).
2. Dissect the common, profunda, and superficial femoral arteries bilaterally.
3. Make arteriotomies bilaterally.
4. Perform distal thrombectomies.
5. Pass catheters proximal, simultaneously, and extract the thrombus.
6. Close the arteries.
7. Assess distal perfusion.
8. Assess the legs for compartment syndrome.

NOTE THIS VARIATION
- The femoral arteriotomies are made transverse if an embolic process is suspected and longitudinal if aortoiliac occlusive disease is suspected.

COMPLICATIONS
- Bleeding.
- Hematoma.

J.J. Hoballah and C.E.H. Scott-Conner (eds.), *Operative Dictations in General and Vascular Surgery*, DOI 10.1007/978-1-4614-0451-4_177,
© Springer Science+Business Media, LLC 2012

- Ongoing ischemia.
- Compartment syndrome.
- Limb loss.
- Renal failure.
- Death (due to underlying illness).

TEMPLATE OPERATIVE DICTATION

Preoperative diagnosis: Bilateral lower-extremity ischemia.
Procedure: Aortobiiliac thromboembolectomy.
Postoperative diagnosis: Same.
Indications: This is a ___-year-old *male/female* presenting with bilateral cold pulseless extremities of ___-h duration. On physical examination, the patient had no palpable femoral pulses and no Doppler signals in either lower extremity. Motor and sensory examination revealed sensation and motor function to be *normal/ diminished/absent*. The patient was given 10,000 U of heparin when ischemia was identified. The patient *had/had no* documented femoral and pedal pulses prior to current presentation.

There was fresh thrombus extracted from the distal aorta and bilateral iliac arteries. There was good back-bleeding from the profunda and superficial femoral arteries bilaterally. The patient had palpable DP and PT pulses bilaterally at the termination of the procedure.

Description of procedure: The procedure was performed under *general/local* anesthesia. The patient was placed supine on the operating table and appropriate monitoring lines and catheters were placed. The patient had received 10,000 U of heparin prior to arriving at the operating room. The chest, abdomen, femoral regions, and lower extremities were prepped and draped in standard sterile fashion. (The chest, abdomen, and lower extremities need to be included in the sterile field in case an axillary femoro-femoral bypass is necessary.)

Bilateral vertical femoral incisions were made, two finger breadths lateral to the pubis. The subcutaneous tissue was dissected with ligation and division of small vessels and lymphatics and the common, profunda, and superficial femoral arteries were dissected free bilaterally. Each vessel was double looped using a vessel loop. A transverse arteriotomy was made over the origin of the profunda. *(Longitudinal arteriotomies were made as there was a concern that there is chronic aortoiliac occlusive disease and a bypass may need to be done.)* There was good back-bleeding from the profunda femoris and superficial femoral artery and these vessels were controlled using vascular clamps.

Number 5 Fogarty thromboembolectomy catheters were then passed proximally into the aorta from both femoral arteries, simultaneously. The catheters were inflated simultaneously and withdrawn. This was repeated until all thrombus was extracted. The inflow was tested and noted to be brisk. *(An adequate inflow could not be obtained, and an axillary femorofemoral bypass was needed.)* The common femoral arteries were then clamped. The arteriotomies were then closed using interrupted 6-0 prolene sutures. *(If longitudinal arteriotomies were performed, the vessel should be closed with a vein/Dacron/PTFE patch.)* Flow was established to the lower extremities bilaterally. The patient had palpable PT and DP pulses bilaterally.

The legs were assessed for compartment syndrome *clinically/ with pressure device and fasciotomies were/were not necessary.*

Thrombin-soaked Gelfoam was placed over the suture lines until hemostasis was obtained. Bleeding from the subcutaneous tissue was controlled with electrocautery. The wound was closed using multiple layers of 3-0 Vicryl sutures. The skin incisions were closed using 4-0 absorbable monofilament sutures.

The patient tolerated the procedure well and was taken to the intensive care unit in stable condition.

NOTES

Chapter 178

Lower-Extremity Thromboembolectomy

Jason Chiriano, D.O. and Theodore H. Teruya, M.D.

INDICATION

- Acute lower-extremity ischemia secondary to embolism or thrombotic event.
- DIAGNOSIS
- Acute onset of pain, pallor, paresthesia, poikilothermia, and paralysis in any extremity.
- Complete pulse/Doppler exam.
- Differentiate between embolic vs. thrombotic etiology:
  - Embolism more likely with normal pulse exam on opposite extremity, history of aneurysm, or cardiac arrhythmia.

ESSENTIAL STEPS

1. Identify the likely site of obstruction based on history and physical examination.
   - Most common site is in distal common femoral artery at bifurcation of superficial and deep femoral artery.
   - Second most common site is at distal popliteal artery.
2. Complete dissection of either the common femoral artery from the inguinal ligament to the bifurcation, or the below-knee popliteal artery to the origin of the anterior tibial artery and tibioperoneal trunk (if inadequate thromboembolectomy from the femoral approach).
   - Longitudinal groin cut down most common, however, transverse incision may be adequate if pure embolic disease is strongly suspected.

J.J. Hoballah and C.E.H. Scott-Conner (eds.), *Operative Dictations in General and Vascular Surgery*, DOI 10.1007/978-1-4614-0451-4_178,
© Springer Science+Business Media, LLC 2012

3. Obtain proximal and distal control with vessel loops at the site through which the thromboembolectomy will be performed.
4. Make arteriotomy with an 11 blade scalpel – transverse if vessel is healthy, longitudinal if there is atherosclerotic disease that may require endarterectomy.
5. Catheter thromboembolectomy – must make continual passes with gentle inflation until two sequential returns of balloon catheter with no thrombus and adequate pulsatile inflow/brisk back-bleeding.
   • Iliac arteries – #5 fogarty catheter.
   • Superficial femoral/popliteal arteries – #4/#5 fogarty catheter.
   • Profunda femoris artery – #3/4 fogarty catheter.
   • Tibial arteries – #2/#3 fogarty catheters.
6. Arteriotomy closure – primary if transverse, patch if longitudinal.
7. Assess distal perfusion – if adequate Doppler signals/palpable pulses terminate procedure, otherwise perform intraoperative angiogram (see adjunct procedures/technical notes).
8. Consider need for four compartment fasciotomy – prolonged ischemia time over 4 h, degree of preoperative ischemia, presence of overt compartment syndrome.

ADJUNCT PROCEDURES

1. Perform intraoperative angiogram through either a micropuncture dilator or small 20 g angiocatheter in the common femoral artery if no signals at the end of case.
2. Consider bolus of TPA (tissue plasminogen activator) – if no signals at end of case and angiogram suggests residual thrombus. Inject through sheath or catheter. Dose: 2–10 mg.
3. Bolus of vasodilator – Papaverine – 10–60 mg, Nitroglycerin 500–1,500 μg. Use if no signals and angiogram suggests severe spasm of tibial vessels.
4. Angiojet Device/Trellis – mechanical thrombectomy devices for retained clot.
5. Over the wire fogarty balloon catheters for residual thrombus or further embolization during procedure.
6. Consider bypass procedure if severely diseased vessels and unable to establish flow to the foot.

TECHNICAL NOTES

1. Preoperative imaging for suspected embolic disease is rarely needed. Patients should be expedited to the operating room as quickly as possible.
2. When exposing the below knee popliteal artery it is necessary to identify and ligate the anterior tibial vein to fully expose the origin of the anterior tibial artery. Individual tibial artery thrombectomy is necessary.
3. If there are no signals at end of case pedal cut down procedures are helpful to perform retrograde thrombectomy with #2/3 fogarty catheters for retained tibial thrombus.
4. If after all above fails to restore flow to foot, terminate procedure and take to ICU for further care. Severe spasm of the tibial arteries is the norm not the exception, and signals are often present within 24 h of the operation.
5. Avoid amputation at the same setting unless absolutely necessary, such as the following:
   • Severe reperfusion syndrome.
   • Non-salvageable limb with severe rhabdomyolysis leading to renal failure.

COMPLICATIONS

■ Bleeding.
■ Infection.
■ Ongoing ischemia.
■ Compartment syndrome.
■ Reperfusion syndrome.
■ Limb loss.
■ Death.

TEMPLATE OPERATIVE DICTATION

Preoperative diagnosis: Acute *right/left upper/lower*-extremity ischemia.

Procedure: (1) *Right/Left iliofemoral* thrombectomy. (2) *Right/left popliteal-tibial* thrombectomy.

Postoperative diagnosis: Same.

Indications: The patient is a ___- year-old *male/female* who developed acute onset of *right/left* foot pain at rest. Physical examination revealed a pulseless, cool foot. Sensory and motor function were *present/diminished/absent*. The patient received 10,000 U of heparin intravenously at that time. The patient had *well-known/no prior history* of claudication, rest pain, non healing ulcers, or gangrene. Additionally, the patient had *well-known history/no prior history* of atrial fibrillation/congestive heart failure/myocardial infarction.

Operative findings: *There was fresh thrombus in the right iliac, common femoral, superficial femoral, and profunda femoris arteries. After the iliofemoral thrombectomy, the patient had no Doppler signals at the ankle. An arteriogram demonstrated occlusion of the below-knee popliteal artery. Popliteal and tibial artery thrombectomy was then performed. There was dense old clot in the anterior and posterior tibial arteries. There was fresh thrombus in the tibioperoneal trunk and peroneal arteries. After tibial thrombectomy the patient had biphasic/triphasic Doppler signals (or palpable pulses) at the ankle in the posterior tibial/anterior tibial/peroneal arteries.*

Alternate findings:

- There was severe atherosclerotic disease in the distal external iliac artery and common femoral/superficial femoral artery/profunda femoris artery/popliteal artery that required endarterectomy.
- There were no signals at the end of case after tibial thrombectomy requiring pedal vessel exposure and retrograde tibial thrombectomy.

Description of procedure: The procedure was performed under *general/local* anesthesia (may start under local for femoral thromboembolectomy). The patient was placed in the supine position, and the abdomen and lower extremities were prepped and draped in the standard fashion. Perioperative antibiotics were administered.

A *vertical/transverse* skin incision was made over the femoral artery. The subcutaneous tissue was dissected with cautery and veins and lymphatics were ligated and divided as necessary. The common femoral artery was dissected free and small side branches were controlled. The proximal common femoral artery was controlled with a vessel loop at the level of the inguinal ligament. The profunda femoral artery was dissected free and controlled with a vessel loop. The superficial femoral artery was then dissected free and controlled in the same manner.

The patient was given 100 U/kg of heparin intravenously. After 3 min, a transverse arteriotomy was created on the common femoral artery using a #11 blade scalpel. The arteriotomy was extended using angled Pott's scissors. (Use longitudinal arteriotomy if artery is diseased). A balloon catheter thrombectomy of the profunda was successfully performed using a #3 Fogarty catheter. The superficial femoral artery was cleared of thrombus using a #4 Fogarty catheter. There was good back-bleeding at this point from the superficial femoral and profunda femoris arteries. The #4 Fogarty catheter was then passed retrograde into the iliac artery and thrombus was removed with the establishment of excellent pulsatile inflow. The arteriotomy was then closed using interrupted 6-0 prolene sutures. (Use patch angioplasty with a longitudinal arteriotomy). Excellent Doppler signals in the DP and PT were noted.

If no DP, PT Doppler signals: A continuous-wave Doppler was then used to insonate the tibial vessels. There were no Doppler signals at the ankle at this time. An excellent popliteal Doppler signal was noted. Intraoperative arteriography was performed using a 20-gauge angiocatheter inserted into the common femoral artery. The proximal common femoral artery was clamped. Contrast was injected and fluoroscopy was utilized. The angiogram demonstrated that the superficial femoral artery was widely patent, with an abrupt occlusion of the distal popliteal artery.

A medial incision was made below the knee, 1.5 cm posterior to the medial margin of the tibia. The subcutaneous tissue and fascia were divided. The gastrocnemius muscle was retracted posteriorly. The popliteal artery was palpated and dissected free from the accompanying vein and nerve. The vein was retracted posteriorly. The artery was controlled proximally and distally; the dissection was carried out beyond the origin of the anterior tibial artery. The anterior tibial vein was dissected free and ligated proximally and distally and divided. The anterior tibial artery and the tibioperoneal trunk were controlled with vessel loops. A transverse/longitudinal incision was then made in the popliteal artery, and extended with angled Pott's scissors. There was pulsatile inflow. A #2/#3 Fogarty catheter was then carefully passed into the anterior tibial artery and thrombus was withdrawn with the balloon partially inflated. This was repeated until all of the thrombus was removed. The posterior tibial and peroneal arteries were then cleared of thrombus in the same manner. There was excellent back-bleeding from the tibial arteries at this point.

The popliteal artery was then closed primarily/by patch angioplasty with 6-0/7-0 prolene suture. The vessels were back-bled and flushed prior to completing the repair. The clamps were removed. Doppler was again used to insonate the PT and DP arteries at the ankle. There were good triphasic (biphasic, monophasic) signals at this time.

If still no signals in the foot: A continuous-wave Doppler was then used to insonate the tibial vessels. There were no Doppler signals at the ankle at this time. An excellent popliteal Doppler signal was noted. Intraoperative arteriography was repeated. The angiogram showed widely patent femoral/popliteal and proximal filling of (AT/PT/Peroneal) with abrupt occlusion in the calf.

A longitudinal incision was made in the dorsum of the foot near the ankle. Dissection was carried through the subcutaneous fat and extensor retinaculum. The extensor hallucis and extensor digitorum muscles were retracted and the dorsalis pedis artery was visualized. The artery was dissected away from the veins and controlled with vessel loops proximally and distally. A transverse arteriotomy was made in the artery and a #2/#3 fogarty catheter was passed retrograde passed the origin of the anterior tibial artery. Thrombus was removed with the balloon partially inflated with the return of pulsatile inflow. The catheter was then gently passed antegrade with the removal of a small amount of thrombus. Manual compression of the foot was used to remove additional thrombus. There was good back-bleeding at this point. The artery was then closed with interrupted 7-0 prolene suture. The artery was back-bled and flushed prior to completion of repair.

A longitudinal incision was then made posterior to the medial malleolus. The dissection was carried down through the subcutaneous fat and crural fascia. The posterior tibial artery was visualized and dissected away from the vein. It was controlled with vessel loops proximally and distally. Thrombectomy was then performed in a similar fashion to the dorsalis pedis artery, with the removal of thrombus and establishment of pulsatile inflow and brisk back-bleeding. The artery was repaired with interrupted 7-0 prolene suture. Prior to the completion of repair, the artery was back-bled and flushed. Doppler was again used to insonate the PT and DP arteries at the ankle. There were good triphasic (biphasic, monophasic) signals at this time.

The leg muscle compartments were assessed for the need for fasciotomy.

The incisions were closed using multiple layers of 3-0 braided absorbable sutures and the skin was closed using 4-0 monofilament absorbable sutures.

The patient tolerated the procedure well was extubated and transported to the postanesthesia care unit in stable condition. The patient had triphasic (biphasic, monophasic) Doppler signals in the foot on arrival to PACU.

Chapter 179
Upper-Extremity Thromboembolectomy

Jamal J. Hoballah, M.D., M.B.A.

INDICATION

- Acute upper-extremity ischemia secondary to embolism or thrombotic event.

ESSENTIAL STEPS

1. Identify the likely site of obstruction, based on history and physical exam.
2. Obtain proximal and distal control.
3. Circumferential dissection of the brachial artery at the antecubital fossa.
4. Circumferential dissection of the origin of the radial and ulnar arteries.
5. Make arteriotomy (transverse vs. longitudinal).
6. Catheter thromboembolectomy (avoid overdistension and repeated passes).
7. Artery closure (primary vs. patch).
8. Assess distal perfusion.
9. Evaluate the arm for compartment syndrome.

NOTE THESE VARIATIONS

- The brachial artery can be exposed through a transverse or S-shaped skin incision overlying the anticubital fossa.
- Dissection of the origin of the radial and ulnar arteries is optional.

J.J. Hoballah and C.E.H. Scott-Conner (eds.), *Operative Dictations in General and Vascular Surgery*, DOI 10.1007/978-1-4614-0451-4_179,
© Springer Science+Business Media, LLC 2012

COMPLICATIONS

- Bleeding.
- Infection.
- Ongoing ischemia.
- Compartment syndrome.
- Limb loss.

TEMPLATE OPERATIVE DICTATION

Preoperative diagnosis: Upper-extremity ischemia; right brachial artery and radial and ulnar artery occlusions.

Procedure: Brachial, ulnar, and radial artery thromboembolectomy.

Postoperative diagnosis: Same.

Indications: The patient is a ___-year-old *male/female* who developed acute onset of *right/left*-upper extremity pain, with bluish discoloration. The patient was found to have a pulseless, cool hand. Sensory and motor function were *present/diminished/absent*. The patient received 10,000 U of heparin intravenously ___ min prior to the start of the procedure. The patient had no prior history of hand pain, nonhealing finger ulcers, or gangrene. The patient has a history of *atrial fibrillation/congestive heart failure/myocardial infarction*. Duplex evaluation revealed a clot in the brachial, ulnar, and radial arteries. The risks and benefits of the procedure were explained to the patient, who elected to proceed with surgical intervention.

Description of procedure: The procedure was performed under *local/axillary block/general* anesthesia. With the patient in the supine position, the *right/left* upper extremity was prepped and draped in the usual sterile fashion. The skin over the antecubital space was infiltrated with *1.0/0.5%* lidocaine. A 5-cm skin incision overlying the antecubital fossa was then performed and deepened through the subcutaneous tissue and fat. The biceps aponeurosis was incised over the brachial pulse. The brachial artery was circumferentially dissected to its bifurcation into the ulnar and radial arteries. The patient was already receiving heparin anticoagulation. The brachial artery was controlled with silastic vessel loops and a transverse arteriotomy was performed. Clot was extruded and good inflow was established. A #2/3 Fogarty catheter was then introduced into the ulnar artery, and thromboembolectomy of the ulnar artery was performed until no clot could be retrieved and a good back-bleeding was established. The same was then performed to the radial artery. Thorough irrigation with heparinized saline was then performed. The arteriotomy was closed using *6-0/7-0* *interrupted/running* sutures. At the completion of the procedure, there was evidence of palpable pulse in the *radial/ulnar* artery with excellent signals in the radial and ulnar arteries. The suture line was hemostatic. The wound was then irrigated with antibiotic solution and closed using 3-0 Vicryl for the subcutaneous tissue and 4-0 monocryl for the skin.

The patient tolerated the procedure well and was transferred to the postanesthesia care unit in stable condition.

Section **XIX**

Aneurysmal Disease

Chapter 180
Thoracoabdominal Aortic Aneurysm Repair

John W. York, M.D. and Samuel R. Money, M.D.

INDICATIONS

- All symptomatic or ruptured thoracoabdominal aneurysms (THAAs) or type I, II, III, or IV greater than 5.5 cm in suitable open surgical candidates.
- THAA secondary to chronic dissection greater than 5 cm.

ESSENTIAL STEPS

1. Double-lumen endotracheal intubation.
2. Spinal drainage.
3. Right lateral decubitus thoracoabdominal positioning.
4. Thoracoabdominal incision terminating over appropriate interspace (type IV: eighth to ninth interspace; types I, II, and III: fifth interspace).
5. Large aneurysms may require two intercostal incisions.
6. Peritoneum left intact with retroperitoneal exposure.
7. Intra-abdominal contents reflected to the right.
8. Large crossing branch of the left renal vein identified and divided.
9. Left ureter identified and protected.
10. Costal margin divided at the level of the appropriate interspace.
11. Low circumferential (radial) division of the muscular portion of the diaphragm to the hiatus.
12. Systemic heparinization.
13. Proximal aortic control.
14. Distal abdominal *aorta/iliac* control.

J.J. Hoballah and C.E.H. Scott-Conner (eds.), *Operative Dictations in General and Vascular Surgery*, DOI 10.1007/978-1-4614-0451-4_180,
© Springer Science+Business Media, LLC 2012

15. Aortotomy beginning in the abdominal segment of the aorta.
16. Aortotomy extended cephalad and posterior to avoid injury to the visceral vessels.
17. Visceral back-bleeding controlled with Fogarty balloons (if necessary).
18. Proximal aortic anastomosis completed in end-to-end fashion.
19. Visceral patch anastomosis using Crawford technique.
20. Sequential removal of clamps.
21. Left renal anastomosis via 6-mm graft sidearm constructed if necessary.
22. Distal aortic anastomosis.
23. Flow verified in the visceral, renal, and lower extremities by *palpation/Doppler*.
24. Thoracostomy tubes (×2) placed.
25. Hemostasis achieved.
26. PTFE membrane closure over the graft.
27. Chest and abdomen closed.

NOTE THESE VARIATIONS

- In type IV, the visceral vessels may all be incorporated within the proximal anastomosis. However, this may be associated with future patch aneurysmal dilatation.
- In the remaining types, the proximal anastomosis is performed separately first and then the visceral vessels are reimplanted as an island of aortic wall that contains all the visceral orifices. If the aneurysmal disease is such that the left renal orifice is not in close proximity to the other visceral vessels, the right renal, superior mesenteric, and celiac orifices are usually reimplanted together on the same island. The left renal is reimplanted separately or via a graft sidearm.
- A spinal catheter for drainage is usually inserted preoperatively and kept for 48 h postoperatively.
- Cannulas may be placed in the femoral artery and veins and the patient connected to a perfusion pump in complex cases to maintain visceral, pelvic, and distal perfusion.

COMPLICATIONS

- Death.
- Hemorrhage.
- Myocardial infarction.

- Spinal cord ischemic paralysis.
- Intestinal ischemia.
- Renal failure.
- Limb loss.
- Prolonged ventilator dependence.
- Wound infection/dehiscence/hernias.

TEMPLATE OPERATIVE DICTATION

Preoperative diagnosis: Thoracoabdominal aortic aneurysm (type _____).

Procedure: Thoracoabdominal aortic aneurysm repair.

Postoperative diagnosis: Same.

Indications: This is a ___-year-old _male/female_ with ___-cm thoracoabdominal aortic aneurysm. Preoperative cardiac risk stratification performed preoperatively. Risks and benefits of the procedure were explained to the patient, who agreed to proceed with surgical intervention.

Description of procedure: After induction of general anesthesia using a double-lumen endotracheal tube, and the establishment of spinal drainage, the patient was positioned in a modified right lateral decubitus position. The patient was then sterilely prepped and draped in the usual fashion from the left shoulder down to the knees including the groins bilaterally. An incision beginning 3 cm to the left of the midline, below the umbilicus, was made in a curvilinear fashion extending cephalad over the ___ interspace and continuing posterior to the midline. Cautery was used to divide the subcutaneous tissues and fascia. A plane was carefully created between the peritoneum and transversalis fascia along the left flank. This plane was extended superiorly and posteriorly toward the midline. The abdominal contents in the peritoneal cavity were swept anteriorly and to the right. This dissection was continued until the inferior surface of the diaphragm was encountered. Cautery was used to divide the external intercostal muscles and preparations were made to enter the chest. The chest was entered through the ___ interspace. Care was taken to avoid the neurovascular bundle within the interspace. The costal margin of the rib was divided with a rib cutter. A small segment of this rib was excised. The fibers of the diaphragm were divided with cautery in a radial fashion. A small rim of the diaphragm was left intact so as to facilitate closure and postoperative function of the diaphragm. Either side of the diaphragm was marked with interrupted sutures of different colors so as to assist closure at the conclusion of the case. A rib retractor was placed, as well as a self-retaining retractor in the abdomen. The abdominal contents in the peritoneal sac were bluntly dissected free and swept anteriorly, exposing the length of the abdominal aorta. Proximal control was obtained above the aneurysm. At this point, via gentle blunt and sharp dissection a red rubber catheter was passed circumferentially around the aorta proximally. Inferiorly, the left iliac artery was encircled with a Rummel tourniquet. The right iliac artery was slotted on either side so that a clamp could be placed there. Retroperitoneal fatty tissue surrounding the abdominal aorta was carefully dissected away from the posterior portion of the aorta. The origin of the left renal artery was identified. The left retroaortic ileolumbar vein was identified and divided between silk ligatures. Anesthesia administered lasix and mannitol to promote diuresis. Heparin, 5,000 U, was administered intravenously. An appropriately sized (22–32 mm) coated Dacron graft was selected. After approximately 3–5 min and appropriate reduction of systemic blood pressure, the iliac arteries were occluded distally. The proximal aorta was occluded with a vascular occlusive clamp. An arteriotomy was created with a #11 blade through the aneurysm. This was extended cephalad with a large Mayo scissor until healthy aortic tissue was identified. The aortic lumen was dissected free of thrombotic material and debris. The origins of the celiac, superior mesenteric, and right and left renal arteries were identified/*and were controlled with balloon catheters*.

[Choose one:]

If type IV: The visceral and renal vessels were in close proximity to each other and the aneurysm neck. The proximal end of the graft was spatulated and the proximal anastomosis was performed in an end-to-end fashion incorporating the orifices of the celiac, superior mesenteric, and both renal arteries. The anastomosis was constructed with a 0-prolene suture with pledgets at the first and last stitches. After completion of the proximal anastomosis, the vascular clamp was moved from the proximal aorta onto the graft.

If types I, II, or III: The proximal end of the graft was spatulated and the proximal anastomosis was performed in an end-to-end fashion with a 0-prolene suture with pledgets at the first and last stitches. After completion of the proximal anastomosis, the vascular clamp was moved from the proximal aorta onto the graft.

Alternative 1: The visceral and both renal vessels were in close proximity to each other and a Carrel patch was fashioned to incorporate all of them. A matching elliptical segment of the graft opposing the visceral/renal patch was excised. The anastomosis between the graft and the patch was performed using 0-prolene sutures.

***Alternative 2:** The celiac, superior mesenteric, and right renal arteries were in close proximity to each other and a Carrel patch was fashioned to incorporate these three vessels. A matching elliptical segment of the graft opposing the visceral/renal patch was excised. The anastomosis between the graft and the patch was performed using 0-prolene sutures. The left renal artery was flushed with iced/heparinized saline solution and was reimplanted into the graft/a separate side limb of the graft via a preconstructed 6-mm Dacron sidearm graft.*

Care was taken to identify intercostal arteries. *Large intercostal arteries that were found in the lower portion of the chest/upper portion of the abdomen were incorporated into either the proximal or visceral anastomosis.* After the anastomosis, several pledgeted sutures were used where appropriate for controlling bleeding from the visceral patch. On completion of the visceral anastomosis, the aorta was allowed to bleed antegrade to remove clot and debris. An occlusive clamp was then placed across the end of the graft distal to the visceral anastomosis. The suture line was tested. When secure, the proximal clamp was released. Hemostasis was achieved with pledgeted sutures. The arteriotomy was then extended to an area just above the aortic bifurcation. The graft was cut to the correct length and spatulated appropriately. The distal end-to-end anastomosis was performed with running 3-0 prolene sutures. Pledgeted sutures were used for hemostasis along the suture line. Prior to completion of the distal anastomosis, the graft was bled antegrade and the iliac arteries were back-bled. Anesthesia then administered sodium bicarbonate. The anastomosis was completed and the three anastomoses checked for hemostasis. Protamine was then administered. A thin PTFE cardiac membrane was used to facilitate closing the aneurysm sac over the graft. The diaphragm was reconstructed using non-absorbable interrupted vertical mattress sutures. The ribs were reapproximated with double rib sutures of #2 absorbable suture. The pericostal muscles were approximated in two layers using a running 2-0 Vicryl suture. The anterior abdominal wall was reapproximated in two layers using a running 1-0 looped PDS suture. Before closure of the chest, two chest tubes, a 28-French straight and a 28-French angled, were placed exiting through the anterior axillary line through separate stab incisions. The chest tubes were anchored in place with silk sutures. The subcutaneous tissue was approximated using a running 3-0 Vicryl suture. The skin was approximated with a 4-0 Vicryl subcuticular closure, both in the chest and abdomen. At the conclusion of the case, distal perfusion in the feet and the lower extremity was evaluated and there was no evidence of compromised flow.

The patient tolerated the procedure well and was taken to the intensive care unit in stable condition.

NOTES

Chapter 181

Thoracic Endovascular Repair (TEVAR) for Thoracic Aortic Aneurysm

Parth B. Amin, M.D.

Preoperative diagnosis: Thoracic aortic aneurysm.
Postoperative diagnosis: Same.
Procedure: Placement of thoracic aortic stent graft (*with carotid-subclavian bypass/transposition*).
Complications: None.
Condition: Stable to ICU.
Indications for procedure: Patient is a ___ -year-old male/female with findings of a symptomatic/asymptomatic thoracic aortic aneurysm. After assessment of symptoms, size of aneurysm, and observation with serial imaging, a thorough discussion of treatment options was discussed with the patient. (Coverage of the left subclavian artery and need for carotid/subclavian bypass/transposition was also discussed). The risks of paraplegia, bleeding, stroke, and death were discussed at length and patient.
Description of procedure: Preoperative lines and spinal drain was placed by anesthesia. EEG monitoring was performed. Preoperative antibiotics were administered. In the supine position, the patient was then prepped and draped in a sterile fashion from the chin to the knees. *If carotid subclavian bypass*: A left supraclavicular incision was performed. This was deepened through the skin, subcutaneous tissue, and platysma. The scalene fat pad was identified. The phrenic nerve was then identified anterior to the anterior scalene muscle. With the sternocleidomastoid retracted medially, sharp dissection was used to divide the anterior scalene while protecting the phrenic nerve. The thoracic duct was also

J.J. Hoballah and C.E.H. Scott-Conner (eds.), *Operative Dictations in General and Vascular Surgery*, DOI 10.1007/978-1-4614-0451-4_181,
© Springer Science+Business Media, LLC 2012

protected and identified. The subclavian artery was dissected circumferentially and control obtained with vessel loops. The carotid artery was then exposed and controlled with vessel loops. After administration of 5,000 units of heparin an activated clotting time was sent. A test clamp of the common carotid was performed showing no EEG changes. After clamping of the common carotid and the subclavian, an 8-mm ringed PTFE graft was used to perform a standard 6-0 prolene running anastomosis from the common carotid, on the left side to the subclavian artery. The PTFE graft and was flushed, back bled and forward bled and clamps were removed from the common carotid. The EEG showed no changes during this time. The wound itself was then irrigated out and closed in multiple layers with 3-0 vicryl followed by 4-0 monocryl.

Attention was then turned to the bilateral groins. A transverse incision was made one fingerbreath inferior to the inguinal ligament. This was deepened through the skin, subcutaneous tissue, and femoral sheath. The common femoral was identified and sharp dissection used to circumferentially expose the CFA. Vessel loop was placed around the vessel. The same exposure was used on the left side as well. A 4-French micropuncture wire was then used to gain access to the CFA, and exchanged for a 6-French sheath under fluoroscopy. A glidewire and omniflush marking catheter then placed into the aortic arch. An arch aortogram was performed with additional steep left oblique views. Measurements of the aortic diameter and landing zone were taken and noted to be as follows _____. The distance from the left subclavian was also noted as follows_____. A 6-French sheath was then placed into the left CFA with advancement of a glidewire into the arch. A repeat measurement of the proximal neck was then undertaken and compared to the preoperative computed tomography images. Using these measurements, a _____ × _____ stent graft was chosen. The device was flushed with heparinized saline. The right glidewire was exchanged for an Amplatz SuperStiff and the marking catheter placed through the left side. A repeat heparin bolus was administered to keep the ACT above 250 s. The delivery sheath for the Endoprosthesis was placed through the right CFA and observed under fluoroscopy. Once it was in the thoracic aorta, reperat angiogram was performed to evaluate the proximal neck and the distal landing zone. The graft was then deployed just (proxima/distal) to the left subclavian. (A second graft was deployed distally with ____ cm of overlap). Balloon dilation was performed with a Coda balloon. Completion angiogram was performed showing good filling of the left common carotid and no endoleak. Multiple projections were used to confirm the findings. The catheters and wires were removed, the sheaths removed and access sites closed with running 6-0 prolene suture. The groin wounds were irrigated out and closed in multiple layers of 3-0 vicryl followed by a 4-0 subcuticular closure. Patients pedal pulses/signals were unchanged from preop. The patient was extubated, found to be moving all extremities, and taken to ICU in critical condition.

Chapter 182

Creation of Iliac Conduit Prior to Tevar/Evar

Sung Woon Chung, M.D., and Jamal J. Hoballah, M.D., M.B.A.

INDICATION

- Iliac anatomy that precludes insertion of a large aortic device through the femoral/iliac artery.

ESSENTIAL STEPS

1. 10-cm oblique skin incision mid-distance between the costal margin and the anterior superior iliac crest.
2. Division of the external, internal oblique muscles and the transversalis abdominal fascia.
3. Dissection in the retroperitoneum with mobilization of the peritoneal contents medially.
4. Exposure and control of the common, internal, and external iliac arteries.
5. Heparinization: 75 UI/kg.
6. Applying vascular clamps on the common, internal, and external iliac arteries.
7. Performance of another angiogram under magnification.
8. Creation of a 12-mm arteriotomy in the external/common iliac artery.
9. Construction of an anastomosis with a 10-mm Dacron graft.
10. Exposure of the common femoral artery through a transverse inguinal incision.
11. Creation of a tunnel from the retroperitoneum to the inguinal incision.
12. Passage of the graft in the tunnel.

J.J. Hoballah and C.E.H. Scott-Conner (eds.), *Operative Dictations in General and Vascular Surgery*, DOI 10.1007/978-1-4614-0451-4_182,
© Springer Science+Business Media, LLC 2012

NOTE THIS VARIATION

- The iliac conduit may be ligated at the end of the procedure or anastomosed to the common femoral artery in the presence of severe iliac occlusive disease.

COMPLICATION

- Bleeding/disruption of the anastomosis while passing or removing the aortic device.

TEMPLATE DICTATION

Preoperative diagnosis: Performance of TEVAR/EVAR in the presence of small/occluded external iliac arteries.

Procedure: Creation of iliac artery conduit.

Postoperative diagnosis: Same.

Indications: The patient has a thoracic/abdominal aortic aneurysm and is a candidate for endovascular treatment. His iliac arteries were of a *small size/occluded* not allowing the passage of the stent graft necessitating the construction of a conduit to the common iliac artery.

Details of the operation: With the patient in the supine position and after induction of general anesthesia, the abdomen and chest were prepped and draped in the usual sterile fashion. A transverse incision was then performed over the lateral aspect of the flank. This was deepened through the external and internal oblique muscles. The transverse fascia was then incised. The retroperitoneum was entered and the peritoneal contents were mobilized medially exposing the iliac vessels. The external iliac artery was then identified and encircled with a vessel loop. Dissection proximally was performed until the mid-level of the common iliac artery. The take-off of the internal iliac artery was also identified and controlled. The patient was then given 5,000 units of IV Heparin and the common, internal, and external iliac arteries were clamped. A 12–15 mm arteriotomy was then performed in the common iliac artery. A size 10-mm diameter Dacron graft was then obtained and beveled to match the opening in the common iliac artery. The anastomosis was then conducted using a 4-0 Prolene running suture. At the completion of the anastomosis there was evidence of excellent hemostasis. The graft was flushed. A transverse incision was then made in the groin and the common femoral artery was dissected. The graft was then tunneled from the retroperitoneal space into the inguinal incision. The wound was packed with a lap pad and the procedure was then continued for the endovascular *thoracic/abdominal* aortic aneurysm repair.

Chapter 183

Percutaneous Fenestration and Stenting of Complicated Acute Type B Aortic Dissections

Mel J. Sharafuddin, M.D.

INDICATION

■ Evidence of end organ malperfusion as a result of branch vessels static or dynamic occlusion caused by a descending aortic dissection flap.

ESSENTIAL STEPS

1. Initial evaluation requires demonstration of the upper and lower limits of the dissection flap and the characteristics of each branch vessel obstruction.
2. Intravascular Ultrasound (IVUS) is invaluable in assessing the location of the guidewires whether in true or false lumen. IVUS also is an excellent supplement to pressure measurements in determining the effectiveness of the therapy. Angiography alone is often deceptive. The pressurization of the true or false lumen with contrast may distort the in vivo position of the intimal flap.
3. Proper selection of the access vessels based on individual dissection patterns is critical. Often access to the right brachial artery is needed if true lumen access from the femoral arteries is compromised by the dissection flap.
4. Anticoagulate with IV heparin sulfate (100 U/kg).
5. Access and verify position of the guidewire in the true lumen using transesophageal echo or intravascular ultrasound.

J.J. Hoballah and C.E.H. Scott-Conner (eds.), *Operative Dictations in General and Vascular Surgery*, DOI 10.1007/978-1-4614-0451-4_183,
© Springer Science+Business Media, LLC 2012

6. Position guidewire in the false lumen either by puncture of the intimal flap or through a separate access or natural fenestration.
7. Controlled balloon dilatation of the intimal flap, or tearing if using the snare or retrograde approaches.
8. Reimage dissection flap after each intervention to confirm true lumen re-pressurization.
9. Stenting of branch vessels that continue to have dissections extending into them.

NOTE THESE VARIATIONS
■ Three options for fenestration:
   ○ Trans-intimal puncture – Described under operative dictation.
   ○ Snaring of the guidewire across an existing fenestration. By passing a guide wire through a defect in the flap, then snaring from the false lumen and pulling a cut through the flap may be created.
   ○ Retrograde fenestration using a Sheath. Through a single sheath access is obtained into both the true and false lumens using two separate wires. A long sheath is then advanced over these two wires to the level of the infrarenal aorta creating a tear in retrograde fashion.

COMPLICATIONS
■ Aortic Rupture.
■ Propagation of dissection flap.
■ Embolization.
■ Failure to reperfuse target vessels.

TEMPLATE OPERATIVE DICTATION
Preoperative diagnosis: Malperfusion secondary to descending aortic dissection.
Procedure: (1) Thoracic endograft of acute aortic dissection, (2) percutaneous fenestration of intimal dissection flap, (3) celiac artery stenting, (4) intravascular ultrasound of the aorta, (5) aortogram, (6) selective mesenteric arteriogram, and (7) open access to right femoral artery (unilateral).
Postoperative diagnosis: Malperfusion secondary to descending aortic dissection.
Indications: This ___-year-old *male/female* patient presented with severe back and abdominal pain. Computed tomographic angiography demonstrated a dissection within the descending aorta.

The visceral vessels were originating from either the true or false lumen as follows: _____. There is evidence of malperfusion of the *renal and or visceral vessels* due to *renal insufficiency or abdominal pain and elevated white blood cell count and rising acidosis.*

Description of procedure: The procedure was performed under *general/spinal/epidural* anesthesia. The patient was positioned on the operating table in a supine position. The right arm and bilaterally groins were prepped and draped in a sterile fashion.

The right common femoral artery is exposed through an oblique incision just above the inguinal crease. Arterial access is established from both common femoral arteries (CFAs). The left-sided access was obtained percutaneously. If there was no palpable pulse, an ultrasound-guided puncture was performed. Soft-tip J wires are advanced to the level of the aortic valve. 7-F sheaths are placed into the groins. An intravascular ultrasound catheter is advanced from the left groin to the level of the left subclavian artery. The position of both wires with respect to the intimal flap is then confirmed. The position of the intimal flap and its relationship to the visceral vessels is documented. The locations of any large fenestrations were noted.

The visceral vessels are confirmed by ultrasound to be originating from the true lumen which is compressed. The celiac appears partially dissected. There is a large fenestration just distal to the left subclavian artery extending 3 cm.

A straight exchange catheter is placed over the right-sided guidewire. True lumen pressure measurements are made at the level of the visceral vessels. This catheter is then used to exchange to a stiff Amplatz wire to the level of the aortic valve. The femoral sheath is exchanged to large bore sheath appropriate for the thoracic endograft device. Based on computed tomographic estimations of the normal size aorta for this patient an endograft that is closest to the diameter is chosen. Oversizing was avoided. The graft is delivered to the level of the subclavian and deployed. The stent graft was NOT balloon dilated after deployment. Over the wire a pigtail catheter is placed and flush aortogram performed. The IVUS catheter wire and device on the left are withdrawn below the level of the graft and advanced into the arch. Repeat IVUS of the aorta is performed. The fenestration appears completely covered by the stent graft. The true lumen is pressurized and appears larger than prior to the deployment of the stent graft to the level of the diaphragm. Yet, the visceral vessels which continue to arise from the true lumen are still compressed. The decision is made to fenestrate the infrarenal aorta.

Through the right femoral access sheath a Rösch-Uchida transjugular liver access needle sheath is advanced over the Amplatz wire to the level of the infrarenal aorta based on IVUS within the true lumen. The level of puncture should allow enough room from the needle to be safely passed in to the false lumen. Under fluoroscopic and intravascular US control, the needle assembly was positioned until it could be clearly seen indenting the intimal flap. The puncture is created from the true to the false lumen using a 5-F catheter and 20-G. Nitinol needle. The stylet is removed leaving the inner catheter in place. Through the catheter a stiff guidewire is advanced well into the false lumen. A straight catheter was then placed into the false lumen over the guidewire. False lumen pressure measurements were made. Arteriography confirmed no extravasation of contrast. An amplatz stiff guidewire is then advanced through the straight catheter into the false lumen. A small diameter 4- to 6-mm balloon is then advanced under fluoroscopic and IVUS guidance to the level of the fenestration. Dilatation is performed to allow advancement of the larger diameter balloon for final fenestration. A large diameter 15- to 20-mm balloon is then advanced to the level of the fenestration and a slow dilation is performed to profile. If the balloon needed to be repositioned it was deflated fully prior to manipulation to prevent advancement of the intimal flap into branch vessels or injury to the aortic wall itself. The IVUS catheter which lies in the true lumen is then exchanged to a straight catheter and pressure measurements in to the true and false lumens are made simultaneously. A gradient less than 5 mmHg between true and false lumens denoted success.

The IVUS catheter is then placed back to the level of the left subclavian artery and the aorta is again reassessed. The celiac artery is noted to continue to be compressed by the false lumen. The superior mesenteric artery and renal vessels appear to have adequate luminal diameter. Through the left femoral access a short LIMA 7-F guiding catheter is used to cannulate the celiac artery. Selective lateral arteriography confirms true lumen access. A 0.018 in. wire is placed into the celiac artery. An 8-mm balloon expandable stent was then deployed at the level of the ostial extending 1–2 mm into the aorta. Completion arteriography demonstrated patency of the celiac artery.

The sheaths are removed. The right femoral artery is repaired with 5-0 prolene and the wound closed in layers. A percutaneous closure device is used to close the left femoral artery access site.

ANGIOGRAM SUPERVISION AND INTERPRETATION

1. **Flush aortogram:** Pigtail is placed at the level of the supraceliac aorta within the true lumen based on IVUS findings. An anterioposterior arteriogram reveals aortic dissection to the level of the iliac arteries, with unrestricted flow into the common femoral arteries. The right renal artery does not opacify, the left renal fills well with no evidence of stenosis. A lateral projection demonstrates a small true lumen with obstructed flow into the celiac and SMA arteries.

2. **Thoracic stent endograft:** A 26 mm × 10 cm thoracic endograft was deployed at the level of the left subclavian artery. This was not angioplastied. Completion arteriogram demonstrated filling of true lumen with retrograde filling of the false lumen from fenestrations occurring below the level of the diaphragm.

3. **Aortic balloon angioplasty:** After an intimal puncture was created with Rösch-Uchida transjugular liver access needle a 6-mm angioplasty balloon was used to the predilate the fenestration initially. A 15-mm balloon is used to angioplasty the intimal puncture site. This is inflated to profile.

4. **Selective mesenteric arteriogram:** The celiac artery was selectively cannulated with a guiding catheter. Arteriography revealed a comprised ostia with otherwise unobstructed flow in to the celiac artery and its branches.

5. **Celiac artery balloon angioplasty:** An 8 mm × 15 mm balloon expandable stent was deployed at the origin of the celiac artery with 2 mm into the aorta. Post-stenting angiography revealed wide patency of the celiac artery and no evidence of distal embolization.

NOTES

Preoperative Imaging

Contrast CT scan of the chest, abdomen and pelvis with 3-mm increments and 3D reconstruction.

Anatomic Requirements

Nonthrombosed false lumen.
Access to true lumen either from brachial or femoral arteries.

Contraindications

New dense neurologic deficit.
Chronic dissections.
Evidence of aortic rupture or leak.

Chapter 184

Elective Transabdominal Replacement of Infrarenal Abdominal Aortic Aneurysm

Jamal J. Hoballah, M.D., M.B.A.

INDICATIONS

- Diameter >5.5 cm in men, 5.0 cm in women.
- Rapid growth >1 cm in 1 year.
- Distal embolization.
- Tenderness.

ESSENTIAL STEPS

1. Midline xiphoid to pubis incision.
2. Abdominal exploration for unexpected findings.
3. Retract the transverse colon anteriorly and to the right.
4. Retract the splenic flexure posteriorly and laterally.
5. Divide the peritoneal periaortic attachment of the duodenum.
6. Wrap the small bowel in a wet towel and retract to the right.
7. Incise the retroperitoneum overlying the aorta and continue proximally.
8. Identify the left renal vein.
9. Dissect the aortic aneurysm neck and prepare it for clamping.
10. Incise the retroperitoneum overlying the aorta and continue distally.
11. Expose the right common iliac artery and its bifurcation.
12. Dissect the right external and internal iliac arteries and prepare them for clamping.

J.J. Hoballah and C.E.H. Scott-Conner (eds.), *Operative Dictations in General and Vascular Surgery*, DOI 10.1007/978-1-4614-0451-4_184,
© Springer Science+Business Media, LLC 2012

13. Incise the peritoneal attachments of the sigmoid colon to the lateral abdominal wall.
14. Reflect the sigmoid medially and expose the left external iliac artery.
15. Extend the dissection to expose the left common iliac artery and its bifurcation.
16. Dissect the left external and internal iliac arteries and prepare them for clamping.
17. Anticoagulate with heparin 75–100 U/kg and wait 5 min.
18. Cross-clamp the external and internal iliac arteries, and then the aorta.
19. Enter the aneurysm and remove aneurysmal content.
20. Oversew bleeding lumbars and control the inferior mesenteric artery (IMA).
21. Prepare the proximal neck for construction of the anastomosis.
22. Construct the proximal anastomosis and check for hemostasis.
23. Construct the right distal anastomosis and check for hemostasis.
24. Perfuse into the internal iliac artery first, and then the external iliac artery.
25. Repeat the same on the left.
26. Check sigmoid viability.
27. Re-evaluate hemostasis.
28. Close the aneurysm wall.
29. Close the abdomen.
30. Recheck distal pulses.

NOTE THESE VARIATIONS

- Endovascular repair (EVAR) is typically offered first as an option if the anatomy is appropriate.
- When constructing the proximal anastomosis, the aneurysm neck can be completely transected or Td off, leaving the posterior wall intact.
- The distal anastomosis is carried at the aortic bifurcation or iliac level depending on the distal extent of the aneurysmal disease.
- Every attempt is made to reperfuse at least one hypogastric vessel. The IMA is reimplanted if there is concern regarding the adequacy of the pelvic reperfusion.

COMPLICATIONS

- Bleeding.
- Myocardial infarction.
- Pneumonia.
- Renal failure.
- Wound infection.
- Wound dehiscence.
- Limb ischemia.
- Bowel ischemia.
- Buttock ischemia.
- Spinal cord ischemia.

TEMPLATE OPERATIVE DICTATION

Preoperative diagnosis: *Asymptomatic/tender* abdominal aortic aneurysm.

Procedure: Replacement of *infrarenal/juxtarenal* abdominal aortic aneurysm with *tube/bifurcated* graft.

Postoperative diagnosis: Same.

Indications: This is a ___-year-old *male/female* with an *asymptomatic/tender* abdominal aortic aneurysm measuring ___ cm. The risks of rupture and surgical intervention were discussed with the patient and *he/she* elected to undergo surgical intervention. The patient was not deemed to be a good candidate for EVAR.

Description of procedure: The patient was placed supine on the operating table. *His/her* arms were *tucked in/placed at 80°*. Normal bony prominences were padded. Anesthesia placed appropriate lines and induced and intubated the patient without complications. A Foley catheter was then placed under sterile technique. The patient's anterior abdomen and both lower extremities were circumferentially prepped and draped in the usual sterile fashion. Preoperative antibiotics were administered prior to skin incision.

The skin incision was then made from the subxiphoid to the suprapubic region. The subcutaneous tissue was divided with electrocautery. The linea alba was exposed and incised. The peritoneum was elevated and entered sharply. The abdominal wall incision was then extended to the full length of the skin incision.

There was *no/moderate number of* adhesions requiring lysis.

Abdominal exploration revealed *no/the following* incidental findings (detail).

The transverse colon was then elevated superiorly out of the wound, wrapped in a moist towel. A moist rolled lap pad was placed in the bed of the splenic flexure of the colon, which was retracted laterally and posteriorly. The remainder of the small bowel was then deflected to the right, exposing the aortic aneurysm. Sharp dissection of the ligament of Treitz and the distal fourth portion of the duodenum allowed further exposure of the aneurysm and retraction of the small bowel to the right. The small bowel was then wrapped in a moistened towel and held in place using an Omni retractor.

The retroperitoneum overlying the aorta was incised and continued proximally to the level of the left renal vein. *The inferior mesenteric vein was encountered, ligated, and divided.* The lymphatics overlying the aortic neck were ligated and divided.

The abdominal aortic aneurysm neck was then sharply dissected.

The infrarenal neck appeared to be adequate for clamping and constructing the proximal anastomosis.

The infrarenal neck appeared to be inadequate for clamping and constructing the proximal anastomosis. Further mobilization of the left renal vein was performed. The left gonadal, lumbar, and adrenal veins were ligated and divided. The left renal vein was circumferentially mobilized and retracted proximally, exposing the renal arteries. The suprarenal aorta was sharply dissected and appeared adequate for clamping.

The dissection was then carried out in the pelvic region for exposure of the iliac arteries.

The retroperitoneum overlying the aorta was incised distally, exposing the right common iliac artery and its bifurcation. The right external and internal iliac arteries were dissected and prepared for clamping. The right ureter was identified and protected.

The peritoneal attachments of the sigmoid colon to the lateral abdominal wall were incised. The sigmoid colon was reflected medially, exposing the left external iliac artery. The dissection was extended proximally, exposing the left common iliac artery and its bifurcation. The left external and internal iliac arteries were dissected and prepared for clamping. The left ureter was identified and protected.

Heparin 75–100 U/kg and mannitol 12.5 g were administered intravenously. After 5 min from the heparin administration, the external arteries were cross-clamped, followed by the internal iliac arteries and then the aorta.

The aneurysm wall was then incised longitudinally on its anterior aspect, keeping to the right of the origin of the inferior mesenteric artery. The aneurysm cavity was entered and the aneurysm content and debris removed. The IMA had pulsatile back-bleeding and was oversewn with 2-0 silk sutures/*the IMA had sluggish back-bleeding and was controlled with a double-looped silastic tape*. The bleeding lumbar arteries and middle sacral artery were oversewn with figure-of-eight 2-0 silk sutures.

The aneurysm neck was then prepared for the construction of the proximal anastomosis. The incision in the aorta was carried to the level of the neck of the aneurysm. The incision was then Td off on each side of the neck, leaving the posterior wall intact/*transecting the posterior wall*.

A *20 × 10/18 × 9/16 × 8 Dacron/PTFE* graft was then soaked in antibiotic solution. The body of the graft was trimmed for the proximal anastomosis. The anastomosis was constructed in a running fashion using 3-0 prolene sutures. At the completion of the suture line, the sutures were tied and the anastomosis checked for hemostasis. Hemostasis was *adequate/except for a suture line bleeding controlled with an interrupted mattress suture/needle hole bleeding controlled with the topical application of Gelfoam soaked with thrombin*.

Attention was focused on the iliac anastomoses.

The right side was performed first. The incision in the right common iliac artery was carried beyond the aneurysmal disease. The incision was then Td off on each side, leaving the posterior wall intact/*transecting the posterior wall*.

The right limb of the graft was then sized and cut. The anastomosis was then performed with 4-0 prolene running sutures. Prior to completing the anastomosis the iliac clamps were released, allowing for back-bleeding of the right external and internal iliac arteries. The aortic clamp was released for forward-flushing of the graft. The anastomosis was copiously irrigated with heparinized saline solution. The clamps were then released, allowing flow into the internal iliac artery first, followed by the external iliac artery. The right femoral artery was palpated and had a strong pulse.

Attention was then focused on the left iliac anastomosis. An incision in the left common iliac artery was carried beyond the aneurysmal disease. The incision was then Td off on each side, leaving the posterior wall intact/*transecting the posterior wall*.

The left limb of the graft was then tunneled *through/anterior to* the left common iliac artery and then sized and cut. Again, this was done in similar fashion with 4-0 prolene running sutures. Prior to completing the anastomosis, the graft limb was forward-flushed and the anastomosis back-bled and copiously irrigated with heparin saline solution. The anastomosis was then completed and blood flow resumed first into the internal iliac artery, followed by the external iliac artery. The left femoral artery was palpated and had a strong pulse.

The aneurysm lumen was reinspected. Hemostasis was *adequate/bleeding from a lumbar artery was identified and was controlled with figure-of-eight 2-0 silk sutures*.

The IMA was re-evaluated. There was evidence of good back-bleeding and good Doppler signals in the sigmoid mesentery. The IMA was oversewn with a 3-0 prolene sutures/*there was poor back-bleeding and poor Doppler signals in the sigmoid mesentery. IMA reimplantation was performed. The IMA was prepared by creating a circular button of aortic wall around the orifice of the IMA. An eversion endarterectomy of the orifice was performed. A partially occluding clamp was then applied to the aortic graft. An incision was then created in the graft and the anastomosis to the IMA was performed using 4-0 prolene running sutures. After the completion of the anastomosis there was evidence of good Doppler signals in the sigmoid mesentery*.

Reinspection of all the suture lines was performed and revealed adequate hemostasis.

The field was then irrigated with antibiotic solution.

The redundant aneurysm wall was then sutured over the aortic graft using 3-0 Vicryl suture, minimizing the dead space between the aortic graft and the aortic wall.

The retroperitoneum was then closed with 3-0 Vicryl in a running fashion.

The bowel was then placed back in the anatomic position.

Abdominal wall closure was then performed with *running/interrupted* 0 prolene sutures.

The wound was reirrigated, dried, and the skin edges opposed with skin staples.

The peri-incisional prep and drape were cleaned and dried, followed by 4×4 gauze, silk tape.

The feet were inspected and there was evidence of strong Doppler signals.

The patient tolerated the procedure well, was awakened, and was taken to the *postanesthesia care unit/intensive care unit* in stable condition.

Chapter 185

Left Posterolateral Retroperitoneal Abdominal Aortic Aneurysm Repair

Dale Maharaj, M.D. and R. Clement Darling III, M.D.

INDICATIONS

- As for the conventional transperitoneal approach – especially if juxtarenal, for reoperative aortic procedures, inflammatory aneurysms, aneurysms associated with a horseshoe kidney.
- Particularly useful in patients with previous transperitoneal procedures and in obese patients.

COMPLICATIONS

- Hemorrhage.
- Graft thrombosis.
- Trash foot.
- Spinal ischemia.
- Splenic injury.
- Ureteric injury.
- Flank bulge/hernia.
- Intercostals neuralgia.
- Anastomotic pseudoaneurysm.

ESSENTIAL STEPS

1. Incise skin and muscle obliquely between tenth and eleventh interspace.
2. The posterior peritoneum and posterior Gerota's fascia are retracted anteriorly, medially and cephalad.
3. Obtain distal arterial control before proximal (iliac or femoral).

J.J. Hoballah and C.E.H. Scott-Conner (eds.), *Operative Dictations in General and Vascular Surgery*, DOI 10.1007/978-1-4614-0451-4_185,
© Springer Science+Business Media, LLC 2012

4. Anticoagulate with heparin after dissection and just prior to clamping.

5. If the right common or external iliac segments are involved, a right suprainguinal counterincision is made for access to the external iliac, or vertical groin incisions for access to the femoral vessels.

6. Identify and clamp the common iliac arteries.

7. The neck of the aneurysm is located using the following landmarks – the left crus of the diaphragm, the lumbar branch of the left renal vein, and the left renal artery.

8. Ligate the lumbar branch of the left renal vein. Retract the left kidney and peritoneum medial, cephalad, and anterior.

9. The non-aneurysmal neck of the aorta is cross-clamped.

10. The lumbar and inferior mesenteric arteries can be controlled from outside the aneurysm sac, or suture ligated from within.

11. The aneurysm sac is opened and any residual back-bleeders are oversewn with 3/0 polypropylene.

12. The proximal anastomosis is performed with 3/0 polypropylene continuous suture.

13. The distal aortic, iliac, or femoral anastomoses are performed either in an end-to-end or inn an end-to-side configuration as dictated by the anatomy.

14. Assess the anastomotic sites and secure hemostasis.

15. Inspect spleen and descending colon via a small peritoneal window.

16. Close the wound.

OPERATIVE NOTE

Preoperative diagnosis	Suprarenal/infrarenal AAA or aortoiliac aneurysm (R or L iliac involvement)	
Procedure	Aneurysmorraphy with a tube/bifurcation graft	
	Distal anastomosis to	Aorta
		Right common iliac/external iliac/ femoral
		Left common iliac/external iliac/ femoral
	PTFE	Dacron
Postoperative diagnosis	Same	

Indications	____-year-old man/woman with:
	Symptomatic/asymptomatic/ruptured ____cm AAA found on
	Duplex/angiography/MRA
	Diameter ____cm

Description of the procedure: The patient was placed on a bean bag in the right lateral decubitus position with the left shoulder elevated to 45° and the left thigh elevated 15 in. above the horizontal plane (corkscrew).

The table was extended to open the space between the costal margin and the iliac crest.

The procedure was performed under general endotracheal anesthesia.

The abdomen, flank, and both groins were prepped and draped in a standard surgical fashion.

An oblique incision was made extending from the posterior axillary line to the lateral border of the rectus muscle, through the tenth or eleventh interspace.

The incision was deepened through the muscle layers with electrocautery.

The retroperitoneal space was entered and the peritoneum and Gerota's fascia were retracted anterior and cephalad. Care was taken not to retract too vigorously on the cephalad retractor to prevent splenic trauma. The fascia is left intact on the left psoas muscle.

Exposure was maintained using a Buckwalter self-retaining retractor.

30 U/kg of heparin was administered intravenously just before clamping.

The right and left common iliac arteries were dissected and cross-clamped using a double rubber and/or a straight Cooley clamp.

The aneurysm neck was identified. This was facilitated by division of the lumbar branch of the left renal vein.

Circumferential control of the proximal aorta was achieved and the aorta was cross-clamped above the level of the aneurysm neck using a Fogarty clamp or a large DeBakey aortic clamp.

The inferior mesenteric and the lumbar vessels were clip ligated before opening the aneurysm sac.

The sac was then opened using electocautery and the back-bleeding lumbar arteries were oversewn with 3/0 polypropylene suture.

The aorta was then transected at the level of the aneurysm neck.

A 16-mm PTFE tube/bifurcation graft was sutured to the proximal cut end of the aorta using a 3/0 poly propylene continuous suture.

A second vascular clamp was placed on the graft, and the proximal clamp on the aorta was opened to assess for bleeding along the suture line, especially posteriorly. Hemostasis was confirmed.

The lumen of the graft then irrigated with heparinized saline.

The distal graft was anastomosed to the aorta (iliacs or femorals) in an end-to-end (end-to-side) fashion using 3/0 (5/0) polypropylene suture.

The common iliacs were unclamped sequentially and allowed to back-bleed, thus confirming good hemostasis at the distal suture line.

The external iliacs were Dopplered and excellent flow signals were noted bilaterally.

A 4-cm window was created in the peritoneum to assess for splenic injury and colonic ischemia. The spleen and the left colon were normal and the peritoneum was closed with 3/0 polypropylene.

Hemostasis was ensured.

The muscle was closed in three layers using 0 polypropylene or #1 PDS suture continuously.

The skin was closed with staples.

Sterile dressings were applied.

Adequate circulation to both feet was assessed.

The patient was taken to the recovery room in stable condition.

Chapter 186

Endovascular Abdominal Aortic Aneurysm Repair with the Gore Excluder Endograft

Cassius Iyad Ochoa Chaar, M.D., M.S. and Michel S. Makaroun, M.D.

INDICATIONS
- Infrarenal abdominal aortic aneurysm (AAA).
- Iliac artery aneurysm.

ESSENTIAL STEPS
1. Use general anesthesia or alternatively regional block in well-chosen patients.
2. Puncture both femoral arteries using micropuncture kit.
3. Advance a 0.035-in. starter wire and exchange to 8-Fr sheaths to start a tract.
4. Place Prostar (Abbott) sutures in the femoral arteries and exchange to short 11-Fr sheath on the contralateral side. On the ipsilateral side use a 180-cm superstiff Amplatz wire through the Prostar device and insert an 18-Fr sheath, 30 cm in length. If you are using a 31-mm main body endograft you need to use a 20-Fr sheath.
   - (Note: Use a Lunderquist wire in cases of severe iliac tortuosity)
   - (Steps 1–3 are used preferentially to perform percutaneous EVAR. As an alternative, the common femoral arteries can be exposed through transverse groin incisions prior to sheath placement)
5. Heparinize the patient with one bolus of 100 U/kg. There is no absolute need for ACT monitoring.

J.J. Hoballah and C.E.H. Scott-Conner (eds.), *Operative Dictations in General and Vascular Surgery*, DOI 10.1007/978-1-4614-0451-4_186,

6. Pass a 5-Fr pigtail marker catheter over guide wire through the contralateral artery.

7. Obtain aortogram and pelvic angiogram with a power injection of intravenous contrast. A 15-ml injection at a rate of 15 ml/s is usually adequate. Less contrast volume can be used with smaller channels and renal compromise or this step can be completely avoided if needed.

8. Measure the length of the aorta from the lowest renal artery to the ipsilateral common iliac artery bifurcation. This will determine the length of the endograft needed. If you are hesitating between two lengths, choose the longer one as you will lose length through the body of the AAA especially if you cross the legs of the endograft. You should aim to cover down to the iliac bifurcation.

9. Prepare the appropriate device. The diameter should have been chosen by evaluating the preoperative computerized tomography (CT) scan.

10. Advance the ipsilateral sheath as far into the aorta as possible.

11. Insert the main body of the excluder endograft through the ipsilateral femoral sheath and position in the infrarenal aorta.

12. Orient the endograft under fluoroscopy to the desired position. Crossing the limbs is usually a good option. It is also preferable to have the contralateral gate slightly anterior in order to facilitate subsequent cannulation.

13. Obtain a repeat aortogram orthogonal to the neck with magnification for final positioning. A 15° cranial angulation is usually required even in the absence of angulation of the neck of the aneurysm. A left anterior oblique (LAO) of 10–15° can better visualize the origins of the renal arteries in most cases. This however should be guided by the origin of the renal arteries on the CT scan.

14. Mark the lowest renal artery and pull the pigtail into the aorta.

15. Position the proximal marker of the endograft right under the lowest renal artery.

16. Pull back the long sheath to the light-colored shaft marker on the delivery device to expose the endograft completely in the aorta.

17. Loosen the deployment knob and exert a continuous pull to deploy the main body.

18. Confirm the position of the endograft with fluoroscopy.

19. Introduce a 180-cm stiff 0.035-in. Glidewire (Terumo) from the contralateral side and retrieve the pigtail catheter.
20. Use an angled 5-Fr selective catheter (e.g., KMP from Cook) and a torque device to cannulate the contralateral gate.
21. Confirm the position in the endograft either by twirling the angled catheter without the wire or use of a balloon.
22. Introduce a superstiff 180 cm 0.035 Amplatz wire through the selective catheter into the descending thoracic aorta.
23. Place pigtail catheter in the contralateral limb up to the long radiopaque marker of the main body proximally.
24. Obtain a retrograde iliac angiogram from the short iliac sheath and mark the iliac bifurcation and the distance to the gate.
25. Choose and prepare the contralateral limb.
26. Replace the short 11-Fr sheath with a 30-cm long 12-Fr sheath, or a larger sheath if a large limb is desired. Advance the sheath into the contralateral gate.
27. Insert the contralateral limb of the endograft to the level of the graft bifurcation 3 cm cephalad to the ring marker.
28. Pull back the long sheath to the light-colored shaft marker on the delivery device.
29. Loosen the deployment knob and exert a continuous pull to deploy the endograft.
30. Balloon angioplasty the neck, the sealing zones of the iliac limbs and the zone of overlap between the main body and the contralateral iliac limb.
31. Obtain completion angiogram and confirm the absence of endoleaks.
32. Remove sheath and catheters and reverse the heparin with protamine.
33. Close arteriotomies with Prostar sutures and skin with 4-0 polysorb. Alternatively, the arteriotomies can be closed with 5-0 prolene and the skin and the subcutaneous in the standard surgical manner.

COMPLICATIONS

- Early: Bleeding, iliac artery dissection or rupture, distal embolization, kinking, systemic complications.
- Late: Endoleak, Aneurysm rupture, migration, limb thrombosis, structural graft failure, graft infection.

TEMPLATE OPERATIVE DICTATION

Preoperative diagnosis: Infrarenal AAA.

Postoperative diagnosis: Same.

Procedure: (1) Percutaneous puncture of both common femoral arteries and placement of sheaths. (2) Advancement of catheter into the aorta. (3) Aortogram and pelvic angiogram. (4) Supervision and Interpretation (S&I). (5) Endovascular repair of abdominal aortic aneurysm with a bifurcated modular Excluder prosthesis (S&I). (6) Closure of femoral arteries.

Surgeon:

Anesthesia:

Indications: This ___-year-old *male/female* was found to have an asymptomatic, ___-cm infrarenal AAA suitable for endovascular repair on CT scan.

Description of procedure: The patient was placed in the supine position on the operating table. The procedure was performed under *general endotracheal/regional* anesthesia. A Foley catheter and arterial line were placed for monitoring. The abdomen and both groins were prepped and draped in the standard sterile fashion.

Prophylactic intravenous antibiotics were given prior to skin incision.

The common femoral arteries were accessed using a Seldinger technique. A starter wire was advanced into the aorta and an 8-Fr sheath was placed on each side. Prostar sutures were deployed in both femoral arteries and tagged outside the punctures. An 18-Fr sheath was placed on the right and an 11-Fr sheath on the left. The patient was heparinized (mention dose).

(For open access: The common femoral arteries were dissected bilaterally through transverse incisions and controlled below the inguinal ligament.)

A 5-Fr marker pigtail catheter was advanced to the level of the renal arteries, and an aortogram and pelvic angiogram were obtained. Single renal arteries were noted on both sides (or alternatively describe the anatomy of the renal arteries). The SMA was patent. The aneurysm starts 15 mm below the renal arteries and ends at the bifurcation (describe other anomalies, branches, involvement of the iliac arteries...). The length of the aorta from the lower renal artery to the right common iliac artery bifurcation was measured.

A ___×___mm, ___cm Gore Excluder endograft was prepared and advanced through the right sheath into the infrarenal aorta under fluoroscopy. Final positioning was obtained with serial injections at the level of the renals under magnification. The sheath was pulled back and the device deployed at the desired location.

The pigtail catheter was exchanged over a 0.035-in stiff glidewire to a 5-Fr KMP catheter. The contralateral gate was cannulated. The marker pigtail catheter was reintroduced through the left femoral sheath over an Amplatz wire and a retrograde left iliac angiogram was obtained to mark the common iliac artery bifurcation and confirm the length of the desired limb. A ____mm × ___cm contralateral limb was prepared. The 11-Fr sheath was exchanged for a 30-cm long 12-Fr sheath which was advanced into the contralateral gate. The limb was introduced and deployed at the graft bifurcation. A 14 mm×4 cm balloon was used to secure the overlap zone while a large compliant balloon was used to mold the endograft in the neck, and both iliac sealing zones.

A completion angiogram was obtained. It showed good position of the endograft with complete exclusion of the aneurysm. There were no apparent endoleaks. The wires, catheter, and sheaths were withdrawn. The arteriotomies were closed with the Prostar sutures and the closure was hemostatic. The skin was closed using a 4-0 Vicryl U-stitch. The heparin was reversed with protamine (mention dose). The patient tolerated the procedure well and was taken to the postanesthesia care unit in stable condition.

(For a cut down, the common femoral artery was repaired with a 5-0 prolene suture. Hemostasis was assured and the wounds were closed using 3-0 Vicryl sutures. The skin was closed with a subcuticular suture).

Chapter 187
EVAR Using the Powerlink Device

Parth B. Amin, M.D.

INDICATIONS

- Asymptomatic 5.5 cm or greater infrarenal aneurysm in male.
- 5.0 cm infrarenal aortic aneurysm in female.
- Contained rupture in hemodynamically stable patient.

ESSENTIAL STEPS

1. Examine femoral and lower extremity pulses preoperatively.
2. Measure length, diameter, and angulation of infrarenal aortic neck.
3. Determine size of landing site for device.
4. Femoral cutdown on side of device introduction (ipsilateral side).
5. Percutaneous access on contralateral side with 9-F sheath (contralateral side).
6. Biplanar aortogram.
7. Delivery of 180 cm wire from contralateral sheath to ipsilateral cutdown site through dual-lumen catheter, with assistance of snare catheter.
8. Place stiff wire access through ipsilateral side through skive on dual-lumen catheter.
9. Heparinize patient. Send ACT. Re-bolus heparin if inadequate.
10. Placement of Endologix Powerlink Device over stiff wire.

J.J. Hoballah and C.E.H. Scott-Conner (eds.), *Operative Dictations in General and Vascular Surgery*, DOI 10.1007/978-1-4614-0451-4_187,
© Springer Science+Business Media, LLC 2012

11. Deploy contralateral limb.
12. Bring entire device over iliac bifurcation.
13. Deploy main body of graft from distal to proximal, readjusting device as necessary.
14. Deploy ipsilateral limb of graft.
15. Remove catheter and wires.
16. Close arteriotomy.
17. Close groin in multiple layers.
18. Remove access sheath.
19. Hold pressure/use automatic closure device.

NOTE THESE VARIATIONS
- Need for extension cuffs proximally.
- Need for additional iliac limbs.
- Preoperative coiling for feeder vessel.

COMPLICATIONS
- Endoleak.
- Stent-graft migration.
- Percutaneous access site pseudoaneurysm.

OPERATIVE TEMPLATE
Preoperative diagnosis: Infrarenal abdominal aortic aneurysm.
Procedure: EVAR using Endologix Powerlink stent graft.
Postoperative diagnosis: Same as above.
Indications for procedure: Patient is a ____-year-old (male/female) with a history of (asymptomatic/symptomatic) abdominal aortic aneurysm. After noting appropriate anatomy for EVAR, and risks/benefits of open vs. endovascular repair, patient decided upon endograft placement.
Description of procedure: After correct patient and procedure to be performed was noted and preoperative IV antibiotics were administered, the patient was prepped and draped in a sterile fashion. A (right/left) femoral artery cutdown was performed sharply after which blunt and sharp dissection was used to encircle the SFA, profunda, and common femoral artery with vessel loops. On the contralateral (right/left) side, a 9-F catheter was inserted percutaneously, under fluoroscopic guidance. 5,000 units of heparin were then administered intravenously.

An 8-F sheath was then inserted through ipsilateral CFA. A pigtail catheter was inserted above the renal arteries over a guidewire and an aortogram was performed using ___ cc of contrast. An EnSnare catheter was advanced through the CFA at the cutdown site and used to snare the 180-cm 0.035" guidewire which had already been advanced through the 9-F sheath on the contralateral limb.

The dual-lumen (Endologix) catheter was then advanced from the 9-F sheath to the ipsilateral side and the skive marker was positioned just over the bifurcation. An Amplatz Super Stiff 0.035" wire was then advanced through the ipsilateral side of the dual-lumen (Endologix) catheter such that it exited the catheter through the skive and into the thoracic aorta. The dual-lumen catheter was then removed.

The 19-F stent-graft delivery system for the (graft size) was then loaded onto an Amplatz Super Stiff 0.035" wire and placed through a transverse arteriotomy into the (right/left) common femoral artery. The contralateral limb markers were identified under fluoroscopic guidance and the Powerlink catheter was then unsheathed. The contralateral iliac limb was then released and pulled down to sit right at the bifurcation. The main body of the graft was then deployed from bottom to top. Lastly, the ipsilateral iliac limb was deployed. Additional extensions were used proximal.

The Powerlink catheter was then removed, followed by removal of guidewired. The arteriotomy in the (right/left) common femoral artery was closed with interrupted 6-0 prolene suture. The groin was closed in three layers with 2-0 vicryl, followed by 3-0 vicryl, and 4-0 monocryl suture for the skin. The 9-F sheath was removed and manual pressure held for 20 min on the access site. Sterile dressings were placed on the wounds and patient was taken to recovery. All counts were correct.

Chapter 188

Endovascular Abdominal Aortic Aneurysm Repair with the Cook Zenith or Zenith Flex Endograft

Fady F. Haddad, M.D. and Jamal J. Hoballah, M.D., M.B.A.

INDICATIONS

- Infrarenal abdominal aortic aneurysm (AAA) >5.5 cm (nonruptured) in men 5.0 cm in women, enlarging AAA >4.0 cm (grown >5 mm in 6 months), Common Iliac artery Aneurysm.
- Anatomic exclusions:
  Neck:
  - Infrarenal neck length <15 mm.
  - Diameter >32 or <18 mm.
  - Neck angulation >60° relative to aneurysm long axis.
  - Neck angulation >45° relative to suprarenal aorta.
  - Inverted funnel.
  - Circumferential thrombus.
  Iliacs:
  - Iliac fixation site >10 mm in length and <20 mm in diameter.

ESSENTIAL STEPS

1. General or Regional Anesthesia in well-selected patients.
2. Prepare surgical field as for an open repair (from nipples to knees).
3. Expose and control of the common femoral arteries through small transverse inguinal incisions (or alternate vessels: iliac conduit if needed).
4. Introduce size 7 French sheath in each common femoral artery.

J.J. Hoballah and C.E.H. Scott-Conner (eds.), *Operative Dictations in General and Vascular Surgery*, DOI 10.1007/978-1-4614-0451-4_188,
© Springer Science+Business Media, LLC 2012

5. Anticoagulate with IV heparin sulfate (100 U/kg) (keep ACT ~300 throughout the case).

6. Introduce guide wires (started, J or hydrophilic) into the thoracic aorta under fluoroscopic guidance bilaterally. Exchange with stiff 260-cm guide wires, *Lundquist (alternatively Amplatz)* through diagnostic catheters on the site selected for main device insertion.

7. Place pigtail or straight marked diagnostic catheter into the infrarenal aorta via the contralateral side.

8. Confirm the level of the renal arteries and measure the distance to the aortic bifurcation to verify that the contralateral gate will open few centimeters proximal to the aortic bifurcation with angiography (15 cc/s for 20 cc).

9. Prep the main device and flush with heparinized solution. Appropriately orient the device and position of the contralateral gate and check mark.

10. Remove the ipsilateral sheath and insert main device over the stiff guide wire to the level of the renal arteries while maintaining the desired orientation of the device.

11. Position proximal markers (top of fabric) at the approximate desired location (just below lowest renal artery).

12. Tilt the Image intensifier cephalad to align markers, accommodating for common anterior angulation of the neck.

13. Repeat the angiogram (15 cc/s for 15 cc) under a magnified view to mark the position of the renal arteries.

14. Using continuous fluoroscopy begin deployment of the Zenith graft at the desired level until the first two stents are opened and a diamond shape stent is seen. At this point, one can still readjust position of the device.

15. Confirm endovascular graft position to the renal arteries by angiography (15 cc/s for 15 cc) and then retract the contralateral catheter to the aortic bifurcation level.

16. Complete the deployment just until the contralateral limb is opened.

17. Access the contralateral limb using floppy wires and directional catheters.

18. Confirm wire position within the graft by coiling the wire and then by angiography using a straight diagnostic catheter.

19. Release and push the cap covering the suprarenal stent only 2–3 mm to allow visualization of the renal arteries while perform an angiogram for final confirmation of the

level of deployment in relationship to the renal arteries (optional) (refer below to variations).

20. Push the cap to the level of the diaphragm thus fully deploying the suprarenal stent (advance the top cap 1–2 cm beyond the deployed stent).

21. Advance the straight catheter and wire into the thoracic aorta from the contralateral leg.

22. Replace the wire with a stiff 260-cm Amplantz or Lunderquist wire.

23. Place a marking catheter over the wire.

24. Perform an angiogram through the contralateral sheath to document the origin of the hypogastric artery.

25. Select the contralateral limb size based on the measured length from the contralateral gate to the internal iliac (keeping in mind a 1–1.5 stent overlap into the main body contralateral leg).

26. Prep the contralateral limb.

27. Remove the 7 French sheath and insert the device with the contralateral limb.

28. Deploy the graft under continuous fluoroscopic guidance overlapping the gate completely.

29. Retrieve the nose cone with the delivery system under fluoroscopic control.

30. Complete the deployment of the ipsilateral limb.

31. Release the last trigger wire (holding the graft to the delivery system).

32. Advance the gray pusher on the ipsilateral side to the level of the cap and allow it to dock into the cap (suprarenal stent cover) and retrieve the cap under continuous fluoroscopic control.

33. Place marking catheter and perform retrograde angiogram to identify the origin of the ipsilateral hypogastric artery and verify the selected ipsilateral limb.

34. Prep the ipsilateral limb and introduce into the main device sheath.

35. Deploy the ipsilateral limb at the desired location (keep in mind 1–3 stent overlap with the main body ipsilateral limb).

36. Mold junction and attachment sites with appropriately sized Coda balloon.

37. Place pigtail catheter into the aorta above the stent graft.

38. Evaluate graft position, patency, and the presence of endoleaks by angiography.

39. Remove catheters, sheaths, and wires sequentially.

40. Close arteriotomies.
41. Confirm hemostasis.
42. Check distal pulses.
43. Close the wounds.

NOTE THIS VARIATION

■ An additional size 5 French sheath may be placed in the contralateral femoral artery or through the left brachial artery through which a straight diagnostic catheter can be parked above the renals to provide continuous evaluation on the level of the renal arteries prior to final deployment of the suprarenal fixation stent.

COMPLICATIONS

■ Early: mal deployment, coverage of the renal arteries, renal failure, bleeding, iliac artery dissection or rupture, distal embolization, kinking, systemic complications.
■ Late: Endoleak, Aneurysm rupture, migration, limb thrombosis, structural graft failure, graft infection.

TEMPLATE OPERATIVE DICTATION

Preoperative diagnosis: Infrarenal AAA.
Postoperative diagnosis: Same.
Procedure: (1) Exploration of bilateral common femoral arteries. (2) Advancement of catheter into the aorta. (3) Aortogram and pelvic angiogram. (4) Supervision and Interpretation (S&I). (5) Endovascular repair of abdominal aortic aneurysm with a bifurcated modular Zenith endoprosthesis. S&I (6) Repair of femoral arteries.
Surgeon:
Anesthesia:
Indications: This ___-year-old *male/female* was found to have an asymptomatic, ___-cm infrarenal AAA suitable for endovascular repair on CT scan.
Description of procedure: The patient was placed in the supine position on the operating table. The procedure was performed under *general endotracheal/regional* anesthesia. A Foley catheter and arterial line were placed for monitoring. The abdomen and both groins were prepped and draped in the standard sterile fashion.

Prophylactic intravenous antibiotics were given prior to skin incision.

The common femoral arteries were exposed through small transverse inguinal skin incisions Using Seldinger technique, a size 7 French sheath was introduced in each common femoral artery. The patient was anticoagulated with IV heparin sulfate (100 U/kg). Floppy guide wires were introduced into the thoracic aorta under fluoroscopic guidance bilaterally. On the *right/left side (Main body side)* the floppy wire was exchanged with a stiff 260-cm guide wires *Amplatz/Lundquist* through diagnostic catheters. A *pigtail/straight* marked diagnostic catheter was introduced into the infrarenal aorta via the contralateral side. An aortogram was performed confirming the level of the renal arteries and the distance from the lowest renal artery to the aortic bifurcation was measured. The main device was prepped with heparinized saline solution and appropriately oriented under fluoroscopy. The ipsilateral sheath was removed and the main device inserted over the stiff guide wire to the level of the renal arteries while maintaining the desired orientation of the device. A repeat angiogram (15 cc/s for 15 cc) under a magnified view was performed and the position of the renal arteries was marked. Using continuous fluoroscopy deployment of the Zenith graft was started at the desired level (with the top markers just below the lowest Renal artery) until the first two stents are opened and a diamond shape stent is seen. The endovascular graft position to the renal arteries was confirmed appropriate again by repeat angiography (15 cc/s for 15 cc). *The diagnostic catheter was pulled back to the aortic bifurcation level.* The deployment was continued until the contralateral limb was fully opened. The gate of the contralateral limb was cannulated using a glide wire and a *multipurpose/KMP/cobra/double curve* directional catheters. The wire was allowed to coil inside the body of the graft suggesting its position inside the graft. An MP catheter was introduced over the wire and an angiogram was obtained further confirming the intra graft position of the catheter. The cap covering the suprarenal stent was released and pushed forward by only 2–3 mm. An angiogram through the MP catheter confirmed appropriate position of the graft in relationship to the renal arteries. A j wire was placed again in the graft and allowed to loop again. The cap was then advanced to the level of the diaphragm thus fully deploying the suprarenal stent. The straight catheter and the wire were then advanced into the thoracic aorta. The wire was exchanged with a stiff 260-cm *Amplantz/Lunderquist* wire. A marking catheter was advanced over the wire and a retrograde angiogram through the contralateral sheath was performed documenting the origin of the hypogastric artery. The length from the contralateral gate to the internal iliac artery was measured and the appropriate contralateral limb measuring ___ was selected. The contralateral limb was prepped. The 7 French sheath was then removed and the device with the contralateral limb inserted into the desired location. The graft limb was deployed under continuous fluoroscopic guidance overlapping the gate completely (1–1.5 stent overlap). The nose cone was retrieved and the delivery system was removed under fluoroscopic control. Attention was then directed to the ipsilateral limb where the deployment of the main graft body was completed.

After releasing the pin-vice, the gray pusher on the ipsilateral side was advanced to the level of the cap and allowed to dock into the cap (suprarenal stent cover) under continuous fluoroscopic control and the cap retrieved. The marking catheter was introduced into the main graft body and a retrograde angiogram was performed to identify the origin of the ipsilateral hypogastric artery. The distance from the ipsilateral gate to the origin of the internal iliac artery was measured and the appropriate ipsilateral graft limb was selected (Size___). The ipsilateral limb was prepped with heparinized saline and introduced through the main device sheath. The ipsilateral limb was deployed at the desired location (*with___number of stents overlap with the main body, recommended 1–3*). The cone and delivery systems were retrieved. The infrarenal attachment site as well, the graft junctions and the distal attachment sites were molded using a Coda balloon.

A pigtail catheter was introduced into the aorta above the stent graft and an angiogram was performed. This revealed appropriate placement of the graft with patent limbs and no evidence of type 1 or 3 endoleaks. *There was evidence of type I, III endoleak necessitating reinsertion of the Coda Balloon and remolding of the junction and attachment site. There was evidence of type 2 endoleak which will be monitored.*

All catheters, sheaths, and wires were removed sequentially. The arteriotomies were closed using 5-0/6-0 Prolene interrupted/continuous sutures. Hemostasis was secured. The distal pulses were present. Heparin was reversed *(or not)* using protamine sulfate. The subcutaneous tissue was closed with 3-0 Vicryl sutures and the skin was closed with 4-0 Monocryl subcuticular sutures. The patient was transferred to the recovery room in a stable condition.

Chapter 189

Endovascular Aneurysm Repair (Talent-Bifurcated Graft)

F. Ezequiel Parodi, M.D. and Murray L. Shames, M.D.

INDICATIONS

- Infrarenal abdominal aortic aneurysm (AAA) >5 cm (nonruptured), enlarging AAA >4.0 cm (grown >5 mm in 6 months).

ESSENTIAL STEPS

1. Access and control of the common femoral arteries (or alternate access vessels).
2. Anticoagulate with IV heparin sulfate (100 U/kg).
3. Access the artery and exchange floppy guide wires with stiff guide wires *Amplatz, Lundquist* through diagnostic catheters, into the thoracic aorta under fluoroscopic guidance.
4. Select the *femoral/iliac* artery (healthiest, straightest, longest) for main device insertion.
5. Insert a 6-French sheath into the contralateral side over the guide wire.
6. Place pigtail or straight diagnostic catheter into the infrarenal aorta via the contralateral side.
7. Confirm level of the renal arteries and the renal to ipsilateral hypogastric artery length with angiography (15 cc/s for 30 cc).
8. Insert main device over stiff guide wire to the level just above the renal arteries and appropriately orient the device, using radiopaque markers.

J.J. Hoballah and C.E.H. Scott-Conner (eds.), *Operative Dictations in General and Vascular Surgery*, DOI 10.1007/978-1-4614-0451-4_189,
© Springer Science+Business Media, LLC 2012

9. Repeat the angiogram (15 cc/s for 15 cc) under a magnified view to mark the position of the renal arteries.

10. Using continuous fluoroscopy begin deployment of the Talent graft just above the desired level; after the first two stents are opened, gently pull device distally to desired level. Top of figures of 8 should be just below the renal arteries.

11. Confirm endovascular graft position by angiography (15 cc/s for 15 cc).

12. Complete graft deployment.

13. Retract the pigtail catheter into the aneurysm over a guide wire.

14. Retrieve the nose cone, remove the delivery system and place a 14-French sheath.

15. Access the contra lateral limb using floppy wires and directional catheters.

16. Confirm wire positions within the graft using a pigtail catheter or angiogram.

17. Measure length from the contralateral gate to the internal iliac artery using marker pigtail and a retrograde angiogram.

18. Exchange the pigtail catheter to stiff wire.

19. Remove the 6-French sheath and insert the device with the contralateral limb.

20. Deploy the graft under continuous fluoroscopic guidance overlapping the gate completely.

21. Retrieve the nose cone, remove the delivery system under fluoroscopic control and place 14-French sheath.

22. Mold junction and attachment sites with appropriately sized (based on artery diameter) balloons as needed (Reliant).

23. Place pigtail catheter into the aorta above the stent graft.

24. Evaluate graft position, patency, and the presence of endoleaks by angiography.

25. Remove catheters, sheaths, and wires sequentially.

26. Close arteriotomies.

27. Confirm hemostasis.

28. Check distal pulses.

29. Close the wounds.

NOTE THIS VARIATION

■ In the presence of common iliac arteriomegaly, the procedure is modified to avoid an endoleak. One option is to use a flared iliac extension. Another option is to embolize the internal iliac artery and extend the iliac limb into the external iliac artery, which is typically free of aneurysmal disease.

COMPLICATIONS

- Arterial injury (dissection, disruption, thrombosis, embolization).
- Graft migration.
- Type I or III endoleaks.
- Renal failure.

TEMPLATE OPERATIVE DICTATION

Preoperative diagnosis: Infrarenal AAA.

Procedure: Endoluminal repair of AAA using Talent endovascular graft.

Postoperative diagnosis: Infrarenal AAA.

Indications: This ___-year-old *male/female* patient was found to have an *asymptomatic/symptomatic* ___-cm infrarenal AAA. Preoperative imaging was reviewed and the patient is a good candidate for endovascular repair.

Description of procedure: The procedure was performed under *general/spinal/epidural* anesthesia. The patient was positioned on the operating table in a supine position. A prophylactic intravenous antibiotic (Ancef) was administered. The patient was prepped and draped in the standard fashion. A *longitudinal/oblique* incision was made at the level of the inguinal ligament and carried down to the common femoral artery bilaterally. The common femoral arteries were dissected and encircled with vessel loops proximally and distally.

The anesthesia team administered 100 U/kg or 5,000 U of heparin sulfate. The distal vessel loops were cinched down and clamped. The common femoral artery was accessed using the Seldinger needle a *Bentson/Glide* wire passed under fluoroscopic guidance into the thoracic aorta and was then exchanged through a catheter for Amplatz (or other still) wire. On the side of the contralateral limb a wire was similarly placed, 6-French introducer sheath was advanced and through it a graduated pigtail catheter was positioned at the level of the renal arteries. On the ipsilateral limb, a 6-mm arteriotomy was performed. The Talent stent graft was flushed and advanced over the ipsilateral guide wire to above the level of the renal arteries. The graft was oriented using the radiopaque markers. All the manipulations were performed under fluoroscopic guidance. An angiogram was performed under magnification and the renal arteries were marked on the screen. The device was positioned slightly proximal to the desired landing zone and deployment started. Once the first two stents were opened, the device was gently pulled down to the desired level making sure the figures of 8 were just below the renal arteries. Repeat arteriogram assured proper infrarenal positioning. Deployment was continued until the device was fully deployed. The contralateral pigtail catheter was straightened with a wire and pulled into the aneurysm sac. The ipsilateral device was retrieved without difficulty. The pigtail catheter was exchanged for a directional catheter. Under continuous fluoroscopy the contralateral limb was cannulated with a floppy wire and the catheter advanced into the proximal aorta. The diagnostic catheter was again exchanged for the pigtail to assure an intragraft position. A retrograde angiogram was performed to locate the contralateral hypogastric artery and select the contralateral limb. Once the appropriate limb extension was selected the pigtail was exchanged for a stiffer wire and the delivery system with the contralateral limb was advanced into the gate of the main device. Under continuous fluoroscopy the limb deployed overlapping the gate. The delivery system was retrieved and a 14-French sheath was placed. The pigtail catheter was then reintroduced over a guide wire and positioned proximal to the device. An angiogram was performed to assess for endoleaks and confirm positioning. The endovascular repair was free of stenoses, kinks, or endoleaks. All catheters and sheaths were carefully removed while observing the patient's vital signs. Finally, the wires were removed and the arteriotomies closed with 5-0 prolene sutures. The vessels were flushed prior to closure. Once hemostasis was confirmed the wounds were copiously irrigated and closed in layers with running sutures.

Examination of distal pulses confirmed no change from preoperative assessment.

Dressings were applied.

The patient tolerated the procedure well and was taken to the postanesthesia care unit in stable condition.

ANGIOGRAM SUPERVISION AND INTERPRETATION

1. *Flush aortogram:* A pigtail catheter is seen at the level of the renal arteries. *Single/multiple* renal arteries are present bilaterally. No significant disease is present in either renal artery. An aneurysm is seen originating distal to the renal arteries. The iliac arteries are free of significant disease. Both internal iliac arteries are patent.

2. *Level of deployment:* The Talent stent graft has a suprarenal stent, figures of 8 mark the beginning of the graft, they should be positioned below the renal arteries. There is no evidence of stenosis, kinks, or endoleaks. The renal, internal iliac arteries are widely patent. There is no evidence of stenosis or dissection in either external iliac artery.

NOTES

Preoperative Imaging

Contrast CT scan of the abdomen and pelvis with 3-mm increments and 3D reconstruction.

Selective use of contrast angiography.

Anatomic Requirements

Proximal healthy aortic neck ³10 mm in length.

Proximal aortic diameter 18–32 mm.

Iliac artery diameter 8–22 mm.

Contraindications

Neck angulation >60°

Presence of thrombus at landing sites

Severe bilateral iliac occlusive disease (or lumen less than 7 mm).

Severe iliac artery tortuosity and calcification.

Necessary Equipment

X-ray compatible operating table.

Angled C-arm with:

- High-resolution fluoroscopy.
- High-definition angiography.
- Digital subtraction capabilities.

Power injector.

Seldinger needles.

Selection of 0.035″ guide wires (Bentson, Glide, Amplatz, Lundquist).

Selection of catheters (MPA, graduated pigtail, Cobra, SOS, Simmons)

Arterial sheaths (6–14 F).

Talent endovascular graft with the necessary extension limbs and cuffs.

Angioplasty balloons (Reliant).

Cell saver unit (optional).

Additional Aortic Endografts

Excluder endovascular graft (W.L. Gore and Associates, Flagstaff, AR).

Zenith endovascular graft (Cook Medical, Bloomington, IN).

IntuiTrack (Endologic, Irvine, CA).

Specific devices have different steps that should be included in the dictations.

Chapter 190
Internal Iliac Artery Embolisation

Jamal J. Hoballah, M.D., M.B.A.

INDICATIONS
- Dilated common iliac artery in the presence of otherwise suitable anatomy for EVAR.
- Internal iliac artery aneurysm.
- Pelvic bleeding following pelvic fracture.

ESSENTIAL STEPS
1. Percutaneous access of the contralateral femoral artery.
2. Placement of a size 5 French sheath.
3. Introduce a wire followed by Omni Flush Catheter into the aorta.
4. Perform an aortogram with iliac runoff and confirm the iliac pathology.
5. Crossing from the contralateral iliac artery into the ipsilateral common iliac artery where the interior iliac artery is to be embolized.
6. Changing the projection to an LAO/RAO oblique.
7. Replacement of the size 5 French sheath with a size 6 guiding catheter or a long 5 French (Balkin) sheath.
8. Canalization of the ipsilateral internal iliac artery.
9. Advancement of a size 5 French catheter into the internal iliac artery at the level of embolization. Insertion of Volcano/Nester Coils into the internal iliac artery preserving flow in the distal branches.
10. Packing the coils into internal iliac artery without spilling into the common or external iliac artery.

J.J. Hoballah and C.E.H. Scott-Conner (eds.), *Operative Dictations in General and Vascular Surgery*, DOI 10.1007/978-1-4614-0451-4_190,
© Springer Science+Business Media, LLC 2012

11. Angiogram completion angiogram.
12. Reversal of anticoagulation and removal of the sheath.

NOTE THIS VARIATION

■ Occasionally access into the internal iliac artery may be achieved through an ipsilateral approach other types of embolization devices with a retrievable option (Amplantzar Vascular Plug) also available and have been successfully used for occluding the internal iliac artery.

COMPLICATIONS

■ Extension of the coil into the common iliac artery.
■ Migration of the coils into the external iliac artery.
■ Access site bleeding.
■ Pelvic ischemia.
■ Buttock claudication.
■ Sexual dysfunction.

TEMPLATE OPERATIVE DICTATION

Preoperative diagnosis: Common iliac artery aneurysm extending into the iliac bifurcation in a patient who is otherwise a good candidate for EVAR/internal iliac artery aneurysm/persistent pelvic bleeding in a patient with pelvic fractures follow blunt trauma.

Procedure: Aortogram with iliac runoff; *Right/left* internal iliac artery embolization.

Postoperative diagnosis: Same.

Indications: The patient is a ___-year-old *male/female* with a large abdominal aortic aneurysm and aneurismal dilatation of the common iliac artery extending into the iliac bifurcation. The patient is otherwise a good candidate for EVAR. Embolization of the internal iliac artery is indicated to provide a suitable landing zone for the EVAR limb into the external iliac artery. The contralateral iliac artery is patent without any significant pathology. The patient has been informed of the risks and benefits the embolization of the internal iliac artery, and has agreed to the procedure.

Description of procedure: The patient was brought to the angiography suite and was placed in the angiography table in the supine position. The right and left groins were prepped and draped in the usual sterile fashion. The contralateral groin was infiltrated with 1% Lidocaine and the common femoral artery was accessed using a Seldinger technique. A size 5 French sheath was inserted in the common femoral artery and a glide wire was advanced in to the aorta. An Omni flush catheter was then advanced into the aorta and an aortogram with iliac runoff was obtained delineating the anatomy. The *Omni flush/Cobra* catheter was then used to cross over to the contralateral common iliac artery. The 5-French sheath was then replaced by a size *5/6 French guiding catheter/5 Balkin sheath*. The tip of the sheath was parked in the common iliac artery just proximal to the take off of the internal iliac artery. A *right/left anterior oblique RAO/LAO* projection was then obtained and another angiogram was performed delineating the orifice of the *right/left* internal iliac artery. Using an *MP/angle glade/catheter/ cobra catheter* the internal iliac artery was accessed with a 0.035 hydrophilic glide wire and the catheter was advanced into the distal segment of internal iliac artery. An angiogram through the *MP/ angle glade/catheter/cobra catheter* was obtained further documenting its position and its relationship to the common iliac artery and internal iliac artery branches. A Size 10 Tornado coil was then introduced and deployed into the desired location in the internal iliac artery preserving the collateral of the internal iliac artery. Multiple coils were introduced until the entire iliac artery was filled and packed with coils. An angiogram was then performed documenting absence of any spillage of coils into the common iliac or external iliac arteries. The catheter, wires and sheath were then removed after the patient's anticoagulation was reversed with Protamine sulfate. The sheath was removed and pressure was applied to the groin.

NOTES

Chapter 191

Transabdominal Replacement of Ruptured Infrarenal Abdominal Aortic Aneurysm

Jamal J. Hoballah, M.D., M.B.A.

INDICATIONS
- Abdominal pain.
- Hypotension.
- Shock.

ESSENTIAL STEPS
1. Large-bore intravenous lines.
2. Prepping and draping prior to induction of general anesthesia.
3. Midline xiphoid to pubis incision.
4. Incise the triangular ligament and mobilize the left lobe of the liver to the right.
5. Incise the lesser omentum and retract the stomach to the right.
6. Divide the right crus of the diaphragm.
7. Supraceliac aortic cross-clamping.
8. Retract the transverse colon anteriorly and to the right.
9. Retract the splenic flexure posteriorly and laterally.
10. Divide the peritoneal periaortic attachment of the duodenum.
11. Wrap the small bowel in a wet towel and retract to the right.
12. Incise the retroperitoneum overlying the aorta and continue proximally.
13. Identify the left renal vein.

J.J. Hoballah and C.E.H. Scott-Conner (eds.), *Operative Dictations in General and Vascular Surgery*, DOI 10.1007/978-1-4614-0451-4_191,
© Springer Science+Business Media, LLC 2012

14. Dissect the aortic aneurysm neck and prepare it for clamping.
15. Clamp the infrarenal aorta and release supraceliac clamp.
16. Incise the retroperitoneum overlying the aorta and continue distally.
17. Expose the proximal right common iliac artery.
18. Expose the proximal left common iliac artery.
19. Cross-clamp the right and left common iliac arteries.
20. Enter the aneurysm and remove aneurysmal content.
21. Oversew bleeding lumbars and control the inferior mesenteric artery (IMA).
22. Prepare the proximal neck for construction of the anastomosis.
23. Construct the proximal anastomosis and check for hemostasis.
24. Prepare the aortic bifurcation for the distal anastomosis.
25. Construct the distal anastomosis.
26. Perfuse into the right common iliac artery with manual compression of the right external iliac artery.
27. Check for femoral pulse.
28. Repeat the same on the left.
29. Check sigmoid viability.
30. Re-evaluate hemostasis.
31. Close the aneurysm wall.
32. Close the abdomen.
33. Recheck distal pulses.

NOTE THESE VARIATIONS

- Endovascular repair (EVAR) may be offered first in institutions with appropriate resources and expertise if the anatomy is appropriate.
- Proximal aortic control is typically obtained at the supraceliac level. This can be achieved blindly or under direct visualization.
- Tube replacement is most expedient and is usually attempted unless the iliac aneurysmal disease is extensive and the aortic bifurcation does not allow such a reconstruction.

COMPLICATIONS

- Bleeding.
- Myocardial infarction.
- Pneumonia.

- Renal failure.
- Wound infection.
- Wound dehiscence.
- Limb ischemia.
- Trash foot.
- Bowel ischemia.
- Buttock ischemia.
- Spinal cord ischemia.

TEMPLATE OPERATIVE DICTATION

Preoperative diagnosis: Ruptured abdominal aortic aneurysm (AAA).

Procedure: Replacement of ruptured infrarenal abdominal aortic aneurysm with tube graft.

Postoperative diagnosis: Same.

Indications: This is a ___-year-old *male/female* with *abdominal pain/back pain/hypotension/tender pulsatile abdominal mass* and the presumptive diagnosis of a ruptured AAA. The risks of nonoperative management and surgical intervention were discussed with the patient and *he/she* elected to undergo surgical intervention.

Description of procedure: The patient was placed supine on the operating table. The arms were placed at 80° and the anesthesia team placed large-bore intravenous lines and monitoring lines. Normal bony prominences were padded. A Foley catheter was then placed under sterile technique. The patient's anterior abdomen and both upper thighs were prepped and draped in the usual sterile fashion.

Preoperative antibiotics were administered prior to skin incision.

The patient was induced and intubated.

Immediately thereafter, the skin incision was made from the subxiphoid to the suprapubic region. The subcutaneous tissue was then divided with electrocautery. The linea alba was exposed and incised. The peritoneum was elevated and entered sharply. The abdominal wall incision was then extended to the full length of the skin incision.

[Choose one:]

If supraceliac control under direct visualization: The triangular ligament of the liver was incised and the left lobe of the liver was mobilized to the right; the lesser omentum was incised and the stomach retracted to the left; the right crus of the diaphragm was divided; the supraceliac aorta was dissected and cross-clamped.

If supraceliac control without direct visualization: The lesser omentum was incised and the supraceliac aorta was palpated, dissected blindly, and cross-clamped.

The transverse colon was then elevated superiorly out of the wound, wrapped in a moist towel. A moist rolled lap pad was placed in the bed of the splenic flexure of the colon, which was retracted laterally and posteriorly. The remainder of the small bowel was then reflected to the right, exposing the aortic aneurysm. Sharp dissection of the ligament of Treitz and the distal fourth portion of the duodenum allowed further exposure of the aneurysm and retraction of the small bowel to the right. The small bowel was then wrapped in a moistened towel and held in place using an Omni retractor.

The retroperitoneum overlying the aorta was incised and continued proximally to the level of the left renal vein. The inferior mesenteric vein was encountered, ligated, and divided.

The abdominal aortic aneurysm neck was then sharply dissected, avoiding any injury to the left renal vein. The infrarenal aorta was clamped and supraceliac clamp released.

The dissection was then carried out in the pelvic region for exposure of the iliac arteries.

The retroperitoneum overlying the aorta was incised distally, exposing the proximal right and left common iliac arteries and avoiding any injury to the iliac veins. The common iliac arteries were then cross-clamped.

The aneurysm wall was then incised longitudinally on its anterior aspect, keeping to the right of the origin of the IMA. The aneurysm cavity was entered and the aneurysm content and debris removed. The IMA had pulsatile back-bleeding and was oversewn with 2-0 silk sutures/*the IMA had sluggish back-bleeding and was controlled with a double-looped silastic tape*. The bleeding lumbar arteries and middle sacral artery were oversewn with figure-of-eight 2-0 silk.

The aneurysm neck was then prepared for the construction of the proximal anastomosis. The incision in the aorta was carried to the level of the neck of the aneurysm. The incision was then Td off on each side of the neck, *leaving the posterior wall intact/transecting the posterior wall.*

A *20/18/16 Dacron/PTFE* graft was then soaked in antibiotic solution. The body of the graft was trimmed for the proximal anastomosis. The anastomosis was constructed in a running fashion using 3-0 prolene sutures. At the completion of the suture line, the sutures were tied and the anastomosis checked for hemostasis. Hemostasis was adequate/*except for a suture line bleeding controlled with an interrupted mattress suture/needle hole bleeding controlled with the topical application of Gelfoam soaked with thrombin.*

Attention was focused on the distal anastomosis.

The aortic bifurcation was prepared for the distal anastomosis. The incision in the aorta at the level of the aortic bifurcation was

Td off on each side, *leaving the posterior wall intact/transecting the posterior wall*.

The graft was then sized and cut. The anastomosis was then performed with 3-0 prolene running sutures. Prior to completing the anastomosis the iliac clamps were released, allowing for back-bleeding of the iliac arteries. The aortic clamp was released for forward-flushing of the graft. The anastomosis was copiously irrigated with heparinized saline solution and the sutures tied. The aortic clamp was released, allowing blood flow into one common iliac artery at a time. The flow was directed first into the internal iliac and then into the external iliac artery by manually compressing the external iliac artery/*common femoral artery* when the common iliac artery was initially perfused. Strong palpable pulses were noted in both femoral arteries.

The aneurysm lumen was reinspected. Hemostasis was adequate/*bleeding from a lumbar artery was identified and was controlled with figure-of-eight 2-0 silk sutures*.

The IMA was re-evaluated.

If good IMA back-bleeding: *There was evidence of good back-bleeding from the IMA and good Doppler signals in the sigmoid mesentery. The IMA was oversewn with a 3-0 prolene suture.*

If poor IMA back-bleeding: *There was poor back-bleeding from the IMA and poor Doppler signals in the sigmoid mesentery. Because the patient was hemodynamically stable, the IMA was reimplanted.*

Reinspection of all the suture lines was performed and revealed adequate hemostasis.

The field was then irrigated with antibiotic solution.

The redundant aneurysm wall was then sutured over the aortic graft using 3-0 Vicryl sutures, minimizing the dead space between the aortic graft and aortic wall.

The retroperitoneum was then closed with 3-0 Vicryl in a running fashion.

The bowel was then placed back in the anatomic position.

Abdominal wall closure was then performed with *running/interrupted* 0 prolene sutures.

The wound was reirrigated, dried, and the skin edges opposed with skin staples.

The peri-incisional prep and drape were cleaned and dried, followed by 4×4 gauze, silk tape.

The feet were inspected and there was evidence of strong Doppler signals in the pedal arteries.

The patient tolerated the procedure well and was awakened and taken to the *postanesthesia care unit/intensive care unit* in stable condition.

NOTES

Chapter 192

Endovascular Repair of Ruptured Abdominal Aortic Aneurysms

Manish Mehta, M.D., M.P.H.

INDICATIONS

- Ruptured abdominal aortic aneurysm.
- Ruptured aortoiliac aneurysm.

ESSENTIAL STEPS

1. Once the diagnosis of ruptured abdominal aortic aneurysm (AAA) is made, patients need expeditious transfer from the emergency room (ER) to the operating room (OR) that is well equipped for both endovascular and open surgical repair.

2. All hemodynamically stable patients should undergo preoperative CTA. In patients with preexisting renal insufficiency, limited contrast or non-contrast thin axial CT images (0.625 mm) can be obtained. Standardized protocols should be developed to expedite patient transfer from the ER to the OR that are time sensitive and allow for CT in all patients with ruptured AAA.

3. All hemodynamically unstable patients, when preoperative CT is prohibitive, if endovascular abdominal aortic aneurysm repair (EVAR) is attempted, intraoperative aortic neck measurements can be accessed by intravascular ultrasound, or routine arteriography. If angiography is used, one needs to oversize the stent grafts 20–30%, to compensate for possible underestimation of the aortic neck diameter on angiography.

J.J. Hoballah and C.E.H. Scott-Conner (eds.), *Operative Dictations in General and Vascular Surgery*, DOI 10.1007/978-1-4614-0451-4_192,
© Springer Science+Business Media, LLC 2012

4. Patient positioning and prep should be ideal for both EVAR and possible conversion to open surgical repair, this includes a patient in supine position, left arm tucked, right arm out for arterial and venous access (at the discretion of anesthesiologist), and prep from above the xiphoid to mid-thigh level.

5. Femoral artery access via cut down or percutaneous approach is up to the discretion of the individual surgeon/interventionalists. Most reports of ruptured EVAR are via femoral artery cut down. We reserve percutaneous access for patients who are truly hemodynamically unstable; when general anesthesia induction might result in the loss of sympathetic tone and hemodynamic collapse.

6. In hemodynamically unstable patient – Access the femoral artery; needle, floppy wire, guide catheter, stiff wire exchange, 12–18 Fr sheath placement, aortic occlusion balloon advancement to the supraceliac aorta and inflation. Subsequent contralateral femoral access; appropriate sheath placement (18–24 Fr), angiography, and EVAR.

7. In hemodynamically stable patients – Access the femoral artery; needle, floppy wire, guide catheter, stiff wire exchange, 12–18 Fr sheath placement, angiography, and EVAR.

8. If aortic occlusion balloon is needed, advanced a 30–40 cm, 12 Fr or greater sheath up to the aortic neck, advance the occlusion balloon, and during the aortic occlusion balloon inflation, maintain forward traction on the femoral sheath and the aortic balloon catheter to support the balloon catheter and prevent occlusion balloon prolapse into the AAA.

9. During EVAR, identify appropriate proximal and distal landing zones, and in cases of aortoiliac aneurysms when internal iliac artery occlusion with stent graft extension to the external iliac artery is needed, get stent graft proximal fixation and seal before dealing with the internal iliac arteries.

10. During EVAR, prior to the deployment of the stent graft, if aortic occlusion balloon is needed to maintain hemodynamic stability, one needs to identify proximal landing zone, deflate and remove the occlusion balloon, deploy the stent graft, reposition the aortic occlusion balloon from within the ipsilateral main body up to the stent graft

main body/aortic neck and reestablish balloon inflation. This would allow time for further EVAR steps including contralateral gait cannulation, iliac stent graft extensions, or conversion of bifurcated stent graft into aortouniiliac devices.

11. In hemodynamically unstable patients, one could consider primary use of aortouniiliac stent grafts with the femoral bypass, and contralateral common iliac occlusion.

12. Generally, management of ruptured EVAR revolved around the patient's hemodynamic status, and during the course of the procedure, the surgeon/interventional-ists, the anesthesiologist, and the OR staff need to be in continuous communication regarding the patient's hemodynamic status. Furthermore, one should anticipate frequent use of aortic occlusion balloon as needed during the course of the procedure.

13. With few exceptions, highlighted above, the remainder of the ruptured EVAR procedure is similar to standard elective EVAR procedure.

VARIATIONS

- Similar to open surgical ruptured AAA repair, we do not anticoagulated the patient during ruptured EVAR, and utilize frequent sheath flush techniques to limit thromboembolic complications.

- Management of variations during ruptured EVAR is dependent of the patient's hemodynamic status during presentation and during the course of the procedure as described above. Other variations to consider include the use of brachial access for occlusion balloon placement, which today is really of historic importance, and rarely needed; however when needed, one needs to be familiar with these techniques.

- In cases when percutaneous access is obtained for ruptured EVAR, one has to decide on preclosure techniques versus percutaneous access and subsequent femoral cut down and direct femoral artery repair. We have generally reserved the percutaneous access for hemodynamically unstable patients and in such cases we have generally avoided preclose techniques to further expedite rupture EVAR, and subsequent to the completion of the procedure, perform femoral artery cut down, and direct repair.

COMPLICATIONS

- Standard complications include cardiac, respiratory, renal insufficiency, ischemic colitis, lower extremity thromboembolism, and ischemia. Certainly ongoing bleeding and hypotension should be evaluated by repeat CT scan, and managed as indicated based on finding of the CT scan.

- Life threatening complications include abdominal compartment syndrome. Risk factors for abdominal compartment syndrome include (1) massive blood transfusion requirement, (2) use of aortic occlusion balloon, (3) coagulopathy in the perioperative period. One needs to assess for abdominal compartment syndrome frequently during the procedure, and in the presence of one or more of the above risk factors, should consider decompression laparotomy. Bladder pressure measurements can be useful for the diagnosis of abdominal compartment syndrome, and generally speaking, bladder pressures of greater than 35 mmHg should indicate one for the presence of abdominal compartment syndrome.

DICTATION

Procedure: Ruptured EVAR.
Preoperative diagnosis: Ruptured Abdominal Aortic Aneurysm.
Postoperative diagnosis: Ruptured Abdominal Aortic Aneurysm.
Surgeon/Interventionalist:
Anesthesia type:
Estimated Blood Loss:
Fluids:
Intraoperative Complications:
Patient Presentation: Patient is an XX-year-old gentleman who presents with sudden onset of abdominal pain, back pain, hypotension, has abdominal aortic pulsatility, and a CT scan indicates a ruptured abdominal aortic aneurysm. Appropriate risk benefits and alternatives were explained to the patient and family. They understand the procedure, and we are planning on endovascular abdominal aortic aneurysm repair, possible open surgical repair.
Procedure:
1. Bilateral femoral artery cut down.
2. Introduction of bilateral catheters into aorta with interpretation.
3. Endovascular aneurysm repair using two docking limb modular bifurcated stent graft with interpretation.

4. Distal stent graft extension, right common iliac artery with interpretation.
5. Additional distal stent graft extension left common iliac artery with an interpretation for endoleak.

Completion arteriogram indicates adequate proximal distal fixation of the stent graft just below the lower most renal arteries and bilateral common iliac arteries. No type one or type three endoleak is noted. Both renal arteries and both internal iliac and external iliac arteries are well perfused and both limbs of the stent graft are widely patent.

Patient was prepped and draped in a routine fashion, bilateral femoral cut downs were made, fascia was dissected, and femoral arteries were isolated.

A 19-gauge needle was used to puncture right common femoral artery. Benson wire was advanced into the aorta with a Berenstein catheter which was exchanged for a stiff wire, over which an 18-Fr sheath was advanced and placed into the abdominal aortic aneurysm. Similarly, from the left a 19-gauge need, Benson wire, and Berenstein catheter was used to cannulate the abdominal aorta, Benson wire was exchanged for a stiff wire, over which an 18-Fr sheath was advanced and placed into the abdominal aortic aneurysm. Marker flush catheter was advanced up to the juxtarenal aorta. Aortogram was done. Findings indicated abdominal aortic aneurysm with rupture, patent visceral vessels, patent bilateral renal arteries, adequate infrarenal aortic neck for endovascular aneurysm repair, aneurysm extends to the aortic bifurcation. Patent bilateral external, internal, and common iliac arteries.

Endovascular abdominal aortic aneurysm repair. Patient became hemodynamically unstable, therefore from the right femoral approach over a stiff wire an aortic occlusion balloon (you could use any of the occlusion balloons available in the USA, they are Reliant, Equalizer, Corda, and Q50), was used and placed up to the supraceliac level and inflated. Patient regained hemodynamic stability, from the left femoral approach, a stent graft was advanced and placed just below the lower most renal artery, from the sheath that was used to support the balloon catheter from the right femoral artery an arteriogram was done to mark the level of the aortic neck and the lower most renal artery. Prior to deployment of the stent graft, the occlusion balloon was deflated and removed, the stent graft was deployed just below the lower most renal artery. From the ipsilateral stent graft side, the occlusion balloon was advanced and placed up to the aortic stent graft main body within the aortic neck and the occlusion balloon was reinflated to maintain hemodynamic stability. From the contralateral side, the contralateral gait was cannulated using a guide catheter and a glide wire. Arteriogram and catheter manipulations were done to assess adequate cannulation of the gait.

Additional iliac stent graft extensions were advanced and placed proximally within the stent graft contralateral gait, and distally in the common iliac artery and deployed. The occlusion balloon was deflated. Patient remained hemodynamically stable.

Bilateral pelvic arteriograms were done. Two additional distal stent graft extensions were needed in the right and left common iliac arteries. Two additional stent graft extensions were advanced on the right and left part proximally within the prior stent graft limbs, distally in the native right and left common iliac arteries and deployed.

A compliant balloon was used to mold the proximal fixation site, all stent graft overlap sights and the common iliac landing zones. Completion arteriogram was done with a catheter at the juxtarenal aorta from within the stent graft, findings indicated the following:

Adequate placement of the stent graft.

Exclusion of the ruptured abdominal aortic aneurysm.

Preservation of flow to both renal arteries, both internal iliac and external iliac arteries, and both limbs of the stent graft.

During the entire procedure, the abdomen was assessed repeatedly for the development of abdominal compartment syndrome and bladder pressures were measured.

In case of no signs or symptoms of development of abdominal compartment syndrome: All catheters, wires, and sheaths were drawn back and removed. Bilateral femoral arteriotomies were closed primarily. Anterior and retrograde arterial flushes were done appropriately prior to the completion of closure. Good Doppler signal and pulses were noted on both arteriotomy closures. Complete hemostasis was obtained, both groin incisions were closed in two layers. Dressings were applied.

In case of development of abdominal compartment syndrome or signs of development of abdominal compartment syndrome with abdominal distention, pulmonary compromise, elevated peak and plateau pressures, and sustained hypotension: Midline laparotomy was made, fascia was dissected, and the abdominal cavity was entered. The retroperitoneum was NOT explored. The abdominal cavity was left open with dressing placed to suction. Patient was resuscitated. Femoral sheaths were removed, bilateral femoral arteriotomies were closed, anterior and retrograde arterial flushes were done appropriately. Good Doppler signal and pulses were noted after arteriotomy closures. Both groin incisions were closed in two layers. Dressings were applied, patient tolerated the procedure well.

Chapter 193

Open Repair/Ligation of Splenic Artery Aneurysm

Houssein Haidar Ahmad, M.D. and Jamal J. Hoballah, M.D, M.B.A.

INDICATIONS

- Asymptomatic splenic artery aneurysm in a child-bearing age female patient.
- Asymptomatic splenic artery aneurysm and planned liver transplantation.
- Asymptomatic splenic artery aneurysm greater than 2 cm.
- Asymptomatic splenic artery false aneurysm and chronic pancreatitis.
- Symptomatic splenic artery aneurysm.

ESSENTIAL STEPS

1. Left subcostal or chevron incision.
2. Access to lesser sac through the gastrohepatic ligament.
3. Exposure of the celiac artery and its three branches: left gastric, splenic, and common hepatic arteries.
4. Oversewing of the splenic aneurysm after proximal and distal control.
5. Check the viability of the spleen.
6. Secure hemostasis.
7. Closure in layers.

NOTE THESE VARIATIONS

- The procedure may be approached through a midline or subcostal incision.
- Splenic artery aneurysms may be approached anteriorly or laterally.

J.J. Hoballah and C.E.H. Scott-Conner (eds.), *Operative Dictations in General and Vascular Surgery*, DOI 10.1007/978-1-4614-0451-4_193,
© Springer Science+Business Media, LLC 2012

- Anterior approach through the gastrocolic or gastrohepatic ligament provides good exposure for aneurysms in the proximal third. The lateral approach provides exposure to aneurysms in the mid and distal part of the splenic artery.
- Access to the lesser sac through the gastrohepatic ligament allows excellent exposure for proximal control of the celiac, common hepatic and origin of the splenic artery without disruption of any collaterals.
- The lateral retroperitoneal approach after medial visceral rotation allows exposure of most of the splenic artery.
- Open surgical approaches may include: Trans-aneurysmal arterial ligation, Proximal and distal splenic artery ligation with or without resection of the aneurysm; Partial or total splenectomy/distal pancreatectomy with removal of the aneurysm for distal splenic aneurysms.
- Aneurysm resection with primary anastomosis is occasionally possible. Interposition graft insertion has been described but rarely indicated.

COMPLICATIONS

- Post-embolization syndrome.
- Splenic infarct.
- Splenic abscess.
- Pancreatic injury and leak.

TEMPLATE OPERATIVE DICTATION

Preoperative diagnosis: Splenic artery aneurysm.
Procedure: Ligation of splenic artery aneurysm.
Postoperative diagnosis: Splenic artery aneurysm.
Indications: This_____ year-old male/female patient presenting with *symptomatic/asymptomatic splenic artery aneurysm.* Evaluation revealed a saccular/fusiform splenic aneurysm with/without other abnormalities. The patient was not a candidate for endovascular treatment. The risks and benefits of the surgical options were discussed with the patient and *he/she* elected to proceed with surgical intervention.

Description of the procedure: With the patient in the supine position and after induction of general anesthesia, the abdomen was prepped and draped in the usual sterile fashion.

A left subcostal incision was then performed starting from the lateral edge of the right rectus muscle and extending toward the left subcostal region. The anterior rectus sheaths, the right and left rectus muscles and the posterior rectus sheaths were divided and the abdominal cavity was entered. A quick exploratory laparotomy was performed and revealed no pathology except for the splenic artery aneurysm.

Attention was then directed to the lesser omentum. The gastro-hepatic ligament was divided and the lesser sac was entered. The area of the common hepatic artery was identified and the common hepatic artery was circumferentially dissected. The dissection was progressed proximally until the origin of the splenic artery was identified. Further dissection proximally revealed the celiac artery and the origin of the left gastric artery. The celiac artery was then circumferentially dissected and controlled. Attention was then carried to the origin of the splenic artery. The latter was sharply dissected. The dissection progressed distally toward the aneurysm. The overlying tissues were identified and divided. It was felt at this stage that the best would be to oversew the aneurysm rather than to construct a bypass. The splenic artery was clamped proximally and the aneurysm was entered. The distal end was controlled with finger pressure and followed by a oversewing with a 2-0 Prolene suture. The proximal end was transected and oversewn with a running suture of 4-0 Prolene.

Thorough irrigation was then performed. The hemostasis was secured. The spleen was checked and was viable due to flow from the short gastrics.

The wound was then closed №1-Prolene sutures en mass closure. Skin approximated with 4/0 monocryl in subcuticular fashion. The patient tolerated the procedure well and transferred to the postanesthesia care unit in stable condition.

Chapter 194
Replacement of Common Femoral Aneurysm with PTFE Graft

Jamal J. Hoballah, M.D., M.B.A.

INDICATIONS

- Large asymptomatic femoral aneurysm.
- Tissue loss.
- Gangrene.
- Rest pain.
- Disabling claudication.

ESSENTIAL STEPS

1. Expose the proximal common femoral artery.
2. Expose the superficial and profunda femoris arteries.
3. Anticoagulate.
4. Construct the proximal anastomosis.
5. Construct the distal anastomosis.
6. Check for hemostasis.
7. Wound closure.
8. Pulses re-evaluation.

NOTE THIS VARIATION

- Occasionally, the femoral aneurysm extends beyond the femoral bifurcation. In this situation, the distal anastomosis is constructed to the superficial femoral artery and the profunda femoris artery is reimplanted into the side of the graft.

J.J. Hoballah and C.E.H. Scott-Conner (eds.), *Operative Dictations in General and Vascular Surgery*, DOI 10.1007/978-1-4614-0451-4_194,
© Springer Science+Business Media, LLC 2012

COMPLICATIONS
- Bleeding.
- Gangrene.
- Thrombosis of graft.
- Infection.
- Myocardial infarction.

TEMPLATE OPERATIVE DICTATION

Preoperative diagnosis: *Asymptomatic ___-cm femoral aneurysm/ symptomatic ___-cm femoral aneurysm with right/left leg-disabling claudication. Right/left foot rest pain. Right/left foot/toe ulcerations/ gangrene.*

Procedure: Replacement of *right/left* common femoral artery aneurysm with 8-mm *PTFE/Dacron* graft.

Postoperative diagnosis: Same.

Indications: The patient is a ___-year-old *male/female* with an *asymptomatic ___-cm femoral aneurysm/symptomatic ___-cm femoral aneurysm with right/left leg-disabling claudication, right/left foot rest pain, right/left foot/toe ulcerations/gangrene.*

Preoperative evaluation revealed a *right/left* common femoral aneurysm with reconstitution of the profunda and superficial femoris arteries.

The risks and benefits of aneurysm replacement and nonoperative management were explained to the patient and *he/she* elected to undergo surgical intervention.

Description of procedure: The procedure was performed under *general/spinal/epidural* anesthesia. The patient was placed supine on the operating table. The arms were *tucked in/placed at 80°*. Normal bony prominences were padded. The anesthesia team placed appropriate lines. A Foley catheter was placed under sterile technique. The patient's lower abdomen and both lower extremities were circumferentially prepped and draped in the usual sterile fashion. Preoperative antibiotics were administered prior to skin incision.

A *vertical/curvilinear* skin incision overlying the right common femoral artery pulse was made. The incision was deepened through the subcutaneous tissues with electrocautery. The encountered lymphatics were ligated and divided. The common femoral artery aneurysm was then exposed. The dissection was extended proximally to the inguinal ligament, exposing the most distal part of the external iliac artery, which was sharply dissected circumferentially. Attention was then focused on the distal end of the aneurysm. The superficial femoral and profunda femoris arteries were exposed and circumferentially dissected. The external iliac, superficial femoral, and profunda femoris arteries were encircled with silastic vessel loops. Minor branches of the common femoral artery were identified and spared.

The patient was given 75–100 U/kg of heparin intravenously and, after allowing it to circulate for 3–5 min, vascular clamps were applied on the external iliac, superficial femoral, and profunda femoris arteries. The aneurysm was opened longitudinally and the arteriotomy was extended proximally and distally. Toward the proximal neck of the aneurysm, the incision was Td off, transecting the posterior wall 1–2 cm distal to the vascular clamp. Similarly, toward the distal neck of the aneurysm the arteriotomy was carried in a T shape, transecting the posterior wall 1–2 cm proximal to the origin of the superficial and profunda femoris arteries. An *8/10*-mm *PTFE/Dacron* graft was used to replace the aneurysm. An end-to-end proximal anastomosis was constructed between the graft and the transected distal end of the external iliac artery with a running *5-0/6-0 prolene/Gortex* suture. The anastomosis was then completed and checked for hemostasis, which was adequate/*revealed needle hole bleeding that was controlled with the application of Gelfoam soaked with thrombin*. The graft was then transected to the appropriate length and its distal end was spatulated to match the common femoral bifurcation. An end-to-end distal anastomosis was constructed with a running *5-0/6-0 prolene/Gortex* suture. Prior to the completion of the anastomosis, forward-bleeding of the graft and back-bleeding of the superficial and profunda femoris arteries were performed. The sutures were then tied and the clamps released. The suture lines and the wounds were then rechecked for hemostasis. There were good *Doppler signals/palpable pulses* in the foot and a good augmentation of the signal with compressing and releasing the PTFE graft. The wounds were all irrigated with antibiotic solution. The subcutaneous tissue in the groin wound was closed in two layers of 3-0 Vicryl sutures. The skin was closed with staples.

The patient tolerated the procedure well and was transferred to the postanesthesia care unit in stable condition.

NOTES

Chapter 195

Ligation of Popliteal Aneurysm: Femoropopliteal/Tibial Reversed Vein Bypass

Jamal J. Hoballah, M.D., M.B.A.

INDICATIONS

- Asymptomatic popliteal aneurysm.
- Tissue loss.
- Gangrene.
- Rest pain.
- Disabling claudication.

ESSENTIAL STEPS

1. Expose the popliteal artery below the knee.
2. Expose the inflow femoral vessels.
3. Expose/harvest/reverse the greater saphenous vein (GSV).
4. Expose the popliteal artery above the knee through the GSV vein harvest incision.
5. Create graft tunnel.
6. Construct the proximal anastomosis.
7. Check graft for hemostasis.
8. Pass graft through the tunnel.
9. Ligate the proximal and distal necks of the aneurysm.
10. Construct the distal anastomosis.
11. Completion angiogram.
12. Wound closure.
13. Pulses re-evaluation.

J.J. Hoballah and C.E.H. Scott-Conner (eds.), *Operative Dictations in General and Vascular Surgery*, DOI 10.1007/978-1-4614-0451-4_195,
© Springer Science+Business Media, LLC 2012

NOTE THESE VARIATIONS

- Endovascular treatment with stent graft placement may be offered in select patients with appropriate anatomy.
- If the popliteal aneurysm is extremely large, causing significant venous compression, it may be accessed through a posterior approach with the patient in a prone position.
- The bypass can be constructed using a reversed (as described here), nonreversed or in situ technique.
- The proximal anastomosis can be performed at various sites depending on the anatomy.
- The site of the distal anastomosis is dictated by the aneurysmal disease and degree of distal embolization. If the distal anastomosis is to the popliteal artery, it is usually performed in an end-to-end manner. Alternatively, the anastomosis is conducted in an end-to-side manner with ligation of the popliteal artery proximal to the anastomosis.

COMPLICATIONS

- Bleeding.
- Gangrene.
- Thrombosis of graft.
- Infection.
- Myocardial infarction.

TEMPLATE OPERATIVE DICTATION

Preoperative diagnosis: Asymptomatic ___-cm popliteal aneurysm/symptomatic ___-cm popliteal aneurysm with right/left leg-disabling claudication. Right/left foot rest pain. Right/left foot/toe ulcerations/gangrene.

Procedure: Ligation of right/left popliteal artery aneurysm; femoropopliteal/tibial reversed/nonreversed/in situ bypass.

Postoperative diagnosis: Same.

Indications: The patient is a ___-year-old male/female with an asymptomatic ___-cm popliteal aneurysm/a symptomatic ___-cm popliteal aneurysm with right/left leg-disabling claudication, right/left foot rest pain, right/left foot/toe ulcerations/gangrene.

Preoperative evaluation revealed a right/left popliteal aneurysm with a patent popliteal artery and good tibial runoff/occluded popliteal artery with reconstitution of the anterior tibial/posterior tibial/peroneal artery.

The risks and benefits of aneurysm ligation and bypass and nonoperative management were explained to the patient, who elected to undergo surgical intervention.

Description of procedure: The procedure was performed under *general/spinal/epidural* anesthesia. The patient was placed supine on the operating table. The arms were *tucked in/placed at 80°*. Normal bony prominences were padded. The anesthesia team placed appropriate lines. A Foley catheter was placed under sterile technique. The patient's lower abdomen and both lower extremities were circumferentially prepped and draped in the usual sterile fashion. Preoperative antibiotics were administered prior to skin incision.

A 10- to 12-cm longitudinal skin incision was performed 1–2 cm posteromedial and parallel to the tibia. The incision was deepened through the subcutaneous tissue, exposing the fascia. The fascia was incised and the popliteal space was entered. A self-retaining retractor was applied, retracting the gastrocnemius muscle posteriorly and laterally. The tendons of the semimembranosus and semitendinosus muscles were divided to further facilitate the exposure. The popliteal vessels were identified. A 2-cm segment of the most distal popliteal artery was sharply dissected.

Attention was then directed to the groin. A vertical curvilinear skin incision overlying the right common femoral artery was made extending down the upper medial thigh along the preoperatively mapped GSV. The incision was deepened through the subcutaneous tissues with electrocautery. The encountered lymphatics were ligated and divided. The common femoral artery was then exposed and sharply dissected circumferentially. The dissection was extended proximally to the inguinal ligament and distally to include the superficial femoral and profunda femoris arteries. The common femoral, superficial femoral, and profunda femoris arteries were encircled with silastic vessel loops. Minor branches of the common femoral artery were identified and spared.

The GSV was then identified. The vein was exposed from the saphenofemoral junction to the *mid/lower leg through one continuous incision/multiple incisions separated by skin bridges*. Dextran–heparin–papaverine solution was infused into the GSV through a blunt needle that was placed in a side branch in the most distal aspect of the vein. The GSV was harvested and its tributaries ligated with 3-0 silk ties.

The above-knee popliteal artery was then exposed through the bed of the harvested GSV. The skin incision above the knee was deepened through the subcutaneous tissue, exposing the adductor tendon anteriorly and the sartorius muscle posteriorly. The fascia between these two muscles was incised and the popliteal fossa entered. A self-retaining retractor was placed deeper in the wound and the popliteal artery was palpated and exposed. A 2-cm segment of the proximal popliteal artery was sharply dissected.

A tunnel was then created using a *Zepplin/Kelly weck/Gortex* tunneler. The tunnel was *subcutaneous/subfascial* parallel to the course of the GSV to the level of the exposed popliteal artery.

The patient was given 5000 U of heparin intravenously. The GSV was transected at the saphenofemoral junction and its stump suture ligated with 2-0 silk sutures. The distal end was double ligated and transected.

The common femoral artery, profunda, and superficial femoral artery were clamped. A longitudinal arteriotomy in the common femoral artery was performed and extended with Pott's scissors for 1 cm. The vein was then reversed and its distal end was incised along its posterior wall/*incorporating a side branch creating a T junction shape*. The proximal anastomosis was constructed between the spatulated vein and the femoral arteriotomy with a running *5-0/6-0* prolene suture. Prior to completing the suture line, back-bleeding, forward-flushing, and irrigation of the anastomosis with heparinized solution was performed. The anastomosis was then completed and checked for hemostasis, which was adequate. The flow through the vein was checked and was pulsatile. The end of the vein was ligated with a 2-0 silk tie. The vein was rechecked for hemostasis. The vein was then passed distended through the tunnel, avoiding any twists. The popliteal artery was then suture ligated proximal and distal to the aneurysm using *2-0/3-0 silk/prolene* sutures.

Attention was then focused on the construction of the distal anastomosis. A Yasargil clip was applied on the popliteal artery at the level of its trifurcation. The popliteal artery was transected distal to the ligature. The distal end was incised along its anterior surface for 1 cm. The vein was then transected at the appropriate length. An end-to-end anastomosis was then performed between the distal end of the vein bypass and the popliteal artery using *5-0/6-0* prolene sutures.

Prior to the completion of the anastomosis, forward-bleeding of the graft and back-bleeding of the tibial arteries was performed. The sutures were then tied and the clamps released. A 20-gauge angiocatheter was then introduced into the vein graft near the proximal anastomosis and an intraoperative arteriogram was performed. This revealed a widely patent anastomosis and no evidence of filling defects or kinks. The angiocatheter was removed and its puncture site repaired with a 6-0 prolene suture. The suture lines and wounds were then rechecked for hemostasis. There were good *Doppler signals/palpable pulses* in the foot and a good augmentation of the signal with compressing and releasing the vein graft. The wounds were all irrigated with antibiotic solution. The subcutaneous tissue in the groin wound was closed in two layers of 3-0 Vicryl sutures. The fascia overlying the sartorius muscle and in the popliteal space was approximated with 3-0 Vicryl sutures. The skin was closed with staples.

The patient tolerated the procedure well and was transferred to the postanesthesia care unit in stable condition.

Chapter 196
Endovascular Treatment of Popliteal Artery Aneurysm

Jamal J. Hoballah, M.D., M.B.A.

INDICATIONS
- Asymptomatic popliteal artery aneurysm greater than 2 cm in diameter in the presence of suitable anatomy.
- Symptomatic popliteal artery aneurysm in the presence of suitable anatomy.

ESSENTIAL STEPS
1. Preoperative evaluation by CT angiography to determine suitable anatomy (2 cm landing zones and preferably two tibial vessel runoff).
2. Antegrade Percutaneous access of the ipsilateral common femoral artery or under local anesthesia expose the ipsilateral superficial femoral artery.
3. Place a 5-French sheath.
4. Obtain an angiogram to further document the suitable anatomy.
5. Exchange the 5-French sheath into an 8-French sheath.
6. Anticoagulate with intravenous heparin 75–100 IU/kg to keep ACT greater than 250 s.
7. Evaluate the landing zones if intravascular ultrasound (IVUS) is available.
8. Advance a glide wire into a tibial artery and then exchange into a stiff straight wire (260 cm).
9. Obtain another angiogram with the stiff wire through the aneurysm and re-assess the anatomy.

J.J. Hoballah and C.E.H. Scott-Conner (eds.), *Operative Dictations in General and Vascular Surgery*, DOI 10.1007/978-1-4614-0451-4_196,
© Springer Science+Business Media, LLC 2012

10. Select the desired dimensions of the endoprosthesis (Upsizing by 10% and avoid excessive upsizing to prevent infolding of the graft).
11. Mark the desired landing zones distally and proximally on the screen and using bony landmarks or roadmap.
12. Introduce the endoprosthesis to the desired location.
13. Obtain another angiogram to re-confirm desired landing location.
14. Deploy the endoprosthesis.
15. Remove the delivery system.
16. Perform balloon angioplasty to mold/iron the endoprosthesis at the landing sites.
17. Completion angiogram to check for endoleak or the need for another extension.
18. Remove the sheath and close the puncture site with a closure device if performed percutaneously or with interrupted prolene sutures if performed using an open superficial femoral artery exposure.

NOTE THESE VARIATIONS

- Proper patient selection based on suitable anatomy is essential to the success of the procedure. If poor distal runoff or short landing zones, or presence of significant compression symptoms, an open repair is preferable especially if the patient is not a high medical risk for open procedure.
- Access to the femoral vessel may be performed percutaneously or through an open approach. Due to the large size sheath, an open exposure of the superficial femoral artery under local anesthesia allows easy access and closure of the puncture side. If a percutaneous approach is used, a closure device should be considered for closing the puncture side to avoid excessive manual compression that may occlude the endoprosthesis or cause groin complications.
- Various stent grafts are endoprostheses are available on the market.
- It is preferable to avoid using multiple endoprostheses. However, if there is significant discrepancy between the diameter of the distal landing zone and the proximal landing zone, two stents grafts may be needed. The distal endoprosthesis is first deployed. The second endoprosthesis is then docked inside the distal with a good 2- to 3-cm overlap.
- The patient is usually started on dual antiplatelet therapy with Aspirin and Clopidogrel prior to the procedure.

Clopidogrel is usually maintained for 3 months postoperatively and Aspirin indefinitely.

COMPLICATIONS
- Thrombosis of endoprosthesis.
- Endoleak.
- Distal Embolization.
- Bleeding.
- Gangrene.

TEMPLATE OPERATIVE DICTATION
Preoperative diagnosis: Asymptomatic ___-cm popliteal aneurysm/symptomatic ___-cm popliteal aneurysm with right/left leg-disabling claudication. Right/left foot rest pain. Right/left foot/toe ulcerations/gangrene.

Procedure: Endovascular repair of *right/left* popliteal artery aneurysm using a _____ *Viaban/Fluency/Other* endoprosthesis.

Postoperative diagnosis: Same.

Indications: The patient is a ___-year-old male/female with an asymptomatic ___-cm popliteal aneurysm/a symptomatic ___-cm popliteal aneurysm with right/left leg-disabling claudication, right/left foot rest pain, right/left foot/toe ulcerations/gangrene.

Preoperative evaluation revealed a *right/left* popliteal aneurysm with *a patent popliteal artery and good tibial runoff* and reconstitution of the *anterior tibial/posterior tibial/peroneal artery*. The landing zones were deemed appropriate for endovascular treatment.

The risks and benefits of endovascular aneurysm aneurysm repair and alternatives with bypass and nonoperative management were explained to the patient, who elected to undergo endovascular intervention.

Description of procedure: The procedure was performed under *local monitored* anesthesia. The patient was placed supine on the operating table. The arms were *tucked in/placed at 80°*. Normal bony prominences were padded. The anesthesia team placed appropriate lines. A Foley catheter was placed under sterile technique. The patient's lower abdomen and both lower extremities were circumferentially prepped and draped in the usual sterile fashion. Preoperative antibiotics were administered prior to skin incision. The patient has been on dual antiplatelet therapy with Aspirin and Clopidogrel.

Alternative 1 Using a Seldinger technique and under ultrasound guidance, the common femoral artery was punctured in an antegrade manner. The wire was advanced into the superficial femoral artery.

The micropuncture sheath was then exchanged into a size 5-French sheath.

Alternative 2: The skin over the course of the proximal superficial femoral artery was infiltrated with 1% lidocaine. A 7-cm longitudinal incision was performed over the upper thigh and deepened through the subcutaneous tissue and fat. The superficial femoral artery was identified along the lower border of the sartorius muscle and was dissected for a 5-cm segment. Using sledinger technique a 5-French sheath was inserted.

Angiography through the sheath was performed delineating the location of the aneurysm and its proximal and distal landing zones. The anatomy appeared to be appropriate for endovascular graft treatment. The patient was given 75–100 IU of heparin intravenously to keep the activated clotting time (ACT) greater than 250 s. The 5-French sheath was exchanged for a size 8 French sheath. *The intravascular ultrasound IVUS was introduced and the landing zones were evaluated and confirmed to be appropriate.* The superficial femoral artery/popliteal artery diameter were measured proximal and distal to the aneurysm. A glidewire was then introduced and manipulated through the aneurysm and advanced to the tibial arteries. The wire was then exchanged to an 260-cm Amplatz/straight tip stiff wire. A repeat angiogram was then performed with the stiff wire in place. The proximal and distal landing zones were marked using a *Glow 'N Tell tape/erasable marker on the screen/and bony landmarks.* The appropriate size stent graft was selected. A size ____mm x ____cm *Viabahn/Fluency* graft was then introduced over the wire to the area of the aneurysm. The stent graft was then placed at the appropriate location. After an additional angiogram was performed to further confirm the appropriate position, the stent graft was deployed. The delivery system was then removed. A size ____mm × ____cm balloon was then used to mold each landing zone to maximize the apposition of the graft against the arterial wall. The balloon was then removed. An angiography was then performed and revealed proper placement with no evidence of any Type I endoleak. There was no need for any additional extension limbs.

Alternative 1: The sheath was then removed and a closure device (Perclose was used to close the puncture side).

Alternative 2: The sheath was removed and the puncture hole in the superficial femoral artery was closed with interrupted 5-0 Prolene sutures. The wound was then closed with 3-0 absorbable sutures (Vicryl) for the subcutaneous tissue and 4-0 absorbable subcuticular sutures (Monocryl) for the skin.

The patient tolerated the procedure well and was transferred to the recovery room in good condition with excellent distal pulses and no complications.

NOTES

Section XX

Venous Disorders

Chapter 197

Stripping of the Greater Saphenous Vein and Stab Avulsion of Branch Varicosities

Michael S. Connors III, M.D. and Samuel R. Money, M.D.

INDICATIONS

- Pain.
- Fatigue.
- Bleeding.
- Ulcerations.
- Cosmesis.

ESSENTIAL STEPS

1. Mark the varicose veins preoperatively with the patient upright.
2. Incise the skin over the saphenofemoral junction.
3. Identify and ligate the greater saphenous vein at the saphenofemoral junction.
4. Ligate all branches draining into the greater saphenous vein at the saphenofemoral junction.
5. Incise over the greater saphenous vein *at/below* the *knee/ankle*.
6. Pass vein stripper from the greater saphenous vein from below *knee/ankle* to the groin.
7. Pull stripper from the groin, avulsing the greater saphenous vein.
8. Incise the skin over the marked varicose vein tributaries.
9. Identify the varicose vein and avulse in both proximal and distal directions with a *hemostat/crochet* hook.
10. Assess hemostasis, close the wound, and then wrap the lower extremity with cotton gauze followed by an Ace

J.J. Hoballah and C.E.H. Scott-Conner (eds.), *Operative Dictations in General and Vascular Surgery*, DOI 10.1007/978-1-4614-0451-4_197,
© Springer Science+Business Media, LLC 2012

bandage (start at foot and wrap proximal to the most cephalic incision site).

NOTE THESE VARIATIONS

- Endovascular laser or radiofrequency ablation has replaced stripping of the greater saphenous veins in many practices and will be described in Chapter 198, endovenous ablation of varicose veins.
- Stripping of the greater saphenous vein from the ankle to the groin is associated with saphenous nerve injury because of the adherence of the saphenous nerve to the vein in the lower leg. This can be avoided by stripping the vein from just below the knee to the groin.
- If the greater saphenous vein is not varicosed and the saphenofemoral junction is competent, the greater saphenous vein is not stripped and only stab avulsion of the branch varicosities is performed.

COMPLICATIONS

- Infection.
- Bleeding.
- Saphenous nerve injury.

TEMPLATE OPERATIVE DICTATION

Preoperative diagnosis: Varicose veins of the *right/left* lower extremity.

Procedure: *Right/left* lower-extremity greater saphenous vein stripping and stab avulsion of varicose veins.

Postoperative diagnosis: Same.

Indications: This is a ___-year-old *male/female* with a history of varicose veins involving the *right/left* lower extremity. The patient has been complaining of pain, fatigue, bleeding, and ulcerations and is nonresponsive to compression therapy. *The veins are being excised for cosmetic purposes.* Preoperative lower-extremity duplex revealed no DVT and *competent/incompetent* saphenofemoral junction.

Description of procedure: After the induction of *general/epidural/ spinal* anesthesia, the patient was positioned supine with both legs elevated. The patient was sterilely prepped and draped in the usual fashion from the tip of the toe up to the umbilicus. A primary incision was made in the *right/left* inguinal crease overlying the saphenofemoral junction. This was identified as being 1 cm medial and 1 cm inferior to the femoral artery pulse. The subcutaneous tissue was divided with electrocautery. The greater saphenous vein was identified and traced proximally toward the saphenofemoral junction. Multiple (ordinarily five) venous tributaries were divided with 3-0 silk ligatures. The greater saphenous vein was doubly ligated at its origin with a 2-0 silk ligature. The distal ligature was not tied; however, it was left in position.

[Choose one:]

If stripping to knee level: A second incision was made a few centimeters below the knee. The subcutaneous tissue was divided and the saphenous vein identified, then circled proximally and distally with 3-0 silk ties. This time the distal ligature was secured and the proximal ligature left in position.

If stripping to ankle level: A second incision was made at the ankle/approximately one finger breadth anterior and superior to the medial malleolus. The subcutaneous tissue was divided and the saphenous vein identified, then circled proximally and distally with 3-0 silk ties. This time the distal ligature was secured and the proximal ligature left in position. Care was taken to avoid injury to the saphenous nerve (which lies in close proximity to the vein at this position).

A small transverse venotomy was created with a #11 blade. The stripping wire was inserted and passed proximally toward the groin without difficulty. The greater saphenous vein was then divided completely at the groin, allowing the vein stripping wire to exit. Prior to removal the stripping wire was secured at both ends with the 2-0 silk ties that had been left in position. The greater saphenous vein was then stripped from distal to proximal with pressure being exerted as the vein was stripped. At this point, hemostasis was controlled by elevation and pressure. Small incisions, approximately 2–4 mm, were created over the preoperative marked areas using a #11 blade. A *small crochet hook/or mosquito hemostat* was used to avulse these veins. The veins were pulled both proximally and distally. After hemostasis was obtained, the wounds were irrigated copiously. The wound in the groin was closed in multiple layers with 3-0 absorbable sutures followed by a running 4-0 subcuticular stitch. The wounds where the stab avulsions occurred were closed with steristrips. The wound at the *ankle/below-knee* incision was closed with a 4-0 *absorbable suture/ steristrips*. All wounds were sterilely dressed with gauze, then a doubly applied 4-in. Ace bandage was placed on the lower leg beginning at the head of the metatarsals. This was concluded by a 6-in. Ace bandage on the upper leg.

The patient tolerated the procedure well and was taken to the postanesthesia care unit in stable condition.

NOTES

Chapter 198
Endovenous Ablation of Varicose Veins

Dale Maharaj, M.D., Kathleen J. Ozsvath, M.D., and R. Clement Darling III, M.D.

INDICATIONS

- As for the conventional sapheno-femoral or sapheno-popliteal ligations, particularly in the redo patient with previous groin dissection. Particularly useful in patients with lower calf perforators with skin changes, and in obese patients.

COMPLICATIONS

- Hemorrhage.
- Bruising.
- Phlebitis.
- Deep venous thrombosis.
- Paresthesia.
- Skin burns.

ADVANTAGES

- No incisions, minimal scaring, and less chance of surgical site infection.
- Can be done under local anesthesia.
- Can be done with active ulcer.
- Can ambulate right away.

ESSENTIAL STEPS

1. Preoperative ultrasound vein mapping and marking of the vein to be ablated, including the sapheno-femoral (SFJ) or sapheno-popliteal junctions (SPJ) and perforators.

J.J. Hoballah and C.E.H. Scott-Conner (eds.), *Operative Dictations in General and Vascular Surgery*, DOI 10.1007/978-1-4614-0451-4_198,
© Springer Science+Business Media, LLC 2012

2. Prevention of vasospasm when performing the percutaneous access.
3. Trendelenberg position when accessing and reverse Trendelenberg when ablating.
4. Ensure that fiber tip is exposed, and not within the sheath when ablating.
5. Ensure that the tip of the laser is distal to the first tributaries at the sapheno-femoral junction.
6. Aim for a laser energy delivery of 90 J/cm.
7. Apply compression after procedure and ambulate immediately.

OPERATIVE NOTE

Preoperative diagnosis: Rt/Lt Sapheno-femoral incompetence; Sapheno-popliteal incompetence; Perforator incompetence.
Procedure: Rt/Lt; Endovenous ablation under local anesthesia.
Postoperative diagnosis: Same.
Indications: ___-year-old man/woman.

Painful varicose veins/ankle edema/stasis dermatitis/non-healing ulcer.

Duplex scan revealed reflux at the sapheno-femoral, sapheno-popliteal, or perforator incompetence.

Description of the procedure: Vein mapping was performed with the patient standing. Attention was paid to marking the SFJ/SPJ/perforators.

The patient was placed in the reverse-Trendelenberg position.

The Rt/Lt lower limb was prepped and draped in a standard surgical fashion.

Under ultrasound guidance, the GSV/SSV was accessed using a 14G, 70-mm percutaneous entry needle, and the intravascular position was confirmed by "flashback."

The ultrasound transducer was placed at the SFJ and a 035″ J-guidewire was inserted into the vessel utilizing the standard Seldinger technique and directed to the common femoral vein via the GSV.

The catheter sheath assembly was fed over the guidewire into the vessel and positioned under ultrasound guidance just distal to the first tributary at the SFJ (e.g., 2 cm from the SFJ).

The laser fiber tip was advanced into the sheath up to the first "site-mark."

The sheath was then withdrawn to the second "site-mark."

The patient was placed in the Trendelenberg position and suction applied to the three-way stopcock using a 20-ml syringe.

Tumescent anesthesia was administered in the perivenous space with 500 ml of saline containing 50 ml of 1% lidocaine (with 10 ml of sodium bicarbonate) via direct visualization with ultrasound.

The sheath positioning was confirmed under ultrasound, with the fiber tip located approximately 1–2 cm below the saphenofemoral junction.

Laser safety goggles were used.

The fiber was attached to the laser consol and the aiming beam confirmed the position of the laser fiber tip.

The laser was set in the continuous mode at 14 W (or lower depending on area to be ablated).

The sheath and fiber were withdrawn at the rate of 1–2 mm/s for the first 5–10 cm of the vessel, and then 2–3 mm/s for the remainder of the treated segment.

Confirmatory ultrasound was then performed documenting a successfully ablated vein, and no deep venous thrombosis.

The limb was wrapped with an ace bandage and a Class II compression hose was placed on the patient.

The patient was ambulated immediately (if no general anesthesia/conscious sedation was used).

For Perforator Ablation (pathologic perforator associated with CEAP>4): Under duplex guidance, a 21G venous access needle was inserted into the perforator.

A 10 cm × 4F Introducer Sheath was directed into the subfascial plane over an 0.018″ Guidewire.

A 400 mm Optical Fiber was then inserted into the sheath and the tip was directed to 1 cm from the deep vein and perforator junction.

Tumescent local anesthesia was injected into the perforator perivenous area.

The laser was set in continuous mode at 5 W and the perforator was ablated.

Chapter 199

Femorofemoral Vein Bypass (Palma Procedure)

Munier M.S. Nazzal, M.D.

INDICATIONS

- Persistent isolated unilateral iliac/common femoral vein occlusion in patients with severe venous insufficiency unresponsive to conservative therapy.
- Evidence of hemodynamic or venographic stable occlusion over 1 year.
- Venous claudication unresponsive to conservative therapy in active patients.
- Patient with progressive swelling of the leg secondary to external compression that is not relieved by conservative therapy.

ESSENTIAL STEPS

1. Bilateral vertical groin incision to expose the femoral veins.
2. Exposure of the contralateral greater saphenous vein down to the knee.
3. Dissection of the contralateral greater saphenous vein at the saphenofemoral junction, preserving all tributaries.
4. 180° exposure of the anterior wall of the ipsilateral common femoral vein.
5. Suprapubic tunnel formation.
6. Check the tunneled saphenous vein for twisting or kinking.
7. Heparinization of the patient.

J.J. Hoballah and C.E.H. Scott-Conner (eds.), *Operative Dictations in General and Vascular Surgery*, DOI 10.1007/978-1-4614-0451-4_199,
© Springer Science+Business Media, LLC 2012

8. End-to-side anastomosis of the saphenous vein to the common femoral vein.
9. Closure of the groin and thigh incisions in layers.

NOTE THIS VARIATION

- Femorofemoral venous bypasses can also be constructed using prosthetic conduits with adjunctive arteriovenous fistulae.

COMPLICATIONS

- Thrombosis.
- Wound complications.
- Lymph leak.

TEMPLATE OPERATIVE DICTATION

Preoperative diagnosis: *Left/right* lower-extremity *swelling/claudication/venous ulcer* with iliofemoral vein occlusion.

Procedure: Cross-femoral venous bypass (Palma procedure).

Postoperative diagnosis: Same.

Indications: This is a ___-year-old *male/female* who presented with *swelling/claudication/venous ulcer* for about ___ years, not responding to conservative therapy.

Description of procedure: The patient was placed in a supine position. The procedure was performed *under general/epidural/spinal* anesthesia. The abdomen and both lower extremities were prepped and draped in the usual fashion.

A vertical incision was made in the contralateral groin. The saphenofemoral junction was exposed. All tributaries of the greater saphenous vein at the junction were isolated and preserved.

The greater saphenous vein was exposed from the groin down to the knee using small interrupted incisions. The affected groin was incised vertically down to the femoral veins. The common femoral vein and deep femoral vein were exposed.

The anterior surface of the common femoral vein was dissected, exposing the anterior 180° of the vein.

Patency of the common femoral vein was confirmed by palpation and Doppler flow.

A suprapubic subcutaneous tunnel was made between the two groin incisions using a tunneler that was left in place.

Length of the saphenous vein needed for bypass was confirmed.

Hemostasis was secured.

The saphenous vein was isolated and dissected out of the thigh. The distal transected saphenous vein was ligated with silk 0-0. The saphenous vein was distended carefully with heparinized solution to check for leaks.

The patient was heparinized (100 U/kg bolus) intravenously.

The saphenous vein was passed distended through the tunnel with care to avoid any twisting or kinking

A U-shaped vascular clamp was applied to the recipient common femoral vein. A vertical venotomy was made using a #11 blade and extended with Pott's scissors. An anastomosis was constructed between the end of the saphenous vein and the side of the common femoral vein using 6-0 prolene. A duplex scan was obtained to confirm patency of the saphenous graft and the femoral vein.

Hemostasis was secured.

Wounds in the donor thigh were closed in two layers. A closed suction drain was left in both groin incisions. The vertical groin incisions were closed in three layers: The fascia and subcutaneous layers with Vicryl 3-0 continuously and the skin with staples. Dressings were applied.

The patient tolerated the procedure well, recovered from anesthesia, and was taken to the postanesthesia care unit in stable condition.

NOTES

Chapter 200

Venous Thrombectomy for Iliofemoral DVT Using Mechanical Devices and Lysis

Chad Laurich, M.D.

INDICATION

- Acute iliofemoral DVT with symptoms <14 days, good functional status, life expectancy >1 year who have a low risk of bleeding.

ESSENTIAL STEPS

1. Define the extent of thrombus preoperatively via duplex or CT.
2. Prevent PE with systemic anticoagulation if not contraindicated, vena cava filter or balloon occlusion during thrombectomy, positive end expiratory pressure during thrombectomy.
3. Access femoral vein percutaneously.
4. Cross thrombus with wire and perform mechanical, pharmacomechanical, or catheter-directed thrombolysis directly to the area of thrombus.
5. If catheter-directed thrombolysis performed, plan repeat venography within 24 h.
6. Perform completion venography to ensure adequate results and evaluate for venous outflow stenosis.

NOTE THESE VARIATIONS

- Access may be from the popliteal vein with the patient prone if thrombus extends down the femoral vein.

J.J. Hoballah and C.E.H. Scott-Conner (eds.), *Operative Dictations in General and Vascular Surgery*, DOI 10.1007/978-1-4614-0451-4_200,
© Springer Science+Business Media, LLC 2012

- Angioplasty/stenting may be necessary if underlying iliac stenosis identified.
- For free floating IVC thrombus, a vena cava filter may be placed or occlusive balloon placed from the contralateral side for use during mechanical thrombolysis to prevent emboli.
- Multiple thrombolysis devises/catheters are available including, but not limited to, the Angiojet (Possis Medical, Minneapolis, MN), EKOS EndoWave (Bothell, WA) system, and Trellis catheter (Bacchus Vascular, Santa Clara, CA).
- Thrombolytic agent may be infused through both the thrombolysis catheter and the sheath.
- Venous outflow stenosis must be treated with angioplasty/stenting if found after thrombolysis.

COMPLICATIONS
- Bleeding.
- Non-resolution of thrombus.
- Embolization.
- Recurrence.

TEMPLATE OPERATIVE DICTATION
Preoperative diagnosis: Acute iliofemoral DVT.
Procedure: Venous thrombectomy with mechanical device *with/ without* lysis.
Postoperative diagnosis: Same.
Indications: The patient is a ___-year-old *male/female* presenting with *right/left* lower extremity swelling and pain. Preoperative duplex evaluation is consistent with *right/left* iliofemoral DVT. The patient has been informed of the risks and benefits of venous thrombectomy and thrombolysis and wishes to undergo the procedure.
Description of procedure: The patient was brought to the operating room and placed in supine position. Prophylactic antibiotics were administered. The patient was fully anticoagulated and maintained on an unfractionated heparin drip *or was administered a therapeutic (1 mg/kg) does of low molecular weight heparin*. The *right/left* groin and leg were prepped and draped in the usual sterile fashion. Monitored anesthesia care was provided and local anesthetic (1% Lidocaine) was infiltrated into the skin and subcutaneous tissues around the femoral vein.

Percutaneous access was achieved in the common femoral vein with a micropuncture kit using ultrasound and fluoroscopic guidance. A 5-mm nick was made in the skin with an 11 blade and a 6-Fr sheath was placed using Seldinger technique. Venography was performed and the area of thrombus confirmed. An angled Glidewire and straight Glide catheter were used to cross the area of occlusion. The Glidewire was exchanged for a Benson wire (Amplatz wire or stiff Glidewire may be used as well) and the 6-Fr Angiojet catheter was placed. A balloon catheter was passed from a contralateral percutaneous access site and inflated in the inferior vena cava above the thrombus to protect against embolization. Multiple passes of the Angiojet were performed. Venography revealed removal of a significant portion of clot. A ___ cm multi-side hole thrombolysis catheter was then placed across the area of thrombus and rt-PA infusion was initiated at a rate of 0.5 *mg/h*. The catheter was secured to the skin with a 2-0 silk stitch and a dressing applied.

For pulse spray technique: After access, the Angiojet catheter was placed across the thrombus and rt-PA was pulse injected into the thrombus with a total of 5–20 mg of rt-PA. The 6-Fr catheter was left in place and secured with a 2-0 silk stitch for planned venography with repeat treatment, if necessary, within 24 h.

For isolated segmental pharmacomechanical thrombolysis technique: After access, the Trellis catheter was placed into the thrombus with the proximal balloon positioned at the most proximal edge of the thrombus. The balloons were inflated and rt-PA was infused, while the catheter ran for 15 min with the aspiration of thrombus. The catheter was repositioned and the infusion/aspiration cycle was repeated until the entire area of occlusion had been treated. A ___ cm multi-side hole thrombolysis catheter was then placed across the area of residual thrombus and rt-PA infusion was initiated at a rate of 1 mg/h. The catheter was secured to the skin with a 2-0 silk stitch and a dressing applied.

The patient tolerated the procedure well and was taken to the postanesthesia care unit in stable condition.

Chapter 201

Endovenous Recanalization for Chronic Occlusion or Stenosis, May-Thurner Syndrome

Chad Laurich, M.D.

INDICATION

- Chronic stenosis or obstruction of the femoroiliocaval venous outflow tract.

ESSENTIAL STEPS

1. Access the femoral vein with ultrasound guidance.
2. Perform venography and/or intravascular ultrasound to define the severity and length of stenosis.
3. The full area of disease must be defined and treated with stenting.
4. Predilation is performed; serial dilatations may be necessary in occluded segments.
5. Large diameter stents are used (14–16 mm) in the common and external iliac veins.
6. Post-stent dilatation is performed with appropriately sized (14–16 mm) balloons.
7. Completion venography/intravascular ultrasound evaluation confirms successful results.

NOTE THESE VARIATIONS

- Patients may present with iliofemoral DVT and require pharmacomechanical lytic therapy and/or catheter-directed lytic therapy prior to intervention with angioplasty and stenting.

J.J. Hoballah and C.E.H. Scott-Conner (eds.), *Operative Dictations in General and Vascular Surgery*, DOI 10.1007/978-1-4614-0451-4_201,
© Springer Science+Business Media, LLC 2012

- Intravascular ultrasound or venography may be used exclusively for the procedure, but intravascular ultrasound is considered more sensitive and its use highly encouraged.
- The popliteal vein may be used for access, if necessary.
- Serial dilations may be necessary for initial catheter placement.
- For proximal common iliac lesions, it is necessary to extend the stent well into the inferior vena cava to prevent recurrent stenosis.
- For chronic occlusions, multiple maneuvers with soft and stiff wires supported by guide catheters may be necessary to cross the occlusion.
- If a long-segment stenosis is present, it is acceptable to extend the stents across the inguinal ligament to the common femoral vein (to just above the greater saphenous, circumflex and profunda vein tributaries).

COMPLICATIONS

- Bleeding.
- Early thrombotic events.
- Late recurrence.

TEMPLATE OPERATIVE DICTATION

Preoperative diagnosis: Chronic obstruction of the left iliofemoral venous outflow tract.

Procedure: Intravascular ultrasound evaluation with venography and endovenous balloon angioplasty/stenting of left iliac veins.

Postoperative diagnosis: Same.

Indications: The patient is a ___-year-old *female/male* who presents with *previous DVT and/or lower extremity swelling and pain* that is refractory to conservative management. Evaluation with IVUS and venography with possible balloon angioplasty and stenting is indicated. The patient has been informed of the risks and benefits of the procedure and wishes to proceed.

Description of Procedure: The patient was brought to the endovascular suite, placed in supine position and *general endotracheal anesthesia was induced or monitored anesthesia care with local anesthetic was provided*. Prophylactic antibiotics were administered. The *right/left* groin and leg were prepped and draped in the usual sterile fashion.

The *left* femoral vein was accessed distal to the obstruction with a micropuncture kit using ultrasound guidance. An *8–12*-Fr sheath was then placed using Seldinger technique. 5,000 units of unfractionated heparin was given intravenously. Venography was performed with multiple oblique projections (0, 45, and 60°) and an area of stenosis was visualized in the common iliac vein with numerous pelvic collaterals. An angled glidewire and straight glide catheter were used to cross the femoral and iliac veins into the inferior vena cava. Intravascular ultrasound was performed and confirmed the findings with a greater than 50% stenosis in the common iliac vein, with the extension of stenosis into the proximal external iliac vein.

Balloon angioplasty was performed with a *14–16 mm* balloon over a stiffened Glidewire to predilate the stenosis. A self-expanding *14–16 mm* bare metal stent was placed across the stenosis, extending from the external iliac vein to the inferior vena cava. *If two stents are necessary due to the length of involvement*: A 14-mm stent was placed distally in the external iliac artery and a 16-mm stent was placed proximally in the common iliac vein with extension into the inferior vena cava and sufficient overlap of the stents to prevent separation. Balloon angioplasty was performed inside the stent(s) with a *14–16 mm* balloon and the proximal end was overexpanded slightly to "flare" it in the inferior vena cava.

Completion venography and evaluation with intravascular ultrasound revealed widely patent iliac veins with decreased flow through collaterals. All catheters and wires were removed and the sheath was removed after the activated clotting time was <180 s.

The patient tolerated the procedure well with no apparent complications and was taken to the postanesthesia care unit in stable condition.

Chapter 202
Inferior Vena Cava Filters

F. Ezequiel Parodi, M.D. and Murray L. Shames, M.D.

INDICATIONS

Absolute

- Deep venous thrombosis or documented thromboembolism in a patient who has a contraindication to anticoagulation.
- Recurrent thromboembolism despite adequate anticoagulation.
- Complications of anticoagulation that required discontinuation of therapy.
- Immediately after pulmonary embolectomy.
- Failure of another form of caval interruption, demonstrated by recurrent pulmonary thromboembolism.

Relative

- A large free-floating iliofemoral thrombus demonstrated on venography in a high-risk patient.
- A propagating iliofemoral thrombus despite adequate anticoagulation.
- Chronic pulmonary embolism in a patient with pulmonary hypertension and cor pulmonale.
- A patient who has occlusion of more than 50% of the pulmonary vascular bed and would not tolerate additional thromboembolism.
- Presence of recurrent septic embolism.
- Patient at high risk for DVT/PE with contraindications for prophylactic anticoagulation.

J.J. Hoballah and C.E.H. Scott-Conner (eds.), *Operative Dictations in General and Vascular Surgery*, DOI 10.1007/978-1-4614-0451-4_202,
© Springer Science+Business Media, LLC 2012

ESSENTIAL STEPS

Femoral Approach

1. Local anesthesia over the femoral vein (right usually used).
2. Percutaneous puncture of the common femoral vein with Seldinger needle.
3. Place guide wire into the vena cava under fluoroscopic guidance.
4. Sequential dilation of the tract.
5. Place marker pigtail catheter in the inferior vena cava.
6. Venogram to identify the renal veins and assess the diameter of the vena cava.
7. Place provided sheath into the vena cava to the level of the lowest (left) renal vein.
8. Insert filter into sheath, with tip of filter to be distal to the lowest renal vein.
9. Withdraw sheath to expose filter.
10. Deploy filter under continuous fluoroscopy.
11. Completion venogram.
12. Remove sheath and hold pressure on the puncture site for 10–15 min to obtain hemostasis.

Jugular Approach

1. Local anesthesia over the internal jugular vein (usually right).
2. Percutaneous puncture of the internal jugular vein with Seldinger needle.
3. Place guide wire into the vena cava under fluoroscopic guidance.
4. Sequential dilation of the tract.
5. Place marker pigtail catheter in the inferior vena cava.
6. Venogram to identify the renal veins and assess the diameter of the vena cava.
7. Place provided sheath into the vena cava to the level of the lowest (left) renal vein.
8. Insert filter into sheath, with top of filter to be distal to the lowest renal vein.
9. Withdraw sheath to expose filter.
10. Deploy filter under continuous fluoroscopy.
11. Completion venogram.
12. Remove sheath and hold pressure on the puncture site for 10–15 min to obtain hemostasis.

NOTE THIS VARIATION

- The procedure may be performed through a femoral or jugular approach, using various filters.

COMPLICATIONS

- Vena cava perforation.
- Filter misplacement (cephalad to the renal veins, in an iliac vein, tilt).
- Acute or late filter thrombosis.
- Access site bleeding/hematoma.

TEMPLATE OPERATIVE DICTATION

Preoperative diagnosis: Recurrent pulmonary embolus.
Procedure: Vena cava filter placement (*jugular/femoral* approach).
Postoperative diagnosis: Recurrent pulmonary embolus.
Indications: The patient is a ___-year-old *male/female* with recurrent pulmonary emboli despite *adequate anticoagulation/significant DVT* and contraindications for anticoagulation. The patient has been informed of the risks and benefits of inferior vena cava filter placement and has agreed to the procedure.
Description of procedure:

[Choose one:]

If femoral approach: The patient was placed on the operating table in a supine position. The *right/left* groin was prepped and draped in the standard fashion. Using 1% lidocaine, the area overlying the common femoral vein was anesthetized. (Intravenous sedation was administered by the anesthesia staff if needed.) The common femoral vein was punctured with the Seldinger needle and a guide wire placed into the vena cava to the level of the second lumbar vertebrae under fluoroscopic guidance. A pigtail catheter was placed into the vena cava over a guide wire. Contrast venography was performed and there was no thrombus within the vena cava or iliac veins. The vena cava is ___ mm in diameter. The renal veins and iliac veins confluence is identified and marked on the screen. The tract was serially dilated over the guide wire and the provided sheath placed into the vena cava under fluoroscopy. The sheath was flushed with heparin solution. The device was inserted over the wire into the sheath and positioned below the lowest renal vein. The sheath was withdrawn, exposing the filter. With continuous fluoroscopic imaging, the filter was deployed in the infrarenal vena cava. Completion venogram shows good filter position within the vena cava without thrombus formation. The device and sheath were removed and 15 min of pressure applied to the puncture site for hemostasis. Dressings were applied.

The patient tolerated the procedure well and was taken to the postanesthesia care unit in stable condition.

If jugular approach: The patient was placed on the operating table in a supine position. The right neck was prepped and draped in the standard fashion. Using 1% lidocaine, the area overlying the internal jugular vein was anesthetized. Intravenous sedation was administered by the anesthesia staff. The internal jugular vein was punctured with the Seldinger needle and a guide wire placed into the vena cava to the level of the second lumbar vertebrae under fluoroscopic guidance. A pigtail catheter was placed into the vena cava over a guide wire. Contrast venography was performed and there was no thrombus within the vena cava or iliac veins. The vena cava is ___mm in diameter. The renal veins and iliac veins confluence was identified and marked on the screen to identify the renal veins and assess the diameter of the vena cava. The tract was serially dilated over a guide wire and the provided sheath placed into the vena cava under fluoroscopy. The sheath was flushed with heparin solution. The device was inserted over the wire into the sheath and positioned distal to the lowest renal vein. The sheath was withdrawn, exposing the filter. With continuous fluoroscopic imaging, the filter was deployed in the infrarenal vena cava. Completion venogram shows good filter position within the vena cava without thrombus formation. The device and sheath were removed and 15 min of pressure applied to the puncture site for hemostasis. Dressings were applied.

The patient tolerated the procedure well and was taken to the postanesthesia care unit in stable condition.

RADIOLOGY SUPERVISION AND INTERPRETATION
1. *Venogram:* Venogram, no intraluminal thrombus noted.
2. *Completion venogram:* Interval placement of inferior vena caval filter device caudad to renal veins. Device is in good position, no evidence of tilt or adherent thrombus.

Section XXI

Creation of Arteriovenous
Fistulae for Dialysis

Chapter 203
Radiocephalic Arteriovenous Fistula for Hemodialysis

Christopher Bunch, M.D.

INDICATION
- End-stage renal disease requiring hemodialysis.

ESSENTIAL STEPS
1. Evaluate the cephalic vein with duplex scan unless good quality and continuity to the upper arm clearly established by physical exam.
2. Allen test.
3. Regional/local anesthesia.
4. *Transverse incision overlying the artery and vein/longitudinal incision between the artery and vein.*
5. Develop skin flaps.
6. Identify and mobilize 2 cm of the radial artery.
7. Identify and mobilize the vein.
8. Obtain proximal and distal control.
9. Longitudinal arteriotomy.
10. *End-to-side/side-to-side* anastomosis to the vein.
11. Check for thrill, distal pulse.
12. Check hemostasis.
13. Close the incision.

NOTE THESE VARIATIONS
- Skin incision is tailored depending on the location of the vein relative to the artery.

J.J. Hoballah and C.E.H. Scott-Conner (eds.), *Operative Dictations in General and Vascular Surgery*, DOI 10.1007/978-1-4614-0451-4_203,
© Springer Science+Business Media, LLC 2012

- The anastomosis may be performed in a side-to-side or end-to-side configuration.

COMPLICATIONS
- Failure to achieve sufficient arterialization of venous network.
- Steal syndrome.
- Bleeding.
- Occlusion.
- Infection.

TEMPLATE OPERATIVE DICTATION

Preoperative diagnosis: End-stage renal disease requiring chronic hemodialysis.

Procedure: *Left/right* wrist arteriovenous fistula for hemodialysis.

Postoperative diagnosis: Same.

Indications: This ___-year-old *male/female* developed end-stage renal disease due to ___, requiring *(anticipated)* need for chronic hemodialysis. Arteriovenous fistula was chosen to provide access. Risks and benefits were explained to the patient and *he/she* elected to undergo the procedure.

Description of procedure: The patient was brought to the operating room and placed in the supine position. Following induction of *regional* anesthesia, the patient's right arm was prepped and draped in the usual sterile fashion. A *transverse/longitudinal* incision was made adjacent to the radial artery and cephalic vein in the wrist. The cephalic vein was identified. This measured approximately ___ mm in diameter. It was dissected at a large branch point. *Several small tributaries were ligated with 4-0 silk.* The vein was mobilized and secured with silastic loops. Next, the radial artery was identified and dissected. The artery measured approximately ___ mm in diameter and was without significant atherosclerotic disease. The artery was mobilized proximally and distally for a 2-cm segment *and several small tributaries were ligated with 4-0 silk and divided.* The vein was brought adjacent to the artery and appeared to lie comfortably without tension or kinking.

The artery was controlled proximally and distally with silastic loops and an anterolateral arteriotomy was made using a #11 blade scalpel. The artery was then locally heparinized.

[Choose one:]

If end-to-side configuration: The distal vein was ligated and the vein divided with proximal control. The end of the vein was then opened and spatulated.

If side-to-side configuration: A similar length venotomy was made on the corresponding portion of the cephalic vein.

The arteriovenous anastomosis was then performed using a running 7-0 prolene suture. Following completion of the anastomosis, vascular control appeared excellent. Excellent flow was established through the fistula, and a strong distal pulse was palpable within the radial artery.

Hemostasis was achieved with electrocautery and 4-0 silk ties. The wound was irrigated and the subcutaneous tissues were reapproximated using interrupted 3-0 Vicryl sutures. The skin was closed with *3-0 nylon vertical mattress sutures/a subcuticular closure/other*. A dry sterile dressing was applied.

The patient tolerated the procedure well and was taken to the postanesthesia care unit in stable condition.

NOTES

Chapter 204
Creation of Brachiocephalic Fistula

Christopher Bunch, M.D.

INDICATION
- End-stage/impending end-stage renal disease.

ESSENTIAL STEPS
1. Skin incision over the antecubital fossa.
2. Expose and circumferentially dissect the cephalic vein.
3. Expose and circumferentially dissect the brachial artery.
4. Anticoagulate with IV heparin.
5. Transect the vein.
6. Construct the anastomosis.
7. Check for thrill and distal radial and ulnar pulses.

COMPLICATIONS
- Infection.
- Bleeding.
- Thrombosis of fistula.
- Finger/hand ischemia.
- Nerve injury.
- Steal syndrome.

TEMPLATE OPERATIVE DICTATION
Preoperative diagnosis: End-stage renal artery disease.
Procedure: Creation of brachiocephalic arteriovenous fistula.
Postoperative diagnosis: Same.

J.J. Hoballah and C.E.H. Scott-Conner (eds.), *Operative Dictations in General and Vascular Surgery*, DOI 10.1007/978-1-4614-0451-4_204,
© Springer Science+Business Media, LLC 2012

Indications: The patient is a ___-year-old *male/female with an end-stage/impending end-stage renal artery disease*. The risks of the procedure were discussed with the patient and *he/she* elected to undergo surgical intervention.

Description of procedure: The patient was positioned supine with the arm outstretched to near 90°. The procedure was performed under *local/axillary block/general anesthesia*. The right upper extremity was prepped and draped in the usual sterile fashion.

The skin over the antecubital fossa was infiltrated with 0.5% lidocaine.

A 6-cm transverse skin incision was then performed over the antecubital fossa. The cephalic vein was identified and encircled with a vessel loop. The vein was dissected for a segment of 5 cm. The dissection was carried as distally as possible through that incision.

Attention was then directed to the brachial artery. The tendonous aponeurosis of the biceps muscle was incised. The location of the brachial artery was identified by palpation. The soft tissue over the brachial artery was then incised and the brachial artery was identified and encircled with a vessel loop.

The patient was given 3,000 U of heparin intravenously.

The cephalic vein was then ligated at its most distal end. Yasargil clips were applied on the brachial artery and a 6-mm incision in the anterior wall of the brachial artery was performed. The cephalic vein was then gently curved and allowed to lie over the arteriotomy. The end of the vein was spatulated to match the size of the arteriotomy.

The anastomosis was then performed using a *5-0/6-0* prolene running suture. At the completion of the suture line, the brachial artery was forward-flushed and then allowed to backbleed. The cephalic vein was also allowed to backbleed. The anastomosis was irrigated with heparinized solution. The sutures were then tied and the suture line evaluated for hemostasis, which was adequate.

There was evidence of an excellent thrill in the cephalic vein. There was evidence of strong palpable pulses in the brachial, radial, and ulnar arteries at the wrist. There was no evidence of any kinks.

The wound was then irrigated with antibiotic solution.

The subcutaneous tissue was closed with 3-0 Vicryl and the skin closed with 4-0 subcuticular monocryl sutures. There was evidence of an excellent thrill in the cephalic vein after wound closure.

The patient tolerated the procedure well and was taken to the postanesthesia care unit in stable condition.

Chapter 205

Creation of Brachiobasilic Fistula: Basilic Vein Transposition

Mazen M. Hashisho, M.D.

INDICATION
- End-stage/impending end-stage renal disease.

ESSENTIAL STEPS
1. Skin incision over medial aspect of the upper arm from the antecubital fossa to the axilla.
2. Expose and circumferentially dissect the basilic vein and ligate its branches.
3. Expose and circumferentially dissect the brachial artery at the antecubital fossa.
4. Create a subcutaneous tunnel from the axilla to the antecubital fossa.
5. Anticoagulate with IV heparin.
6. Transect the vein at the antecubital fossa.
7. Pass the vein distended in the tunnel.
8. Construct the anastomosis.
9. Check for thrill and distal radial and ulnar pulses.
10. Close the wounds.

NOTE THIS VARIATION
- When the basilica vein is smaller than 4 mm, the procedure may be performed in two stages. First, brachiobasilic fistula is created at the elbow. The vein is then transposed or superficialized when it grows or matures usually 6 weeks later.

J.J. Hoballah and C.E.H. Scott-Conner (eds.), *Operative Dictations in General and Vascular Surgery*, DOI 10.1007/978-1-4614-0451-4_205,
© Springer Science+Business Media, LLC 2012

COMPLICATIONS
- Infection.
- Bleeding.
- Thrombosis of fistula.
- Finger/hand ischemia.
- Nerve injury.
- Steal syndrome.

TEMPLATE OPERATIVE DICTATION
Preoperative diagnosis: End-stage renal artery disease.
Procedure: Creation of brachiobasilic arteriovenous fistula.
Postoperative diagnosis: Same.
Indications: The patient is a ___-year-old *male/female with an end-stage/impending end-stage renal artery disease*. The cephalic vein was unavailable. The risks of the procedure were discussed with the patient and *he/she* elected to undergo surgical intervention.
Description of procedure: The procedure was performed under *axillary block/general anesthesia*. The patient was positioned supine with the arm outstretched to near 90°. The right upper extremity was prepped and draped in the usual sterile fashion.

A longitudinal skin incision was performed in the upper arm over the previously mapped basilic vein. The incision was deepened down through the subcutaneous tissue and fat, and the basilic vein was identified at the level of the antecubital fossa. The basilic vein was encircled with a vessel loop. The vein was then dissected proximally all the way up to the axilla and its branches were isolated, ligated, and divided. The overlying nerve branches were preserved. The basilic vein was dissected free from the antecubital fossa to the axilla.

Attention was then directed to the brachial artery in the antecubital fossa. The brachial artery was palpated and the soft tissue overlying it was incised. The brachial artery was exposed and encircled with a vessel loop. A 2-cm segment of the brachial artery was then circumferentially dissected.

A curved tunneler was then used to create a tunnel along the anterior aspect of the upper arm from the axillary fossa to the antecubital area in a position that will facilitate venipuncture.

The patient was given 3,000 U of heparin intravenously.

The basilic vein was then ligated as distally as possible in the antecubital fossa and divided. The basilic vein was then introduced in the tunnel in a distended form, avoiding any kinks or twists.

Yasargil clips were then applied on the brachial artery and a 6-mm incision was then performed in its anterior wall. The end of the basilic vein was then spatulated to match the size of the arteriotomy.

An anastomosis was then created between the end of the vein and the arteriotomy using a *5-0/6-0* prolene running suture. At the completion of the procedure, the basilic vein was allowed to backbleed and the brachial artery was forward-flushed and backbled. The anastomosis was irrigated with heparinized saline. The sutures were tied and the suture line was checked for hemostasis, which was adequate.

There was an excellent thrill in the vein and the vein was readily palpable under the skin. Hemostasis was then ensured. There was evidence of an excellent pulse in the radial and ulnar arteries at the wrist. The wounds were irrigated and then closed with 3-0 Vicryl for the subcutaneous tissue.

The skin was closed with 4-0 monocryl subcuticular sutures.

The patient tolerated the procedure well and was transferred to the postanesthesia care unit in stable condition.

Chapter 206
PTFE Forearm Graft for Hemodialysis

Mazen M. Hashisho, M.D.

INDICATIONS
- End-stage renal disease requiring hemodialysis.
- Inability to construct primary arteriovenous fistula.

ESSENTIAL STEPS
1. Map the vein and artery.
2. *Regional/local* anesthesia.
3. *Transverse incision overlying the artery and vein/longitudinal incision between the artery and vein.*
4. Develop flaps.
5. Identify the artery and mobilize.
6. Ligate the small tributaries if necessary.
7. Obtain proximal and distal control with silastic loops.
8. Identify the vein and mobilize.
9. Similarly ligate the small tributaries and obtain proximal and distal control.
10. Create a 2-cm transverse skin incision in the distal forearm.
11. Create skin flap and a pocket for the loop part of the graft.
12. Create a tunnel and pass the graft in the tunnel.
13. Longitudinal arteriotomy.
14. Anastomose spatulated end of the graft to the side of the artery.
15. Anastomose spatulated end of the graft to *side/end* of the vein.

J.J. Hoballah and C.E.H. Scott-Conner (eds.), *Operative Dictations in General and Vascular Surgery*, DOI 10.1007/978-1-4614-0451-4_206,
© Springer Science+Business Media, LLC 2012

16. Check for thrill, distal pulse.
17. Check hemostasis.
18. Close the incision.

NOTE THESE VARIATIONS

- Size and type of graft vary.
- Location on forearm varies.
- May perform the arterial or venous anastomosis first.
- The venous anastomosis may be performed using a side-to-side or end-to-side configuration.

COMPLICATIONS

- Steal syndrome.
- Bleeding.
- Occlusion.
- Infection.

TEMPLATE OPERATIVE DICTATION

Preoperative diagnosis: End-stage renal disease requiring chronic hemodialysis.

Procedure: Creation of *left/right* forearm loop hemodialysis PTFE graft.

Postoperative diagnosis: Same.

Indications: This ___-year-old *male/female* developed end-stage renal disease due to ___, *requiring/anticipating* need for chronic hemodialysis. Because of *inadequate veins/previous surgery/other*, PTFE graft from *brachial/other* artery to *basilic/cephalic/other* vein was chosen.

Description of procedure: The patient was brought to the operating room and placed in the supine position. Following induction of *regional* anesthesia, the patient's *left/right* arm was prepped and draped in the usual sterile fashion. A transverse incision was made *(specify location or locations)*.

The brachial artery was identified, gently dissected, and encircled with silastic loops. A second incision was then made over the *cephalic/basilic* vein and the vein similarly dissected and encircled. A 2-cm transverse skin incision in the distal forearm was performed.

A skin flap was developed, creating a pocket for the loop part of the graft.

The tunneling device was then passed between these incisions. A ___ *(specify type, length, and caliber)* graft was passed through the tunnel, taking care to avoid kinking or twists. The graft was irrigated with heparinized saline solution.

Proximal and distal arterial control was then obtained and an anterior arteriotomy was made. The artery was irrigated with heparinized saline solution. An end PTFE to side artery anastomosis was then performed, using a running 6-0 prolene suture. Upon the completion of the anastomosis, two *Bulldog/Fogarty* clamps were placed on the PTFE graft just distal to the anastomosis, and vascular control of the artery was released to reestablish flow to the hand.

Attention was directed to the vein. Proximal and distal control was obtained and an anterolateral venotomy was made. The vein was then irrigated with heparinized saline solution. The end of the PTFE graft was then cut in a beveled fashion at the appropriate length. An end PTFE graft to side vein anastomosis was then performed, using a running, 6-0 prolene suture. Following the completion of the anastomosis, vascular control was released and flow was established through the graft. *Papaverine was injected into the adventitia/the native vessels.*

There was an excellent distal pulse in the artery and a strong thrill in the vein. Hemostasis was achieved and the wound irrigated. The subcutaneous tissues were reapproximated using interrupted 3-0 Vicryl sutures. The skin was reapproximated using *3-0 nylon in a vertical mattress fashion/subcuticular suture/other.*

A dry sterile pressure dressing was applied.

The patient tolerated the procedure well and was taken to the postanesthesia care unit in stable condition.

NOTES

Chapter 207

Creation of Upper-Arm Prosthetic Arteriovenous Grafts

Christopher Bunch, M.D.

INDICATIONS

- End-stage/impending end-stage renal disease.
- Inability to construct a native autogenous fistula.

ESSENTIAL STEPS

1. Skin incision over medial aspect of the upper arm at the axilla.
2. Expose and circumferentially dissect the basilic vein.
3. Skin incision over the antecubital fossa.
4. Expose and circumferentially dissect the brachial artery.
5. Create a subcutaneous tunnel from the axilla to the antecubital fossa.
6. Anticoagulate with IV heparin.
7. Construct an end-to-side anastomosis between the graft and the brachial artery.
8. Pass the graft in the tunnel.
9. Construct the anastomosis between the graft and the basilica vein.
10. Check for thrill and distal radial and ulnar pulses.
11. Close the wound.

COMPLICATIONS

- Infection.
- Bleeding.
- Thrombosis of fistula.

J.J. Hoballah and C.E.H. Scott-Conner (eds.), *Operative Dictations in General and Vascular Surgery*, DOI 10.1007/978-1-4614-0451-4_207,

- Finger/hand ischemia.
- Nerve injury.

TEMPLATE OPERATIVE DICTATION

Preoperative diagnosis: End-stage renal artery disease.
Procedure: Creation of brachiobasilic arteriovenous fistula.
Postoperative diagnosis: Same.
Indications: The patient is a ___-year-old *male/female with an end-stage/impending end-stage renal artery disease*. The cephalic vein was unavailable. The risks of the procedure were discussed with the patient and *he/she* elected to undergo surgical intervention.
Description of procedure: The procedure was performed under *axillary block/general anesthesia*. The patient was positioned supine with the arm outstretched to near 90°. The upper extremity was prepped and draped in the usual sterile fashion.

A 5-cm skin incision was then performed over the medial aspect of the upper arm toward the axilla. The incision was deepened down through the subcutaneous tissue and fat. The basilic vein was identified and circumferentially dissected and encircled with a vessel loop. A 4-cm segment of the basilic vein was circumferentially dissected.

A 3-cm longitudinal incision was then performed over the antecubital fossa. The aponeurosis of the biceps muscle was incised and the brachial artery was palpated and its location determined. The soft tissues over the brachial artery were incised and the brachial artery was circumferentially dissected and encircled with a vessel loop. A 3-cm segment of the brachial artery was circumferentially dissected.

A curved tunneler was then used to create a subcutaneous tunnel connecting the incision in the antecubital fossa to the incision in the axilla. The tunnel was created in the anterior aspect of the upper arm to facilitate puncture for dialysis.

The patient was given 3,000 U of heparin intravenously.

Yasargil clips were then applied on the brachial artery and a 6-mm incision was performed in the anterior wall of the brachial artery. The end of a 6-mm PTFE graft was spatulated to match the size of the arteriotomy. An anastomosis was then performed between the end of the PTFE graft and the arteriotomy using a 6-0 prolene running suture. Forward- and backbleeding from the brachial artery was performed. The anastomosis was then irrigated with heparinized saline. The sutures were tied and the anastomosis was checked for hemostasis, which was adequate. Flow was allowed to resume through the brachial artery. The PTFE graft was then introduced in the tunnel distended, avoiding any kinks or twists.

Attention was then directed toward the basilic vein. The basilic vein was then controlled with Yasargil clips, and a 1-cm incision was then created in the vein. The PTFE graft was measured to length and was transected in an oblique fashion to match the size of the venotomy. An anastomosis was then created between the end of the PTFE graft and the venotomy using a 6-0 prolene running suture. At the completion of the anastomosis, backbleeding from the venous side and forwardbleeding from the graft were performed. The sutures were tied and the anastomosis checked for hemostasis, which was adequate. Flow was allowed in the arteriovenous graft.

There was evidence of excellent thrill in the basilic vein and Doppler signals. There was also evidence of palpable pulses in the radial and ulnar arteries at the wrist. The suture lines were checked again for hemostasis, which was adequate. Hemostasis in the soft tissues was secured and the wound was then closed using 3-0 Vicryl for subcutaneous tissue and 3-0 monocryl subcuticular sutures for the skin.

The patient tolerated the procedure well and was transferred to the postanesthesia care unit in stable condition.

NOTES

Chapter 208
Distal Revascularization and Interval Ligation (DRIL)

Simon Roh, M.D.

INDICATION
- Ischemic steal syndrome related to a functioning dialysis access graft or fistula.

ESSENTIAL STEPS
1. Exposure of fistula.
2. Exposure of the outflow artery for the construction of the distal bypass anastomosis 1–2 cm distal to the access anastomosis.
3. Exposure of the inflow artery for the construction of the proximal bypass anastomosis at greater than or equal to 7 cm from the access anastomosis.
4. Harvesting an appropriate length greater saphenous vein.
5. Creation of a tunnel from the proximal anastomosis to the site of the fistula.
6. Anticoagulation with IV Heparin sulfate at 50 UI/kg.
7. Construction of the proximal anastomosis.
8. Passing the graft in the tunnel.
9. Construction of the distal anastomosis.
10. Ligation of artery distal to the access anastomosis.
11. Check for flow using ultrasound Doppler.
12. Closure.

J.J. Hoballah and C.E.H. Scott-Conner (eds.), *Operative Dictations in General and Vascular Surgery*, DOI 10.1007/978-1-4614-0451-4_208,
© Springer Science+Business Media, LLC 2012

NOTE THESE VARIATIONS

- DRIL may be performed for various upper extremity AV fistulas as well as lower extremity AV fistulas, although very rarely needed for distal radiocephalic fistulae.
- DRIL was designed to overcome the limitations of fistula plication, a technique where by the lumen of the first few centimeters of the fistula is narrowed to increase the outflow resistance in the fistula.
- The site of the proximal anastomosis in the inflow vessel may be exposed by extending the incision at the level of the fistula proximally for 7 cm or by creating a new incision 7–10 cm proximal to the level of the fistula.

COMPLICATIONS

- Vascular injury (dissection, thrombosis, perforation, and embolization).
- Distal limb ischemia (embolization and thrombosis).
- Damage to surrounding neurovascular structures.

TEMPLATE OPERATIVE DICTATION

Preoperative diagnosis: *Right/left* upper extremity ischemic steal syndrome related to a functioning arteriovenous fistula.

Procedure: Distal revascularization with interval ligation of *radial/brachial* artery.

Postoperative diagnosis: *Right/left* upper extremity ischemic steal syndrome related to a functioning arteriovenous fistula.

Indications: This ___-year-old *male/female* patient was found to have a *right/left* upper extremity ischemic steal syndrome related to a functioning *right/left radial/brachial cephalic/basilic/axillary* arteriovenous fistula.

Details of operation: The patient was brought to the operating room and placed on the operating table in the supine position. The *right/left* arm was stretched out in a 90° fashion, prepped with povidone–iodine solution, and draped in the standard fashion. A time-out was called consisting of identifying the correct patient, procedure, antibiotics, and ASA class. General anesthesia was induced along with endotracheal intubation.

The area over the arteriovenous fistula was palpated and an incision was made providing sufficient exposure of the fistula. The incision was deepened down to the access vessels using electrocautery. Hemostasis was achieved. The *radial/brachial cephalic/basilic/axillary* arteriovenous fistula was identified and was found to have good flow with ultrasound Doppler. *The radial/brachial* artery was exposed for a 2 cm distance distal to the fistula for creation of the distal anastomosis.

The incision was extended proximally for 10 cm/A 4 cm skin incision was then performed 10 cm proximal to the site of the fistula. The radial/brachial artery was exposed 7–10 cm proximal to the fistula site and dissected circumferentially in preparation for the proximal anastomosis of the bypass. Attention was then directed to the upper thigh where the greater saphenous vein was previously mapped. The greater saphenous vein was harvested for an appropriate 12 cm segment. A subfascial tunnel was then created from the level of the proximal radial/brachial artery. The patient was anticoagulated with intravenous heparin at 50 UI/kg. The proximal radial/brachial artery was then clamped and a 1 cm arteriotomy was created. The vein was reversed and its end was spatulated to match the arteriotomy. An end-to-side anastomosis was then constructed using 5-0 Prolene suture. The vein was then passed distended in the tunnel. The point for the distal bypass anastomosis was identified 1–2 cm distal to the arteriovenous fistula on the *radial/brachial* artery. Vascular/Yasargil clamps were placed on the distal *radial/brachial* artery. A longitudinal arteriotomy was made over the *radial/brachial* artery and a side-to-end anastomosis was constructed with the distal end of a saphenous vein graft. A 2-0 silk suture was used to ligate the *radial/brachial* artery between the access anastomosis and distal bypass anastomosis.

Yasargil clamps were removed and ultrasound Doppler was used to verify good flow through the fistula and bypass graft. Hemostasis was checked. The subcutaneous tissues were approximated with multiple interrupted 3-0 Vicryl sutures and the skin was closed with 4-0 Monocryl in a running subcuticular fashion.

The patient tolerated the procedure well and was transferred to the postanesthesia care unit in stable condition. There were no complications.

NOTES

Anatomic Requirements
Steal syndrome resulting from functional arteriovenous fistula.

Necessary Equipment
Yasargil clamps.
11 and 15 blade knives.
Debakey forceps.
Electrocautery.
Sutures.
Greater saphenous vein graft.

Chapter 209
Revision Using Distal Inflow (RUDI)

Simon Roh, M.D.

INDICATION

- Ischemic steal syndrome related to a functioning dialysis access graft or fistula.

ESSENTIAL STEPS

1. Exposure of the fistula.
2. Exposure of the artery distal to the fistula and identification of its bifurcation.
3. Exposure of one of the bifurcation arteries which will serve as the new distal inflow of the fistula and preparing it for the construction of the proximal bypass anastomosis.
4. Harvesting an appropriate length greater saphenous vein.
5. Anticoagulation with IV Heparin sulfate at 50 UI/kg.
6. Construction of the proximal anastomosis.
7. Ligate/transect the fistula at its origin.
8. Construction of the distal anastomosis.
9. Check for flow using ultrasound Doppler.
10. Closure.

NOTE THESE VARIATIONS

- Revision using distal inflow (RUDI) may be performed using either the radial or ulnar artery as the source for distal inflow.
- The distal anastomosis may be constructed using end-to-end or end-to-side configuration.

J.J. Hoballah and C.E.H. Scott-Conner (eds.), *Operative Dictations in General and Vascular Surgery*, DOI 10.1007/978-1-4614-0451-4_209,
© Springer Science+Business Media, LLC 2012

COMPLICATIONS

- Vascular injury (dissection, thrombosis, perforation, embolization).
- Distal limb ischemia (embolization, thrombosis).
- Damage to surrounding neurovascular structures.

TEMPLATE OPERATIVE DICTATION

Preoperative diagnosis: *Right/left* upper extremity ischemic steal syndrome related to a functioning arteriovenous fistula.

Procedure: RUDI from *radial/ulnar* artery.

Postoperative diagnosis: *Right/left* upper extremity ischemic steal syndrome related to a functioning arteriovenous fistula.

Indications: This ___-year-old *male/female* patient was found to have a *right/left* upper extremity ischemic steal syndrome related to a functioning *right/left radial/brachial cephalic/basilic/axillary* arteriovenous fistula.

Details of operation: The patient was brought to the operating room and placed on the operating table in the supine position. The *right/left* arm was stretched out in a 90° fashion, prepped and draped in the usual sterile fashion. A timeout was called consisting of identifying the correct patient, procedure, antibiotics, ASA class. General anesthesia was induced along with endotracheal intubation.

The area over the arteriovenous fistula was palpated and an incision was made providing sufficient exposure of the fistula. Incision was deepened down to the access vessels using electrocautery. Hemostasis was achieved. The *radial/brachial cephalic/basilic/axillary* arteriovenous fistula was identified and was found to have good flow with ultrasound Doppler.

The brachial artery distal to the fistula was exposed to its bifurcation. The radial/ulnar artery was selected as the new distal inflow site. A 2 cm segment of the radial/ulnar artery was further dissected and prepared for the creation of the proximal anastomosis. The distance between the fistula and the new inflow site was approximately 4–5 cm necessitating a vein segment to connect the fistula to the new distal inflow. A 5 cm segment of right/left greater saphenous vein was harvested from the thigh. The patient was administered Heparin Sulfate 50 UI/kg intravenously. Yasargil/bulldog clamps/vessel loops were applied on the radial/ulnar artery. A 6 mm arteriotomy was created. An end-to-side anastomosis was created between the harvested vein and the radial/ulnar artery. The anastomosis was checked for hemostasis which was adequate. A 2-0 Silk tie was used to ligate the arteriovenous fistula at its origin.

Yasargil clamps were applied on the fistula. A 6–10 mm incision was performed in the fistula distal to the ligature./*The harvested vein segment was measured to the appropriate length and an end-to-side anastomosis was then created between the harvested vein and the fistula./(Alternative) An end to side The fistula was transected distal to the ligature. An end-to-end anastomosis was created between the vein and the fistula*

The Yasargil clamps were removed and ultrasound Doppler was used to verify good flow through the distal inflow graft and fistula, as well as the distal portions of the *radial/ulnar* artery and the palmar arch. Hemostasis was checked. The subcutaneous tissues were approximated with multiple interrupted 3-0 Vicryl sutures and the skin was closed with 4-0 Monocryl in a running subcuticular fashion.

The patient tolerated the procedure well and was transferred to the postanesthesia care unit in stable condition. There were no complications.

NOTES

Anatomic Requirements

Steal syndrome resulting from functional arteriovenous fistula.

Chapter 210

Pharmacologic/Mechanical Lytic Therapy for Occluded Dialysis Access

Eanas S. Yassa, M.D.

INDICATION
- Acute occlusion of dialysis access graft or fistula.

ESSENTIAL STEPS
1. Determine if dialysis access is via PTFE graft or autogenous fistula. If graft, determine if loop configuration.
2. Rule out any signs of infection at potential percutaneous access site.
3. Confirm the patient is physiologically appropriate for percutaneous mechanical or pharmacologic thrombectomy.
4. Examine access for pseudoaneurysms.
5. Secure antegrade access via arterial limb of dialysis graft/fistula.
6. Venogram – note location of any stenoses.
7. Anticoagulate with IV Heparin Sulfate (2,000–5,000 units typically).
8. Exchange angiogram catheter for 6- or 7-French sheath (usually, though different devices call for differing sheath sizes).
9. Advance a 0.035 in. steerable guidewire to occlusion site.
10. Remove thrombus with device of choice, brought into position over guidewire.
11. Exchange thrombectomy device over guidewire for angioplasty balloon.
12. Treat noted venous stenoses.

J.J. Hoballah and C.E.H. Scott-Conner (eds.), *Operative Dictations in General and Vascular Surgery*, DOI 10.1007/978-1-4614-0451-4_210,
© Springer Science+Business Media, LLC 2012

13. Insertion of a second vascular access via micropuncture kit, retrograde from the venous limb toward the arterial anastomosis.
14. Exchange micropuncture sheath for 6- or 7-French working sheath.
15. Dislodge any arterial plugs (an organized densely packed collection of red blood cells and fibrin plug).
16. Remove sheaths and obtain hemostasis.

NOTE THESE VARIATIONS

- Diagnostic venogram may reveal a severe proximal venous stenosis that may preclude removal of thrombus and will need to be treated prior to thrombus removal – mechanical thrombectomy techniques include:
  - Balloon thromboaspiration – use of a Fogarty type balloon to coax thrombus toward sheath through which thrombus is subsequently aspirated.
  - Amplatz mechanical thrombectomy device (Microvena Corp, White bear Lake, MN).
  - Hydrolser Catheter (Cordis Endovascular, Warren, NJ).
  - Possis AngioJet (Possis, Minneapolis, MN).
  - Oasis Catheter (Boston Scientific, Natick, MA).
  - Gelbfish Endovac (Neovascular Technologies, Brooklyn, NY).
  - Trerotola device (Arrow International, Reading, PA).
  - Akonya Eliminator Plus (IDev Technologies, Houston, TX).
- If occlusion is unable to be adequately treated by thrombectomy device, usually secondary to inability to re-cannulate lumen using guidewire, recombinant tissue plasminogen activator (tPA) can be administered directly at thrombus site for later maceration using angioplasty balloon or sheath can be left in place and tPA instilled at site of occlusion.
- If mechanical thrombectomy is not an option, tPA can be injected into the graft and allowed to act for 30 min prior to starting the procedure, which can then be supplemented by pulse spray injection of tPA inside the occluded graft.

COMPLICATIONS

- Venous/arterial endothelial injury and dissection.
- Vessel rupture with balloon dilatation.
- Embolization of small fragments into the distal arterial circulation *or* into central venous circulation.

- Excessive blood loss from inattention to appropriate manual pressure with sheath exchanges or prolonged activation of aspiration arm on mechanical thrombectomy devices.

CONTRAINDICATIONS

- Local infection at access site.
- Immature fistulae or one never having previously been used for dialysis access.
- Large pseudoaneurysms at the cannulation sites.
- Patient physiology unable to tolerate possibility of embolism of small thrombus particles to lungs – i.e., Significant left or right heart failure, pulmonary hypertension, presence of right-to-left shunt.
- *Relative contraindication:* Significant clot burden (suggested as >100 cc).

TEMPLATE OPERATIVE DICTATION

Preoperative diagnosis: Occluded dialysis access *graft/fistula.*

Procedure: Percutaneous *mechanical/pharmocomechanical/ pharmacologic* thrombectomy or thrombolysis.

Postoperative diagnosis: Same.

Indications: This ___-year-old *male/female* patient was found to have an acutely occluded dialysis access *graft/fistula.* Preoperative ultrasound confirmed absence of flow and the patient is a good candidate for attempt at percutaneous repair.

Description of procedure: The procedure was performed under *regional/local* anesthesia. The patient was positioned on the hybrid table in a supine position with affected extremity extended on an arm board/*exposed for imaging.* A prophylactic intravenous antibiotic for coverage of skin flora was administered. The extremity was prepped and draped in the standard sterile fashion.

A percutaneous access site was selected *for loop configuration grafts, access is obtained at the apex of the loop pointing toward the venous anastomosis/for autogenous fistulae the access is in the fistula just distal to the anastomosis.* Access is obtained via micropuncture kit . Once access is confirmed, a guidewire is advanced beyond the occlusion and an angiographic catheter is exchanged for the micropuncture sheath over a guidewire. A venogram to include the central venous circulation is obtained. Location of the thrombus and any other significant stenoses are noted. *If venous outflow cannot be traversed or recannulated and/or no other obstruction explains fistula failure, the procedure is aborted or tPA therapy is initiated.*

IV heparin is administered for therapeutic anticoagulation. Over a wire, the angiographic catheter is exchanged for a working sheath (typically 6–8 French depending upon device to be used). The mechanical thrombectomy device is advanced to the level of the thrombosis. The device is activated. Care is taken to monitor blood loss if there is a suction or evacuator port. Once the thrombus has been removed, attention is turned toward treatment of underlying venous stenosis. A repeat angiogram is performed to verify any stenoses previously obscured by presence of thrombus. An angioplasty balloon is selected to be 10–20% greater in the diameter than adjacent vessel diameter. The balloon is advanced to the site of stenosis and inflated to approximately 20 atm using a 1/2 strength contrast mixture to observe dilatation under fluoroscopy.

A second micropuncture is made to access the arterial limb of the anastomosis. *In a loop configuration graft the arterial stick is also at the apex with sheaths oriented in a "crossing" fashion/ in an autogenous fistula the site of access is at the venous limb and directed retrograde.* Attention is then turned toward dislodgement of the arterial plug. A fogarty (or other compliant balloon) is advanced under fluoroscopic guidance beyond the arterial anastomosis. It is partially inflated and pulled across the anastomosis while the degree of inflation is continually adjusted. Once dislodged, the arterial plug is allowed to pass into venous circulation *(in situations of compromised pulmonary reserve, the plug can attempt to be aspirated through the sheath in the same manner as the venous thrombus. In these situations, it may also be prudent to delay treatment of venous stenoses until after the arterial plug is retrieved).*

Completion fistulagram is performed via the antegrade sheath. Return of palpable thrill is documented. The sheaths are withdrawn. Access site hemostasis is obtained by *manual pressure (if autogenous fistula)/by placement of superficial figure-of-eight/purse-string stitch of nonabsorbable monofilament (typically 3-0 or 4-0 PDS) in the skin overlying the access site but not incorporating the underlying PTFE graft.* Sterile dressing is applied.

The drapes were drawn at the patient was transferred to the postanesthesia recovery unit in stable condition after tolerating the procedure well.

Section **XXII**

Sympathectomy

Chapter 211
Supraclavicular Cervical Sympathectomy

Mario Martinasevic, M.D.

INDICATIONS

- Hyperhidrosis.
- Posttraumatic pain (frostbite).
- Raynaud's syndrome.
- Nonhealing finger ulcerations with nonreconstructable vessels.

ESSENTIAL STEPS

1. General anesthesia with a double-lumen endotracheal tithe.
2. Barber chair position.
3. Transverse skin incision two finger breadths above the clavicle starting at the lateral border of the sternocleido-mastoid muscle.
4. Scalene fat pad mobilized.
5. Anterior scalene muscle and the phrenic nerve identified.
6. Anterior scalene muscle divided.
7. Transverse process of the sixth cervical vertebra identified.
8. The nerve roots of the brachial plexus identified and protected.
9. The middle scalene muscle identified and divided from its attachments to the first rib.
10. The pleura bluntly dissected away.

J.J. Hoballah and C.E.H. Scott-Conner (eds.), *Operative Dictations in General and Vascular Surgery*, DOI 10.1007/978-1-4614-0451-4_211,
© Springer Science+Business Media, LLC 2012

11. The thoracic sympathetic chain identified and its level determined by counting down from the first rib at the apex of the thoracic cavity.
12. A segment of thoracic sympathetic chain from T2 to the T4 ganglion excised.
13. Hemostasis and closure.

NOTE THIS VARIATION

- Cervical sympathectomy can also be performed under thoracoscopic guidance.

COMPLICATIONS

- Chylous fistula.
- Phrenic nerve injury.
- Horner's syndrome.
- Pneumothorax.

TEMPLATE OPERATIVE DICTATION

Preoperative diagnosis: *Hyperhidrosis/causalgia/Raynaud's syndrome/finger ulceration.*

Procedure: *Right/left/bilateral* cervical sympathectomy.

Postoperative diagnosis: Same.

Indications: The patient is a ____-year-old *male/female with right/left/bilateral upper-extremity hyperhidrosis/causalgia/nonreconstructable ischemia.* The risks and benefits of cervical sympathectomy were discussed with the patient, who elected to undergo surgical intervention.

Description of procedure: The patient was placed in a supine position. The procedure was performed under general anesthesia with a double-lumen endotracheal tube (which is preferred). The neck was extended and rotated to the *right/left.* The neck, chest, and *right/left* arm were all prepped and draped in a sterile fashion. A transverse skin incision was made two finger breadths above the clavicle starting at the lateral border of the sternocleidomastoid muscle. This was carried down through the platysma muscle. The scalene fat pad was exposed and the cutaneous nerves divided. The scalene fat pad was then retracted laterally. The anterior scalene muscle was then exposed. The phrenic nerve was identified and retracted. The anterior scalene muscle was then divided from its attachments to the first rib. The muscle was retracted superiorly and the dissection was carried down to the level of the transverse process of the sixth cervical vertebra. The nerve roots of the brachial plexus were identified. The middle scalene muscle was identified and divided from its attachments to the first rib. The nerve roots were protected during this procedure at all times. The pleura was bluntly dissected away, avoiding any penetration into the pleural space. The thoracic sympathetic chain was then identified and its level determined by counting down from the first rib at the apex of the thoracic cavity. The sympathetic chain was encircled with a silastic loop. A segment of thoracic sympathetic chain from T2 to the T4 ganglion was excised. The stellate ganglion was preserved. The wound was inspected for hemostasis. The fat pad was placed overlying the brachial plexus nerve roots. The platysma was closed with 3-0 Vicryl. The skin was closed with subcuticular sutures.

The patient tolerated the procedure well, was extubated, and was taken to the postanesthesia care unit in stable condition.

NOTES

Chapter 212
Thoracoscopic Sympathectomy

Pierre Sfeir, M.D.

INDICATIONS
- Upper limb hyperhydrosis.
- Raynaud disease.
- Reflex sympathetic dystrophy.
- Angina pectoris.

ESSENTIAL STEPS
1. Preoperative CXR.
2. Double-lumen endotracheal intubation.
3. Lateral decubitus position.
4. Appropriate operating table flexion.
5. Axillary sandbag.
6. Make 1 cm skin incision in the mid-axillary line over the fourth intercostals space.
7. Insert 10-mm trocar followed by a thoracoscope.
8. Insert 5-mm port under vision along the third intercostal space and anterior axillary line.
9. Insert another 5-mm port along the third intercostal space and the posterior axillary line.
10. Identify the main sympathetic chain.
11. Identify important collateral fibers.
12. Identify and preserve the stellate ganglion.
13. Ablate or resect appropriate levels.

J.J. Hoballah and C.E.H. Scott-Conner (eds.), *Operative Dictations in General and Vascular Surgery*, DOI 10.1007/978-1-4614-0451-4_212,
© Springer Science+Business Media, LLC 2012

14. Hemostasis.
15. Chest drainage.
16. Wound closure.

NOTE THESE VARIATIONS
- Chest drainage is optional.
- Excision or interruption of the sympathetic chain are both acceptable options.

COMPLICATIONS
- Thermal injury to the stellate ganglion resulting in Horner's syndrome.
- Bleeding from posterior thoracic wall veins.
- Injury to intercostals or intercostobrachial nerves.

TEMPLATE OPERATIVE DICTATION
Preoperative diagnosis: Palmar hyperhydrosis.
Procedure: Thoracoscopic sympathectomy.
Postoperative diagnosis: Same.
Indications: This is a ___-year-old *male/female* presenting with incapacitating palmar hyperhydrosis that was resistant to all conservative measures. The procedure along with its risks and alternatives was described to the patient in details.
Description of procedure: The patient was taken to the operating room and the side of the surgery was verified. In the supine position, general endotracheal anesthesia with a double-lumen tube was induced. The patient was then put in the *left/right* lateral decubitus position with appropriate flexion of the table to maximize the intercostal spaces. The chest was then scrubbed and draped in the usual fashion. The lung was deflated and the table was tilted forward to enhance exposure of the posterior chest wall by letting the deflated lung naturally fall downward. A 1 cm skin incision was made in the mid-axillary line over the fourth intercostal space. With blunt dissection, the pleural space was entered over the rib. A 10-mm trocar was then introduced followed by the thoracoscope. A second 5-mm port was then inserted under vision along the third intercostal space and anterior axillary line. A third port was introduced at the same level along the posterior axillary line. Quick exploration of the chest cavity did not reveal any gross abnormality. The fat pad on the neck of the first rib, overlying the stellate ganglion was identified along with the upper thoracic sympathetic chain beneath the parietal pleura. The latter was then

incised and the nerve dissected and elevated with a hook at the neck of the third rib. All communicating rami were divided up to the level of the second rib. Above the second ganglion, the chain was clipped and divided. Electrocautery was not used to avoid injury to the stellate ganglion by the transmitted current. Distally, the nerve was transected below the third ganglion. The specimen was sent to pathology. Hemostasis was secured. A 20 F chest tube was left along the chest apex through the 1 cm incision. The trocars were then removed and the lung reinflated. The wounds were closed with subcuticular fine absorbable monofilament. Steri-strips were applied.

The patient tolerated the procedure well, was extubated on the table and was transferred to the postanesthesia care unit in stable condition.

NOTES

Chapter 213
Lumbar Sympathectomy

Mario Martinasevic, M.D.

INDICATIONS
- Causalgia.
- Posttraumatic pain (frostbite).
- Hyperhidrosis.
- Vasospastic disorder.
- Combine with arterial reconstruction.
- Nonhealing ulcers in inoperable arterial occlusive disease.

ESSENTIAL STEPS
1. General anesthesia.
2. Supine position.
3. Skin incision from the edge of the rectus toward the midpoint between the lower costal margin and the *anterior/ superior* iliac spine.
4. The external oblique incised and spread.
5. The internal oblique aponeurosis incised and spread.
6. The transversalis fascia incised and the peritoneum swept medially to expose the psoas muscle.
7. The ureter identified and retracted medially and protected.
8. The inferior vena cava dissected away from the psoas muscle and retracted medially (only on the right side).
9. The sympathetic chain was exposed and retracted on a nerve hook.

J.J. Hoballah and C.E.H. Scott-Conner (eds.), *Operative Dictations in General and Vascular Surgery*, DOI 10.1007/978-1-4614-0451-4_213,

10. A segment of lumbar sympathetic chain from the L2 to L3 ganglion excised.
11. Hemostasis and closure.

COMPLICATIONS
- Postsympathectomy neuralgia.
- Retrograde ejaculation (if bilateral may be as high as 50%).

TEMPLATE OPERATIVE DICTATION
Preoperative diagnosis: *Causalgia/hyperhidrosis/nonhealing foot ulcers.*
Procedure: *Right/left/bilateral* lumbar sympathectomy.
Postoperative diagnosis: Same.
Indications: The patient is a ____-year-old *male/female with right/left/bilateral causalgia hyperhidrosis/ischemic leg.* The risks and benefits of lumbar sympathectomy were discussed with the patient and *he/she* elected to undergo surgical intervention.
Description of procedure: The patient was placed in the supine position. The procedure was performed under *general/spinal/endotracheal anesthesia.* The abdomen was prepped and draped in the usual sterile fashion.

An 8- to 10-cm skin incision was made from the edge of the rectus toward the midpoint between the lower costal margin and the anterior superior iliac spine. The incision was carried through the subcutaneous tissue. The external oblique was incised and spread. The internal oblique aponeurosis was incised and spread in the direction of its fibers. The transversalis fascia was incised and the peritoneum was swept medially to expose the psoas muscle. The ureter was identified and retracted medially and kept out of harm's way. The inferior vena cava was dissected away from the psoas muscle and retracted medially with minimal dissection (only on the right side). The sympathetic chain was exposed and retracted with a nerve hook. The nerve was dissected proximally and distally, exposing a ganglion at approximately the L2–L3 level. A 2.5-cm section of the nerve was clipped proximally and distally with metal clips. The nerve specimen was resected and sent to pathology, which confirmed it to be a nerve and ganglion. Hemostasis was secured. The incision was closed by approximating the transversalis muscle and the internal oblique with #1 PDS and the external oblique with 0 prolene. The skin was approximated with staples.

The patient tolerated the procedure well, was extubated, and was taken to the postanesthesia care unit in stable condition.

Section **XXIII**

Amputations

Chapter 214
Above-Knee Amputation

Maen S. Aboul Hosn, M.D.

INDICATIONS
- Nonhealing below-knee amputation.
- Ischemic leg with nonreconstructable occlusive disease.
- Ischemic leg in a nonambulatory patient with knee contracture.
- Trauma.
- Life-threatening infections.
- Phlegmasia.

ESSENTIAL STEPS
1. Outline with a marking pen the anterior and posterior skin flaps. (The flaps are usually equal in size, with a fish mouth pattern.)
2. Incise the skin and subcutaneous tissues down to the fascia.
3. Ligate and divide the greater saphenous vein on the medial aspect of the thigh.
4. Divide the fascia and the muscles at the same level as the skin flaps.
5. Locate the superficial femoral/proximal popliteal artery and vein on the deep posteromedial aspect of the thigh. Suture ligate the artery and vein individually.
6. Locate the sciatic nerve posterior to the femoral/popliteal vessels.
7. Pull, ligate, and divide the sciatic nerve.

J.J. Hoballah and C.E.H. Scott-Conner (eds.), *Operative Dictations in General and Vascular Surgery*, DOI 10.1007/978-1-4614-0451-4_214,
© Springer Science+Business Media, LLC 2012

8. Make a circular incision in the periosteum of the femur and free the periosteum proximally.
9. Divide the femur with a saw at least 5 cm proximal to the level of the soft-tissue transaction.
10. File any sharp bony edges.
11. Close the periosteum over the transected femur.
12. Approximate the deep investing fascia of the anterior and posterior muscles flaps with interrupted absorbable sutures.
13. Close the skin with interrupted nonabsorbable sutures/staples.

NOTE THIS VARIATION
■ A circular incision can be performed and the skin edges are trimmed during closure to avoid any dog-ears.

COMPLICATIONS
■ Infection.
■ Nonhealing of amputation site.
■ Bleeding.
■ Phantom pain.

TEMPLATE OPERATIVE DICTATION
Preoperative diagnosis: *Ischemic/gangrenous/trauma* with severe soft-tissue injury to the *right/left* leg.
Procedure: Above-knee amputation.
Postoperative diagnosis: Same.
Indications: The patient is a ____-year-old *male/female* with *nonhealing below-knee amputation/ischemic leg with nonreconstructable occlusive disease/ischemic leg in a nonambulatory patient/trauma/life-threatening leg infection/phlegmasia.* The risks of surgical intervention were discussed with the patient and *he/she* elected to undergo surgical intervention.
Description of procedure: The procedure was performed under *general/spinal/epidural/sciatic nerve block* anesthesia. The patient was placed supine. The *right/left* lower extremity was prepped and draped in the usual sterile fashion. An occlusive dressing was applied to the leg tip to the level of the knee.

Anterior and posterior skin flaps were outlined with a marking pen 5–10 cm proximal to the knee joint.

The skin incision was then performed and deepened through the subcutaneous tissue until the muscular fascia was identified.

The greater saphenous vein was identified, ligated with 2-0 silk ties, and divided.

The muscle groups over the anterior and medial thighs were divided with electrocautery at the same level of the skin incision. The neurovascular bundle was identified on the medial aspect of the thigh. The popliteal artery and veins were isolated and suture ligated with a 2-0 silk ligature. The sciatic nerve was pulled, ligated with a 2-0 silk tie, and divided. The posterior thigh muscles were then divided with electrocautery. Once the muscle groups were circumferentially divided, the periosteum was incised and elevated approximately 5 cm proximally off the femur. The femur was divided with an *electric/Gigli* saw. The proximal end of the transected femur was smoothed with a file. The amputation stump was irrigated copiously with antibiotic solution. Hemostasis was secured. The periosteum was closed with a running 3-0 Vicryl suture over the transected femur. The fascia of the thigh muscles was closed with interrupted 3-0 Vicryl sutures. The skin was approximated with interrupted 3-0 *nylon sutures/skin staples* and dressed with 4×4 gauze, Kerlix, and an Ace bandage.

The patient tolerated the procedure well and was taken to the postanesthesia care unit in stable condition.

NOTES

Chapter 215
Below-Knee Amputation

Maen S. Aboul Hosn, M.D.

INDICATIONS

- Nonhealing transmetatarsal amputation.
- Ischemic foot with nonreconstructable occlusive disease.
- Ischemic foot in a nonambulatory patient.
- Trauma.
- Life-threatening foot infections.

ESSENTIAL STEPS

1. Outline, with a marking pen, the skin incisions. (The anterior skin incision is made 10–12 cm below the tibial tuberosity and extends medially and laterally toward the edges of the gastrocnemius muscle. The posterior skin incision creates a posterior flap that extends 10–12 cm distal to the anterior incision.)
2. Incise the skin and subcutaneous tissues down to the fascia.
3. Ligate and divide the greater and short saphenous veins on the medial and posterior aspects of the leg, respectively.
4. Divide the fascia and the muscles at the same level of the anterior skin incision.
5. Divide the muscles in the anterior and lateral compartments.
6. Ligate the anterior tibial vessels.
7. Divide the interosseous membrane.
8. Incise the tibial periosteum at the same level of the skin and muscle division.

J.J. Hoballah and C.E.H. Scott-Conner (eds.), *Operative Dictations in General and Vascular Surgery*, DOI 10.1007/978-1-4614-0451-4_215,
© Springer Science+Business Media, LLC 2012

9. Strip the tibial periosteum proximally for 2 cm.
10. Divide the tibia with an anterior bevel.
11. Expose and transect the fibula with a bone cutter or Gigli saw 2 cm proximal to the tibial division.
12. Transect the soleus obliquely and the gastrocnemius muscle at the same level as the posterior flap.
13. Ligate and oversew any bleeding soleal veins and posterior tibial and peroneal vessels.
14. File any sharp bony edges.
15. Approximate the fascia of the anterior and posterior muscles flaps with interrupted absorbable sutures.
16. Close the skin with interrupted nonabsorbable sutures/staples.

NOTE THIS VARIATION

■ Various types of flap coverage may be used to construct a below-knee amputation. The technique described herein utilizes a longer posterior flap and is the most commonly used.

COMPLICATIONS

■ Infection.
■ Nonhealing of amputation site.
■ Bleeding.
■ Phantom pain.

TEMPLATE OPERATIVE DICTATION

Preoperative diagnosis: *Ischemic/gangrenous/trauma with severe soft-tissue injury to the right/left lot.*
Procedure: Below-knee amputation.
Postoperative diagnosis: Same.
Indications: The patient is a ____-year-old *male/female* with *nonhealing transmetatarsal amputation/ischemic foot with nonreconstructable occlusive disease/ischemic foot in a nonambulatory patient/trauma/life-threatening foot infection.* The risks of surgical intervention were discussed with the patient and *he/she* elected to undergo surgical intervention.
Description of procedure: The procedure was performed under *general/spinal/epidural/sciatic nerve block* anesthesia. The patient was placed supine. The *right/left* lower extremity was prepped and draped in the usual sterile fashion. An occlusive dressing was applied to the foot up to the level of the ankle.

Anterior and posterior skin incisions were outlined with a marking pen. The anterior skin incision was made 12 cm below the tibial tuberosity and extended medially and laterally toward the edges of the gastrocnemius muscle. The skin incision was then extended distally on either side parallel to the tibia for 12–15 cm, creating a posterior flap. The skin and subcutaneous tissues were incised down to the fascia. The greater and short saphenous veins on the medial and posterior aspects of the leg, respectively, were ligated and divided. The fascia and the muscles were then divided with the electrocautery at the same level of the anterior skin incision. The muscles in the anterior and lateral compartment were divided, exposing the anterior tibial vessels, which were ligated and divided. The interosseous membrane was then incised. The tibial periosteum was incised circumferentially with the electrocautery at the same level of the skin and muscle division. Using a periosteal elevator, the tibial periosteum was stripped proximally for 2 cm. The tibia was then transected with a *Gigli/electric* saw 2 cm proximal to the skin incision with an anterior bevel. The fibula was then exposed, dissected circumferentially, and transected with a *bone cutter/Gigli* saw 2 cm proximal to the tibial division. The amputation was then completed with an amputation knife, transecting the soleus muscle obliquely and the gastrocnemius muscle at the same level as the posterior flap. Bleeding soleal veins and posterior tibial and peroneal vessels were clamped and oversewn with 2-0 silk sutures. Sharp bony edges were then filed, eliminating any bony prominences over the anterior aspect of the tibia. The fascia of the anterior and posterior muscle flaps were approximated with interrupted absorbable sutures. The skin was approximated with *interrupted 3-0 nylon sutures/skin staples* and dressed with 4×4 gauze, Kerlix, and an Ace bandage.

The patient tolerated the procedure well and was taken to the postanesthesia care unit in stable condition.

NOTES

Chapter 216
Transmetatarsal Foot Amputation

Jamal J. Hoballah, M.D., M.B.A.

INDICATIONS
- Multiple-toe gangrene/chronic osteomyelitis of metatarsal heads.

ESSENTIAL STEPS
1. Noninvasive vascular testing suggests transmetatarsal amputation is likely to heal.
2. Mark the skin and the shape of the desired plantar flap.
3. Perform a transverse skin incision over the level of the midmetatarsal bones.
4. Deepen the incision to the bone.
5. Elevate the periosteum 1.5 cm proximal to the level of the skin incision.
6. Divide the bone.
7. Bend the divided bones and create the plantar flap.
8. Secure hemostasis.
9. Irrigate the wound.
10. Close the skin without tension.

NOTE THESE VARIATIONS
- Depending on the extent of tissue loss, a transmetatarsal amputation can be an open amputation which will be closed later with a skin graft, or a closed amputation as described in this chapter.

J.J. Hoballah and C.E.H. Scott-Conner (eds.), *Operative Dictations in General and Vascular Surgery*, DOI 10.1007/978-1-4614-0451-4_216,
© Springer Science+Business Media, LLC 2012

COMPLICATIONS

- Nonhealing amputation site.
- Infection.

TEMPLATE OPERATIVE DICTATION

Preoperative diagnosis: *Multiple-toe gangrene/infection of metatarsal heads.*

Procedure: Transmetatarsal forefoot amputation.

Postoperative diagnosis: Same.

Indications: This is a ___-year-old *male/female with multiple gangrenous/infected toes.* Noninvasive testing with toe pressure and transcutaneous oxygen tension suggested good skin perfusion. The risks and benefits of surgical intervention were discussed with the patient and *he/she* elected to undergo the procedure.

Description of procedure: The procedure was performed under *regional/general anesthesia.* The *right/left foot* was prepped and draped in a sterile fashion. A skin incision was then performed at the level of the midmetatarsal level and then extended on the sides of the foot and the plantar aspect of the foot at the level of the metatarsophalyngeal joints. The incision was deepened to the level of the bone. The periosteum was then elevated with a periosteal elevator. The bone was then transected at the midmetatarsal level, 1.5 cm proximal to the level of the skin incision. The divided bones were then reflected up and the amputation completed at the level of the plantar flap. Hemostasis was then secured and the wound was irrigated with saline solution. The skin was then closed with interrupted sutures of 4-0 nylon.

The patient tolerated the procedure well and was taken to the postanesthesia care unit in stable condition.

Chapter 217

Transmetatarsal (Ray) Toe Amputation

Jamal J. Hoballah, M.D., M.B.A.

INDICATION

- Toe gangrene/chronic osteomyelitis extending to the metatarsophalangeal joint or metatarsal head.

ESSENTIAL STEPS

1. Noninvasive vascular testing suggesting healing of toe amputation is likely.
2. Perform the skin incision (shape varies between toes; refer to variations).
3. Divide all attached tendons.
4. Elevate the periosteum to the level of the amputation.
5. Divide the bone.
6. Close the skin without tension.

NOTE THIS VARIATION

- For the first and fifth toes, an elliptical incision at a 30° angle to the longitudinal axis of the toe is made. For the second, third, and fourth toes, a circular incision is made at the metatarsophalyngeal level and then extended on the dorsal aspect of the foot along the axis of the metatarsal bone.

COMPLICATIONS

- Nonhealing amputation site.
- Infection.

J.J. Hoballah and C.E.H. Scott-Conner (eds.), *Operative Dictations in General and Vascular Surgery*, DOI 10.1007/978-1-4614-0451-4_217,
© Springer Science+Business Media, LLC 2012

TEMPLATE OPERATIVE DICTATION

Preoperative diagnosis: *Toe gangrene/infection.*

Procedure: Toe amputation.

Postoperative diagnosis: Same.

Indications: This is a ___-year-old *male/female* with a *gangrenous/ infected* toe extending to the proximal phalanx. Noninvasive testing with toe pressure and transcutaneous oxygen tension suggested good skin perfusion. The risks and benefits of surgical intervention were discussed with the patient and *he/she* elected to undergo the procedure.

Description of procedure: The procedure was performed under *regional/general* anesthesia. The *right/left foot* was prepped and draped in a sterile fashion. *An elliptical skin incision was then performed at the level of the metatarsophalyngeal joint at 30° to the longitudinal axis of the metatarsal bone. A circular incision was performed at the metatarsophalyngeal level and extended on the dorsal aspect of the foot along the metatarsal bone.* The incision was deepened to the level of the bone, dividing all tendinous attachments. The periosteum overlying the metatarsal bone was then elevated with a periosteal elevator. The bone was then transected at the *distal/mid/proximal* metatarsal level, 1.5–2 cm proximal to the level of the skin incision. Hemostasis was then secured and the wound was irrigated. The skin was then closed with interrupted sutures of 4-0 nylon.

The patient tolerated the procedure well and was taken to the postanesthesia care unit in stable condition.

Chapter 218

Transphalyngeal Toe Amputation

Jamal J. Hoballah, M.D., M.B.A.

INDICATION
- Toe gangrene/chronic osteomyelitis.

ESSENTIAL STEPS
1. Noninvasive vascular testing suggesting healing of toe amputation is likely.
2. Perform an elliptical skin incision perpendicular to the axis of the toe.
3. Elevate the periosteum to the level of the amputation.
4. Divide the bone.
5. Close the skin without tension.

COMPLICATIONS
- Nonhealing amputation site.
- Infection.

TEMPLATE OPERATIVE DICTATION
Preoperative diagnosis: *Toe gangrene/infection.*
Procedure: Toe amputation.
Postoperative diagnosis: Same.
Indications: This is a ___-year-old *male/female* with a *gangrenous/infected* toe. Noninvasive testing with toe pressure and transcutaneous oxygen tension suggested good skin perfusion. The risks and benefits of surgical intervention were discussed with the patient and *he/she* elected to undergo the procedure.

J.J. Hoballah and C.E.H. Scott-Conner (eds.), *Operative Dictations in General and Vascular Surgery*, DOI 10.1007/978-1-4614-0451-4_218,
© Springer Science+Business Media, LLC 2012

Description of procedure: The procedure was performed under *regional/general* anesthesia. The *right/left foot* was prepped and draped in a sterile fashion. A skin incision was then performed at the level of the mid-proximal phalynx. The incision was deepened to the level of the bone. The periosteum was then elevated with a periosteal elevator. The bone was then transected at the proximal phalyngeal level, 1.5 cm proximal to the level of the skin incision. Hemostasis was then secured and the wound was irrigated. The skin was then closed with interrupted sutures of 4-0 nylon.

The patient tolerated the procedure well and was taken to the postanesthesia care unit in stable condition.

NOTES

Section **XXIV**

Miscellaneous Procedures

Chapter 219

Supraclavicular Resection of Cervical Rib/First Thoracic Rib

Ismail Mohamad Khalil, M.D.

INDICATION

- Neurogenic pain/axillary vein compression/axillary artery compression.

ESSENTIAL STEPS

1. Patient in supine position, head of bed elevated 30°. The head and neck are turned to the opposite side.
2. The upper extremity and shoulder are prepped into the field to allow maneuvering the extremity for residual compression after scalenectomy and rib resection.
3. Incision starts 1–2 cm above and parallel to the clavicle. Start medially at the lateral border of clavicular head of sternocleidomastoid muscle and extending laterally parallel to the clavicle for 6–7 cm.
4. The incision is carried through the platysma muscle to expose the scalene fat pad.
5. Mobilization of the scalene fat pad begins at the lateral border of the internal Jugular vein. The use of bipolar cautery is helpful at this stage to control bleeding veins.
6. The fat pad is freed medially, inferiorly, and superiorly then retracted laterally on its pedicle to expose the underlying roots of the brachial plexus. It is then held out in position with a suture and kept moist during the procedure. (The thoracic duct joins the left internal Jugular vein at the base of the neck medially. Meticulous dissection in this region is obligatory to avoid injury to the duct.)

J.J. Hoballah and C.E.H. Scott-Conner (eds.), *Operative Dictations in General and Vascular Surgery*, DOI 10.1007/978-1-4614-0451-4_219,
© Springer Science+Business Media, LLC 2012

7. The Phrenic nerve is clearly visualized within the investing fascia of the scalene anterior muscle.

8. The anterior scalene insertion on the first rib is clearly visualized. It is resected taking special effort to avoid any tension on the phrenic nerve.

9. The omohyoid muscle is seen traversing the field and can be divided.

10. The C5 and C6 roots and the brachial plexus and subclavian artery are observed at the lateral border of the edge of the anterior scalene.

11. The cervical rib and any cartilaginous or fibrous extensions to the first rib or other structures in the thoracic inlet are seen inferior to the subclavian artery.

12. The artery and roots are dissected carefully, avoiding any tension on the nerves.

13. Free the rib, circumferentially starting at its tip in the thoracic inlet, then proceeding posteriorly along its course toward the cervical spine.

14. Resect the rib as far as you can and excise any additional remnants with a bone rongeur.

15. Release any adhesions around the artery and nerve roots.

16. For exposure of the first rib, the above steps are followed. Attention should be paid to avoid injuring the pleura when the inferior border of the rib is being freed. Similarly, the long thoracic nerve should be clearly visualized and protected when the scalene minimus insertion is mobilized.

17. At this stage the rib can be freed, circumferentially, from all facial and periosteal attachments, then resected.

18. The ipsilateral extremity can be manipulated at this stage to ensure that the vessels and roots are not compressed by any residual osseous or facial bands.

NOTE THESE VARIATIONS

- An infraclavicular approach may also be needed to allow further excision of the first rib and additional exposure of the subclavian vein.

- If any repair is required on the subclavian vein and superior vena cava the supraclavicular exposure can be extended to provide adequate exposure.

- After resecting the first rib, the supraclavicular incision is extended medially to the sternal notch. The incision is then continued along the midline of the manubrium sterni then carried laterally into the first rib space (which has been removed). The manubrium is slit for that short segment. The clavicle is kept attached to the segment of the manubrium and the whole trap-door is lifted in one unit exposing the superior mediastinum including the major vessels. This allows control of the axillary-subclavian vein as well as the superior vena cava for any bypass or patching of a narrowed segment of the vein.

COMPLICATIONS
- Injury to the phrenic, long thoracic, intercostals, and brachial plexus nerves.
- Injury to the axillary vein or artery.
- Injury to the thoracic duct.
- Pneumothorax.
- Incomplete rib resection.
- Recurrent symptoms.

TEMPLATE OPERATIVE DICTATION
Preoperative diagnosis: Right/left thoracic outlet syndrome.
Procedure: Supraclavicular resection right/left cervical or thoracic rib.
Postoperative diagnosis: Same.
Indications: The patient is a ____-year-old male/female with symptoms suggestive of thoracic outlet syndrome with neurogenic/venous or arterial compression. The risks and benefits of supraclavicular rib resection were discussed with the patient and he/she elected to undergo surgical intervention.
Description of procedure: After induction of general anesthesia, the patient was placed in the supine position, with the head elevated 30° and tilted to the opposite side of the surgery. The entire ipsilateral extremity is scrubbed and draped in the field to allow full range of motion during the procedure. A transverse incision, 1–2 cm above the clavicle was made starting medially at the lateral border of the clavicular head of the sternocleidomastoid and extended parallel to the clavicle for a distance of 6–8 cm. The incision was deepened through the platysma muscle which was divided. The Scalene fat pad was visualized. Using a bipolar-cautery, the fat pad was mobilized from its medial attachment, starting at the lateral border of the internal Jugular, as well as superiorly and inferiorly. It was retracted laterally on a pedicle, attached to the drapes with a silk suture and covered with moist

gauze. The Scalene anterior muscle came clearly into view with the phrenic nerve traversing its anterior belly. Laterally the brachial plexus roots and the subclavian artery were visualized. The middle scalene formed the lateral border. The cervical rib lied beneath the nerve roots and subclavian artery and was lifting the roots and artery upward. The area was inspected for fibrous or cartilaginous attachments between the rib and adjacent structures. The rib reached to and attached to the first rib with osseous and cartilaginous extensions. Soft tissue surrounding the cervical rib along with its fascia were carefully peeled away, circumferentially, with a small periosteum elevator as far back toward the cervical spine as possible. The rib was excised and any remnants removed with a fine rongeur. Soft tissue bands or adhesions to the artery or root were gently removed. The nerve roots were carefully protected from unnecessary mobilization or manipulation. The first rib was then removed. It was readily palpated in the base of the wound using the scalene attachment as a guide. Attachments of the middle scalene and scalene minimus were resected as well, after carefully guarding the long thoracic nerve. The fascia surround the rib was carefully peeled away circumferentially avoiding injury to the pleura underneath. To excise the rib adequately, it was necessary to divide the intercostals muscles between the first and second ribs. Similarly, medially the subclavious muscle is carefully resected after carefully protecting the subclavian vein. The neurovascular bundle was completely freed.

After resecting the rib and securing hemostasis, the wound was irrigated with saline. There was no evidence of lymph leak or leaks in the pleura. The wound was closed using 3-0 Vicrly for the subcutaneous tissue and 4-0 monocryl for the skin. The wound was covered with a sterile dressing.

The patient tolerated the procedure well and was taken to the postanesthesia care unit in stable condition.

NOTES

Chapter 220
Transaxillary First Rib Resection

William J. Sharp, M.D.

INDICATION
- Neurogenic pain/axillary vein compression/axillary artery compression.

ESSENTIAL STEPS
1. Patient in straight lateral position.
2. Transverse skin incision below the axillary hairline.
3. Deepen the incision straight down to the rib cage.
4. Create an axillary tunnel.
5. Identify the first rib and incise its overlying fascia.
6. Gently push the axillary artery, vein, and brachial plexus toward the roof of the axillary tunnel.
7. Hook the attachment of the anterior scalene muscle to the first rib and divide it.
8. Identify and divide the attachment of the subclavius muscle tendon to the first rib.
9. Divide the intercostal muscles between the first and second ribs.
10. Free the first rib circumferentially from any muscular attachments.
11. Transect the rib anteriorly and posteriorly.
12. Excise additional rib remnants with a bone rongeur.
13. Check for pneumothorax.
14. Close the wound.

J.J. Hoballah and C.E.H. Scott-Conner (eds.), *Operative Dictations in General and Vascular Surgery*, DOI 10.1007/978-1-4614-0451-4_220,
© Springer Science+Business Media, LLC 2012

NOTE THIS VARIATION

- First rib resection can be performed through supra- and infraclavicular incisions or through a transaxillary approach as described in this chapter.

COMPLICATIONS

- Injury to axillary vein, artery.
- Nerve injury: Brachial plexus, intercostobrachial nerve, and long thoracic nerve.
- Recurrent symptoms.
- Pneumothorax.
- Incomplete rib resection.

TEMPLATE OPERATIVE DICTATION

Preoperative diagnosis: *Right/left* thoracic outlet syndrome.
Procedure: Transaxillary *right/left* first rib resection.
Postoperative diagnosis: Same.
Indications: The patient is a ___-year-old *male/female* with symptoms suggestive of thoracic outlet syndrome with *neurogenic/ venous arterial compression*. The risks and benefits of transaxillary first rib resection were discussed with the patient and *he/she* elected to undergo surgical intervention.
Description of procedure: After the induction of general anesthesia, the patient was turned and placed in a straight lateral position with the *right/left* side up. The patient was supported with a beanbag and the contralateral axilla was padded and protected. The entire *right/left* upper extremity and upper chest were prepped and draped in the usual fashion. An assistant was holding the forearm in a double wristlock and elevating the upper extremity from the thorax. A transverse skin incision was made from the anterior edge of the latissimus dorsi muscle to the posterior edge of the pectoralis major muscle over the level of the third rib just below the axillary hairline. The incision was deepened down to the rib cage without angulating up into the axillary fat. The intercostobrachial nerves were identified and were spared and preserved. No accessory intercostobrachial nerves were identified. An axillary tunnel was then created. The first rib was identified. The fascia overlying the first rib was incised and then using a combination of blunt and sharp dissection the subclavian artery, vein, and brachial plexus were peeled off from the attachments to the top of the rib and pushed upward toward the roof of the axillary tunnel. Attention was then directed toward dividing the muscular attachments on the first rib. The anterior scalene muscle was identified, hooked

with a right angle clamp, and then divided while protecting the subclavian artery and vein. The tendon of the subclavius muscle was identified and divided without any injury to the subclavian vein. The intercostal muscles between the first and second ribs were carefully released using a periosteal elevator. A raspatory was also used to free any additional attachments off the first rib superiorly and inferiorly. The intercostal space was then opened and the Sibson's fascia and remnants of the scalene muscles were incised. The first rib was completely freed circumferentially of all attachments from the transverse process of the vertebra posteriorly to the costal cartilage anteriorly, and a rib shears was used to transect the rib on both sides. Once the major portion of the rib was removed the remaining stumps were palpated and shortened using a rongeur. Thorough irrigation was then performed. There was no evidence of any holes in the pleura. The neurovascular bundle was completely freed. The wound was then closed using 3-0 Vicryl for the subcutaneous tissue and 4-0 monocryl for the skin.

The patient tolerated the procedure well and was taken to the postanesthesia care unit in stable condition.

NOTES

Chapter 221

Surgical Repair of Femoral Pseudoaneurysm

Gregory A. Carlson, M.D.

INDICATIONS

- Expanding hematoma following percutaneous femoral puncture.
- Persistent pseudoaneurysm following percutaneous femoral puncture.

ESSENTIAL STEPS

1. Local/general anesthesia.
2. Longitudinal incision over the pseudoaneurysm.
3. Proximal control if easily achievable.
4. Enter pseudoaneurysm and evacuate hematoma.
5. Finger control of bleeding site.
6. Proximal and distal control if arterial wall injury is complex.
7. Repair the femoral artery.

COMPLICATIONS

- Recurrent hematoma.
- Nerve injury.
- Leg ischemia.

TEMPLATE OPERATIVE DICTATION

Preoperative diagnosis: Femoral pseudoaneurysm.
Procedure: Repair of femoral artery and evacuation of groin hematoma.

J.J. Hoballah and C.E.H. Scott-Conner (eds.), *Operative Dictations in General and Vascular Surgery*, DOI 10.1007/978-1-4614-0451-4_221,
© Springer Science+Business Media, LLC 2012

Postoperative diagnosis: Same.

Indications: The patient is a ___-year-old *male/female* who recently underwent a percutaneous femoral puncture for *angiography/ cardiac catheterization.* The patient now has a *large/expanding* groin hematoma, *with hypotension and evidence of significant blood loss. The skin overlying the hematoma is tense and appears compromised.* A pseudoaneurysm has been identified on ultrasound. The risks and benefits of surgical intervention were discussed with the patient and *he/she* elected to undergo surgical intervention.

Description of procedure: The procedure was performed under *local/general* anesthesia. The patient was placed in a supine position. The *right/left* lower extremity was prepped and draped in a sterile fashion.

A longitudinal skin incision was then performed over the hematoma. The hematoma was then entered and the blood clot evacuated. The bleeding point was then controlled with finger pressure. The common femoral artery was then dissected around the injury site proximally and distally for a 3-cm segment. Vascular clamps were then applied on the femoral artery proximal and distal to the puncture site. Back- and forwardbleeding were performed. There was no evidence of any intraluminal clots. The lumen was then irrigated with heparinized saline.

Two interrupted 5-0 prolene sutures were then used to close the arterial wall defect.

The limb was reperfused and hemostasis was secured. The pedal pulses were evaluated by Doppler examination and revealed excellent flow.

A JP drain was placed in the wound and exteriorized through a separate stab incision. The wound was then irrigated and closed with 3-0 Vicryl for subcutaneous tissue and staples for the skin.

The patient tolerated the procedure well and was taken to the postanesthesia care unit in stable condition.

Chapter 222

Ultrasound-Guided Percutaneous Obliteration of Common Femoral Artery Pseudoaneurysm with Thrombin Injection

Jamal J. Hoballah, M.D., M.B.A.

INDICATION
- Persistent large pseudoaneurysm following percutaneous femoral puncture.

ESSENTIAL STEPS
1. Local anesthesia.
2. Duplex identification of the pseudoaneurysm.
3. Introduction of the needle into the pseudoaneurysm.
4. Injection of microairbubbles to further verify the needle tip position.
5. Incremental thrombin injection until no flow is seen in the pseudoaneurysm.

NOTE THIS VARIATION
- Femoral pseudoaneurysms following percutaneous arterial punctures can be left alone (if small), compressed under ultrasound guidance, or injected with thrombin as described in this chapter.

COMPLICATIONS
- Persistent pseudoaneurysm.
- Leg ischemia.
- Femoral artery thrombosis or distal embolization.
- Nerve injury.

1019

J.J. Hoballah and C.E.H. Scott-Conner (eds.), *Operative Dictations in General and Vascular Surgery*, DOI 10.1007/978-1-4614-0451-4_222,
© Springer Science+Business Media, LLC 2012

TEMPLATE OPERATIVE DICTATION

Preoperative diagnosis: Tender *right/left* femoral pseudoaneurysm.

Procedure: Thrombin injection of *right/left* femoral pseudoaneurysm.

Postoperative diagnosis: Same.

Indications: The patient is a ____-year-old *male/female* who recently underwent a percutaneous femoral puncture for *diagnostic angiography/cardiac catheterization*. Duplex ultrasonography revealed a large pseudoaneurysm measuring cm. *Ultrasound compression of the pseudoaneurysm was unsuccessful.* The risks and benefits of intervention were discussed with the patient and *he/she* elected to undergo intervention.

Description of procedure: The procedure was done under local anesthesia. The patient was placed supine. The *right/left* groin was prepped and draped in the usual sterile fashion. The duplex probe was placed in the lateral aspect of the left common femoral artery pseudoaneurysm, revealing a ____-cm pseudoaneurysm with an identifiable neck communicating with the left common femoral artery.

The skin was infiltrated with 1% lidocaine. A 20-gauge spinal needle was introduced into the pseudoaneurysm under ultrasound guidance. The needle tip was visualized penetrating the pseudoaneurysm capsule. A few microbubbles of air were injected through the needle to further confirm its position within the pseudoaneurysm.

The injection solution consisted of thrombin 5,000 U mixed with 5 cc of normal saline. Thrombin was injected at increments of 500 U per injection.

The first injection produced a near obliteration of the pseudoaneurysm. After waiting approximately 2 min, there was some persistent flow within the pseudoaneurysm. Additional increments of 500 U of thrombin were injected, which successfully obliterated the pseudoaneurysm completely. Duplex investigation revealed no evidence of blood flow into the pseudoaneurysm. The needle was removed. The patient had no change in the quality of the pedal pulses following the procedure.

There were no complications.

The patient tolerated the procedure well and was taken to the postanesthesia care unit in stable condition.

Chapter 223

Surgical Repair of Femoral Arteriovenous Fistula

Gregory A. Carlson, M.D.

INDICATION

- Persistent arteriovenous fistula following percutaneous femoral puncture, with *distal ischemia/heart failure.*

ESSENTIAL STEPS

1. Local/general anesthesia.
2. Longitudinal incision over the femoral artery.
3. Proximal arterial control.
4. Distal arterial control.
5. Circumferentially dissect and mobilize the femoral artery.
6. Finger control of bleeding site from venous hole.
7. Repair venous wall defect.
8. Repair arterial wall defect.

COMPLICATIONS

- Nerve injury.
- Leg ischemia.
- Venous thrombosis.

TEMPLATE OPERATIVE DICTATION

Preoperative diagnosis: Femoral arteriovenous fistula.
Procedure: Division of arteriovenous fistula and repair of femoral artery and vein.
Postoperative diagnosis: Same.

J.J. Hoballah and C.E.H. Scott-Conner (eds.), *Operative Dictations in General and Vascular Surgery*, DOI 10.1007/978-1-4614-0451-4_223,
© Springer Science+Business Media, LLC 2012

Indications: The patient is a ___-year-old *male/female* who recently underwent a percutaneous femoral puncture for *diagnostic angiography/cardiac catheterization.* Duplex evaluation revealed the presence of an arteriovenous fistula. The patient had *evidence/no evidence* of *leg swelling and distal ischemia/congestive heart failure.* The risks and benefits of surgical intervention were discussed with the patient, who elected to undergo surgical intervention.

Description of procedure: The procedure was performed under *local/general* anesthesia.

The patient was place in a supine position. The *right/left* lower extremity was prepped and draped in a sterile fashion.

A longitudinal skin incision was then performed over the common femoral artery. The incision was deepened through the subcutaneous tissue and the femoral sheath entered. The common femoral artery was identified at the level of the inguinal ligament and circumferentially dissected and encircled with a vessel loop. The superficial femoral artery was circumferentially dissected and encircled with a vessel loop. The dissection of the superficial femoral artery was extended proximally. The profunda femoris artery was identified and encircled with a vessel loop.

The patient was given 5,000 U of heparin intravenously. The common femoral, superficial femoral, and profunda femoris arteries were then controlled with atraumatic vascular clamps. As the femoral artery was skeletonized, the fistula was encountered. The femoral artery was separated from the femoral vein. The hole in the femoral vein was controlled with the *forceps/finger pressure* and oversewn with a 5-0 prolene suture. Interrupted 5-0 prolene sutures were used to close the hole in the femoral artery. Flow was then resumed into the lower extremity.

Doppler evaluation revealed no evidence of any bruits or fistulae with good arterial signals in the foot.

The wound was then irrigated and closed with 3-0 Vicryl for subcutaneous tissue and staples for the skin.

The patient tolerated the procedure well and was taken to the postanesthesia care unit in stable condition.

Chapter 224
Four-Quadrant Fasciotomy

Jamal J. Hoballah, M.D., M.B.A.

INDICATION

- Status post lower-extremity revascularization with compartmental hypertension.

ESSENTIAL STEPS

1. Longitudinal incision from the upper leg to the ankle 3 cm lateral to the tibia.
2. Skin flaps over the anterior and lateral compartments are created.
3. Longitudinal incision in the fascia of the anterior compartment.
4. Longitudinal incision in the fascia of the lateral compartment.
5. Longitudinal incision from the upper leg to the ankle 3 cm medial to the tibia.
6. The superficial fascia is incised.
7. The soleus muscle is incised longitudinally until the posterior fascia in identified and incised.

NOTE THIS VARIATION

- A four-quadrant fasciotomy can also be performed completely through a lateral approach. This approach will require excision of a large segment of the fibula. The deep and superficial posterior compartments are decompressed through the fibular bed.

J.J. Hoballah and C.E.H. Scott-Conner (eds.), *Operative Dictations in General and Vascular Surgery*, DOI 10.1007/978-1-4614-0451-4_224,
© Springer Science+Business Media, LLC 2012

COMPLICATIONS
- Nerve injury.
- Bleeding.

TEMPLATE OPERATIVE DICTATION

Preoperative diagnosis: Compartmental hypertension of the lower extremity.

Procedure: Four-quadrant fasciotomy.

Postoperative diagnosis: Same.

Indications: The patient is a ___-year-old *male/female* who is status post *right/left* lower-extremity revascularization for acute ischemia. Postoperatively, the patient was noted to have pain with increasing leg swelling. Compartment pressures were obtained and were elevated greater than 35 mmHg.

Description of procedure: The procedure was performed under general anesthesia. The patient was placed supine. The *right/left* lower extremity was prepped and draped in the usual sterile fashion.

A longitudinal incision was then performed over the lateral aspect of the leg 3 cm lateral and parallel to the tibia. The incision was deepened through the subcutaneous tissue until the fascia was identified. Skin flaps were created on either side of the incision to expose the anterior and lateral compartments. The fascia overlying the anterior compartment was then incised and the incision carried along the entire length of the skin incision. The same was performed over the lateral compartment. The underlying muscles were released and appeared to bulge through the fascial incisions.

Attention was then turned to the medial compartment. A medial skin incision was then performed a few centimeters below the knee and extending down to 5 cm above the ankle. The incision was deepened down to the subcutaneous tissue until the fascia was identified. The superficial fascia was then divided, releasing the superficial posterior compartment. The soleus muscle was then incised with electrocautery until its posterior fascia was identified. The posterior fascia was then incised with the electrocautery along most of the length of the incision, freeing the deep posterior compartment.

Thorough irrigation was then performed and hemostasis was secured. The wounds were then covered with Vaseline Xeroform gauze. He/she had excellent signals in the foot. The patient was taken to the postanesthesia care unit in stable condition.

Chapter 225
Split-Thickness Skin Graft

Jamal J. Hoballah, M.D., M.B.A.

INDICATION
- Open wound, primary closure not possible.

ESSENTIAL STEPS
1. Prepare the open wound and debride any nongranulating areas.
2. Identify the donor site.
3. Harvest the skin using the dermatome.
4. Mesh the skin graft.
5. Apply the skin graft over the wound and trim the edges.
6. Staple the skin graft.
7. Apply an occlusive immobilizing dressing.

COMPLICATIONS
- Failure of the skin graft to take.
- Donor site infection.

TEMPLATE OPERATIVE DICTATION
Preoperative diagnosis: Open wound (specify location).
Procedure: Split-thickness skin graft from *thigh/abdomen* to open wound (specify location).
Postoperative diagnosis: Same.
Indications: This is a ___-year-old *male/female* with an open wound over ___. The wound has a good granulation base and

J.J. Hoballah and C.E.H. Scott-Conner (eds.), *Operative Dictations in General and Vascular Surgery*, DOI 10.1007/978-1-4614-0451-4_225,
© Springer Science+Business Media, LLC 2012

is not amenable to primary closure. A split-thickness skin graft was recommended. The risks and benefits of the procedure were explained to the patient, who agreed to proceed with the surgical procedure.

Description of procedure: The patient was placed in a supine position. *General/regional* anesthesia was induced. The *lower abdomen/upper thigh* and the wound area was prepped and draped in the usual sterile manner. The wound was then prepared and the granulation tissue gently scraped using a #10 blade. Using an electric dermatome a skin segment measuring ___ cm × ___ cm was harvested. The skin graft was then meshed at 1:1.5 ratio. The skin graft was then applied over the wound and the excessive skin trimmed. The skin was then stabilized to the wound using staples. The skin graft was then covered with a porous Vaseline gauze dressing. A cotton ball dressing was applied over the Vaseline gauze and secured using *tie over silk sutures/Ace bandages.* A tegaderm dressing was applied over the donor site.

The patient was taken to the postanesthesia care unit in stable condition.

Chapter 226
Temporal Artery Biopsy

Jean Salem, M.D. and Jamal J. Hoballah, M.D., M.B.A.

INDICATION
- Tissue diagnosis to rule out Giant cell/temporal arteritis.

ESSENTIAL STEPS
1. Incise the skin and subcutaneous tissue over the temporal artery.
2. Identify and dissect the temporal artery located in the superficial layers of the superficial temporal fascia.
3. Suture/ligate the proximal and distal portions of the isolated artery.
4. Remove the ligated vessel.
5. Secure hemostasis.
6. Close the wound.

NOTE THESE VARIATIONS
- Biopsy is done on the side of most pain and/or tenderness. If there is no difference, the most easily palpable artery is chosen.
- The artery is usually mapped out by palpation. Rarely Doppler-Ultrasound is needed to locate the artery. Duplex may reveal a thickened artery with a Halo sign.
- Temporal artery biopsy may be contraindicated in the presence of internal carotid occlusion as it may play an important collateral role.

J.J. Hoballah and C.E.H. Scott-Conner (eds.), *Operative Dictations in General and Vascular Surgery*, DOI 10.1007/978-1-4614-0451-4_226,

COMPLICATIONS

- Wound infection.
- Hematoma formation.
- Incisional alopecia.
- Injury to the branches of the auriculotemporal or facial nerves.

TEMPLATE OPERATIVE DICTATION

Preoperative diagnosis: Temporal arteritis.
Procedure: Temporal artery biopsy.
Postoperative diagnosis: Same.
Indications: This ___-year-old *male/female* has *new-onset headache/jaw claudication/loss of visual acuity and diplopia/erythrocyte sedimentation rate greater than 50 mm/h* with *right/left* temporal artery *tenderness to palpation/reduced pulsation*. The patient has been informed that a temporal artery biopsy is required to confirm the diagnosis of temporal arteritis before starting steroid therapy. The risks of the procedure were explained to the patient who elected to proceed with the biopsy.

Description of procedure: The patient was placed in the supine position with the head turned so the operative side is up. The *right/left* temporal area was prepped and draped in the usual sterile fashion. Local anesthetics (1% Lidocaine) without epinephrine to minimize arterial spasm were injected using a 27-gauge needle. A 3.5 cm incision was made directly over the artery through the skin and subcutaneous tissue using a #15 blade scalpel. The temporal artery was identified in the superficial layers of the superficial temporal fascia. Blunt dissection with a hemostat was performed parallel to the vessel to avoid tearing it. Electrocautery was used for hemostasis. The dissection proceeded beneath the vessel so that a hemostat was passed below it. After the vessel was isolated, 4-0 silk sutures were passed around the proximal and distal portions of the isolated artery and tied. Branches of the main artery were also ligated. The vessel was then transected. After ensuring hemostasis, the subcutaneous tissues were closed using interrupted 5-0 Vicryl sutures. The skin was closed with a running subcuticular 6-0 Vicryl sutures. Steri-strips were applied over the wound and covered with sterile dressings.

The patient tolerated well the procedure.

The specimen was spread over an applicator stick and submitted in saline solution to the pathologist.

Index

J.J. Hoballah and C.E.H. Scott-Conner (eds.), *Operative Dictations in General
and Vascular Surgery*, DOI 10.1007/978-1-4614-0451-4
© Springer Science+Business Media, LLC 2012